Genetic Manipulations with Plant Material

NATO ADVANCED STUDY INSTITUTES SERIES

A series of edited volumes comprising multifaceted studies of contemporary scientific issues by some of the best scientific minds in the world, assembled in cooperation with NATO Scientific Affairs Division.

Series A: Life Sciences

Volume 1 – Vision in Fishes: New Approaches in Research
    edited by M. A. Ali

Volume 2 – Nematode Vectors of Plant Viruses
    edited by F. Lamberti, C. E. Taylor, and J. W. Seinhorst

Volume 3 – Genetic Manipulations with Plant Material
    edited by Lucien Ledoux

Volume 4 – Phloem Transport
    edited by S. Aronoff, J. Dainty, P. Gorham, L. M. Srivastava,
    and C. A. Swanson

Volume 5 – Tumor Virus–Host Cell Interaction
    edited by Alan Kolber

The series is published by an international board of publishers in conjunction with NATO Scientific Affairs Division

A	Life Sciences	Plenum Publishing Corporation
B	Physics	New York and London
C	Mathematical and Physical Sciences	D. Reidel Publishing Company Dordrecht and Boston
D	Behavioral and Social Sciences	Sijthoff International Publishing Company Leiden
E.	Applied Sciences	Noordhoff International Publishing Leiden

Genetic Manipulations with Plant Material

Edited by
Lucien Ledoux
Molecular Genetics
Department of Botany
University of Liège
Liège, Belgium

PLENUM PRESS • NEW YORK AND LONDON
Published in cooperation with NATO Scientific Affairs Division

Library of Congress Cataloging in Publication Data

Nato Advanced Study Institute on Genetic Manipulations with Plant Material, Liège, 1974.
    Genetic manipulations with plant material.

    (Nato advanced study institutes series: Series A, life sciences; v. 3)
    "Published in cooperation with NATO Scientific Affairs Division."
    Includes bibliographical references and index.
    1. Plant genetics—Congresses. 2. Genetic engineering—Congresses. I. Ledoux, Lucien.
II. North Atlantic Treaty Organization. Division of Scientific Affairs. III. Title. IV.
Series.
QH433.N22 1974   581.1'5   75-12547
ISBN 0-306-35603-1

Lectures presented at the 1974 NATO Advanced Study Institute on Genetic
Manipulations with Plant Material, held in Liège, Belgium, Summer 1974

© 1975 Plenum Press, New York
A Division of Plenum Publishing Corporation
227 West 17th Street, New York, N.Y. 10011

United Kingdom edition published by Plenum Press, London
A Division of Plenum Publishing Company, Ltd.
Davis House (4th Floor), 8 Scrubs Lane, Harlesden, London, NW10 6SE, England

Preface

Mankind, throughout history, has strived to improve his food sources. By means of slow and empirical selections, it has been possible to greatly increase both quantity and quality of plant crops. This procedure has brought the most useful cereals to a state of refinement that seems to be difficult to further improve by the same methodology.

Indeed, natural sexual mechanisms were always used to cross closely related sexually and genetically compatible organisms; the selection procedure consisted of isolating the most promising progenies. Obviously, by this way, plants could only share preexisting genetic pools.

On the other hand, the last decade has seen drastic modifications of the experimental plant sciences, with the appearance of new technological possibilities.

Because of this profound reshaping of our experimental approaches, other means can now be realistically envisaged in order to achieve similar or even higher goals.

It is, for instance, possible to attempt completing sexual crosses (where both male and female gametes bring together the genetic informations necessary for growth and development of the offspring) by parasexual means by which novel genetic informations could possibly be added to the heritage.

At the limit, such genetic manipulations could enable man to create plants capable of producing new substances characteristic of unrelated plants or, more generally, of other living organisms.

Even if these possibilities might appear quite remote, the interest of Scientists has been awaken and, indeed, several attempts to such genetic manipulations have already been made.

When we organized, in 1970, a first NATO Course on "Uptake of genetic informations by living materials" (North Holland Cy. 1972), about 100 research workers showed interest in the matter. We were somewhat surprised, this time, to receive several hundred enquiries. This fact clearly indicates the actual spreading of interest in the field.

It should also be added that these new approaches become available at a time characterized by a renewed interest for the plant material and for its fundamental aspects. In fact, plants appear to have a biological complexity intermediate between that of micro-organisms and that of aniamls; they also show very interesting properties such as the regeneration of whole organisms from frag-mented tissues. Because of that, they do attract a growing number of Biologists.

Several approaches to genetic manipulations are being used by different groups. In addition to attempts to correct inborn errors or deficiencies of metabolism by using purified DNA and/ or viruses, attempts have been made to introduce novel genetic traits via the same agents. The keenest interest is centered around manipulations with protoplasts or haploid variants, de-differentiated callus tissues and pollen grains. No doubt that these new methods will greatly help analysi'ng developmental problems and fundamental genetic aspects. Very likely also they will enable developing new biochemical genetics.

The aim of the present Course was to bring together crop scientists, plant and microbial geneticists, molecular biolo-gists, plant physiologists, tissue culture morphologists and to have them review, compare and discuss techniques, materials, results and outlook for the near future.

The lectures were therefore planned to cover most of the related fields of interest, going from the simplest to the com-plex and mixing theoretical and technological informations.

Needless to say that nothing definitive was achieved by the meeting, but a better comprehension of the problems, diffi-culties and results developed in a challenging atmosphere.

It is clear that a long way remains to be travelled before the dreams of today can be explored and analysed. It is however hoped that we won't have to wait long before part of them be turned into tomorrow's reality.

Acknowledgements

Many people contributed to the organisation of this meeting. In particular, I am grateful to Profs. D. Hess and A. Tomasz who functioned with me in the Scientific Committee and to Drs.P.

Charles, R. Loppes, P. Lurquin, R. Matagne and M. Mergeay who helped me to organize this Course.

In that respect, thanks are due to many members of the University Staff for their valuable assistance before and during the Course and to several members of the Centre d'Etudes de l'Energie Nucléaire for their very efficient help.

L. LEDOUX

Contents

Analysis of Microbial Genome Structure   1
   T. Mojica-A

The Mechanism of Competence for DNA Uptake
      and Transformation 27
   A. Tomasz

Integrated and Free State of Plasmids 45
   J. Schell

F-Prime Manipulations of Possible Interest
      to Plant Biologists 59
   T. Mojica-A

Interallelic Complementation in the Study
      of Gene Action 77
   R. F. Matagne and R. Loppes

Principles of Genetic Regulation in Lower
      and Higher Plants 89
   R. Loppes and R. F. Matagne

The Enzymology of Nitrogen Fixation 107
   J. Postgate

The Physiology and Genetics of Nitrogen Fixation 123
   J. Postgate

Molecular Biology of the Genus Agrobacterium 135
   J. De Ley

Crown Gall: A Model for Tumor Research
      and Genetic Engineering 141
   R. A. Schilperoort and G. H. Bomhoff

The Role of Plasmids in Crown Gall Formation
     by A. Tumefaciens 163
  J. Schell

Genetic Mechanisms in Differentiation and Development 183
  G. P. Redei

Plant Cell Cultures: Present and Projected
     Applications for Studies in Cell Metabolism 211
  H. E. Street

Plant Cell Cultures: Present and Projected
     Applications for Studies in Genetics 231
  H. E. Street

Heterogeneous Associations of Cells Formed *in vitro* 245
  P. S. Carlson and R. S. Chaleff

Plant Regeneration and Chromosome Stability
     in Tissue Cultures 263
  Wm. F. Sheridan

Single Cell Culture of an Haploid Cell: The Microspore 297
  C. Nitsch

Plant Protoplasts as Genetic Systems 311
  E. C. Cocking

Induction of Auxotrophic Mutations in Plants 329
  G. P. Redei

In vitro Selection for Mutants of Higher Plants 351
  R. S. Chaleff and P. S. Carlson

Isozymes and a Strategy for Their Utilization in
     Plant Genetics: Genetic and Epigenetic Control 365
  M. Jacobs

Isozymes and a Strategy for Their Utilization in
     Plant Genetics: Isozymes as a Tool in Plant Genetics . . 379
  M. Jacobs

Physico-Chemical Aspects of Chromatin and
     Chromosome Structure 391
    E. Fredericq

Isolation and Gradient Analysis of DNA 405
  P. Charles

Use of Molecular Sieving on Agarose Gels to Study
    DNA Uptake by Chlamydomonas Reinhardi 429
  P. F. Lurquin and R. M. Behki

Molecular Hybridization and Its Application to
    RNA Tumor Virus Research 449
  M. Janowski

DNA-Hybridization Studies of the Fate of Bacterial
    DNA in Plants 461
  A. Kleinhofs

Fate of Exogenous DNA in Plants 479
  L. Ledoux

DNA Mediated Genetic Correction of Thiamineless
    Arabidopsis Thaliana 499
  L. Ledoux, R. Huart, M. Mergeay, P. Charles,
  and M. Jacobs

Uptake of DNA and Bacteriophage into Pollen and
    Genetic Manipulation 519
  D. Hess

Theoretical and Comparative Aspects of Bacteriophage
    Transfer and Expression in Eukaryotic Cells
    in Culture 539
  P. M. Gresshoff

Studies on the Use of Transducing Bacteriophages as
    Vectors for the Transfer of Foreign Genes to
    Higher Plants 551
  H. Smith, R. A. McKee, T. H. Attridge, and G. Grierson

COMMUNICATIONS

A *uvr* Mutation That Enhances the Transformation
    Frequency by Intergenetic CNA in *B. subtilis* 565
  K. Matsumoto, H. Takahashi, and H. Saito

Studies on Protease Sensitive Transfecting DNA
    of Bacillus Phage 566
  H. Hirokawa

Genetic Control of D.Amino Acid Metabolism in
    Gram-Negative Bacteria 567
  W. Walczak, J. Wild, K. Krajewska-Grynkiewicz, and
  T. Klopotowski

Regulation of Development in Fission Yeast 569
    J. M. Meade

In Vitro Growth and Polyphenol Production by Tissue
    Cultures of Datura and Cassia 570
    A. Mekta, K. Venkatasubbaiah, and R. Shah

Properties of 5-Bromodeoxyuridine-Resistant Lines of
    Higher Plant Cells in Liquid Cultures 571
    K. Ohyama

Respiration and Nitrogen Nutrition of Carrot
    Callus Cultures 572
    G. H. Craven

Quantitative Mutagenesis in Soybean Suspension Cultures . . . 574
    Z. R. Sung, J. Smith, and E. R. Signer

Protoplast Isolation from Leaves of C3, C4 and C.A.M.
    Plants and Biochemical Activities 575
    M. Gutierrez, S. B. Ku, and G. E. Edwards

Anther Derived Plants from Digitalis Purpurea 576
    G. Corduan and C. Spix

Mutations Obtained from Anther Derived Plants
    of Hyoscyamus Niger 578
    G. Corduan

Ribonucleic Acid Synthesis in Plants 579
    D. Grierson

Fate of Homologous DNA in Seedlings of Matthiola Incama . . . 581
    V. Hemleben

DNA Synthesis and Bacterial Contamination in Plants 582
    M. Delseny

Mitochondrial Nucleic Acids from Parthenocissus
    Tricuspidata Cells 583
    F. Vedel, F. Quetier, and J. M. Grienenberger

Involvement of Nucleic Acids and Microtubules in
    Ciliogenesis: Implications for Cytoplasmic
    Inheritance 584
    J. K. Kelleher

Methyl 4-Chloroindolyl-3-Acetate in Pea and Barley 585
    K. C. Engvild

Evidence for a Proposed Function of DNA as Transducer
    Acting at the Cell Surface 586
    B. L. Reid

Genome Activation During Seed Germination 588
    M. Dobrzanska-Wiernikowska

PARTICIPANTS 589

INDEX 597

ANALYSIS OF MICROBIAL GENOME STRUCTURE

T. MOJICA-A

Cell Biochemistry, Radiobiology Department
Centre d'Etude de L'Energie Nucléaire
B-2400 MOL, Belgium

I. INTRODUCTION

It might appear meaningless for a group of distinguished plant biologists to hear about the genetic manipulations with the evolutionarily distant microbes. It is conceivably possible, however, to draw some morals from the concepts of bacterial genetic transfer and recombination and the possibilities the systems offer for a great deal of fine genetic manipulations. These potentialities have permitted the understanding of a host of fundamental molecular biological processes, long before the sexual biology and mechanisms of transfer and recombination began to be understood.

It is not my intention to make plant biologists envious but rather to set down the guidelines and principles of microbial genetic systems as known to date. It should be kept in mind that this type of guidelines is not to be taken as literally applicable to higher organisms. It would be rather surprising to find that the same mechanistical events apply, although the reasoning and logistics could be applicable. Scientific literature does indeed show many examples where wrong assumptions of this type have been made. As an example, and to not go too far, it was assumed that integration of bacteriophage lambda into the bacterial chromosome, used the same mechanism and the same recombinational machinery as "general" recombination. This, of course, it's not the case.

This is not meant to be an exhaustive review of the field, but rather an outline of methodologies and rationales of genetic analysis in micro-organisms. Throughout, "bacteria" is taken to mean *Escheria coli* and some of its related, sexually adept cousins such as *Salmonella typhimurium*,unless otherwise explicitly indicated.

1

II. CHARACTERISTICS OF BACTERIA

Bacteria are unicellular organisms that share the following characteristics :
1. They are genetically HAPLOID and as a rule contain a single chromosome
2. The intracellular POOLS of metabolites are SMALL such that on removal of the metabolite source, at best a few cell divisions can occur
3. Cell populations are large. It is possible to handle more than 10^{10} cells/ml.
4. Bacterial populations are homogeneous at least in the sense that they do not differentiate.
5. The generation time is very short. For *E. coli*, it ranges from 20 min to about 60 min. Moreover rate of growth can be experimentally controlled.
6. There is very little, if any, COMPARTAMENTALIZATION.

In addition to these, inherent characteristics of bacteria, it is worthwhile to mention that, it is relatively simple to synchronize and clone bacterial populations and that there are three fairly well understood modes of genetic transfer : CONJUGATION, TRANSDUCTION and TRANSFORMATION.
These systems were first described for 3 different bacterial species. Since then, genetic transfer in bacterial systems has fallen under one or other of the existing headings. It is to be expected that newly discovered systems will fall into one of these three categories, since it is hard to visualize how bacteria can exchange genetic material by a mode other than cell-to-cell contact (conjugation), via a virus (transduction) or by naked DNA (transformation). Transformation will not be considered here.

The characteristics outlined above made bacteria keenly genetically tractable. Genetic tractability, in turn, makes bacteria the chosen material in a great deal of studies of fundamental biological problems.

Presently, *E. coli* is the only whole organism which lends itself to the following combination of genetic manipulations :
a) Efficient mutagenesis both on a random basis and for any desired, specific, small region of the chromosome.
b) Genetic mapping at the level of the chromosome.
c) Genetic mapping at the level of the small transducing fragment (40-80 genes).
d) Genetic mapping at the level of the gene and the codon.
e) Dominance and complementation studies for essentially any chromosomal region with a whole battery of available or easily-obtainable episomes.
f) Directed transposition, deletion and fusion of genetic elements.

g) Many-fold enrichment of specific genes for essentially any desired chromosomal region.
h) Analysis of hybrid "recombinants" with *E. coli* one one side and
other, sexually adept, enteric bacteria on the other.

   I will elaborate, below, on these points, except points d, e,
f, and g, which will be covered somewhere else in this volume.
Emphasis will be put on hybrid analysis because the system could be
of considerable theoretical interest to those bent on genetic manipulations with plant materials. In addition, brief mention of particular problems in the analysis of genome structure of bacteriophage and
fungi will be made.

   More detailed analysis of the topic can be found in the excellent
treatise by Hayes (1968) for bacteria and bacteriophage and by Finchan
and Day (1971) for fungi.

III. MUTAGENESIS

   The role that mutations and mutagenesis has played in our understanding of genetics and particularly of the nature of the gene its
perhaps becoming part of popular wisdom. The mechanism of mutagenesis
has been recently reviewed (Drake, 1969), and will not be dealt with
here. Bacteria are available for mutagenesis with a variety of physical and chemical agents, and regarding the chromosomal specificity of
the "mutant" product, mutagenesis can be considered as being random
and site-specific.

   The most common mutant phenotypes are auxotrophs (requiring or
responding to particular metabolites), fermentation mutants (unable
to grow on particular carbon sources), conditional lethal mutants
depending on particular growth conditions (temperature-sensitive, cold
sensitive), mutants resistant to certain metabolites (with alterations
in the regulation of the affected pathways or in the machinery for
macromolecular synthesis and function. (see Umbarger, 1971 ; Weisblum and Davies, 1968), and bacteriocins and bacteriophages (usually
with altered cell surface).

A. RANDOM MUTAGENESIS

   Random mutagenesis refers to the inability to predict the chromosomal location of mutated genes with known selectable phenotypes.

   For the experimental methodology for random mutagenesis and enrichment, see Miller (1972). The rationale of random mutagenesis resides in the fact that the probability for any gene to mutate in the
presence of a mutagen is: a) enhanced as compared to the probability

of spontaneous mutation and b) equal for any gene with respect to the others. The second parameter depends on the size of the gene and on the number of gene-copies in the population (Cerdà-Olmedo et al. 1968).

Final mutant yield is greatly improved by the long-used procedures of enrichment. Fundamentally, mutant-enrichment consists of selectively killing non-mutant cells (parental) by the use of bacteriocidal agents (e.g. penicilline, ampicillin) that only affect actively growing cells, by transfering mutagenized stock to conditions in which mutant cells cannot grow (e.g. high temperature, minimal salts medium) and killing parental cells with the antibiotic. The use of selective "assay" media permits the enhanced recovery of particular mutant phenotypes wherever it is possible to place mutagenized stock under conditions in which the desired mutant phenotypes does not grow while not only the parental but also all other (or most of them) mutant phenotypes do grow, followed by "enrichment" as mentioned above.

The potentialities of random mutagenesis for genetic and biochemical studies are clearly obvious. Perhaps the only limitation consists of the impossibility to recognize certain mutant (e.g. lethal) phenotypes.

A system of random mutagenesis first described by Taylor (1963) consists in the use of phage mu, which is able to integrate (Boram and Abelson, 1971) into the bacterial chromosome, with no preference for a specific site (Taylor, 1963), thus, occasionally disrupting genes or gene arrangements and producing mutant phenotypes. The insertion of phage mu often produces polar effects in the disrupted operon (Nomura and Engbaenk, 1972).

The principles of random mutagenesis, as outlined, are valid with certain limitations, for bacteriophage (see below) and for fungi (Fincham and Day, 1971).

B. SITE SPECIFIC MUTAGENESIS

Site-specific mutagenesis has been of tremendous importance in the analysis of genome structure in bacteria, and refers to the ability to predict the chromosomal location (within a gene or a small chromosomal segment) of mutated genes with selectable phenotypes.

Direct selection, for mutants in specific genes, relies heavily on the use of antibiotics and other antimetabolites. When a cell population is asked to grow in the presence of a particular toxic anti-metabolite, usually, the genetic choices to achieve such a response are limited, such that only cells with mutations in specific genes will be able to grow. The following cases are given as examples :

In *S. typhimurium*, mutants able to grow in the presence of 1,2, 4-triazole carry mutations in the *cysK* gene (Hulanicka and Klopotowski 1972; Hulanicka et al., 1974). Thymine-requiring mutants screened for resistance to trimethoprime in the presence of thymine carry mutations in the *thyA* gene (e.g. see Miller, 1972). Strains resistant to spectinomycin and other similar antibiotics are mutated in a cluster of ribosomal genes (Weisblum and Davies, 1968). Rifampicin resistance is controlled by an RNA polymerase gene (Jacobson and Gillespie, 1971). Selection for resistance to phage T1 in *E. coli* leads to mutations in the *tonB* locus (Yanofsky and Lennox, 1959), in some cases these mutations extend (deletions) to the nearby *trp* operon, producing tryptophan requirement (Gratia, 1966). Similarly, selection for *leu*+ of *leu-500*, a promoter mutation, in *S. typhimurium* leads to mutations in the *supX* gene and sometimes to deletions covering *trp* and/or *cysB* and *pyrF* (Dubnau and Margolin, 1972). "Eduction" of *E. coli* P2-lysogens often leads to deletions of all or part of the *his* operon (Kelly and Sunshine, 1967; Sunshine and Kelly, 1971). More examples can be found in the literature

More important and of wider possible applications is a system originally developed for *B. subtilis* (Anagnostopoulos and Crawford, 1961) and recently extended for other bacteria (Hong and Ames 1971), that consists of using mutagenized transducing phage (or transforming DNA) to repair known mutations (e.g. auxotrophy to prototrophy), and by manipulating experimental conditions, to select mutations with recognizable phenotypes (e.g. temperature sensitivity) linked to the repaired genes.

I would conclude that through a judicious choice of working elements it is possible to construct new strains with almost any desired characteristics.

IV. GENETIC MAPPING AT THE LEVEL OF THE CHROMOSOME

As a general rule, the first step in genetic mapping is mapping at the chromosome level, that is to say, the determination of the position of a genetic marker relative to the position of other known genes. Its counter-part in eukaryotic genetic analysis would be the location of a genetic marker in a particular linkage group.

Genetic mapping at the level of the chromosome is accomplished by conjugation. The reader is referred to some of the excellent books and reviews on the subject : Jacob and Wolman (1961), Hayes (1968), Curtis (1969), to mention just a few and to Miller (1972) for experimental methodology. In bacterial species with no known conjugation system, mapping at the level of the chromosome is carried by physical techniques independent of recombination and described below.

Although conjugation, discovered in 1946, has been widely used in bacterial genome analysis, it is only in recent years that the sexual biology has begun to be understood (Curtiss, 1969). Conjugation, as understood today, is described as a process in which transfer of genetic material from one bacterial strain to another presents the following fundamental features :

a) It depends upon cellular contact between members of the two bacterial strains

b) Transfer of genetic material is non-reciprocal (one-way transfer), from DONOR to RECIPIENT cells, male to female by anthropomorphical analogy. Thus, there are two fundamental mating types (see Curtiss, 1969 and Schell, this volume, for the characteristics of mating types).

c) Donor state is conferred by an extrachromosomal genetic element called F (other episomes are also known to mediate chromosome transfer) or SEX FACTOR (see Schell, this volume, for the molecular biological properties of episomes).
Three types of donors have been described differing in the relationship. Sex factor-chromosome : i) F^+, the sex factor is not integrated into the chromosome, promotes its own transfer at high frequency and chromosome transfer at low frequency. ii) F-prime (F^1), like F^+ except that the sex factor has been altered and carries genetic material acquired from the chromosome. It is diagnosed by high frequency of transfer of the chromosomal genes carried by the sex factor. iii) Hfr, (for High frequency of recombination), refers to an altered sex factor integrated into the bacterial chromosome. Transfer of chromosomal markers occurs at high frequency (a criterion for diagnosis) and transfer of the sex factor occurs very rarely, if ever. Hfr's are the most useful donors for mapping at the level of the chromosome.

d) In addition to being non-reciprocal, conjugal genetic transfer is polarized, that is, in all mating pairs the same end of the donor chromosome (origin) is always the first to penetrate the recipient parent. The polarity of chromosomal transfer by Hfr's depends on the site and orientation of integration of the sex factor. More than 20 different integration sites have been described, and, for each site, two orientations are possible, clockwise and counterclockwise. Under standard conditions the rate of transfer is approximately constant, although chromosome transfer is rarely, if ever, complete. The conjugation system of *Streptomyces coelicolor* differs from that of *E. coli* in that transfer is reciprocal and the chromosome is transferred simultaneously from two different points. It is not clear whether cell fusion occurs (Hopwood, 1967).

As in other systems of genetic transfer, the tendency is towards
haploidy. Partial diploidy is temporary, exogenotic donor genetic
material being incorporated into the recipient chromosome or otherwise "deactivated". This is not true in all cases, however.

The fundamental concepts used in mapping at the level of the
chromosome are the non-completeness, polarity and non-reciprocality
of conjugal transfer. Two main procedures are routinely used :
a) Time of marker-entry or interrupted matings that consist   of
   measuring the kinetics of appearance of donor markers. The key
   features of conjugation here are polarity and the possibility to
   interrupt, experimentally,transfer of donor genes, simply by
   separating mating cells. Thus, with a donor of known "origin"
   is possible to locate the position of a marker, with respect to
   the origin and to other markers, by measuring the "times" at which
   donor markers are transferred. Time of entry mapping is limited
   by inherent procedural errors and by unsynchronized transfer of
   genes.
b) Cotransfer : The frequency of coinheritance of 2 or more donor
   markers is also widely used in preliminary experiments. This
   method has the advantage that standardization of experimental
   conditions need not be rigorous and the disadvantage that the
   degree of accuracy is even lower than in time of entry mapping.
   The interpretation of the results of cotransfer experiments is
   essentially the same as the interpretation of 2-point and 3-
   point transduction crosses (see below).
   Recently, because more and more Hfr strains have become available, procedures for rapid mapping of selectable markers have
   been devised (see for example Low, 1973). These methods make
   use of a large number of donors and are founded on the general
   features of conjugation as outlined above. Conjugation experiments have permitted the construction of a linkage map that is
   circular in accordance to physical maps (Taylor and Trotter, 1972 ;
   Sanderson, 1972 ; Hopwood et al., 1973).
   Mapping at the level of the gene and the codon, as well as dominance and complementation tests in bacteria, that make use of a
   special type of donor strains, will be considered somewhere else
   in this volume.

V. GENOME STRUCTURE REVEALED BY TRANSDUCTION

Once the relative position of a genetic marker has been determined, the usual practice is to refine this position with respect to
other known markers (see Taylor and Trotter, 1972 ; and Sanderson,
1972 ; for transduction maps). This refinent is accomplished by
phage-mediated transduction or by transformation.

Transduction is defined as genetic transfer mediated by phage. A very useful article on transduction is by Hartman (1963) that discussed criteria for the recognition of transduction as well as methods of genetic analysis dependent upon it. A review of transduction mechanisms has recently been published (Ozeki and Ikeda, 1968).

Two phenomenological types of bacteriophages have been described the virulent types such as phage T1 that always kills the host cells and the temperate phage that has two choices upon infection to the bacterial host, it either lysogenizes the cell (A lysogen will thus have its normal genetic complement plus the genetic complement of the lysogenizing phage) or else it grows through a lytic cycle, killing the host.

Clearly, virulent phages are not convenient vectors in transduction, thus most often, transduction is performed using temperate vectors. The general consensus is, however, that all phages are able to mobilize bacterial genes (see for example Drexler, 1970), and as far as transduction analysis is concerned, the choice of temperate vector is purely of experimental convenience. Two experimentally distinct classes of transduction have been recognized : generalized and specialized transduction.
Generalized transducing phages are able to transfer any gene (or virtually so) from a donor (strain in which the phage was previously propagated) to a recipient strain. Specialized transducing phages are able to mobilize only a circumscribed set of genes adjacent to the chromosomal attachment site of the phages. The best known example of special transducing phages is coliphage λ.

Generalized transducing phages on the other hand, mobilize chromosomal regions with no apperent circunscription. They are, however, often able (under certain conditions) to behave as specialized transducing phages. For example, *S. typhimurium* phage P22 has been shown to transduce preferentially the *pro* region (Smith-Keary, 1966) while coliphage P1 can promote specialized transduction of the *lac* region (Luria, Adams and Ting, 1960).
Mapping by generalized transduction completely depends on the concept of co-transduction, obviously, only closely-linked genes (separated by no more than one phage genome equivalent of DNA) can be carried by the same transducing phage. Cotransduction is, of course, in itself diagnostic of close linkage.

Cotransduction is detected by adding phages grown on a donor strain bearing a selectable allele to a recipient strain bearing the counter-selected allele, and testing "transductants" for the presence (or absence) of another (unselected) marker.

For example, we have two strains A^+B^- (donor) and A^-B^+ (recipient), the two strains are crossed by transduction and A^+ transductants are selected under conditions in which the B marker (B^+ or B^-) goes unselected. Transductants are analyzed for the presence of B^- phenotype. If, for example 50 % of A^+ transductants are A^+B^- (like the donor), the frequency of cotransduction of the A^+ and B^- markers is said to be 50 %.

At least two very important parameters will affect the frequency of cotransduction : a) the physical distance between the two loci, this distance will be reflected in the probability that the two loci are included in the same transducing fragment (clearly, if two loci are so far apart that they cannot be included in the same transducing fragment, they cannot be used in transduction analysis). The physical length of the transducing fragment will partially determine the probability for two loci to be in the same transducing fragment. For example in *S. typhimurium* P1 sensitive mutants, P1-mediated cotransduction frequencies for several markers tested are about twice as large as those mediated by P22 (Mojica-a, unpublished). The length of the P1 transducing fragment in *E. coli* is, correspondingly, about twice the length of the P22 transducing fragment in *S. typhimurium*.
b) The second parameter that will affect the frequency of cotransduction is the probability that the two loci are integrated together into the recipient chromosome by appropriately positioned cross-overs. Clearly, this parameter is beyond the control of the investigator, and in at least some cases, the probability of integration is marker-dependent (Lacks, 1966 ; Norkin, 1970), but the nature of the phenomenum is not understood.

Several authors have put forward mathematical equations for the interpretation of transduction data, and for the conversion of genetic cotransduction frequency to actual physical distance. Since the equations are too many and of limited usage, they will not be considered here.

In most cases, two-point transduction crosses, of the type just discussed, have only limited resolution in the ordering of genes in the transducing fragments. Very often it is necessary, in order to sequence genes, to recur to multifactorial transducing crosses, that is to say, crosses involving three or more markers.

The simplest, and in experimental terms most useful, type of multifactorial cross is the so-called three-point cross, in which three markers are involved, one which is selected from the donor while the others (donor and/or recipient) are unselected. As an example, take a donor strain $A^+B^-C^+$ and a recipient strain $A^-B^+C^-$.

The two strains are crossed by transduction with selection for A^+
under conditions such that the B and C markers are unselected.
A^+ transductants are analyzed for the presence of B^+, B^-, C^+ and C^-.
It is asked whether the order of the three loci is ABC or an alternative one. Below are given "typical" results consistent with a given
order (in %) :

Class	Phenotype of transductants	Order I (ABC)	Order II (ACB)	Order III(CAB)
I	$A^+B^+C^+$	2	8	8
II	$A^+B^-C^+$	50	40	50
III	$A^+B^+C^-$	40	50	2
IV	$A^+B^-C^-$	8	2	40

Three-factor transductional crosses rely on the concept of cross-
over frequency, that is to say, the frequency of appearance of recombinants with a particular genetic constitution depends on the number
of cross-overs needed to generate such recombinant. The largest the
number of cross-over needed,the lowest the probability of appearance.
Thus, if order I is correct, $A^+B^+C^+$ recombinants will be the less
frequent one, since the generation of such recombinants requires the
largest number of cross-overs. Similarly, if order II or order III
are correct, the less frequent transductant type will be $A^+B^-C^-$
and $A^+B^+C^-$ respectively.

It is clear, however, that orders ABC and CBA are equivalent in
a three-point cross; thus, transduction resolves the "order" of genes
in the transducing fragment but not the "orientation" of the "transducing fragment" in the chromosome. The uncertainty is resolved either by a) exhaustive transduction tests with different combinations
of markers, like in *E. coli* (Taylor and Trotter, 1972) where most
markers have been shown to be sequentially linked on the chromosome,
or b) by interrupted mating experiments, as described above, like
in *S. typhimurium* (Sanderson, 1972) where most genes do not seem to
be sequentially linked.

In some cases, either one of the alternative solutions might
prove to be inadequate. A third possibility exists, that consists
of the analysis of intergenetic recombinants (see below).

Other functional genetic tests such as complementation and dominance are very often difficult to perform with bacteria, since,
as mentioned above, heterozygosity is not prolonged enough for
tests to be performed. Exceptions are provided by those systems
in which "abortive transduction" occurs, as in the case for the
S. typhimurium-P22 system (Stocker, Zinder and Lederberg, 1953).
Abortive transduction is interpreted as unilinear inheritance of a
transducing fragment, due to preservation without replication of the

inherited fragment. Thus, an abortive transductant is a colony (small) in which one cell (in practice probably more than one, but in any case, very few) at a time harbors the donor fragment, and consequently, is heterozygous for any selected genes.

The test requires a great deal of practice to be performed accurately. Moreover, to my knowledge it does not seem to occur (it has not been detected) in every transduction system analyzed, and, possibly, the presence or absence of abortive transduction depends on the recipient, since no abortive transductants were observed for ten *E. coli* markers tested with P1; on the other hand, abortive transductants were observed in *S. typhimurium* with six (of ten) similar markers tested also with P1 (Mojica-a, unpublished).

VI. INTERGENERIC GENETIC TRANSFER

Intergeneric genetic transfer, in enteric bacteria, was first observed nearly twenty years ago (Luria and Burrons, 1957) and has been extensively used and studied in more recent years (for reviews see Baron et al., 1968 ; Middleton and Mojica-a, 1971). Although it has been studied mostly between *E. coli* and a few *Salmonella* species, it occurs among a variety of bacterial species (Mandel, 1969 ; Jones and Sneath, 1970). The best known system of genetic transfer is mediated by conjugation but it is also known to occur by transduction (Charakbarty and Gunsalus, 1970 ; Mojica-a, unpublished) and by transformation (Beattie and Setlow, 1970 ; Biswas and Ravin, 1971 ; Mergeay et al. 1971 ; Wilson and Young, 1972 ; Harford and Mergeay, 1973).

I will elaborate on the parameters affecting conjugal transfer and fate of the incoming DNA in crosses with *E. coli* donors and *S. typhimurium* recipients. Where appropriate I will comment on other systems of transfer.

Intergeneric transfer began to be understood only in recent years, particularly because it was generally assumed that the parameters acting on intraspecific transfer were the same as those affecting intergeneric transfer.

The main consistent observation was the extremely low recovery of recombinants in conjugal crosses (Mojica-a and Middleton, 1970 and 1971). This low frequency of recovery was generally explained as being a consequence of low homology of the DNA. A detailed analysis of the system revealed that low frequency of recovery is at least due to the action of two main barriers : a) a barrier that affects transfer proper and b) a barrier that affects recombination, maintenance and expression of donor DNA.

The factors affecting transfer proper are at least two :
a) Differences in the cell surface that decreases the frequency of
mating pairs, and is partially corrected by mutations affecting the
structure of the cell wall polysaccharide (Watanabe, Arai and
Hatori, 1970). Mutations affecting other components of the cell
envelope have not been looked for but one can expect to find them.
b) Low homology of the DNA (Mojica-a and Middleton, 1971). This
barrier is partially corrected by the presence of the "leading end"
of the Hfr chromosome, integrated into the recipient chromosome
(Johnson et al., 1964 ; Curtiss, 1969 ; Mojica-a and Middleton,
1971).

Factors that affect the successful recovery of transferred DNA
include : Restriction of newly transferred DNA (see Arber and Linn,
1969, for a review on DNA restriction) that prevents not only recombination but also expression of donor genes (Mojica-a and
Middleton, 1971 ; Mojica-a, unpublished). The restriction barrier
can be removed either by altering the growth conditions of the
recipient (Mojica-a and Middleton, 1971) or by using strains with
impaired restriction systems (Mojica-a, unpublished). Low homology
of the DNA that decreases recombination and increases the availability of the substrate for restriction. This parameter cannot be manipulated and, because of its very nature, intergeneric matings and
analysis of hybrid recombinants are used to study recombinational
homology and evolutionary relatedness (Demerec and New, 1965 ;
Mandel, 1969 ; Jones and Sneath, 1970).

One might predict several fates for the donor DNA in intergeneric
crosses : It will be destroyed by restriction, or other nucleases, in
which case it will no be genetically detectable. It will be maintained in one of several modes (see below) in which case it will be
detectable by genetic means, if it is functional ; otherwise it can
only be detected by physical means In fact, most of the "expected"
exconjugants, based on physical and genetic measurements of DNA
transfer (Mojica-a, unpublished) fail to "appear". This is interpreted to mean that because of lack of homology (and probably other
genetic and physiological factors) most of the donor DNA (under
conditions in which is not restricted) fails to be conserved either
as a true recombinant or as an exogenote. It is a distinct possibility that there exists a minimum size (and/or conformation) requirement
for the conservation (and expression) of exogenotic DNA.

Extensive analysis of a large number of "hybrid recombinants"
(Mojica-a and Middleton, 1972 ; Colson and Colson, 1974) revealed
five distinguishable classes of hybrids as predicted on theoretical
and practical considerations :

Class I : Selected donor DNA becomes integrated into the recipient chromosome to replace exactly the equivalent genetic region of

the female. This class is rare but appears at detectable frequencies.
Class II : Selected donor DNA becomes integrated at a novel site very
near the equivalent recipient DNA.
Class III : Selected donor DNA becomes integrated at a novel site
which involves, in the recombination event the group of recipient genes which contains the allele selected against.
Class IV : Selected donor DNA becomes integrated at a novel site outside the transducing fragment which bears the female allele selected
against. Hybrids with donor DNA integrated at novel sites (Classes
II, III and IV) are also rare but more frequent that those of Class I.
The donor DNA in hybrids of classes I, II, III and IV is presumable
maintained, replicated and expressed with the rest of the recipient
chromosome.
Class V : Selected donor DNA does not become integrated into the female chromosome. This class appear at high frequency, and although
the mode of maintenance, replication and expression is not clearly
understood, in several well characterized cases the donor DNA is in
the form of closed-circular DNA molecules of varying lengths (Leavitt
et al. 1971), moreover, at least in some cases hybrids of this type
carry all or part of the donor sex factor (Johnson et al. 1973), thus,
the donor DNA in those strains is under the control of the sex factor
genetic system.

   A phenomenon, very little understood (presently under experimental scrutiny) and which might turn out to be of considerable importance, is the observation that in certain combinations, conjugal and
transformant hybrids segregate specific adventitious mutations, at relatively high frequency (Mergeay et al., 1971; Mergeay, 1972a and 1972b;
Mojica-a, unpublished). It is not actually known whether the adventitious mutations are really specific in the sense that all the mutations are segregated through exactly the same "mutational" event, but
it is clear that a particular hybrid that shows those adventitious mutations always segregate mutants with the same phenotype, and in the
case of conjugal hybrids, the "mutagenic" event affects always the
same gene. Phenomenologically similar events have been reported in
transformation of the blue-green alga Anacystis nidulans (Herdman,
1973) where the "mutational" events were ascribed to recombination.
It should be kept in mind, however, that donor DNA was homologous
to recipient DNA.

   The reader might legitimately wonder why intergeneric systems
are studied at all. In addition to studies on the definition of
the intergeneric transfer system itself, that yields information on
subtle genetic, anatomical, physiological, operational, formal and
other differences between bacterial species (There might be some
morals here for those interested in genetic manipulations with "higher"
biological systems), intergeneric hybridization has been successfully used as an approach and/or as an alternative means, to study
the following problems :

a) Evolution at the level of DNA (Demerec and New, 1965) by measuring genetic recombinational homologies.

b) Ordering and orientation of nearby genes that are too closely
   linked to be analyzed by conjugation but that are not contrans-
   ducible (Demerec 1965 ; Glatzer et al., 1966 ; Armstrong, 1967).

c) Location of certain wild type genes, for which there are not
   available mutations (lethal or else) or for cases in which mutations are not suitable. The additional concept here is the difference of gene products (between two species) that make them
   discriminable by biochemical techniques. The genes for 30S
   ribosomal proteins (O'Neil et al., 1969), 50S ribosomal proteins
   (Sypherd et al., 1969), polypeptide chain elongation "factors"
   (Gordon et al., 1972) have been located by intergeneric hybridization.

d) Analysis of quaternary protein structure (Lew and Roth, 1971).

e) Dominance of mutant genes with respect to wild type (Ridlle and
   Roth, 1972 ; Wu et al.,1970). Only certain type of hybrids are
   useful for this type of analysis

f) Expression of operons in foreign cytoplasms (Schlesinger and Olsen,
   1968).

g) Mapping of wild type genes for which selection of mutants is either
   impossible or too laborious. For example, genes coding for virulence, pathogenicity and antigenic properties (Sarvas et al.,
   1967 ; Krishnapillai and Karthigasu, 1969 ; Johnson and Baron,
   1969).

Of more recent vintage is a system that utilizes a "transformation"
system in *E. coli* to detect and characterize "hybrid episomes" and
their products (Chang and Cohen, 1974). The construction of episomes
will be described elsewhere in this volume.

I have emphasized the intergeneric transfer system in bacteria, not
only because it has been extremely useful in studying certain fundamental problems, but specially because it might turn out to be useful and important for those inclined to manipulate, genetically,
plants and other higher systems.   Any possible morals are to be
drawn by the interested reader.

VII. OTHER MAPPING PROCEDURES

   The methods of genetic analysis outlined so far depend both on
a system of transfer and on recombination. Genetic analysis by
either transduction or transformation generally yields a series of
"small linkage groups" such that in systems without conjugation
(e.g. the Bacilli) no hard genetic evidence, of a linkage group and

of the relative order of markers, is obtained through recombination, that is to say, mapping at the level of the chromosome, for many markers, is not feasible.

An alternative approach was originally designed for *B. subtilis* by Yoshikawa and Sueoka (1963a) and later confirmed (Dubnau et al., 1967) and extended to other bacterial species (Berg and Caro, 1967 ; Abe and Tomizawa, 1967 ; Cerda-Olmedo, Hanawalt and Guerola, 1968 ; Jyssum, 1969 ; Altenbern, 1968).

The approach depends on the reasoning that, in an exponentially growing culture (synchronized or not), and assuming that chromosome replication begins at a fixed point (as turned out to be the case), there would be more copies of genes lying close to the "replication origin" than of genes at the end ; "intermediate" genes would presumably be present in "intermediate" numbers of copies, such that a gradient of gene copies would appear.

The methodologies utilized for estimating the number of copies, varying with the skill and expertise of the investigators and with the inherent limitations of the bacterial species used, include the following :

a) "Marker frequency" as measured by the frequency of transformation (Yoshikawa and Sueoka, 1963a ; Dubnau et al., 1967). The frequency of transformant donor ability of an exponentially growing culture is compared to that of a stationary phase culture. Marker frequency has also being measured in *E. coli* by means of P1-mediated transduction (Berg and Caro, 1967).

b) "Density transfer" depends on the feasibility of synchronizing bacterial cultures with respect to DNA replication. In one type of experiments bacterial DNA is labelled (D_2O and N^{15}) previous to synchronization and the culture is brought to a light medium (H_2O and N^{14}). At various time-intervals, the DNA is extracted and separated by caesium chloride density gradient centrifugation (see Charles, this volume) into heavy (not replicated) and hybrid (semiconservatively replicated) fractions, which are used separately to transform recipients with respect to various markers (Yoshihawa and Sueoka, 1963b ; Dubnau et al., 1967). In another set of experiments DNA replication is synchronized and cell growth is restarted in the presence of a density label (e.g. 5-bromouracil), at various times labelled DNA is measured by either transformation or transduction, after separation by caesium chloride density gradient centrifugation (Abe and Tomizawa, 1967).

c) "Frequency of mutations" depends on the concept that the mutagen N-methyl-N'-nitro-N-nitrosoguanidine is more effective at the replicating point (Cerda-Olmeda et al., 1968 ; Altenbern, 1968). The frequency of appearance of mutations on a time scale has also been measured in differentially labelled cultures of *E. coli*

(Vielmetter and Messer, 1964).

It seems to me that it is important to emphasize the limitations of these approaches for genetic mapping. First, it should be
kept in mind that bacterial chromosome replication is bidirectional
(Masters and Broda, 1971 ; Harford, 1974) which has to be taken into
consideration in the interpretation of experimental data, and second,
that the assumption that all markers have the same innate probability of transformation and/or transduction, is not correct (see Lacks
1966 ; Norkin, 1970 ; for marker specific affects in recombination).

VIII. ANALYSIS OF VIRAL GENOME STRUCTURE

The next two sections on viruses and fungi are included only
for the sake of completeness and will be very brief.

Viruses make use of either DNA or RNA to store their genetic
information in either single or double stranded form. In DNA viruses,
the genetic information is distributed in a single molecule. There
are some exceptions to this rule. On the other hand, genetic information in RNA-containing viruses is often distributed in more than
one molecule. In such cases, reassortement of genetic markers follows
a pattern similar to that of eukaryotes.

To my knowledge, recombination in RNA containing viruses has
not been detected, on the other hand, DNA viruses often recombine
either using host-recombination systems and/or systems specified
by their own genomes.

For more detailed information on the molecular biology of
bacterial and other viruses, the reader is referred to the monogra-
phies by Stent (1963) and by Luria and Darnell (1967). Other important
reviews should also be consulted (Hershey, 1971 ; Mosig _et al._,
1971
I will comment below on three characteristical features of virus genetics : mutations, recombination and complementation.

A. Viral mutations

The most important and useful type of mutations are the so called
"conditional lethal" mutations, that, as the term indicates, render the
virus unable to propagate under certain conditions. Two types of
"conditional" lethals are available : a) temperature sensitive (or
cold-sensitive) that render the virus unable to reproduce at one
temperature, the non-permissive temperature (high or low) while the
virus is able to reproduce at another temperature, the permissive
temperature (low or high). b) Host-dependent mutations, which are
able to propagate on certain types of host (the permissive host)

while unable to do so in a second host (the non-permissive host). This type of mutations are also called *sus* for suppressor-sensitive or *am* for amber. The first type requires one host and two temperatures while the second type requires two hosts for analysis (Epstein **et al.**, 1963 ; Fenner, 1970).

Clearly, conditional lethal mutations are restricted to genes coding for essential functions. Other type of mutations include virulent mutants, host-range mutants and plaque-type mutants. Of some importance, in the analysis of genome structure of bacteriophages are deletion mutants. Deletion mutants are either viable (deleted for non-essential functions) or defective (deleted for essential functions), maintained in a cryptic lysogenic state. The first types are screened as "heat-resistant" based on the observation that in a phage population, phage particles with less than normal DNA content are more resistant to heat (65°) and to high ionic strength, than wild type (Parkinson and Huskey, 1971). The second types are isolated after induction of an thermosensitive lysogen, as in λ (see Hershey, 1971) or after transduction (Chan and Botstein, 1972).

B. Viral Recombination

Crosses involving viruses are very different from those of cellular organisms. This is so because of the possibility of having many rounds of matings. A few phage particles of two parental viruses may enter a host cell and often hundred and even thousands of progeny particles leave it. A virus cross is thus a problem of population genetics. Mathematical functions have been devised to analyze viral recombination. These functions are of questionable validity since they were based on assumptions that, at best, are hard to justify.

The great majority of mapping studies of viruses have used recombination frequencies representing the crude proportion of recombinants, in respect to a pair of markers, among the total progeny issuing from a cross. Such recombination figures have yielded maps that are both consistent and useful, despite that they are, clearly not true recombination frequencies equivalent to those in cellular organisms. Conditions must be standardized and controls should be rather rigorous.

The most important variables are the multiplicity of infection and the proportion of parental phages ; the number of rounds of matings taking place and the appearance of lysis, that affects the frequency of progeny. The former two are, to a certain extent, under the control of the investigator, while the latter two are, for the most part, beyond the control of the investigator. Further details and references can be found in recent publications (Edgar, 1963 ; Foss and Stahl, 1963 ; Lindhal, 1969, Doermann and Parma, 1967 ; Mosig, 1968; Mosig **et al.**, 1971).

C. Complementation

The rationale, methodology and models of complementations are very elegantly reviewed by Fincham, (1966) and by Matagne (this volume). For our purposes, it will be enough to say that complementation tests with phage "conditional lethal" mutants are not only simple and straightforward but also become a powerful tool of genetic resolution. In practice, it consists of mixing cells with two phage types under non-permissive conditions and assaying the progeny under permissive conditions.

A fairly recent approach to mapping in phages consists of analyzing, with the electron microscope, reannealed DNA molecules, from two different sources (one either a deletion or a phage DNA molecule belonging to another phage "species" (see for example Fiandt et al., 1971). This method, although of limited application, might prove useful with animal and plant viruses, as well as with bacteria.

IX. FUNGAL GENOME STRUCTURE

Genetic analysis in eukaryotic microbes (e.g. fungi) resemble more closely classical genetics of higher organisms than bacteria. There are at least three obvious factors of difference from higher organisms : a) Diploid state is very much circumscribed. b) Genetic characterization of the four products of particular meiosis (tetrad analysis). c) Variability of the genetic complement : haploids, diploids, heterokaryons, dikaryons, aneuploids, are all experimentally feasible for the performance of functional genetic tests (dominance, complementation).

A. The sexual cycle

It might be worthwhile to remember that meiosis, for our purposes, is a reductional division of the chromosome number. Following DNA replication the first meiotic division (equational) takes place followed by the second mitotic division (reductional) that yields haploid "nuclei" which are in turn mitotically divided. In most fungi the four products of a meiosis are recovered in a single ascospore (or basidiospore) which greatly simplifies genetic analysis. In at least some fungi (e.g. neurospora) the nuclei are arranged in "ordered" tetrads which allows for the identification of pre-reductional and post-reductional recombinations.

Linkage maps are usually constructed through the analysis of the products of meiosis. Three types of analysis are feasible : a) ordered tetrads gives the most information due to the possibility to distinguish the pre- and post-reduction of an allelic pair and uses the centromere as an additional marker. b) Unordered tetrads. In some cases the spore arrangements do not allow for conclusions regarding the time of reduction of marker genes, the centromers can

not be used as a marker (e.g. years, basidiomycetes). As an illustration of the limitations of unordered tetrad analysis, is the fact
that single factor crosses (a^+xa) reveal only whether segregation
is reciprocal or non-reciprocal. c) Single strands. In some fungi
(e.g. phycomycetes), tetrad analysis cannot be performed. The isolation and study of single spores remains as a possibility. Since
only one of the four products of meiosis is identified in such case,
this type of analysis has been called single strand analysis.

Linkage between markers refers to the predominance of parental
combinations among the offspring of crosses, i.e. genetic markers
do not recombine at random. Of importance in genetic analysis of
fungi is the occurance of interference, that is the non-random distribution of cross-overs among the four chromatids of the tetrad
Standardization of the experimental conditons is advisable, since
recombination frequencies vary with a number of genetical, physical
and chemical factors.

B. The parasexual cycle

The parasexual cycle (or mitotic recombination), first discovered by Pontecorvo (Pontecorvo **et al.**, 1953) in *Aspergillys nidulans*
and later extended to other microbes, is described as the sequence
of events that leads to the same end product as sexual reproduction
(reassortment of linked and unlinked markers) without the involvement of specialized organs of sexual reproduction or of a regular
alternation of nuclear fusion and meiosis.

The method (probably applicable to any normally haploid fungus
in which diploid strains can be obtained) consists of the selection
of diploid strains, as a first step, followed by the isolation of
vegetative segregants from heterozygous diploids. It is beyond the
scope of this article to describe in detail the events that allow
mapping in fungi through mitotic recombination. Be enough to say
that the system has been successfully used to construct maps, in
several fungi.

C. Conversion or non-reciprocal genetic exchange

First observed in the mid-fifties by Lindegren and his colleagues (Lindegren, 1952) in *Saccharomyces cerevisice* mutant x wild type
crosses, conversion, or non-reciprocal recombination, is defined as
an "abnormal" segregation of nuclei is the ascus. Normal segregation
ratio being 2:2, conversion segregation ratios being most often 3:1
and occasionally 5:3, 7:1, 8:0.

The mechanism of gene conversion is not understood, and conversion is mentioned here, first because it is of academic importance
(it has constituted an obstacle in recombination models) and second

because in intragenic recombinations (fine genetic structure of the gene), most events lead to non-reciprocal segregations.

It is not known whether in bacteria all recombinations are reciprocal or non-reciprocal, or whether some are reciprocal and some non-reciprocal. This is due to the fact that in bacterial crosses, only recombinant types are recovered, in conjugation, for example, both parents are selected against and only certain types of recombinants are recovered. In transduction (and in transformation) only one parent is selected against but reciprocal products of recombination are not recoverable. Some recent evidence indicates that in bacterial recombinations, non reciprocal events are the rule (see Berg and Gallant, 1972).

The difficulty in bacteriophage is compounded by the general difficulties in the handling of bacteriophage crosses mentioned above. It could be, however, experimentally possible to test all products of recombination by single burst analysis. In one studied case, conversion was found (Boon and Zinder, 1971).

More details of fungal genetics can be found in the monography by Fincham and Day (1971).

X. CONCLUDING REMARKS

A review article of this nature is not only circumscribed and non-exhaustive but it also reflects, to a large extent, the personal preferences and expertise of the author and to a certain extent the possible usefulness to the audience. The bias is thus, twofold. I was heavily biased to *E. coli*, not only because of my own experimental and intellectual expertise but also because the genetic tractability of this bacterium has, in terms of research-output, made it a favorite substrate for fundamental genetic, molecular biological and biochemical problems. It is no mystery that *E. coli* is, by far, the best described cellular organism. Although this review is biased to *E. coli*, many of the events that are true for this bacterium are also true for other bacteria. As mentioned above, care should be taken not to make dangerous generalizations and possibly wrong assumptions.

Because of the two fold circumscription of this review, the reader is urged to examine similar reviews with a different flavor (Roth, 1970 ; Hopwood, 1972) and reviews with a different organismic bias (Armstrong et al., 1970) for *B. subtilis* ; Davis and de Serres, 1970, for *Neurospora crassa* Fogel and Mortimer, 1971 ; Hartwell, 1970 ; for *S. cerivissiae* ;Hotchkiss and Gabor, 1970 ; for bacterial transformation ; Holloway et al., 1971 ; for *Pseudomonas* ; Coetzee, 1972 ; for the Proteus group ; Pratt, 1969 ; for single stranded DNA bacteriophages; and Levine et al., 1970 ; for chloroplast genetics), to acquire a more inclusive picture of the field. Miller's book (1972) is a must for methodology of bacterial genetic manipulations, specially since I neglected methodology in favor of conceptual explanations.

It is hoped that plant biologist might draw some morals from this review. I will only mention here that anybody bent to use DNA from bacterial sources for manipulations with higher organisms, must first know the exact location of a particular gene (or set of genes) and its genetic properties.

Acknowledgements

I wish to gratefully acknowledge the encouragement, moral support and comments on the manuscript of P. Charles, P. Lurquin and M. Mergeay.

REFERENCES

ABE, M., and J. TOMIZAWA. (1967). Proc. Nat. Acad. Sci. U.S.A., 58 : 1911-1918.

ALTENBERN, R.A. (1968). J. Bacteriol, 95 : 1642-1646

ANAGNOSTOPOULOS, C., and I.P. CRAWFORD (1961). Proc. Nat. Acad. Sci. U.S.A. 47 : 378-390

ARBER, W. and S. LINN (1969). Annu. Rev. Biochem. 38 : 467 - 500

ARMSTRONG, F.B. (1967). Genetics 56 463 - 466.

ARMSTRONG, R.L., N. HARFORD, R.H. KENNET, M.L. ST. PIERRE, and N. SUEOKA. (1970). In methods in Enzymology VXIIA : 36-59. S. Colowick and N.O. Kaplan Eds.

BARON, L.S., P. Jr. GEMSKI, E.M. JOHNSON, and J.A. WOHLHIETER (1968). Bacteriol. Rev. 32, 362-369

BEATTLE, K.L., and J.K. SETLOW (1970). J. Bacteriol. 104 : 390-400

BERG, C.M. and L.G. CARO (1967). J. Mol. Biol. 29 : 419-431

BERG, D.E., and J.A. GALLANT (1972). Genetics 68 : 457-472

BISWAS, D.G., and A.W. RAVIN (1971). Mol. Gen. Genet. 110 : 1-22

BOON, T., and N.D. ZINDER (1971). J. Mol. Biol. 58 : 133-151

BORAM, W. and J. ABELSON (1971). J. Mol. Biol. 62 : 171-178

CERDA-OLMEDO, E., P.C. HANAWALT, and N. GUEROLA (1968). J. Mol.
        Biol. 33 : 705-719

CHAKRABARTY A.M., and I.C. GUNSALUS (1970). J. Bacteriol. 103 :
        830-832.

CHANG, A.C.Y., and S.N. COHEN (1974). Proc. Nat. Acad. Sci. U.S.A.
        71 : 1030-1034

CHAN, R.K., and D. BOTSTEIN (1972). Virology, 49 : 257-267

COETZEE, J.N. (1972). Annu. Rev. Microbiol. 26, 23-54

CURTISS, R. (1969). Annu. Rev. Microbiol. 23, 69-136

DAVIS, R.H., and F.J. de SERRES (1970), pp. 79-143. In Methods in
        Enzymology XVIIA, S.P. Colowich and N.O. Kaplan (Eds.)
        Academic Press. New York.

DEMEREC, M. (1965), PP. 505-510 in "Evolving Genes and Proteins"
        V. Bryson and H.J. Vogel, eds. Academic Press, New York.

DEMEREC, M., and K. NEW (1965). Biochem. Biophys. Res. Commun. 18 :
        652-655.

DOERMANN, A.H., and D.H. PARMA. (1967). J. Cell. Physiol. 70 supl. 1:
        147-164.

DRAKE, J.H. (1969). Annu. Rev. Genet. 3 : 247-268.

DREXLER, H. (1970). Proc. Nat. Acad. Sci. U.S.A. 66 : 1083-1088

DUBNAU, D., C. GOLDTHWAITE, I. SMITH, and J. MARMUR (1967). J.
        Mol. Biol. 27 : 163-185

DUBNAU, E., and P. MARGOLIN (1972). Mol. Gen. Genet. 117 : 91-112

EDGAR, R.S. (1963). In "Methodology in Basic Genetics", pp. 19-36
        (Ed. W.J. Burdette). Holden-Day, San Fransisco.

EPSTEIN, R.H., A. BOLLE, C.M. STEINBERG, E. KELLENBERGER, E. BOY de
        1a TOUR, R. CHEVALLEY, R.S. EDGAR, S. SLISMAN, G.H. DEN-
        HARDT and G.H. LELAUSIS (1963). Cold Spring Harbor Symp.
        Quant. Biol. 28 : 375-385

FENNER, F. (1970). Ann. Rev. Microbiol. 24 : 297-334.

FIANDT, M., Z. HRADECNA, H.A. LORERON and W. SZYBALSKI (1971). pp.
        329-354 in "The Bacteriophage Lambda". A.D. Hershey Ed.
        Cold Spring Harbor Laboratory, Cold Spring Harbor, New York.

FINCHAM, J.R.S., and P.R. DAY (1971). Fungal Genetics. Blackwell
        Scientific Publications. Third edition. Oxford.

FOGEL, S., and R.K. MORTIMER. (1971). Annu. Rev. Genet. 5 : 219-236

FOSS, H.M., and F.W. STAHL (1963). Genetics 48 : 1659-1672

GLATZER, L., D.A. LABRIE, and F.B. ARMSTRONG (1966). Genetics 54 :
        423-432.

GORDON, J., L.S. BARON, and M. SCHWEIGER (1972). J. Bacteriol.
        100 : 306-312

GRATIA, J.P. (1966). Bikens J. 9 : 77-87

HARFORD N. (1974). (In Press).

HARFORD N., and M. MERGEAY (1973). Mol. Gen. Genet. 120 : 151-155

HARTMAN, P.E. (1963). In "Methodology in Basic Genetics" pp.103-128
        (Ed. W.J. Burdette). Holden-Day, San Fransisco.

HARTWELL, L.H. (1970). Annu. Rev. Genet. 4 : 373-396

HAYES, W. (1968). The Genetics of Bacteria and their Viruses. Black-
        well Scientific Publications. Oxford.

HERDMAN, M. (1973). Mol. Gen. Genet. 120 : 369-378

HERSHEY, A.D. Ed. (1971). The Bacteriphage Lambda. Cold Spring
        Harbor Laboratory. Cold Spring Harbor, New York.

HOLLOWAY, B.W., V. KRISHNAPILLAI, and U. STANISICH (1971). Annu.
        Rev. Genet. 5 : 425-446.

HONG, J. and B.N. AMES (1971). Proc. Nat. Acad. Sci. U.S.A., 68 :
        3158-3162.

HOPWOOD, D.A. (1967). Bacteriol. Rev. 31 : 373 - 403.

HOPWOOD, D.A. (1972). In methods in Microbiol. 7B : 29-158. Norris
        and Ribbons, eds. Academic Press, New York.

HOPWOOD, D.A., F.K. CHATER, J.E. DOWDING, and W. VIVIAN (1973).
        Bacteriol. Rev. 37 : 371-405.

HOTCHKISS, R.D., and M. GABOR (1970). Annu. Rev. Genet. 4 : 193-224.

HULANICKA, M.D., N.M. KREDICH and D.M. TREIMAIN. (1974). J. Biol.
        Chem. 249 : 867-872

HULANICKA, D.M., and T. KLOPOTOWSKI (1972). Acta Biochim. Polon.
        19 : 251-260

JACOB, F., and E.L. WOLLMAN (1961). Sexuality and the Genetics of
          Bacteria. Academic Press. New York.

JACOBSON, A., and D. GILLESPIE (1971). Biochem. Biophys. Res.
          Commun. 44 : 1030-1040

JOHNSON, E.M., W.G. CRAIG, J.A. WOHLHIETER, J.R. LAZERE, R.M.
          SYNENKI, and L.S. BARON (1973). J. Bacteriol. 115 :
          629-634.

JOHNSON, E.M., and L.S. BARON (1969). J. Bacteriol. 99 : 358-359.

JOHNSON, E.M., S. FALKOW, and L.S. BARON (1964). J. Bacteriol. 87
          54-60.

JONES, D. and P.H.A. SNEATH. (1970). Bacteriol. Rev. 34 : 40-81

JYSSUM, K. (1968). J. Bacteriol. 99 : 263-268.

KELLY, B. and M.G. SUNSHINE (1967). Biochem. Biophys. Res. Commun.
          28, 237-243.

KRISHNAPILLAI, V. and K. KARTHIGASU (1969). J. Bacteriol. 97 :
          1343-1351.

LACKS, S. (1966). Genetics 53 : 207-235.

LEAVIT, R.W., J.A. WHOHLHIETER, E.M. JOHNSON, G.E. OLSON and L.S.
          BARON (1971). J. Bacteriol. 108 : 1357-1365

LEVINE, R.P. and U. GOODENOUGH (1970). Ann. Rev. Genet. 4 : 397-408.

LEW, K.K., and J.R. ROTH (1971). Biochemistry 10 : 204-207

LINDEGREN, C.C. (1952). J. Genet. 51 : 625-656

LINDHAL, G. (1969). Virology 39 : 861-866

LOW, B. (1973). J. Bacteriol. 113 : 798-812

LURIA, S.E., J.N. ADAMS, and R.C. TING (1960). Virology 12 : 348-390

LURIA, S.E., and J.W. BURROUS (1957). J. Bacteriol. 74 : 461-476

LURIA, S.E., and J.E. DARNELL (1968). General Virology, 2nd ed.
          Wiley, New York.

MANDEL, M. (1969). Annu. Rev. Microbiol. 23 : 239-274

MASTERS, M. and P. BRODA (1971). Nature New. Biol. 232 : 137-140.

MERGEAY, M. (1971). p. 141-149 in L. Ledoux ed. Uptake of Informative
          Molecules by Living Cells. North-Holland Publishing Company
          Amsterdam.

MERGEAY, M. (1972). Mol. Gen. Genet. 119 : 89-92.

MERGEAY, M., P. CHARLES, R. MARTIN, J. REMY, and L. LEDOUX (1971).
        In : L. Ledoux, Ed. Informative Molecules in Biological
        Systems. North-Holland Pub. Comp.

MIDDLETON, R.B., and T. MOJICA-A (1971). Adv. Genet. 16 : 53-79.

MILLER, J.H. (1972). Experiments in Molecular Genetics. Cold Spring
        Harbor Laboratory. New York.

MOJICA-A, T., and R.B. MIDDLETON (1970). Bacteriol. Proc. p. 22

MOJICA-A, T., and R.B. MIDDLETON (1971). J. Bacteriol. 108 :
        1161-1167.

MOJICA-A, T., and R.B. MIDDLETON (1972). Genetics 71 : 491-505.

MOSIG, G. (1968). Genetics 59 : 137-151.

MOSIG, G., R. EHRING, W. SCHIEWEN and S. BLOCK (1971). Mol. Gen.
        Genet. 113 : 51-91.

MUKAI, F.H., and P. MARGOLIN (1963). Proc. Nat. Acad. Sci. U.S.A.
        50 : 140-148.

NOMURA, M., and F. ENGBAENK (1972). Proc. Nat. Acad. Sci. U.S.A.
        69 : 1526-1530.

NORKIN, L.C. (1970). J. Mol. Biol. 51 : 633-655.

O'NEIL, D.M., L.S. BARON, and P.S. SYPHERD (1969). J. Bacteriol.
        99 : 242-247.

OZEKI, H., and H. IKEDA (1968). Annu. Rev. Genet. 2 : 245-278.

PARKINSON, J.S., and R.J. HUSKEY (1971). J. Mol. Biol. 56 : 369-384

PONTECORVO, G., J.A. ROPER, L.M. HEMMONS, K.D. Mc DONALD and A.W.
        BUFTON (1953). Adv. Genet. 5 : 141-238

PRATT, D. (1969). Annu. Rev. Genet. 3 : 343-362

RIDDLE, D.L. and J.R. ROTH (1972). J. Mol. Biol. 66 : 483-493

ROTH, J.R. (19   . In methods in Enzymology XVIIA : 3 - 35. S. Colo-
        wick and N.O. Kaplan Eds.

SANDERSON, K.E. (1972). Bacteriol. Rev. 36 : 558-586.

SARVAS, M.O., LÜDERITZ and O. WESTPHAL (1967). Ann. Med. Exp. Fenn.
        45 : 117-126.

SCHLESINGER, M.J. and R. OLSEN (1968). J. Bacteriol. 96, 1601-1605.

SMITH-KEARY, P.F. (1966). Genet. Res. 8 : 73-82.

STENT, G.S. (1963). Molecular Biology of Bacterial Viruses. W.H.
        Freeman and Company. San Fransisco.

STOCKER, B.A.D., N.D. ZINDER, and J. LEDERBERG (1953). Gen. Micro-
        biology. 9 : 410-433.

SUNSHINE, M.G., and B. KELLY (1971). J. Bacteriol. 108 : 695-704

SYPHERD, P.S., D.M. O'NEIL, and M.M. TAYLOR (1969). Cold Spring
        Harbor Symp. Quant. Biol. 34 : 77-84.

TAYLOR, A.L. (1963). Proc. Nat. Acad. Sci. U.S.A., 50 , 1043-1051

TAYLOR, A.L., and C.D. TROTTER (1972). Bacteriol. Rev. 36 : 504-524

UMBARGER, H.E. (1971). Adv. Genet. 16 : 119-140.

VIELMETTER, W. and W. MESSER (1964). Ber. d. Bunsengeseltschaft 68 :
        742-743.

WATANABE, T., T. ARAI, and T. HATORI (1970b). Nature (London) 225 :
        70-71.

WEISBLUM, B., and J. DAVIES (1968). Bacteriol. Rev. 32 : 493-528.

WILSON, G.A., and F.E. YOUNG (1972). J. Bacteriol. 111 : 705-716.

WU, Po CHI., P.F. JOHNSON, and A. NEWTON (1970). J. Bacteriol. 103 :
        318-322.

YANOFSKY, C. and E.S. LENNOX (1959). Virology 8 : 425-447.

YOSHIKAWA, H., and N. SUEOKA (1963a). Proc. Nat. Acad. Sci. U.S.A.
        49 : 559-566.

YOSHIKAWA, H., and N. SUEOKA (1963b). Proc. Nat. Acad. Sci. U.S.A.
        49 : 806-813

ZINDER, N.D., and J. LEDERBERG (1952). J. Bacteriol. 64 : 679-699.

THE MECHANISM OF COMPETENCE FOR DNA UPTAKE AND TRANSFORMATION IN PNEUMOCOCCI

Alexander Tomasz*

The Rockefeller University

New York, New York 10021

In the introduction of this paper one should first of all provide some justification for discussing topics in bacterial physiology at a meeting like this, concerned mainly with higher plants. The reason for discussing an aspect of bacterial transformation is that in bacteria considerable amount of information is available about the mechanism of DNA uptake in phenomena leading to genetic change and a brief review of this topic in pneumococci could illustrate with a case history the kinds of ideas, experimental approaches and observations one encounters when working with such a problem. While a "competent" state analogous to that in bacterial transformation has not as yet been detected in eucaryotic cells, biological phenomena involving nucleic acid transport across membranes do exist. The existence of infectious nucleic acid agents implies nucleic acid uptake by the natural hosts of such viroids (1). Lymphoid cells stimulated by phytohemagglutinins are known to secrete DNA into the medium (2) and transport of nucleic acids across intracellular membranes (mRNA through nuclear membrane) must be of frequent occurrence. In addition, it has been suggested that transfection-like phenomena, by uncoated viral genomes, may be responsible for some of the unusual symptoms of some types of viral infections and for the vertical transmission of slow viruses (3). Besides these "natural" phenomena there have been numerous demonstrations of nucleic acid "uptake" by a variety of eucaryotic cells. Reports on the biological activity of such absorbed nucleic acids include initiation of viral infection (4), expression (transcription or translation) of parts of a bacterial genome (5), genetic transformation by homologous (6,7) and even heterologous DNA (8). A sample of the types of systems, methods used and findings claimed may be found in the published proceedings of a recent

symposium on this subject (Informative Molecules in Biological
Systems) (9).

        Our experiments on the mechanism of competence in pneumo-
cocci have been centered around the "competence activator" substance:
a macromolecular agent that can induce the competent state of the
bacteria (10). With this experimental handle we were able to examine quite a few aspects of the mysterious transformable state in
which pneumococci can recognize, adsorb and internalize DNA molecules from their environment and undergo genetic change.

        Over the next pages I shall attempt to briefly review several
aspects of our studies on pneumococcal competence.

Experiments concerning the mechanism of action of activator

        A) Lack of enzymatic activities. The activity of the acti-
vator substance (measured either as the rate of accumulation of
transformable cells or as the rate of acquisition of DNA binding
capacity by the bacteria) has features suggesting an enzyme-like
entity. Thus induction of competence proceeds without a measurable
time lag and shows a saturation kinetics. It has a fairly sharp
pH optimum, it requires mercaptoethanol and the rate increases with
the incubation temperature up to about 39°C. For these reasons we
have done extensive studies to detect in the activator several
types of enzyme activities that one might conceivably associate
with the mechanism of competence. All these experiments yielded
negative results, in spite of the fact that many of the assays used
were bioassays capable of detecting extremely low levels of enzyme
activities. As possible enzyme activities we tested the following:
protease (using as substrate pneumococcal proteins labeled with
radioactive amino acids); RNase (tested by exposing the RNA of
bacteriophage f2 to activator and retitrating the biological
activity afterwards by a transfection assay); DNase (assayed by
testing the effect on the biological titration curve of transforming
pneumococcal DNA); lipolytic action (we used leakage of β-galacto-
sidase from E. coli protoplasts or leakage of hemoglobin from rabbit
red blood cells as assays); autolysin (using pneumococcal cell walls
labeled with high specific activity choline as substrate).

        These experiments had to be performed extremely carefully
since there have been several reports in the literature claiming
the presence of DNase-like (11) or autolysin-like (12) activity in
activator preparations and the somewhat cacophonic name "competase"
has been proposed for the activator in order to emphasize its
enzyme-like properties (13). It seems now that neither one of
these claims could be confirmed and the enzymatic activities reported were due to contamination of the preparations.

        B) The nature of competence induction: the target of the
activator. Since the measurement of transformability involved
three components, the incompetent cell, the activator and the
transforming DNA, it was not immediately obvious whether the

activator interacts with DNA or with the cells. In fact, the stimulation of transfection frequencies by various factors has often
been attributed to their interaction with the donor nucleic acids
(14) and a peculiar, denaturation-like effect of the activator preparations on DNA was claimed by some authors (15). This claim
could not be substantiated, however.

It seems quite clear that the target of the activator is in
the incompetent cell and not in the donor DNA. This conclusion is
based on the following observations: a) induction of transformability is a function of the time of incubation of cells with the
activator; preincubation of DNA (over a ten thousand fold range of
concentrations) with activator for different time periods has no
effect on the frequency of transformation. b) The rate of induction
of competence is a function of the concentrations of the activator
(3rd to 4th order) and of the incompetent cells (1st order) but is
independent of DNA concentration (16). c) Metabolic inhibitors
can completely block acquisition of competence (17). d) It was
found that activator can physically bind to bacteria (18), while
no association between DNA and activator could be detected in
sucrose gradients. e) Possible effects of the activator on several
physical properties of the transforming DNA were tested--all with
negative results. The tests included: determination of effect on
DNA melting and reannealing; on UV absorption spectrum; on the
template properties of DNA in a DNA polymerase reaction; and possible
cosedimentation with DNA in sucrose gradients.

A closer analysis of the interaction between activator molecules and incompetent cells has revealed that the activator can
rapidly attach to bacteria in a process that is only little affected
by variation in pH, temperature or the composition of the medium
(18). Activator attachment could be demonstrated even to cells
killed with formaldehyde or to the genetically incompetent mutant
strain RA7. In addition to physical association with the bacteria,
another consequence of activator attachment was disappearance of
its biological activity. However, brief heating of such "activator-
loaded" bacteria in salt solutions containing mercaptoethanol
resulted in the quantitative recovery of the biological activity in
soluble form. Further studies on activator attachment resulted in
the isolation of the "receptor": it is a heat labile, trypsin
resistant factor, located in the plasma membrane of the cells; it
has an approximate molecular weight of 50,000 daltons and it has
net negative change at physiological pH-s (19).

C. Lack of detectable physiological effects in activator-
treated growing bacteria. The first glimpse at the complexity of
the reaction between cells and activator molecules has come from
experiments designed to detect possible physiological effects of
the activator treatment. The main design of such experiments was
to grow a single culture of bacteria at low pH (in order to prevent spontaneous expression of competence); at a suitable cell

concentration the pH of the culture was shifted to the pH optimum of activation, and half of the culture was treated with activator, while the other half served as control. Under the experimental conditions the treated culture has rapidly (within 10-20 min) become competent (autoradiography with labeled DNA showed that 80-100% of the cells were capable of irreversible DNA fixation). The control culture showed no detectable competence.

We performed a large number of experiments in this system to detect three types of possible physiological effects of activator: i) on the rates of cellular polymer syntheses (RNA, DNA, cell wall, protein); ii) on the rate of turn-over of cellular polymers (i.e. solubilization of DNA, protein, cell wall or lipid label); and iii) possible effects on the general transport--and permeability properties of the cells (K^+ uptake and efflux; "leakage" of such intracellular marker as β-galactosidase, radioactive precursors, such as lysine, phenylalanine, uracil).

All of these experiments yielded negative results (20).

D. Metabolic requirements: protein synthesis, autolysin sensitive equatorial cell wall and active cell wall growth zone. On the other hand, it has become clear that successful activation to competence required that the bacteria performed certain types of synthetic activities during contact with the activator molecules. Specifically, it was found that inhibition of protein or RNA synthesis and the inhibition of the incorporation of nascent teichoic acid units into the cell surface would completely prevent the induction of competence (16,21). Inhibition of DNA synthesis-- on the other hand--had no effect on activation. An additional and dramatic inhibitory effect was noted when bacteria growing in ethanolamine containing medium were tested (22). In this latter case it is known that the cells utilize ethanolamine as a choline analogue and incorporate this abnormal amino alcohol into the cell wall teichoic acid at positions that are normally occupied by choline (23).

It should be emphasized that bacteria inhibited in their protein or cell wall synthesis or bacteria growing on ethanolamine medium would not even show reversible binding of DNA molecules upon treatment with activator. Thus it seemed that the activator controls even this earliest manifestation of cellular competence. Furthermore, the activator-dependent appearance of DNA binding capacity was clearly tied in with complex additional metabolic requirements.

These observations presented--essentially--a threefold puzzle. 1) The role of protein synthesis; 2) the role of continued cell wall synthesis and 3) the need for an autolysin sensitive cell wall. This latter condition has been deduced from the ethanolamine effect. It is known that ethanolamine-grown bacteria synthesize a cell wall that is completely resistant to the action of the endogenous cellular autolysin.

A set of further experiments has succeeded in a somewhat closer definition of these puzzles. It was found that the tryptophan analogue tryptazan was also capable of preventing activation. This antimetabolite is known to allow continued synthesis of peptide bonds and it incorporates into proteins at positions normally occupied by tryptophan. In some cases, such a substitution affects the proteins' biological activity. The inhibition of activation by this analogue showed that successful activation requires the de novo synthesis of a qualitatively correct protein or classes of such protein molecules. Thus the requirement for protein synthesis in activation is not simply a need for nonspecific "growth" or mass increase of the bacteria.

More refined experiments have allowed a closer look at the nature of continued cell wall synthesis also. It was shown that preexisting competence was rapidly lost and rapidly recovered in experiments in which choline incorporation into the cell wall was turned off and then turned on again (21). An equally rapid recovery of competence was also observed when ethanolamine-grown bacteria were given choline and activator: cellular capacity to bind DNA has returned within 5-10 minutes (i.e. within 10% of a bacterial generation time). Parallel experiments have demonstrated that nascent choline molecules incorporate into the cell wall exclusively at an equatorially located growth zone (21). These experiments have bearing on the interpretation of both the need for continuous cell wall synthesis and of the mechanism of ethanolamine inhibition. It seems that a) competence requires an autolysin sensitive (choline containing) wall only at the equatorial zone of the cell surface. b) The need for continuous incorporation of choline seems to reflect a requirement for an active cell wall growth zone.

E. <u>Stages in the expression of competence: temporal order.</u>
The general conclusion from the experiments described thus far was that between the collision of activator molecules with cells and the appearance of DNA binding capacity there is a complex, possibly multistep process. Thus the measurement of activator action by monitoring DNA binding or genetic transformability is an extremely indirect assay. The situation is reminiscent in a sense to the problem of finding the metabolic target of an antibiotic. The identification of such a primary target is a problem quite remote from the relatively easily measurable physiological consequences of action.

In our search for the unknown biochemical target of activator, we tried to untangle stages of the complex process between attachment to the receptors and the manifestations of competent state. It was possible to show that inhibitors of protein synthesis block this process at a different and "earlier" step than inhibition of cell wall synthesis (omission of choline from the medium). Bacteria could be "loaded" with activator in the presence of chloramphenicol. Upon removing extracellular (un-adsorbed) activator it was possible to demonstrate the development of competence upon removal of the block of protein synthesis. Thus the protein synthesis requiring step seems to follow adsorption of activator (16).

During experimentation with protein inhibitors we observed that--similarly to streptococci--pneumococci too show a dramatic agglutination reaction in the competent state. Competent bacteria would clump in low ionic strength--and low pH media, while incompetent cells remain dispersed. It was possible to show that the appearance of agglutination required not only attachment of activator but also a subsequent protein synthesis. In fact agglutination seemed to be caused by a trypsin sensitive substance that is deposited between the plasma membrane and the cell wall of the bacteria (24). It seems likely therefore, that at least one of the products of the protein synthesis essential for competence may be the "agglutinin."

The availability of the agglutination assay made it possible to further resolve the process of competence induction. Treatment of cells with activator in the presence of protein synthesis but in the absence of choline resulted in only a minor inhibition of agglutinin formation while competence (measured as DNA binding capacity) was completely inhibited.

These experiments established a tentative temporal sequence of the events of activation:
1. attachment of activator to receptors
2. protein synthesis (agglutinin)
3. active cell wall growth zone.

It is not clear at what exact stage does the "competence antigen" appear in this process (25,26).

F. Activator-dependent phenomena in cells exposed to abnormal conditions. It is apparent from the foregoing discussion that our attempts to pinpoint the target, i.e. primary biochemical effect of activator have failed. It seems that pneumococci are capable of smoothly accommodating the competent state into their normal physiology without any detectable abnormality that might reveal something about the primary effect of activator. While this was true for bacteria tested in normal growth supporting media, we were struck by the contrasting grossly unique behavior of competent cells in such an abnormal medium as the low ionic strength--low pH solution in which the agglutination assays were performed. Would it be possible that exposure of pairs of activated and non-activated (control) cells to a set of abnormal conditions might exaggerate latent activator-induced lesions in the bacteria? After experi-

menting with several defective growth media, we have stumbled upon
two conditions which have revealed striking differences in the
behavior of competent (activated) versus incompetent cells. One of
the conditions was--in essence--exposure of the activated cells to
a nutritional shift-up and to hypertonic sucrose. The response of
the competent bacteria was a dramatic, rapid and quantitative conversion to protoplasts. The second "exaggerating" condition was
simply transferring the activated cells to a buffered salt solution
(SPA) containing saline, phosphate buffer at pH 7.6, divalent
cations (Ca^{++} and Mg^{++}, each at about 3 mM concentration) and
glucose. Upon incubation in this medium at 30°C the competent
cells rapidly released into the medium a number of intracellular
components, including exonuclease, autolysin, hemolysin, β-galactosidase and intracellular radioactive label (27). The design of the
"exaggerating" strategy is shown in the scheme below:

Phase 1   Phase 2   Phase 3

Growth of culture   In Cd-medium at   Incubate at 30°C in

in C-medium at ⟶   pH 8, 30°C; add   SPA solution

pH 6.6   activator   "Leakage"

                                              Incubate at 37°C in

                                              C-medium containing

                                              20% sucrose

                                              Protoplast formation

Table 1 shows the extent and pattern of leakage.

Table 1. Activator-induced leakage of intracellular components

Strain	Transformants per ml	β-galactosidase	Hemolysin	Exonuclease	Autolysin	^{3}H-uracil
R6 (wild type)						
+ activator	3×10^6	5%	12%	6%	5%	8%
− activator	<300	1	ND	0.5	ND	2
+ activator at pH 6.6	<300	0.8	ND	0.4	0.2	−
+ activator + chloramphenicol	<300	0.9	ND	ND	ND	−
+ activator − choline	<300	1	0.8	ND	0.5	−
RA7 (genetically incompetent)						
+ activator	<300	ND	ND	ND	0.2	−
− activator	<300	ND	1	ND	0.1	−
cw1 (autolysin defective)						
+ activator	6×10^6	ND	0.2	1.2	ND	5
− activator	<300	ND	ND	0.2	ND	0.8

(The leaked enzyme activities are expressed as % of the total
 cellular concentration of the particular enzyme. ND: not
 detectable.)

Table 2 illustrates the parameters of protoplast formation.

Table 2. Activator-induced protoplast formation

Strain	Conditions in phase 2 of experiment	Extent of protoplast formation (% of cells)
R6 (wild type)	+ activator	100
	- activator	0
	+ activator at pH 6.6	1
	+ activator + chloramphenicol	2
	+ activator - choline	0
	+ trypsin-treated activator	0
cells in ethanol-amine medium	+ activator	0
RA7 (genetically incompetent)	+ activator	0
	- activator	0

Several interesting observations are evident from the tables. While both leakage and protoplast formation depend in an absolute manner on the treatment with activator, it is also clear that equally stringent additional requirements exist for these phenomena. Interestingly, these extra requirements are the very ones known as essential for the induction of competent state, i.e. protein synthesis; optimal pH; incorporation of choline; lysis-sensitive cell wall. This finding has two main consequences. First, it reassures one of the specificity of the leakage--and protoplasting phenomena. Second, the fact that all metabolic requirements for competence induction have to be met for both leakage and protoplasting shows that--once again--we picked up phenomena related to the "competent state" (i.e. the end product of activator action) rather than phenomena directly related to the primary target of activator. In other words, the exaggerating conditions amplified some latent or below detection level lesions typical of cells in the competent state. These lesions are: a subcritical cell wall damage and the

lowering of a cellular permeability barrier (leakage). Cell wall
damage seems to be caused by the autolysin (from within), because
of the inhibition of protoplasting in ethanolamine-grown cells.
A modification of the experimental design in the scheme has shown
that autolysin action at the equatorial surface area is sufficient
to induce protoplasting. In the modified experiment we used
choline-pulsed ethanolamine-grown cells; upon activator treatment
normal protoplast formation ensued (27).

As to the nature of the permeability barrier that is lowered
in the competent cells: two observations in Table 2 seem particularly relevant. Among the cell components escaping to the medium
are such normally intramembrane components as β-galactosidase and
phosphorylated uracil compounds. The other important point is the
lack of leakage of macromolecular cell components from the autolysin defective mutant, while this mutant still shows leakage of
low molecular weight uracil compounds. We interpret these findings
the following way: the permeability barrier directly affected by
activator is the plasma membrane. In cells with normal autolysin,
one consequence of the plasma membrane effect is the escape of
autolysin molecules into the periplasmic space from where they
attack the cell walls from within; the resulting increase in wall
porosity would then explain the escape of large molecules from the
periplasmic space (where they leaked, due to the primary membrane
damage) to the outside medium. In the autolysin defective mutant
the low amounts of cellular autolysin are not sufficient to affect
the wall pore-size to cause leakiness of large molecules. One has
to assume that in this bacterium the galactosidase, hemolysin and
exonuclease molecules remain trapped in the periplasmic space.

One should emphasize that we know nothing about the mechanism
by which the exaggerating conditions provoke the phenomena observed.
On the other hand, the nature of the activator dependent defects
are revealing: they imply a latent structural fragility in the
competent state, a fragility that is apparently amplified to
detectable levels by the exaggerating conditions. That this
structural fragility is a specific consequence of the competent
state is documented in a striking manner by the requirement for
activator, the need for protein synthesis and the other correlates
of competence, including genetic capacity. The complete lack of
leakage and lack of protoplasting by the genetically incompetent
(RA7) mutant is particularly noteworthy in this respect. This
mutant is normal as far as its autolysin content is concerned; it
has lysis sensitive, choline containing cell walls; it has normal
complement of nucleases, β-galactosidase and hemolysin; it also
contains receptors for the activator. However, activator treatment
of this mutant does not cause agglutination and none of the exaggerating conditions cause a positive response.

If one accepts the assumption that the exaggerating conditions only amplify latent wall and membrane damage both of which
are characteristic features of the competent state, then one can

construct an interesting working hypothesis for the mechanism of competence. We refer to this hypothesis as the "unmasking" model, and its hypothetical nature should be kept in mind. In essence the model assumes the following sequence of steps in the induction of competence: the combination of activator with the receptor on the plasma membrane causes a destabilization resulting in the escape of several intramembrane components into the periplasmic space. Among those components is the autolysin. It is assumed that the concentration of these autolysin molecules in the periplasmic space is under strict control by the cell because of the potentially lethal activity of these enzymes. On the other hand, all theories concerning the physiological role of these enzymes agree that autolysins must have temporary and cyclic access to the cell wall during the bacterial division cycle. It is tempting to suggest that combination of activator and receptor occurs at a special region of the plasma membrane, in the vicinity of the wall growth zone, e.g. at a mesosomal junction. The activator may then accelerate the normal outward transport of autolysin molecules into the periplasmic space. The consequence of this would be increased activity of autolysins at the growth zone, an activity in excess of what might be needed for the normal mechanism of cell surface expansion. On the other hand, the "excess" activity would provide a sufficient exposure of the plasma membrane (at the equatorial surface area) that membrane bound DNA binding components would be capable of interacting with extracellular DNA molecules. All these phenomena with the exception of DNA binding would occur below the level of detection of experimental techniques, unless one has applied the exaggerating conditions which amplify these processes sufficiently for observation.

The first key assumption of the "unmasking" model is the presumed central role of autolysin as an agent of uncovering DNA binding sites. It should be remembered that a role for autolysin in competence is based primarily on the incompetence of ethanolamine-grown cells. Bacteria grown on this amino alcohol are know to exhibit a whole series of pleiomorphic physiological properties most of which can be explained by the two biochemical level defects in the autolytic system of these bacteria--an autolysin resistant cell wall and an abnormal, inactive autolysin, an L-alanine N-acetyl-muramyl amidase (28).

The existence of the autolysin defective cwl mutant at first glance argues against the autolysin hypothesis. This mutant has only a fraction (about 1%) of the wild type amidase activity and yet, it can be made highly competent in an activator dependent process. However, the "unmasking" model requires only extremely small "wall damage" and the residual level of activity in the mutant may be sufficient.

A critical test of the autolysin is role in competence would require the isolation of temperature sensitive autolysin mutants.

A second key assumption of the "unmasking" model is the notion that the DNA binding sites preexist to competence; they are present in both the incompetent and in the competent bacteria, but only in the latter are they accessible to extracellular DNA molecules.

In the detailed description of the "unmasking" model (27) we proposed that the protein synthesis requiring step in competence may be analogous to the protein synthesis needed for the killing action of cytocidal antibiotics. The mechanism of killing by these antibiotics is known to involve the autolysins (29) and the role of protein synthesis in the killing action is supposed to be via either the synthesis or the transport of autolysin molecules to their physiological sites of action at the cell surface.

G. The nature of DNA receptors on the surface of transformable pneumococci. One of the assumptions implicit in the "unmasking" model for competence is that the DNA binding receptor substance present in competent pneumococci is not at the outermost surface envelope, but beneath it. It has become possible to test this assumption experimentally in the following manner. Competent bacteria were allowed to adsorb DNA in the presence of EDTA (added to prevent escape of the adsorbed molecules inside the cell) (30). Excess, nonradioactive DNA was added next (in order to prevent attachment of further molecules) and then the cell wall of the bacteria was removed by autolysin treatment. It was found that as much as 50 to 80% of the attached molecules fractionated with the protoplasts provided that glucose was present in the adsorption medium. Most of the adsorbed DNA was autolysin sensitive if glucose was omitted. This experiment indicates that most of the DNA binding sites are located on the plasma membrane, at least when the bacteria are provided with an energy source.

The second assumption of the "unmasking" model is that the binding sites for DNA preexist in the incompetent cells. Recent experiments yielded results that are compatible with this assumption.

It was found that--unlike competent cells--incompetent pneumococci do not interact with DNA at all. They do not bind these molecules (not even in a reversible fashion) and they show none of the other activity typical of competent cells, the surface-located nuclease (30). It was possible to induce both of these competence-specific phenomena by physical damage to the cell wall or by lowering the normal ionic strength of the adsorbing medium. Table 3 shows that mechanical disruption (in a Mickle disintegrator), dissection of the equatorial lysis-sensitive cell wall band (with autolysin) (21) or putting the bacteria into low ionic strength media (0.01 M NaCl; 0.01 M potassium phosphate, pH 7.6) was sufficient to eliminate the difference in DNA binding between competent and incompetent cells. Furthermore, there was a great increase in the binding capacity of competent cells, suggesting the presence of a large number of latent DNA binding sites in both kinds of bacteria.

Table 3. Unmasking of DNA binding sites in the incompetent pneumococci

	Total	Nuclease sensitive	Nuclease resistant	Transformants per ml	Surface Nuclease
Competent cells					
in normal ionic strength medium	7,000	3,000	4,000	1.2×10^6	yes
in low ionic strength medium	12,000	7,000	5,000	1.4×10^6	yes
Incompetent cells					
in normal ionic strength medium	620	520	100	ND	ND
in low ionic strength medium	8,400	7,800	600	ND	yes
Competent cells, after disruption	70,000	65,000	(5,000)	–	yes
Incompetent cells, after disruption	71,000	66,000	(5,000)	–	yes
(Mickle disintegrator)					
Incompetent cells, grown in					
ethanolamine medium, pulsed with choline	300	280	20	ND	ND
pulsed with choline and digested with autolysin	4,800	–	–	–	(yes)

(Numbers represent cpm of ^{3}H-DNA bound per 5×10^8 cells or cell equivalents).

If one assumes that the "unmasking" conditions applied in those experiments did not alter the nature of DNA binding in the bacteria, then the results in Table 3 provide indeed experimental confirmation of the assumption that the DNA receptors are "buried" by cell wall material in the incompetent state and that an essential feature of competence induction is the exposure of these receptors. However, the data in Table 3 also add a note of warning. While it is clear that both DNA binding and surface nuclease activity are exhibited by the bacteria in the low ionic strength medium, on the other hand, it is also apparent that the same cells did not transform and that little of the adsorbed DNA has become nuclease resistant--a feature usually interpreted to indicate true intracellular uptake of the molecules. Thus there remains a striking and most essential difference between "unmasking" by activator and "unmasking" by experimental methods and one wonders whether the activator might not also affect the plasma membrane in a more sophisticated and as yet obscure manner?

It is most likely that the "unmasking" model will require serious modifications or it may even have to be abandoned. Nevertheless, we feel that at this stage of our studies on the mechanism of DNA recognition and uptake by cells it serves a very useful function in that it provides a comprehensive summary of experimental findings connected in a functional manner to one another. The model is specific enough in detail to allow the design of a large number of experimentally testable predictions. The model also makes certain predictions about mutations affecting the transformation system. For instance, any mutation in the autolytic system might affect DNA binding. It is possible that the RA7 mutation or the mutation in the so called ntr ("nontransformable") mutants may belong to this class. Other mutants may be affected in the glucose dependent adsorption step (the "noz" mutant of Lacks may belong here) (31). Figure 1 is meant to provide a summary scheme for the unmasking model. The figure shows a cross section of the bacterial surface with the cross-hatched cell wall, the underlying plasma membrane (dash line) and the periplasmic space in between the two. The black beads under the plasma membrane represent DNA binding sites; the dark square represents the receptor for the activator (drawn as a star). Triangles and dots indicate intramembrane markers (autolysin, β-galactosidase) and the circular (and later: "bay"-like) profile on the plasma membrane is standing for a mesosome. In step 1 of the diagram extracellular activator attaches to the receptor causing deformation of the mesosome and leakage into the periplasm (step 2). In step 3, periplasmic autolysin causes wall damage allowing penetration of double stranded DNA (in a glucose dependent process) (steps 4 and 5). Finally, the attached molecules are internalized in a glucose and divalent cation requiring process, with concomitant surface nuclease activity (step 6).

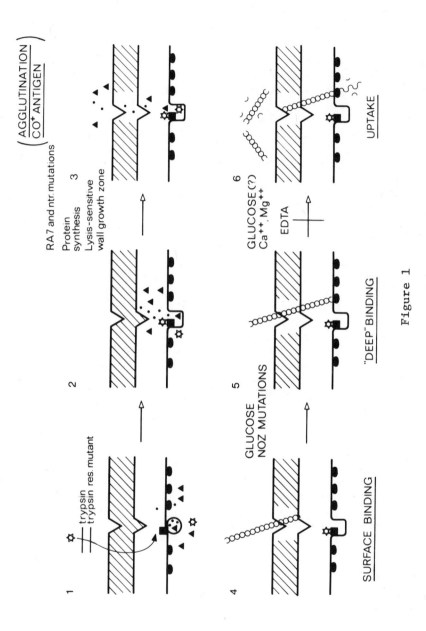

Figure 1

An attractive feature of the "unmasking" model is that it minimizes the number of cellular factors the sole function of which in the cell would be to play a role in genetic transformation. In the "unmasking" model several cellular components with role in the normal physiology of the cell are "exploited" for the additional functions required for the adsorption and uptake of extracellular DNA molecules. Thus the activator-receptor complex may be part of the autolysin transport mechanism; the growth zone of cell wall is--of course--essential for surface enlargement; and it has also been suggested that the DNA binding sites may be enzyme molecules (nucleases) with normal role in the DNA metabolism of the cells (30,31). The active sites of such membrane bound enzymes could provide the specificity required to recognize and capture DNA molecules from the environment.

*Acknowledgement: This review has been written during the tenure of a grant from U.S. Atomic Energy Commission.

References

1. Diener, T.O. (1972). Adv. Virus Res. 17, 295.
2. Rogers, J.C., Coldt, D., Kornfeld, S., Skinner, A. and Valery, R.C. (1972). Proc. Nat. Acad. Sci. US 69, 1685.
3. Herriott, R.M. (1969). Prog. Med. Virol. 11, 1.
4. Crawford, L. Dulbecco, R., Fried, M., Montagier, L. and Stoker, M. (1964). Proc. Nat. Acad. Sci. US 52, 148.
5. Merril, C.R., Geier, M.R. and Petricciani, J.C. (1971). Nature 233, 398.
6. Szybalska, E.H. and Szybalski, W. (1962). Proc. Nat. Acad. Sci. US 48, 2026.
7. Fox, A.S. and Yoon, S.B. (1970). Proc. Nat. Acad. Sci. US 67, 1608.
8. Ledoux, L.G.H., Huart, R. and Jacobs, M. (1971). In Informative Molecules in Biological Systems (ed., L.G.H. Ledoux, North Holland Publishing Company.
9. Informative Molecules in Biological Systems, NATO Symposium, MOL, Belgium (ed., L.G.H. Ledoux, North Holland Publishing Company), (1970).
10. Tomasz, A. (1973). In Membranes and Walls of Bacteria (ed. Leivy, L.) Marcel-Dekker, New York.
11. Kohoutova, M., Brana, H. and Holubova, I. (1968). Bioch. Bioph. Res. Commun. 30, 124.
12. Akrigg, A., Ayad, S.R. and Barker, G.R. (1967). Bioch. Bioph. Res. Commun. 28, 1062.
13. Pakula, P. and Hauschild, A.H.W. (1965). Canad. J. Microbiol. 11, 823.
14. Vaheri, A. and Pagano, J.S. (1965). Virology 27, 434.
15. Lipauska, H., Brana, H. and Kohoutova, M. (1972). Folia

Microbiol. 17, 331.

16. Tomasz, A. (1970). J. Bacteriol. 101, 860.
17. Tomasz, A. and Mosser, T.L. (1966). Proc. Nat. Acad. Sci. US 55, 58.
18. Ziegler, R. and Tomasz, A. (1970). Bioch. Bioph. Res. Commun. 41, 1342.
19. Tomasz, A. (1972). In Biological Membranes (ed. C.F. Fox) Academic Press, p. 311.
20. Tomasz, A. (1971). In Informative Molecules in Biological Systems (ed. L. Ledoux), North Holland Publishers.
21. Tomasz, A., Zanati, E. and Ziegler, R. (1971). Proc. Nat. Acad. Sci. US 68, 1848.
22. Tomasz, A. (1968). Proc. Nat. Acad. Sci. US 59, 86.
23. Mosser, J.L. and Tomasz, A. (1970). J. Biol. Chem. 245, 287.
24. Tomasz, A. and Zanati, E. (1971). J. Bacteriol. 106, 412.
25. Nava, G., Galis, A. and Beiser, S.M. (1963). Nature 197, 903.
26. Tomasz, A. and Beiser, S.M. (1965). J. Bacteriol. 90, 1226.
27. Seto, H. and Tomasz, A. (1975). J. Bacteriol. (in press).
28. Tomasz, A., Westphal, M. Zanati, E. and Briles, E. (1975). J. Supramol. Biol. (in press).
29. Tomasz, A. (1974). Ann. N.Y. Acad. Sci. p. 439.
30. Seto, H. and Tomasz, A. (1974). Proc. Nat. Acad. Sci. US 71, 1493.
31. Lacks, S., Greenberg, B., Carlson, K. (1967). J. Mol. Biol. 29, 327.

INTEGRATED AND FREE STATE OF PLASMIDS

J. SCHELL

Laboratorium voor Genetika

Ledeganckstraat, 35 - GENT
Belgium

I. THE PHENOMENON OF EXTRACHROMOSOMAL INHERITANCE IN BACTERIA

It is a well documented fact that many (if not all) bacteria have but one chromosome (one continuous DNA molecule) forming a single linkage group containing all of the essential genes of the cell. Recently however one has realized that many bacteria in fact contain one or more additional DNA structures usually carrying so called facultative genes that are only essential to the cell's survival under particular circumstances (e.g. antibioticum resistance transfer factors) so that they can be gained or lost without lethal effect for the cell. Furthermore these "extrachromosomal" DNA molecules are usually significantly smaller than the chromosomal DNA.
It should be stressed however that although this distinction between chromosomal and extrachromosomal elements - based on whether the genes they carry are essential or non-essential and whether they consist of large (in the range of 10^8 to 10^9 Dalton) or smaller molecules (in the range $10^6 - 10^8$ Dalton) - is a very useful one, it does not necessarely always applies.
Indeed many extrachromosomal elements are capable of recombination with the chromosome and can thus acquire essential genes. Moreover some extrachromosomal plasmids are known to have sizes in the same range as the chromosome.

I. Definitions and types of extrachromosomal elements

As used most commonly in bacteria the term "extrachromosomal element " is synonymous with the term "plasmid"
i.e. a genetic element that can be perpetuated stably
in the cell separately from the chromosome.
Some of these extrachromosomal elements have the peculiar property that they can become integrated in the
chromosome and are therefore no longer strictly extrachromosomal. Such elements that can exist either as a
free plasmid or occupy a chromosomal site are referred
to as "episomes".

I. 1. A. Temperate phages

   The genomes of some bacteriophages can be maintained
   in the cells of their bacterial hosts without forming
   virus particles. Those bacteria harboring a virus genome are said to be lysogenic and the viral genome in
   these cells is called the "prophage". In all cases
   studied the lysogenic condition is dependant on the
   presence of a phage specific repressor that prevents
   the expression of the viral lytic functions. In general one can distinguish two situations for the prophage :

   1° Covalent insertion in the host chromosome

      In these cases the viral prophage replicates along
      with the rest of the chromosome. If the repressor
      is inactivated (induction) the prophage is excized
      from the chromosome and proceeds to replicate auto-
      nomously and to form new virus particles thereby
      lysing the host cell (lytic cycle). Such temperate
      phages can thus be regarded as episomes, but it
      should be pointed out that they are not really
      true extrachromosomal elements or plasmids because
      they can not persist stably in the autonomous state
      (they lyse their host cells).
      Well known examples of such phages are λ (1) and
      Mu (2) in E.coli.
      Whereas the λ wild-type prophage always occupies a
      given site on the E.coli chromosome, the Mu pro-
      phage can integrate at a large number of different
      sites (3) thereby causing mutations by physically
      separating different parts of the gene in which
      the Mu prophage inserts (Mu stands for mutator).

   2° Prophages as stable extrachromosomal plasmids

      Wild-type phages such as P1 and defective mutants

of phage λ (so called λdv's) (4) are not integrated in the host chromosome and are maintained in
the cells by autonomous replication of the prophage DNA.
Recombination between the prophage genome and the
host chromosome or between the prophage and other
extrachromosomal elements can occur, resulting in
the formation of so called transducing phages that
carry in their genome one or more specific host
genes. Thus one has discovered a P1 recombinant
phage P1Cm1 (5), that can actively grow lytically
but can also lysogenize recipient host cells, by
establishing itself as a plasmid, and then confers
resistance to chloramphenicol to the lysogenic cell.
P1Cm1 carries on its genome genes that confer resistance to chloramphenicol. When this genome replicates actively and forms large numbers of virus
particles, this leads to a very important amplification of the chloramphenicol resistance genes.
Because these phage particles can subsequently lysogenize new recipient bacterial cells and thereby
make them chloramphenicol resistant, this phenomenon of lytic virus growth followed by lysogenisation can result in a very fast and extensive spread
of these bacterial genes throughout the entire population.

I. 1. B. Auto-transmissible (Infectious) Plasmids

Auto-transmissible plasmids have two fundamental properties : they can replicate autonomously in the host
cell and they contain a genetic information that will
enable the cell that carries them to conjugate with
other cells with the result that a copy of the plasmid is transferred from the donor to the receptor cell.
I. 1. B. 1. Different types of transmissible factors
The first transmissible plasmid to be identified was
the F factor of E.coli K12. (For a review see (6)).
This sex-factor or Fertility factor is a typical episome. In the autonomous state, conjugation leads to
transfer of the F factor itself. In the integrated
state conjugation leads to a unidirectional transfer
of the host chromosome. It is the site and the orientation of the insertion of the F factor in the host
chromosome that determines which point of the host
chromosome will enter the receptor cell first and in
which direction (clock - or counter clock wise) the
chromosome will be transferred. So not only is the F
factor itself transmissible but, via the mechanism of

insertion, the F factor can mobilize the host chromosome. When a plasmid has the capacity to mobilize host
chromosome fragments or other non-transmissible plasmids it is said to have sex-factor or fertility factor
activity. Most self-transmissible plasmids studied
thus far appear to have sex-factor activity (see 7)
which would indicate that this is a general property
of transmissible plasmids.

I. 1. B. 1.a. Colicinogenic factors (Col. factors)
Colicins, and in general bacteriocins, are
bactericidal substances, usually proteins,
which are synthesized by certain strains of
bacteria and are active against some other,
usually related strains. The genetic capacity
of a strain to produce a bacteriocin (that
strain is than said to be bacteriocinogenic)
is determined by a bacteriocinogenic factor.
The best studied bacteriocins are the colicins (i.e. bacteriocins produced by Entero-
bactericeae).
The coliconogenic (Col) factors have in many
instances been shown to be carried by plasmids. Col factors are known both on auto-
transmissible and non-auto-transmissible plasmids. All the known auto-transmissible Col
factors exhibit sex-factor activity.
Self-transmissible colicinogenic factors exhibit at least three properties since they
genetically control the production of
1° The colicin protein
2° The specific immunity substance(s) that
protect the colicinogenic strain from the
activity of the homologous colicin (cfr
with the super infection immunity of lysogenic bacteria) and
3° The conjugation apparatus (sex pilus and
the mechanism for the initiation of DNA
replication and transfer).

I. 1. B. 1.b. Resistance transfer factors
These are plasmids that carry genes that confer to the cell resistance to antibacterial
agents such as antibiotics and heavy metals.
The striking aspect of some of these R factors is that some carry resistance to several
different antibacterial agents simultaneously. Multiple drug resistant bacteria thus
occur either because they harbor one R plasmid containing different genes conferring
resistance to different antibiotics, or be-

cause they harbor several different R plasmids each containing genes for resistance to
one or a group of antibiotics.
The drug-resistance genes of R factors usually
produce antibiotic-inactivating enzymes (8).
Resistance to ten or more antibiotics and
other antibacterial agents commonly in use
are known to be specified by genes on R factors (see 8). As was the case for Col factors, both auto-transmissible and non-auto-
transmissible R factors are known. They are
called R(t) and R. And again many of the R(t)
factors are sex-factors since they are known
to be able to mobilize and promote the transfer of fragments of the host chromosome and
of other plasmids.

I. 1. B. 1.c. Fertility factors that have incorporated
essential host genes

Due to the possibility of interaction between
chromosomal and extrachromosomal DNA, essential host genes can become part of a plasmid.
If this plasmid is auto-transmissible these
essential genes can very readily be propagated through the bacterial population. The
integration of host genes into plasmids (or
gene pick-up) can probably occur with all
plasmids. With episomes, such as the F factor, the mechanism of gene pick-up is well
understood. When the sex-factor is inserted
at a given site in the bacterial chromosome
by a single cross-over between the two circular DNA structures (see 6), it is possible
that upon release of the episome from the
chromosome, due to an internal excission
cross-over between two sites on either side
of the inserted sex factor or by one between
a chromosomal site and a homologous region
on the sex-factor, an adjacent bacterial region can be incorporated in the newly crea-
ted sex-factor.

A well documented case is the F-13 merogenote
(9) which has incorporated a very large segment of the host chromosome, having left behind a corresponding deletion in the chromosome of the host cell in which it originated.
Upon transfer of this F-13 to a receptor cell
by conjugation, this receptor cell now becomes
a more or less stable diploid for those host
genes carried by the F-13 factor.

Probably gene pick-up can occur with most plasmids by a mechanism of double cross-over whereby a DNA fragment can be integrated in a
plasmid.

I. 1. B. 1.d. Pathogenic plasmids

Transmissible plasmids have been shown to be
responsible for alpha-hemolysin (Hly) and enterotoxin (Ent) production in certain pathogenic E.coli strains(10) (11).
Recently we have found a large plasmid in
Agrobacterium tumefaciens strains which is involved in the tumor inducing capacity of these
pathogenic bacteria (see 12, and this book :
"The role of plasmids in crown-gall formation
by A.tumefaciens). We do not know yet whether
this plasmid is auto-transmissible or not.

I. 1. B. 2. Classification of auto-transmissible plasmids

It should be stressed here that the fact that we have
described several types of transmissible plasmids
according to their most conspicuous properties (F,
Col, R, etc.) does not mean that these properties
can be used for a natural classification of these
plasmids. In fact these particular properties only
represent a small part of the genetic information of
such plasmids and plasmids of different types are in
fact very closely related. This can easily be demonstrated by the fact that several plasmids with mixed
properties are known such as R-Col (13) and F'-lac-
tetracycline (14).
A more natural classification can be based on the
following properties :

1° Type of sex-pilus : two types of sex-pilus have
been identified (15), they are morphologically
and serologically distinct and differ in their
specificity as receptors for plasmid specific
phages. One type ressembles the prototype of the
F sex factor of E.coli K12 (F-like) and the other
the ColIb-P9 sex pilus (I-like)

2° Repression of fertility : It has been shown that
many sex-factors produce a repressor that specifically represses the expression of the conjugation apparatus (sex pili and transfer of the plasmid) probably via a repressor-operator type mechanism. The original F-factor is a naturally occurring derepressed sex-factor and derepressed mutants
of other sex-factors can be found. The derepressed
F factor however is sensitive to the repressor of
some repressed factors in biplasmid hosts.

The class of R factors able to repress F are called
fi[+] (fertility inhibition) and the others fi[-] (16).
3° Incompatibility and Entry exclusion : It has been
observed that usually two identical plasmids cannot
be maintained stably in the same bacterial host
cell. This plasmid incompatibility is different
from entry exclusion, which is due to a change of
the cell surface of a plasmid containing host
which inhibits the transfer of a related plasmid.
Incompatibility is thought to be the result of a
close interrelationship between the incompatible
plasmids.
Two models have been proposed for plasmid replication and incompatibility : one is based on a
competition for a specific membrane site essential
for replication (17) and the other supposes a specific inhibitor of replication synthesized immediately after initiation of replication and eliminated during the cell growth cycle (18). In a
general way it can be said that most auto-transmissible plasmids are functionally related and
that several groups of genetically related plasmids can be recognized.

I. 1. C. Non-auto-transmissible (non-infectious) plas-
         mids

All these plasmids have in common that they can replicate autonomously but that they cannot promote
their own transfer from one cell to another. For convenience these plasmids can be grouped according to
their best known properties.
I. 1. C. 1. Different types of non-auto-transmissible
            plasmids
The following types are known :
1° Bacteriocinogenic factors several of whom turned
   out to be inducible defective prophages
2° Resistance factors apart from R factors in Entero-
   bactericeae, one has also found such factors in
   Staphylococcal strains (19).
3° Pi-factors : these are non-transmissible plasmids
   found in Salmonella typhimurium (20) after mutagenesis and which appear to be the result of a
   reduplication of a given chromosomal fragment (the
   reduplicated segment is called Pi) followed by the
   apparent attachment of this fragment to a cryptic
   plasmid.
4° Cryptic plasmids. Under this name one can group a
   number of circular DNA plasmids that have been

discovered but for which no host-phenotype is known.
I. 1. C. 2. Mobilization by auto-transmissible factors.
It has often been observed that non-transmissible
plasmids become transmissible provided they are present in a host cell harboring an auto-transmissible
plasmid. It would appear that two distinct mechanisms
can operate to promote this transfer from one cell to
another of non-auto-transmissible plasmids. The same
mechanisms would in fact also be responsible for the
mobilization of host chromosome fragments by transmissible sex-factors.
1° Integration of the non-transmissible element in a
   sex-factor (or vice-versa). The non-transmissible
   element is than transferred as a part of the sex-
   factor.
2° Initiation of transfer probably involves the synthesis and or activation of a sex-factor-deter-
   mined endonuclease specific for a base sequence
   present on a particular strand of the transferred
   DNA. If such a specific base sequence (or one very
   similar to it) were also present on the non-transmissible plasmid (or on the host chromosome for
   that matter) initiation of DNA replication and
   transfer could result.
The functioning of one or the other of these mechanisms can account for some known facts about the
transfer of Rt and R factors. Watanabe and co-workers
(21, 22) have concluded from their work that Rt factors are composed of two linked units : a sex-factor
unit (RTF segment) that controls autonomous replication and conjugal transfer and a unit of drug-resis-
tant genes (r -determinants).
RTF and r units can be either part of the same circular plasmid molecule (monomolecular R factors or plasmid cointegrate see 23) or they can be present on separate plasmids, both of which must be able to replicate autonomously but only one of which needs to have
a RTF unit (multimolecular R factors or plasmid aggregates).
Recently Anderson and co-workers have described cases
that fit such a situation (24).

II. GENERAL PROPERTIES OF PLASMID DNA MOLECULES AND
    METHODS FOR STUDY AND ISOLATION (For a review see 23)

The most important structural features of most of
the plasmids studied thusfar is that they consist
of covalently closed double stranded DNA molecules.
This circular structure of the plasmids plays an

important role in establishing the plasmid DNA as an
autonomous replicating unit (replicon) and, in the
case of episomes, in allowing insertion from one
circular structure in another by a single cross-over
event. Methods for detection, characterization and
isolation of plasmid DNA's are based on either genetical or physico-chemical properties of plasmids or
on a mixture of both.
The genetical methods are based either on the sex-
factor properties of some plasmids or on the demonstration of the absence of linkage between plasmid
determined phenotypes and known chromosomal markers.
The physico-chemical methods are based either on
differences in base-ratio's between plasmid and host
DNA or on the circularity and supercoiled nature of
plasmid DNA (For a more detailed description of some
of these methods see our article in this book en-
titled "The Role of Plasmids in Crown-gall formation
by A.tumefaciens".

III. PLASMIDS AS ELEMENTS OF GENETIC EVOLUTION

In the preceding chapters we have described a number
of ways by which plasmids acquire, amplify and transmit specific genes. We have also briefly indicated
that some episomes can induce mutations by inserting
into genes (e.g. the mutator phage Mu). It is precisely these properties of plasmids that are responsible for the role of plasmids in bacterial evolution.
Plasmids can acquire specific genes (gene pick-up) in
various ways :
1° by insertion into another plasmid or into the chromosome followed by "abnormal" excision (i.e. that
   the excision cross-over involves at least one site
   different from the insertion cross-over)
2° By uptake of another plasmid by insertion not
   followed by excision.
3° By "exchange" recombination involving a double
   cross-over between the plasmid and another genetic
   element.
Plasmids can amplify genes because they are autonomously replicating units (replicons). This is especially evident with transducing temperate phages
(cfr P1Cm1) or with derepressed Col or R factors of
which many copies are present within the same cell.
Plasmids can transmit their genes either by infection
of new hosts (e.g. transducing phages) or by conjugation (e.g. the auto-transmissible plasmids) or
because they are mobilized and co-transferred with

auto-transmissible plasmids.
The plasmid genes can be maintained in the receptor
cells either as autonomous plasmids or they can be
taken up by insertion or exchange recombination in
the chromosome or another resident plasmid.
The mutator phage Mu offers a well documented example
of another way by which plasmids can play a role in
bacterial evolution : when two unrelated DNA molecules, between which no cross-over can normally
occur because of the lack of homology, each contain
an inserted Mu prophage, cross-over can now occur
between them through the respective Mu DNA sequences.
In this way the two DNA molecules can be coupled (25).
Mu dimers can provide yet another way by which two
non-homologous DNA's can be coupled : Mu dimers have
two integration sites. If each of the two integration
sites of one Mu dimer undergoes a cross-over with a
different DNA molecule a coupling results linking
the two non-homologous DNA's with the Mu dimer (26).
The possibility has been raised that certain bacteria
contain very small plasmids which have the property
to randomly insert in other DNA molecules. Non homologous DNA's could than undergo cross-over through
these insertion factors (27).
The main limiting factor to recombination promoted
by these insertion factors or Mu is of course their
presence in the relevant bacterial strains. Indeed
the phage Mu can only penetrate in bacterial strains
that have the required receptors on their cell-sur-
face. A way around this problem is probably provided
by auto-transmissible plasmids with a wide host-range.
An example for this can be found in an R factor first
discovered in Pseudomonas aeruginosa and called RP4.
It has been shown (28) that this plasmid has a very
wide host range since it can be transmitted to various
Enterobacteriaceae (Escherichia, Salmonella, Shigella,
Proteus, Serratia), to Agrobacterium and to Rhizobium.
Recently we (29) have found that a thermo inducible
phage Mu can be integrated in the RP4 plasmid in E.
coli. Upon transfer of this Mu carrying RP4 to different receptor strains it is possible to introduce
phage Mu in these strains.

IV. CIRCULAR DNA IN EUKARYOTIC CELLS

Several types of circular DNA's have been discovered
in Eukaryotic cells. (For a review see ref. 30).
These include :
1° Animal viruses : such as polyoma virus, Simian

virus 40 (SV40) and papilloma virus from rabbit. Both polyoma and SV40 are known to transform certain cell lines and it has been shown that transformed mouse embryo fibroblasts contain up to 20 copies of SV40 DNA per cell. The SV40 and polyoma DNA is covalently linked to the chromosomal DNA of transformed cells.

2° Ribosomal RNA genes in oocytes : deoxyribonuclease sensitive DNA circles of variable contour length (20 to 1000 μ) and containing tandemly arranged repeated copies of the r-RNA genes have been found in the oocytes of Triturus viridescens. They are present in the nucleolar core of the extrachromosomal nuclei found in oocytes.
In view of the wide variation in contour length (and thus in the number of copies of the r-RNA genes) of these circles it can be assumed that they are the result of a gene amplification mechanism whereby the r-RNA genes, on the chromosome are repeatedly copied forming a continuous DNA molecule with tandemly arranged copies of the r-RNA genes. Circles of variable length could than be formed by cross-over between any two gene copies.

3° Mitochondrial DNA : Mitochondria isolated from very diverse organisms (from mammals to insects) contain covalently closed circular DNA's with a contour length of about 5 μ. In yeasts mitochondrial circular DNA appears to be larger (25 μ). Chloroplasts also contain DNA but of a much larger size. This may be the reason why it is difficult to decide whether chloroplasts DNA forms a cova - lently closed circle or not.

References

1. Hershey, A.D. (1971) The bacteriophage lambda. Cold Spring Harbor Laboratory.
2. Taylor, A.L. (1963) Bacteriophage induced mutations in E.coli. Proc. Natl. Acad. Sci. U.S.A. 50, 1043.
3. Boram, W. and Abelson, J. (1971) Bacteriophage Mu integration : On the mechanism of Mu-induced mutations. J. Mol. Biol. 62, 171.
4. Matsubara, K. and Kaiser, A.D. (1968) λ.dv : An autonomously replicating DNA fragment. Cold Spring Harbor Symp. Quant. Biol. 33, 769.
5. Kondo, E. and Mitsuhashi, S. (1964) J. Bacteriol. 88, 1266.

6. Campbell, A.M. (1969) Episomes. Modern perspectives in biology. Harper and Row.

7. Novick,R.P. (1969). Extrachromosomal inheritance in bacteria. Bacteriol. Reviews 33, 210.

8. Davies, J.E. and Rownd, R. (1972). Transmissible multiple drug resistance in Enterobacteriaceae. Science 176, 758.

9. Scaife, J. and Pekhov, A.P. (1964) Deletion of chromosomal markers in association with F-prime factor formation in E.coli. Genet. Res. 5, 495.

10. Smith, H.W. and Halls, W. (1967) The transmissible nature of the genetic factor in E.coli that controls haemolysin production. J. Gen. Microbiol. 47, 153.

11. Smith, H.W. and Halls, W. (1968) The transmissible nature of the genetic factor in E.coli that controls enterotoxin production. J. Gen. microbiol. 52, 319.

12. Zaenen, I., Van Larebeke, N., Teuchy, H., Van Montagu, M. and Schell, J. (1974) Supercoiled circular DNA in crown-gall inducing Agrobacterium strains. J. Mol. Biol. 86, 109.

13. Siccardi, A.G. (1966). Colicin resistance associated with resistance factors in E.coli. Genet. Res. 8, 219.

14. Harada, K., Kameda, M., Suzuki, M., Shigehara, S., Nakajima, T. and Mitsuhashi, S. (1970) Genetic structure of a F-lac-tet factor. Jap. J. Microbiol., 14, 423.

15. Meynell, E., Meynell, G.G. and Datta, N. (1968) Phylogenetic relationships of drug-resistance factors and other transmissible bacterial plasmids. Bacteriol. Rev. 32, 55.

16. Watanabe, T., Nishida, H., Ogata, C., Arai, T. and Sato, S. (1964). Episome mediated transfer of drug resistance in Enterobacteriaceae. VII. Two types of naturally occuring R factors. J. Bacteriol. 88, 716.

17. Jacob, F., Brenner, S., Cuzin, F. (1963) On the regulation of DNA replication in bacteria. Cold Spring Harbor Symp. Quant. Biol., 28, 329.

18. Pritchard, R.H., Barth, P.T., Collins, J. (1969) Control of DNA synthesis in bacteria. Symp. Soc. Gen. Microbiol. XIX, 263.

19. Peyru, G., Wexler, L. and Novick, R.P. (1969) Naturally occuring penicillinase plasmids in Staphylococcus aureus. J. Bacteriol. 98, 215.

20. Ames, B., Hartman, P. and Jacob, F. (1963) Chromoso-
        mal alterations affecting the regulation of
        histidine biosynthetic enzymes in Salmonella.
        J. Mol. Biol. 7, 23.
21. Watanabe, T. (1963). Infective heredity of multiple
        drug resistance in bacteria. Bacteriol. Rev.
        27, 87.
22. Watanabe, I. and Fukasawa, T. (1961) Episome-media-
        ted transfer of drug resistance in Enterobac-
        teriaceae. III. Transduction of resistance
        factors. J. Bacteriol. 82, 202.
23. Clowes, R.C. (1972) Molecular structure of bacterial
        plasmids. Bacteriol. Rev. 36, 361.
24. Anderson, E.S. and Lewis, M.J. (1965) Characteriza-
        tion of a transfer factor associated with
        drug resistance in Salmonella typhimurium.
        Nature 208, 843.
25. De Graaff, J., Kreuning, P.C. and Van de Putte, P.
        (1973) Host controlled restriction and modi-
        fication of phage Mu and Mu-promoted chromo-
        some mobilization in Citrobacter freundii.
        Molec. Gen. Genet. 123, 283.
26. Toussaint, A. and Faelen, M. (1973) Connecting two
        unrelated DNA sequences with a Mu dimer.
        Nature New Biology 242, 1.
27. Starlinger, P. and Saedler, H. (1972) Insertion
        mutations in Microorganisms. Biochemie 54,
        177.
28. Datta, N. and Hedges, R. (1972) "Host ranges of R
        Factors" J. Gen. Microbiol. 70, 453.
29. Van Montagu, M. and Schell, J. (1974) Unpublished
        results.
30. Helinski, D.R. and Clewell, D.B. (1971) Circular
        DNA. Ann. Rev. Biochem. 40, 899.

F-PRIME MANIPULATIONS OF POSSIBLE INTEREST TO PLANT BIOLOGISTS

T. MOJICA-A

Cell Biochemistry, Radiobiology Department

Centre d'Etude de L'Energie Nucléaire, B-2400 Mol,Belgium

I. INTRODUCTION

It seems most probable that the genetic information, in most bacterial species, is stored in a single major linkage group or chromosome, as has been demonstrated for such widely diverse species as
Escherichia coli (Taylor and Trotter, 1972), *Salmonella typhimurium*
(Sanderson, 1972), *Bacillus subtilis* (Dubnau et al., 1967), *Streptomyces coelicolor* (Hopwood et al., 1973) and *Mycoplasma hominis* (Bode
and Morowitz, 1967).

Many types of bacteria are known to have additional facultative
linkage groups, separate from their chromosome and of much smaller
size, which are collectively called extrachromosomal elements or
plasmids. Their formal counterpart in plants are the genomes of intracellular symbionts, mitochondria and chloroplast.

A plasmid is defined as a stably inherited component of the cell
genome, physically separate from the chromosome, and as such, able to
replicate autonomously. In this sense temperate bacteriophages (with
the exception of coliphage P1) are not considered plasmids.

The term episome is used to refer to those activities of a plasmid that are related to the ability of the plasmid to interact with
the host chromosome.

It is generally agreed that plasmids carry genetic determinants
for functions not essential to the cell. While this is the case for
most known plasmids under most experimental conditions; it seems to
me that the circumscription of "essentiality" is not only unne-

cessary but also innacurate. Whether a plasmid is essential or not
depends not only on the plasmid but also on the genetic background
of the host cell and the experimental conditions. For example, an
F-prime lac is essential for a lac⁻ host growing on lactose as sole
carbon source, clearly, the same plasmid is not essential if the
host is lac⁺ and/or another carbon source is available.

A large number of plasmids have been detected in bacteria, and
all those tested consist of circular double-stranded DNA molecules.
The unlikely possibility remains that there may be some plasmids composed of substances other than double-stranded DNA.

This article will deal with some of the possible genetic manipulations, the properties on which they are based, and the uses of
derivatives of the sex factor F. Other episomes are excluded on the
consideration that they are not well explored. The reader is referred to recent reviews that have covered certain areas of extrachromosomal inheritance : Hayes (1968); Campbell (1962 and 1969);
Bradley (1967);Richmond (1968); Novick (1969); Helinski and Clewell
(1971); Clowes (1972); Low (1972); Willets (1972); Helinski (1973);
Schell (this volume); to mention only a few.

Since episomal genetic manipulations lead eventually to the
obtention of highly enriched DNA preparations, of more or less defined genetic content, it is hoped that this paper will be useful
to plant biologists inclined to use bacterial DNA to modify the
genetic information of plants and plant cells (e.g. LEDOUX; HESS;
GRESSHOFF; this volume).

II. MANIPULATIONS WITH F-PRIMES

The sex factor F, the first transmissible plasmid to be identified,
is a small DNA molecule ($\sim 63 \times 10^6$) which, in the F⁺, or autonomous
configuration, normally exists as a covalently closed circle (Sharp
et al., 1972), which can cause its own epidemic spread by the transfer of one of its DNA strands (Vapnek and Rupp, 1970) to recipient
cells (F⁻) by conjugation.

The sex factor can exist in three distinguishable genetic and
physical configurations : F⁺ with only its inherent genetic properties; F-prime, an altered F which carries, in its physical continuity, genetic material acquired from the chromosome; and Hfr, an altered F Factor integrated in the chromosome. In the first two configurations the sex factor replicates autonomously (chromosome-episome
segregation is coordinate, however), while in the latter the sex
factor is replicated with the chromosome.

An important feature is "incompatibility" (Maas, 1963) by which
a resident plasmid "excludes" a superinfecting one, and it is expressed at two levels :
a) Entry (or surface) exclusion, which makes strains carrying an F
   factor (or other plasmid) very poor conjugational recipients
   (Lederberg et al., 1952) probably because conjugational pair
   formation is reduced (Achtman et al., 1971). Surface exclusion
   can be partially abolished by alterations in phenotypic properties of the recipient male (F$^-$-phenocopies) either by growth to
   stationary phase (Hayes, 1968) or by treatment with periodate
   (Sneath and Lederberg, 1961).
b) Even if the entry barrier is removed, two sex factors cannot stably coexist in a cell. Whenever double "males" are selected for,
   the two sex factors have undergone recombination either with each
   other (Press et al., 1971) or with the chromosome (Kaney and Atwood, 1972).

The sex factor and its derivatives, as well as a large variety
of plasmids can be transferred to other bacterial species (Jones and
Sneath, 1970).

The following manipulations will considered below : Construction
of F-primes for almost any desired chromosomal region ; deletion, transposition and fusion of F-primes.

A. Making F-primes

Until not many years ago, the few F-primes available were of "spontaneous" origin, and were (F-prime *lac*, F-prime *gal*, for example) circumscribed to a few chromosomal regions. Because of the spontaneous
origin (they are present in Hfr populations), many clones had to be
tested in order to detect F-prime formation (Berg and Curtiss, 1967)
which probably occurs by rare excision crossovers involving paired
chromosome regions on either side of the integrated sex factor, or
by one involving a chromosomal site and an homologous F region
(Scaife, 1967). Moreover, the independent state was difficult to maintain, since the episome was often lost either by recombination with
the chromosome (due to homology between the chromosome and the equivalent episomal region), or by deletion. Very often the only way to
maintain an F-prime was in a strain carrying a chromosomal deletion
that covered at least the chromosomal genes carried on the episome.
This, clearly, was not only annoying but very limiting.

Nowadays, it is feasible to construct "F-primes" almost at will,
and to maintain the episomal state with not much difficulty. This
possibility came about thanks to the observation of B.Low (1968) that

some recombinationless bacteria, when used as recipients in conjugation with Hfr donors gave rise to unstable "recombinants" that segregate recipient-like clones at high frequency.

The main recombination pathway in *E. coli* is controlled by three
genes : *rec A, rec B, rec C* (See Clark, 1971, for review). B. Low
(1968) found that "recombinants" with *rec B⁻* were recovered at low
frequency (< 10% at wild type) but they were haploid, like recombinants obtained with *rec⁺* bacteria. On the other hand, *rec A* recipients yielded "recombinants" at much lower frequency (0.1 - 1.0 %)
invariably heterozygous for proximal markers, including those nearest
to the Hfr origin. Many Hfr donors were tested, some produced no detectable "recombinants", some produced defective F-merogenotes, and
others produced mostly normal F-primes, of varying size.

The episomal state (merozygosis) is best maintained in a *rec A⁻*
background, in supplemented minimal medium. Alternatively, we have
been succesful in maintaining F-primes of *E. coli* origin in *S. thyphimurium* cytoplasm, where the tendency to recombine is greatly reduced by low homology (Mojica-a, unpublished).

The conclusion of the observations is that it is possible to
"construct" F-primes carrying desired chromosomal genes, by a judicious selection of strains. It is advisable to use an Hfr donor
that injects the "desired" genes early and to use multiply marked recipient strains.

Crosses between two Hfr strains have yielded strains which carry
two integrated factors (Clark, 1963; Kaney and Atwood, 1972). Double-
male strains which have F factors integrated with the same orientation
on the chromosome have been used to donate one of the chromosomal
regions between the F factors to recipient strains and allow selection
of merodiploids (e.g. Clark et al., 1969). This method seems potentially useful particularly for making F-primes carrying chromosomal
regions which are not easily obtained by the method described above.

A third possible method for isolation of F-primes is by transducing small F-prime-forming fragments from an Hfr strain to a recipient (Pittard, 1965). Further details on F-prime-making methodologies
and characteristics, as well as a list of currently-available F-primes
can be found in Low (1972) and Sanderson et al. (1972).

Should plant biologists be interested in transfering F-prime-
borne bacterial DNA to plants, this DNA can be isolated and purified
by segregation into "minicells" (Levy, 1971) or by other methods
(Guerry et al., 1973). It seems to me that since the F-prime DNA molecule is a double-stranded circle; it is possible to study structural and conformational requirements for transfer to higher plants.

B. Deletion

Deletion of parts of an F-prime has often been detected (e.g.
Bastarrachea et al., 1969) either in rec+ (e.g. Cronan Jr. and Godson
1972) or rec A⁻ strains (e.g. Hofnung et al., 1971). One phenotype for
selection of "deleted" F-primes is based on the observation that cells
whose episomes have been shortened, in some cases, grow much faster
than the parental partial diploid (Hofnung, et al., 1971). It is also
possible to devise selection methods, for clones with deleted episomes that depends on the judicious choice of recessive selectable markers and appropriate growth conditions. Since deletion of F-primes
occurs "Spontaneously",the occurrence of such variant diploids can
interfere with accurate complementation and dominance tests.

When a strain harboring an F-prime is used as donor in P1-mediated
transduction, a large family of transductants, carrying "whole" F-primes and "deleted" derivatives of the original F-prime, is produced.
Transductional shortening was first observed by Pittard and Adelberg
(1963) and has been used as a method for detailed deletion mapping
of the ilv operon (Ramakrishnan and Adelberg, 1965; Marsh and Duggan,
1972) of the gal operon and of the sex factor itself (Ohtsubo, 1970).
There is no reason why other regions of the chromosome could not be
manipulated in a similar manner. It is not known whether the shortening event takes place in the donor or in the recipient. A list of
useful shortened episomes has been published (Low, 1972).

A deletion event that "removes" the entire F-prime has been termed
"curing" and is known to occur spontaneously at low rate (Jacob and
Wollman, 1961). The rate of this event is greatly enhanced by exposure of cells to : acridine orange (Hirota, 1960), rifampin (Bazzicalupo and Tocchini-Valentini, 1972); elevated growth temperature
(Stadler and Adelberg, 1972) infection by filamentous phage M13
(Palchoudhury and Iyer, 1971), to sodium dodecyl sulfate (Adachi,et
al., 1972), or to thymine deprivation (Clowes, Moody and Pritchard,
1965). Cell density (low cell density reduces transfer of the episome)
and pH (7.6 for acridine orange curing) appear to be critical factors.
The molecular biological bases of curing are poorly understood, the
situation is further complicated by the existence of F-primes resistant
to curing.

Shortened F-primes are useful for functional genetic tests and
mapping. In manipulations with plant materials it should be possible to answer critical questions as to minimum size and genetic information required for succesful uptake and to elicit biological
responses. Is a "proper" operon sufficient ? Is the presence of
bacterial RNA and/or DNA polymerases (etc.) required for faithful
expression, maintainance and replication of bacterial DNA in plants ?
The thoughtful reader is requested to ask his own relevant questions.

C. Transposition

Transposition refers to the transplant of a group of genes from its wild type chromosomal position to a topologically and genetically different one, such that a transposed group of genes will now be in close linkage with other genes. There is no implication as to whether the transposed genes are duplicated or not.

Genetic transposition in *E. coli*, although known to occur, is rare (De Witt and Adelberg, 1962; Jackson and Yanofsky, 1973). In a strain harboring an F-prime whose replication is thermosensitive ($F_{ts114}lac$) and with a chromosomal region, corresponding to the F-prime, deleted, the F-prime integrated at low frequency at other chromosomal sites(the *lac* genes were thus transposed)(Cuzin and Jacob, 1964). A large number of such transpositions have been analyzed (Beckwith, Signer and Epstein, 1966) and found to be Hfr donors. This method is limited, since it requires strains with deletions.

Of more generalized application is the "directed transposition" technique. The logistics of directed transposition is rather simple and consists of asking a particular cell population to do two things in order to survive.

Since the independent frequency of both events is very low, the cell will, in at least some cases, "perform" a single event that results in both phenotypes. Since the best known case is that of transpositions to the *ton B* locus (Gottesman and Beckwith, 1969), I will use it here as an example.

The *ton B* locus (near ϕ 80 attachment site) controls bacterial sensitivity to phages T1, ϕ 80, to colicins B, I and V; and transport of Fe^{++} (Taylor and Trotter, 1972). Mutations that remove *ton B* activity are resistant to the phages and colicins mentioned, and can be selected by plating cells in the presence of either one of the phages or one of the colicins. In order to avoid selecting mutations at other loci (e.g. *ton A*) it is advisable to select for simultaneous resistance to more than one of the agents mentioned (e.g. phage T1 and colicin V).

A strain harboring an F-prime that carries a set of desired genes (a chromosomal mutation in at least one of the genes should be present, such that only those cells harboring the episome will grow in the absence of the metabolite), and, in addition a temperature-sensitive mutation in the F-factor, such that at high temperature (e.g. 42°) the F-prime character is lost, can be constructed (the temperature sensitive marker of the F-factor can be introduced either by mutagenesis or by recombinations with available temperature-sensitive F-primes (see Gottesman and Beckwith, 1969).

Such strain is placed at 42°, in medium lacking the particular metabolite that is controlled by the episome-borne genes, in the presence of lysates of phage T1 and of colicin V. Surviving colonies are cleaned and tested for the respective characters. Clones in which the integrations of the F-prime occurred at the *ton B* locus are expected to be Hfr's transfering nearby chromosomal genes (on either side) with high frequency (see Mojica-a, this volume).

Transposition of the *lac* genes to the *gal* region has been described (Ippen, Shapiro and Beckwith, 1971) using the same logistics. Inactivation of the *gal T* gene results in resistance to galactose of strains with mutations in the *gal E* gene.

Clearly the system allows for the transposition of episome borne genes to selected sites for which a predictable and detectable phenotype of the strains with inactivated genes is available and not lethal. It should be possible to transpose genes for example to *acr A* or to *bfe*. The *acr A* and *bfe* genes control, respectively, sensitivity to acriflavine, phenetyl alcohol, sodium dodecyl sulfate, and to phage BF23, colicins E1, E2, E3. The reader is invited to browse the recently published genetic maps of *E. coli* (Taylor and Trotter, 1972) and *S. thyphimurium* (Sanderson, 1972) for further possible transposing sites.

As the genetic knowledge of other interesting bacterial species increases it is expected that similar genetic manipulations will become feasible. Transpositions have been used to study operon regulation and for the construction of specialized transducing phages (see below) but they can also be used to study the mechanism of recombination and of the production of deletions and for the study of the genetics of the F factor itself. Transposition might be important to plant biologists as an alternative or additional approach to some of the questions mentioned above.

D. Fusion

A third genetic manipulation with F-prime factors that can also lead to "transposition" of bacterial genes to become in close contact with other bacterial genes and/or attachment sites of specialized transducing bacteriophages, and useful wherever transpositions of the type described above prove to be reactious, is the genetic fusion of F-primes,that originated in studies of incompatibility, recombination and deletion of F factors.

The logistics of fusion is very similar to that of "transpositions". Since it also consists of asking a strain to perform two events in order to survive. Two autonomous F factors cannot normally replicate in

the same *E. coli* cell. One of them will normally be discriminated
against. One of the events a double-male is asked to perform is
to stably maintain the two incompatible episomes. One of the F
factors should carry a temperature-sensitive mutation and one of the
group of markers desired to "fuse", the other should carry the second group of bacterial genes desired to "fuse". Both "donor" and
"recipient" strains should carry chromosomal mutations such that the
presence of the episome can be recognized, and essential for growth
under certain conditions.

In matings performed between two strains with F-primes with the
requisits mentioned above (Press et al., 1971) survivors were recovered at low frequency (about $1/10^3$ recipient cells). Moreover,
about 50% of the survivors behaved as if the two F-primes had
fused to each other. Experiments were performed using *rec A*$^-$ strains
to minimize recombinations of the F-primes with the chromosome.

Electron microscopic measurements of the contour lenghts (Pal-
choudhuri et al., 1972; Willetts and Bastarrachea, 1972) revealed
that fused F-primes are shorter than the sum of the two parental
F-primes. Thus, fusion seems to involve concomitant deletion of some
genetic material, but it is not known whether this deletion is a requirement for stable fusion. Fusion of an F factor with a colicinogenic factor has also been described (Fredericq, 1969), such that it
appears possible to fuse two F factors and to fuse F factors to other
available episomes, if other episomes with the proper genetic configuration are available. In genetic manipulations, fusion of F-primes
is most useful if one of the F-primes carries the attachment site for
a specialized transducing bacteriophage (Press, et al., 1971), such
that new genes become available for specialized transductions and DNA
enrichment (see below).

Fusion of episomes, as described above, is limited to fusion *in
vivo*, which leaves out the possibility of fusing DNA's of non-transmissible plasmids. Of recent vintage is a technique that fuses DNA
molecules *in vitro*. This technique should eventually be useful in
fusing   any two DNA's that can be obtained "pure" in large enough
yields.

The technique makes use of the observation that restriction nucleases (e.g. Eco RI endonuclease) cut the DNA at a few specific sites
on the DNA molecule producing "sticky-ends" (Hedgepeth, et al.,1972)
that can be covalently joined to other DNA molecules, from other sources, treated in the same fashion (Cohen, et al., 1973) generating new
"hybrid" DNA molecules that can form new biologically functional replicons when transferred to *E. coli* by transformation (Cohen,et al.,
1972). Plasmid DNA species generated in this fashion posses genetic
properties and nucleotide base sequences from both of the parent DNA
molecules.

So far, fused DNA molecules from *E. coli* (Cohen, et al., 1973), from *E. coli* and *Staphylococcus* (Chang and Cohen, 1974), and from *E. coli* and *Xenopus laevis* (Morrow, et al., 1974), have been generated. I do not need to point out the possibilities this fusion-transformation system offers for the study of fundamental molecular biological problems in bacteria and for genetic manipulations with higher organisms.

III. MANY FOLD ENRICHMENT OF SPECIFIC DNA'S

The manipulations with episomes described above are useful and important in themselves for the study of specific problems and are also very useful for the generation of specialized transducing phages that in turn can be used for the preparation of enriched, purified, specific DNA's. This purified DNA preparations have been used in studies of regulation of gene expression and protein synthesis *in vitro* (e.g. de Crombrugghe, et al., 1971; Blassi, et al.,1973), they can also be used to study genetic transfer in bacteria and in other biological materials (e.g. Hess; Greshoff; Smith this volume). The methodology for the obtention specialized transducing phages and the purification and handling of purified DNA can be found in Gottesman and Beckwith (1969) and in Miller (1972).

Clearly, the limiting factor is the obtention of specialized transducing phages, since they integrate only at special sites on the bacterial chromosome (see Gottesman and Weisberg, 1971 for review), called the attachment (att) sites, such that specialized transducing phages only cover a small portion of the bacterial chromosome. The most outstanding phage examples are Ø 80, whose att is near *ton B* and λ, whose att is near *gal*. The problem consist then, of shortening the distance between one att and a desired group of genes.

The most generalized and straight forward approach is through transposition of episomal-bound genes and fusion of episomes (when one of the episomes bears the att of a specialized transducing phage. Deletion of episomes thus becomes important, since very often, it is necessary to "remove" genetic material in order to maximize the probability that a particular group of genes falls close to att, after transposition or fusion.

An alternative approach in generating specialized transducing phages, consist of selecting for λ lysogens (Ø80 and other phages should also be useful) with lambda integrated at unusual chromosomal locations in a strain carrying a deletion of the attachment site (Shimada, Weisberg, and Gottesman, 1972). This approach is limited because the phage choices of "integration" sites are limited and, moreover, the sites are not predictable.

IV. FUNCTIONAL GENETIC TESTS

It is often not only desirable but important to know whether a particular mutant is dominant over the wild type or viceversa.

In very general terms, an allele producing an active product, will normally be dominant over an allele producing no product or an inactive one (except when gene dosage is critical). If the mutant allele is dominant over the wild type, it generally indicates qualitative alterations in activity of the gene product.

The analytical power and importance of dominance tests are best exemplified by studies that led to the discovery of positive and negative mechanisms of regulation of gene action (Jacob and Monod, 1961; Sheppard and Englesberg, 1966).

The principle of a dominance test is very simple : the two alleles whose relative dominance is to be tested are introduced into the same cell, the phenotype of the cell is then determined. In *E. coli* and in *S. thyphimurium* F-primes are used for this test (e.g. Riddle and Roth, 1972). In eucaryotic microbes, the test is accomplished by using heterokarions as in *Aspergillus nidulans*. Abortive transduction can be used with some bacteria (Stocker, Zinder and Lederberg,1953).

When different mutations are found to be very close on the genetic map the investigator will usually want to know whether or not they are in the same gene, and what their positions are relative to each other and to nearby chromosomal markers. The methods to answers there questions have been outlined elsewhere (Mojica-a, this volume) : namely, conjugation (interrupted matings) and transduction. Here, I will briefly describe a third possible method of mapping and complementation tests, used in bacteria, that involves the use of F-primes.

The introduction of F-prime factors, and selection for wild type phenotype, with mutations whose phenotypes are recessive in merodiploids can often be used to localize map positions to within a few genes on the chromosome. Mutations with a dominant phenotype can also be localized within a small chromosomal region when $rec\ A^-$ or F-prime donors are crossed with a mutant, and wild type recombinants (often at very low frequency) rather than merodiploids are observed.

When several recessive mutations are localized in a region carried by an F-prime, complementation studies (Fincham, 1966; and Matagne, this volume) can be carried out using the following procedure :

a) Mate F-prime strain with one of the mutant strains to generate a (+)/(−) merodiploid. The use of rec^+ strains is recommended.

b) From the (+)/(−) merodiploid, (−)/(−) segregants are selected by plating out on solid media which allows (−)/(−) and (+)/(−) colonies to grow. Colonies must be tested to distinguish phenotypes,

(-)/(-) segregants are found among (+)/(-) cells at frequencies ranging from 0.1 to 2.0 % (Miller, 1972; Mojica-a, unpublished). Segregants must be checked for donor ability. In this way F-prime strains carrying mutant genes borne on the F factor are generated. These strains are not only important in complementation but also for controls in transfer of episome-bound DNA to "higher" organisms.

c) After one mutant of a group has been put into an F-prime, as described above, it can be mated with all the other mutants of the group. The number of wild type colonies obtained (if any) gives some indication of whether or not the chromosomal and episomal mutations are being complemented. A low number of wild type colonies ($\sim$ 1.0 %) suggests intragenic recombination rather than complementation. Complementation is proved by identifying the two mutant alleles in a putative (+)(-)/(-)(+) merodiploid. The chromosomal mutation is easily checked by "curing" the episome (Hirota, 1960) to an F-segregant and observing the mutant phenotype. The episomal mutation can be detected by back crossing the F-prime factor into the original strain. As mentioned earlier, the use of *rec A*⁻ strains, to avoid recombination and episomal rearrangements, is recommended. It should be emphasized that positive results in complementation are strong evidence for different complementation groups. Negative results, on the other hand, might also be explained by deletions of the F-prime factor. Intracistronic complementation has also been detected with the use of F-prime factors (Garen and Garen, 1963; Perrin, 1963). In a number of cases, mutations which affect the same polypeptide chain have been found to complement. In all cases analyzed, the enzyme involved has been shown to consist of several identical subunits. Enzymes which assemble so as to have both types of mutant chains can often be enzymatically active, while enzymes made of identical mutant chains are inactive.

Other important uses of F-prime factors include the isolation of recessive lethal mutations such as recessive lethal amber and ochre suppressors in essential tRNA genes (Soll and Berg, 1969; Miller and Roth, 1971) mutations in essential genes, such as *rif* (Austin and Scaife, 1970), phage mu-induced polar mutations (Nomura and Engback, 1972), and measurements of gene dosage effects (Stetson and Sommerville, 1971).

V. CONCLUDING REMARKS

I have chosen a group of topics on special manipulations with F-prime factors, not only because these manipulations are of academic interest,and important for bacterial geneticists, but also because I feel that they might become useful for manipulations with plant materials, as more and more is learned about the fundamental molecular biology of plants and other systems. The strong bias towards *E. coli* F-primes should not be taken to indicate that manipulations with other *E. coli* episomes, and with episomes from other sources, are not feasible or useful.

This article is addressed to plant biologists in the hope that they will find it useful. I am aware that many important details were left out and urge the reader to examine the references given, where appropriate.

ACKNOWLEDGEMENTS

I wish to thank P. Lurquin and M. Mergeay for encouragement and for criticisms of the manuscript.

REFERENCES

ACHTMAN M., N. WILLETS, A.J. CLARK (1971).
J. Bacteriol. 106 : 529-538.

ADACHI,H., M. NAKONO, M. INUZUKA and M. TOMOEDA (1972).
J. Bacteriol 109 : 1114-1124.

AUSTIN, S.J., and J.G. SCAIFE (1970).
J. Mol. Biol. 49 : 263-267.

BASTARRACHEA,F., E. TAM and M. GONZALEZ (1969).
Genetics 59 : 153-166.

BAZZICALUPO,P. and G.P. TOCCHINI-VALENTINI (1972).
Proc. Nat. Acad. Sci. U.S.A. 69 : 298-300.

BECKWITH,J.R., E.R. SIGNER and W. EPSTEIN (1966).
Cold Spring Harbor Symp. Quant. Biol. 31 : 393-400.

BERG C.M., and R. CURTIS (1967).
Genetics 56 : 503-525.

BLASSI, F., C.B. BRUNI, A. AVITABILE, R.G. DEBLEY, R.F. GOLDBERGER
and M. MEYERS (1973).
Proc. Nat. Acad. Sci. U.S.A. 70 : 2692-2696.

BODE, H.R. and H.J. MOROWITZ (1967).
J. Mol. Biol. 23 : 191-199

CAMPBELL, A.M. (1962).
Adv. Genet. 11 : 101-145.

CAMPBELL, A.M. (1969).
Harper and Row. New York.

CHANG, A.C.Y., and S.N. COHEN (1974).
Proc. Nat. Acad. Sci. U.S.A. 71 : 1030-1034.

CLARK, A.J. (1963).
Genetics 48 : 105-120.

CLARK, A.J. (1971).
Annu. Rev. Microbiol. 25 : 437-464.

CLARK, A.J., W.K. MAAS, and B. LOW (1969).
Mol. Gen. 105 : 1-15.

BRADLEY, D.E. (1967).
Bacteriol. Rev. 31 : 230-314

CLOWES, R.C. (1972).
Bacteriol. Rev. 36 : 361-405.

CLOWES, R.C., E.E.M. MOODY, and R.H. PRITCHARD (1965).
Genet. Res. 6 : 147-152.

COHEN, S.N., A.C.Y. CHANG, H.W. BOYER and R.B. HELLING (1973).
Proc. Nat. Acad. Sci. U.S.A. 70 : 3240-3244.

COHEN, S.N., A.C.Y. CHANG, and L. HSU (1972).
Proc. Nat. Acad. Sci. U.S.A. 69 : 2110-2114.

de CROMBRUGGHE,B., B. CHEN, W. ANDERSON, P. NISSLEY, M. GOTTESMAN and
I. PASTAN (1971).
Nature, New Biol. 231 : 139-142.

CRONAN, J.E.,Jr., and G.N. GODSON (1972).
Mol. Gen. Genet. 116 : 199-210.

CUZIN, F., and F. JACOB (1964).
C.R. Acad. Sci. 258 : 1350-1352.

DE WITT, S.K. and E.A. ADELBERG (1962).
Genetics 47 : 577-585.

DUBNAU, D., C. GOLDTHWAITE, I. SMITH, and J. MARMUR (1967).
J. Mol. Biol. 27 : 163-185.

FINCHAM, J.R.S. (1966).
W.A. Benjamin, Inc. New York.

FREDERICQ, P. (1969).
In Ciba Foundation Symposium on Bacterial Episomes and Plasmids p. 163-
174, ed. G.E.W. Wolstenholme and M. O'Connon, J. and A. Churchill
London.

GAREN, A. and S. GAREN (1963).
J. Mol. Biol. 7 : 13-22.

GOTTESMAN, M.E., and R.A. WEISBERG (1971).
In A. Hershey (ed.) The Bacteriophage Lambda Cold Spring Harbor Lab.
New York.

GOTTESMAN, S., and J.R. BECKWITH (1969).
J. Mol. Biol. 44 : 117-127.

GUERRY P., D.J. LE BLANC, and S. FALKOW (1973).
J. Bacteriol. 116 : 1064-1066.

HAYES, W. (1968).
The Genetics of Bacteria and their Viruses. Blackwell Scientific
Publications. Oxford.

HEDGEPETH, J., H.M. GOODMAN and H.W. BAYER (1972).
Proc. Nat. Acad. Sci. U.S.A. 69 : 3448-3452.

HELINSKI, D.R. (1973).
Annu. Rev. Microbiol. 27 : 437-480.

HELINSKI, D.R. and D.B. CLEWELL (1971).
Ann. Rev. Biochem. 40 : 899-942.

HIROTA, Y. (1960).
Proc. Nat. Acad. Sci. U.S.A. 46 : 57-64.

HOFNUNG, M., M. SCHWARTZ, and D. HATFIELD (1971).
J. Mol. Biol. 61 : 681-694.

HOPWOOD, D.A., K.F. CHATER, J.E. DOWDING and A. VIVIAN (1973).
Bacteriol. Rev. 37 : 371-405.

IPPEN, K., J.A. SHAPIRO, and J.R. BECKWITH (1971).
J. Bacteriol. 108 : 5-9.

JACOB, F., and J. MONOD (1961).
J. Mol. Biol. 3 : 318-356.

JACOB, F., and E.L. WOLLMAN (1961).
Sexuality and the Genetics of Bacteria. Academic Press. New York.

JACKSON. E.N. and C. YANOFSKY (1973).
J. Bacteriol. 116 : 33-40.

JONES, D., and P.H.A. SNEATH (1970).
Bacteriol. Rev. 34 : 40-81.

LEVY, S.B. (1971)
J. Bacteriol. 108 : 300-308.

LOW, B. (1968).
Proc. Nat. Acad. Sci. U.S.A. 60 : 160-167.

LOW, K.B. (1972).
Bacteriol. Rev. 36 : 587-607.

MARSH, N.J. and D.E. DUGGAN (1972).
J. Bacteriol. 109 : 730-740.

MILLER, C.G., and J.R. ROTH (1971).
J. Mol. Biol. 59 : 63-74

MILLER, J.H. (1972).
Experiments in Molecular Genetics. Cold Spring Harbor Laboratory,
New York.

MORROW, J.F., S.N. COHEN, A.C.Y. CHANG, H.W. BOYER, H.M. GOODMAN
and R.B. HELLING (1974).
Proc. Nat. Acad. Sci. U.S.A. 71 : 1743-174 .

NOMURA, M., and F. ENGBAENK (1972).
Proc. Nat.Acad. Sci. U.S.A. 69 : 1526-1530.

NOVICK, R.P. (1969).
Bacteriol. Rev. 33 : 210-257.

NOVICK, R.P., and D. BOUANCHAUD (1971).
Ann. N.Y. Acad. Sci. 182 : 279-294.

OHTSUBO, E. (1970).
Genetics 64 : 189-197.

PALCHOUDHURY, S.R. , and V.N. IYER (1971).
J. Bacteriol. 106 : 1040-1042.

PALCHOUDHURY, S.R., A.J. MAZAITIS, W.K. MAAS, and A.K. KLEINSCHMIDT
(1972).
Proc. Nat. Acad. Sci. U.S.A. 69 : 1873-1876.

PERRIN, D. (1963).
Cold Spring Harbor Symp. Quant. Biol. 28 : 529-532.

PITTARD, J. (1965).
J. Bacteriol. 89 : 680-686.

PITTARD, J. and E.A. ADELBERG (1963).
J. Bacteriol. 85 : 1402-1408.

PRESS, R., M. GLANSDORFF, P. MINER, J. DE VRIES, R. KADNER, and W.K.
MAAS (1971).
Proc. Nat. Acad. Sci. U.S.A. 68 : 795-798.

RAMAKRISHMAN, T., and E.A. ADELBERG (1965).
J. Bacteriol. 89 : 661-664.

RICHMOND, M.H. (1968).
Adv. Microb. Physiol. 2 : 43-88.

RIDDLE, D.L. and J.R. ROTH (1972).
J. Mol. Biol. 66 : 483-493.

SANDERSON, K.E. (1972).
Bacteriol. Rev. 36 : 558-586.

SANDERSON, K.E., H. ROSS, L. ZIEGLER, and P.H. MAKELA (1972).
Bacteriol Rev. 36 : 608-637.

SCAIFE, J. (1967).
Annu. Rev. Microbiol. 21 : 601-638.

SHARP, P.A., H. MING-TA, E. OHTSUBO and N. DAVIDSON (1972).
J. Mol. Biol. 71 : 471-497.

SHIMADA, K., R.A. WEISBERG, and M. GOTTESMAN (1972).
J. Mol. Bio. 63 : 483-503.

SHEPPARD, D., and E. ENGLESBERG (1966).
Cold Spring Harbor Symp. Quant. Biol. 31 : 345-347.

SNEATH, P.H.A. and J. LEDERBERG (1961).
Proc. Nat. Acad. Sci. U.S.A. 47 : 86-90.

SOLL, L. and P. BERG (1969).
Proc. Nat. Acad. Sci. U.S.A. 63 : 392-399.

STADLER, J. and E.A. ADELBERG (1972).
J. Bacteriol. 109 : 447-449.

STETSON, H., and R.L. SOMMERVILLE (1971).
Mol. Gen. Gen. 111 : 342-351.

STOCKER, B.A.D., N.D. ZINDER, and J. LEDERBERG (1953).
J. Gen. Microbiology. 9 : 410-433.

TAYLOR, A.L., and C.D. TROTTER (1972).
Bacteriol. Rev. 36 : 504-524.

WILLETS, N. (1972).
Annu. Rev. Genet. 6 : 257-268.

WILLETS, N. and F. BASTARRACHEA (1972).
Proc. Nat. Acad. Sci. U.S.A. 69 : 1481-1485.

VAPNEK, D., and W.D. RUPP (1970).
J. Mol. Biol. 53 : 287-303.

INTERALLELIC COMPLEMENTATION IN THE STUDY OF GENE ACTION

R.F. MATAGNE and R. LOPPES[*]

Laboratory of Molecular Genetics, Institute of Botany
University of Liège,
SART TILMAN - B-4000 LIEGE

The present lecture is intended to emphasize some aspects of the interallelic complementation, rather than to present a complete survey of the literature. Examples are only chosen to illustrate certain concepts. This subject has been extensively reviewed by Fincham [1].

COMPLEMENTATION TEST AND THE DEFINITION OF THE CISTRON

Two mutant genomes, or parts of genomes, are said to complement each other if the biochemical function is restored in the heterozygous cell. By the complementation test (also called cis-trans test) the gene can be defined as a function unit.

Let us consider two independent mutations, a and b leading to the same phenotype; genetical analysis revealed that they were closely linked and could be located in the same gene. If they produce a wild phenotype when put in the $trans$ configuration, $i.e.$ if they complement, they are considered as being located in two different genes. If, on the contrary, the $trans$ configuration gives rise to a mutant phenotype (absence of complementation), the two mutations a and b are located in the same gene and affect the same function. This happens for example with the adenine requiring strains ad_8 and ad_{16} in $Aspergillus$ $nidulans$: the $trans$ hetero-zygote $\frac{ad_{16} \quad +}{+ \quad ad_8}$ is mutant whereas the cis configuration $\frac{ad_{16} \quad ad_8}{+ \quad +}$,

[*] Chercheur qualifié du Fonds National Belge de la Recherche Scientifique.

obtained by intragenic recombination, does correspond to the wild phenotype [2].

A gene, so defined from the functional point of view by a *cis-trans* test, was called a cistron [3]; in such a cistron one can find several non complementary mutants, closely linked but separable by recombination.

COMPLEMENTATION BETWEEN MUTATIONS IN THE SAME CISTRON

The Benzer's definition [3] of the cistron greatly clarified the concept of the gene. Nevertheless, exceptions to this definition were rapidly observed in several organisms (*Neurospora*, *Aspergillus*, *Salmonella* or *Escherichia coli*). In many systems indeed, mutants of a same type, mapping in the same short segment of the chromosome, were found to complement, whilst other mutants were non complementary.

Complementation between mutants belonging to the same cistron was depending on which pairs of mutants were combined. This particular type of complementation was called interallelic, intragenic or intracistronic complementation. At the opposite of intergenic complementation where the gene fonction is always restored, a positive interallelic complementation is rare, the absence of complementation between mutants located in the same cistron being the rule. For several genes however, a high frequency of complementation was encountered and a complete lack of non-complementation was even observed among 208 ad_2 mutants of *Saccharomyces* [4]. In fact, the ability to complement seems to be related to the type of mutational alteration and then to depend on the mutagen used.

Is there any relationship between the complementing pattern of the mutants and the genetic map ? Let us consider the example of a series of *pan-2* mutants in *Neurospora* [5] : the order of mutation sites along the chromosome has been determined by recombination (Fig. 1).

Some of them (under the line of genetic map in Fig. 1) complement some others of the series. The complementation relationship can be represented by a diagram (= complementation map) which is often linear but may be circular or become more complex when larger samples of mutants are analyzed [6]. Each line represents a group of mutants which do not complement each other. The absence of overlapping between two lines indicates that each mutant of one group complements any mutant of the other group.

As pointed out by Fincham [1], the comparison of genetic map and complementation map does not allow to subdivide the gene into

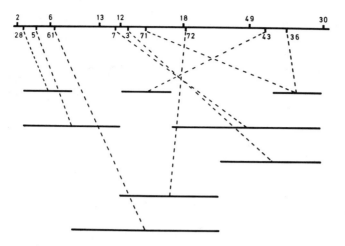

Fig. 1. Genetic map and complementation map of *pan-2* mutants of
Neurospora crassa (from the drawing of Fincham [1] from
the date of case and Giles [5]).

distinct regions. In the example presented in Fig. 1 as in many
other ones, the entire locus behaves as a functional unit. The
best argument to prove that complementation occurred between
mutants located in a unique cistron came from the biochemical
analysis of the mutants : in several systems, it could be demonstrated that the complementing mutants were affecting the activity
of the same enzyme.

A better understanding of the phenomenon of interallelic complementation came from the analysis of the phenotype, and namely
of the properties of the enzyme formed in the diploids.

In general, the complementation between two mutants is not
complete : the phenotype is not truly "wild" and the function is
only partially restored. If, in many cases, the diploids formed
by complementation grow and multiply as the wild strain, the activity of the enzyme in the diploids is often lower than normal.

For example, in different combinations of *Chlamydomonas*
mutants fully defective in argininosuccinate lyase (the last
enzyme in the biosynthetic pathway of arginine), it was found
[7, 8] (table I) that the enzyme activity for various diploids
was ranging from 5 to 39 % of the activity found in the haploid

Table I. - Activity of arginosuccinate lyase and sensitivity to
heat treatment (55° C, 30 min.) in extracts of wild-
type and diploids formed by complementation in *Chlamydomonas* (*Arg 1* mutant is defective in acetylglutamyl-
phosphate reductase; *Arg 7* mutants are defective in
argininosuccinate lyase) (From Loppes *et al.* [7] and
Loppes and Matagne [8]).

Complementing pairs of arginine mutants	Enzyme activity (percent of wild-type)	Enzyme activity after heat treatment (percent of activity at zero time)
Wild-type (haploid)	100	78
Arg 1 x *Arg 7*	45	61
Arg 7 x *Arg 7-2*	19	49
Arg 7 x *Arg 7-7*	20	0
Arg 7 x *Arg 7-8*	16	80
Arg 7-2 x *Arg 7-8*	10	60
Arg 7-3 x *Arg 7-5*	39	10
Arg 7-5 x *Arg 7-7*	8	0
Arg 7-5 x *Arg 7-8*	14	11
Arg 7-7 x *Arg 7-8*	5	0

wild type strain. The diploid strain *Arg 1* x *Arg 7* formed by
intergenic complementation of two mutants defective for two different enzymes had 45 % of the wild type enzyme activity. In none
of these diploids was the growth rate markedly different from that
of the wild strain.

Another important feature is that the enzyme formed by complementation has frequently abnormal properties. In the example
of table I, it can be seen that the stability of the enzyme to
heat varies from one pair of mutants to an other and is lower
than in wild-type, except in one case (diploid *Arg 7* x *Arg 7-8*).
In some cases, the presence of a mutation (*e.g.* 7-7) seems to
confer an increased sensitivity to the enzyme.

In several systems, and for example in a series of *am* mutants
of *Neurospora* lacking glutamate dehydrogenase [9], it could also
be demonstrated that the Michaelis constant of the enzyme formed
by complementation was higher than in the wild type strain, indicating a lower affinity of the enzyme for the substrate.

MECHANISM OF INTERALLELIC COMPLEMENTATION

The question now arises how two mutants, defective for the same enzyme, are able to complement and form an active one.

The possibility has been considered that molecular rearrangement or crossing-over could occur at the template RNA or at the protein level : two abnormal RNA's or proteins could produce normal molecules by recombination. This hypothesis was rapidly ruled out when it was found that the enzymes formed by complementation were in most cases abnormal in their properties.

Complementation between mutants could also originate from the complex nature of the enzyme. If the enzyme is composed of two different polypeptide chains (= heteromultimer), one mutant could supply a normal polypeptide chain and the other mutant another one. In this case, the protein should be specified by two adjacent cistrons and the enzyme formed by complementation should be identical to the wild-type enzyme and be normal in its properties (Fig. 2). This explanation is only valid in a few cases, e.g. for the tryptophane synthetase in *Escherichia coli*, which is an aggregate of two different subunits [10].

As a matter of fact, in many cases, it seems that the enzyme is actually a homomultimer composed of identical subunits, coded by the same structural gene. The alkaline phosphatase produced in *Escherichia coli* is most probably a dimer composed of two identical polypeptide chains [11]; in *Neurospora*, glutamate dehydrogenase is also a homomultimer composed of six identical subunits [12]. Complementation relationships were found between mutants defective for these enzymes. On the basis of the homomultimeric structure of the enzymes, the following hypothesis was proposed [13, 14, 15] : the enzyme formed by complementation is composed of different mutant polypeptide chains correcting each other (Fig. 2). If we assume that the wild-type active enzyme is a dimer (aa), the two mutant enzyme a'a' and a"a" should be inactive but the hybrid enzyme a'a" is expected to display enough activity to restore the wild phenotype. This hypothesis fully agrees with the fact that the enzyme formed by complementation is somewhat abnormal.

The hybrid enzyme hypothesis is also strongly supported by the results of the *in vitro* complementation (see infra) : it became widely accepted when it was demonstrated that a large number of enzymes, perhaps the majority, are composed of several identical subunits (for a review, see [16]).

To explain how the association of two distinct abnormal· subunits can result in the formation of an active form of enzyme, Crick and Orgel proposed [17] that complementation was due to the

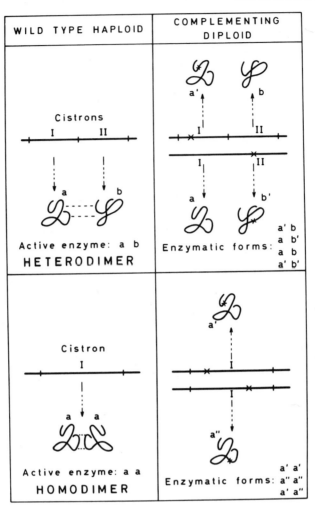

Fig. 2. Complementation between mutants (x) located in two different adjacent cistrons (upper part) or in the same
cistron (lower part) : see text.

correction of the misfolding of one chain by the other. The Crick
and Orgel theory of complementation was used for interpreting complex complementation maps in view to elucidate by this way the
three-dimensional structure of proteins [6, 18]. An example has

been recently given by Korch [19] : from a very detailed complementation map of the *his 1* mutants of *Saccharomyces*, the author
proposed a model for the subunit and for the tertiary and quaternary structure of the enzyme encoded by the gene.

The results concerning the properties of the enzyme formed by
complementation have however to be interpreted with caution.

The abnormal properties of the enzyme formed by complementation are not necessarily the proof that this enzyme is normally
composed of identical subunits. A good example is given by the
complementing mutants of *Escherichia coli*, defective for the β-
galactosidase (Z‾ mutants). Perrin [20] showed that the level of
enzyme activity in diploids for the Lac region was always lower
than in wild-type; moreover, the enzyme in complementing pairs
showed a high sensitivity to heat and a great heterogeneity at
the molecular point of view. Perrin concludes that "the Z region
is expressed by a single product and should be considered as one
cistron". Yet, the more recent studies of Ullmann *et al.* [21]
demonstrate that the Z region is constituted of different cistrons,
coding for different polypeptide chains; most complementing mutants are located in different cistrons. This is surprising since,
in case of intergenic complementation, a normal enzyme is expected.
The explanation lies in the particular structure of β-galactosidase, constituted of 4 identical subunits, each consisting of 2 or
3 non identical chains. If the subunits combine at random to form
the tetramers, a large number of hybrids is expected, only one of
them will have a completely normal structure. This fully agrees
with the Perrin's observation that the enzyme was heterogeneous as
suggested by the shape of the heat denaturation curves.

Choosing between intergenic or interallelic complementation
is not always easy. Nevertheless, a highly probable interpretation
can be drawn when a large number of mutants are analysed. The
general rule is that mutants belonging to different genes always
complement, whereas mutants in the same gene do not.

IN VITRO COMPLEMENTATION

If interallelic complementation occurs through interaction
between the products of the gene, *i.e.* the polypeptide chains, it
should be possible to demonstrate similar interactions *in vitro*.
This has actually been done in various cell free systems, using
crude extracts or purified mutant proteins. By mixing enzymatic
extracts prepared from two mutants, it was possible to recover
some enzyme activity. As pointed out by Fincham [1] there is
often some relation between *in vitro* and *in vivo* complementation :
the pairs of mutants leading to an active enzyme *in vitro* are the

same pairs which complement *in vivo*. Moreover, properties of the
enzymes formed *in vivo* or *in vitro* are similar. An example is given
by the am_1 and am_3 complementing mutants in *Neurospora* [9] both
defective in glutamate dehydrogenase : the enzyme formed by complementation, as well *in vivo* as *in vitro*, has a Michaelis constant 2
to 3 times higher than the wild-type enzyme.

The mechanism of the *in vitro* complementation has been extensively studied by Schlesinger and Levinthal [22]; their results
have fully confirmed the theory of hybrid enzyme formation. We
shall give here some of their data. These authors used mutants of
E. coli defective in alkaline phosphatase. Complementation was
known to occur in this system [23] and moreover, biochemical data
indicated that this enzyme was a homodimer containing zinc [11].
Schlesinger and Levinthal could dissociate the enzyme into monomers
by incubating at pH 4.0. Reassociation of the monomers occurred at
pH 7.8 in the presence of Zn and gave rise to an active enzyme.
They used 2 mutants, U9 and S33, having a low enzyme activity.
When purified monomers of these 2 strains were mixed at pH 7.8, an
active enzyme was formed which had the same rate of sedimentation
in sucrose density gradient as the wild-type enzyme. That the
enzyme formed *in vitro* was an hybrid molecule was confirmed by
electrophoretic analysis : the complementing enzyme had an intermediate position between the two mutant enzymes.

Another interesting result from Schlesinger and Levinthal is
that the dimers are formed by random collisions between free monomers.

If U9 and S33 monomers are mixed in the ratio 1 : 1, one
expects, assuming that association occurs at random : 25 % U9
dimers, 25 % S33 dimers and 50 % of hybrid U9-S33 dimers. In the
same way, a mixture of U9 and S33 monomers in the ratio 9 : 1 one
expects : 2 x 0,1 x 0,9 = 0,18 = 18 % hybrid molecules. By mixing
the monomers in various proportions, the authors obtained various
enzyme activities, corresponding to the quantity of hybrid enzyme.
Assuming that the monomers combine at random, it is possible to
calculate the specific activity of the hybrid enzyme; Schlesinger
and Levinthal found that the specific activity remained constant
whatever was the proportion of the monomers : this was consistent
with the hypothesis that monomers produce dimers by random collisions.

The dissociation-reassociation mechanism described for alkaline phosphate is perhaps not a prerequisite for the formation of
an hybrid enzyme *in vitro*. Coddington and Fincham [24] showed that
an active glutamate dehydrogenase was formed by *in vitro* complementation, without detecting the presence of free subunits at low
pH. They postulated that some exchange of subunits could occur between aggregates, without liberation of free subunits in the solution.

MECHANISM OF COMPLEMENTATION *IN VIVO*

The question arises whether the complementation *in vivo* also occurs by interactions between subunits, to give an hybrid enzyme. In certain systems, it was demonstrated that the enzymes obtained by complementation *in vivo* and *in vitro* can differ in their properties, for example, their sensitivity to heat [25]. This suggests that the process of hybrid enzyme formation in the cells may differ from the complementation mechanism *in vitro*.

An interesting result was obtained by Zipser and Perrin [26] in their complementation studies with *E. coli* mutants defective for β-galactosidase. They found that the Z_1/Z_{178} heterogenote had half of its enzyme activity bound to ribosomes, whereas only 1 % enzyme was bound to ribosomes in wild-type cells. They moreover found that *in vitro* complementation between ribosomes from one mutant (Z_{178}) and a soluble preparation from the other (Z_1) took place much faster than in a mixture of soluble proteins from both mutants.

Similar data were obtained with aspartate transcarbamylase mutants of *Neurospora* [27]. Enzyme activity was recovered after incubation *in vitro* of ribosomes from one mutant with soluble proteins from the other one. Complementation did not occur between ribosomes from both mutants. The enzyme activity remained bound to ribosomes after repeated washings but the nature of the attachment remained obscure. Finally, the enzyme formed by complementation on ribosomes had the same thermosensitivity as the enzyme formed *in vivo* but different from the enzyme formed by complementation between soluble proteins.

These results, if they do not resolve the problem of the mechanism of complementation inside living cells, at least indicate that interaction between polypeptide chains depends not only on their structural conformation but can also be affected by their association with the ribosomes.

NEGATIVE COMPLEMENTATION AND GENE DOSAGE RELATIONSHIPS

If the hypothesis of the conformational correction is true, one can expect that a mutant chain could impose its abnormal folding to another mutant or normal chain in a complex multimer. The complementing enzyme can be less active than the enzyme which is formed by each mutant itself. Such a negative complementation was described between ad_2 mutants of *Saccharomyces* [4]. Similarly, a mutant allele producing an abnormal enzyme might interfere with the formation of a normal enzyme by the wild-type gene. Garen and Garen [23] studied the properties of alkaline phosphatase formed in *P-/P+* heterogenotes of *E. coli*. In some cases, the enzyme was

more thermosensitive in the hybrid than in the wild-type strain;
the inactivation curve, diphasic in its shape, indicated that two
types of proteins were produced : one having the thermostability
of the wild-type enzyme, the other being much more sensitive to
heat.

Zimmerman and coll. [28, 29] extensively studied the enzyme
formed in heterozygotes of *Saccharomyces cerevisiae,* obtained
from crosses between various is_1 mutants (defective in threonine
dehydratase) and the wild-type strain. The enzyme activity was
ranging from 10 to 100 % of the wild-type activity. The apparent
Michaelis constant was increased in many cases and sometimes,
several enzyme forms could be detected. An enzyme with new properties, like resistance to feed-back inhibition, was even found.
These data indicate that hybrid enzymes are probably formed by
interaction between mutant and wild-type subunits.

It is then clear that the dosage between the wild-type and
the mutant gene is not determined by a simple relation. As pointed
out by Zimmerman, a clearcut gene dosis relationship is only expected with genes coding for a monomeric enzyme. If the gene is
coding for a multimer, a clear relation will be observed only with
mutants which do not form a gene product able to combine with an
other subunit. In other cases, the enzyme activity is not determined by a specific allele but by the combination of two alleles :
the total activity will be the sum of the activities present in
the various active hybrid enzymes. For example, in a heterozygote
for a gene coding for a tetramer, the following forms are expected : aaaa, aaaa', aaa'a', aa'a'a', and a'a'a'a'. Assuming that the
subunits combine at random, only 6.25% of the total enzyme corresponds to the wild-type form aaaa. A growth test which is often
used to define a phenotype cannot be used to study a gene dosage
relationship.

In classical genetics, dominance-recessiveness was opposed to
the intermediate behaviour of a certain pair of alleles. Many observations indicate that the intermediate behaviour is very rare.
We moreover observe that the difference between the two homozygous
cells and the heterozygous cells is not necessarily only quantitative since hybrid enzymes can show new properties.

IMPORTANCE OF INTERALLELIC COMPLEMENTATION IN HIGHER PLANTS

Interallelic complementation can only occur in organisms
having a stable diploid phase or an equivalent one : dikaryous,
heterokaryous, heterogenote. Moreover, the enzyme coded by the
involved structural gene must be a multimer. In practice, investigations concerned with interallelic complementation require

the possibility to isolate a relatively high number of mutants all located in the same cistron. The study is more fruitfull when the enzyme coded by the cistron can be determined and analyzed biochemically. This explains why the studies of interallic complementation were mainly confined to microorganisms : *Escherichia coli, Saccharomyces cerevisiae, Schizosaccharomyces pombe, Neurospora, Aspergillus, Coprinus lagopus, Chlamydomonas*. In higher plants, allelic complementation was only obtained with temperature sensitive mutants of *Arabidopsis* [30] and with alcohol dehydrogenase mutants in maize [31].

It is however probable that interallelic complementation plays an important role in Nature. Numerous examples of hybrid enzymes formed by interaction of different natural allels are known. This could be demonstrated by zone electrophoresis techniques, combined with specific staining of certain enzymes, as done by Schwartz [32, 33, 34] on esterase variants in maize. In a plant heterozygote for two allels controlling two electrophoretic variants of esterase, three electrophoretic bands were found : two corresponding to the parent enzymes and a hybrid enzyme, intermediate in position. One can suppose that in many cases, the hybrid enzyme should be advantageous for the cell. This could explain heterosis, *i.e.* the superiority in size and vigor of the heterozygote over the parental homozygotes. A good example of heterosis by interaction of allels was given by Li and Redei [30] in *Arabidopsis*.

As pointed out by Zimmerman and Gunderlach [28], the importance of mutations in diploids has also to be reconsidered. A mutation in one of the two genomes will lead to a heterozygote. The mutated allele will perhaps be completely recessive (= inactive) but most probably, it will lead to a gene product. If the enzyme coded by the gene is a multimer (which seems to be the most frequent situation), the mutant allele will participate to the formation of a new hybrid enzyme and then, to the appearance of a new phenotype. Diploids homozygous might be a good material for isolating, through mutational processes, heterozygotes of practical interest.

REFERENCES

[1] J.R.S. FINCHAM, Genetic complementation, Benjamin Inc. New York, Amsterdam (1966) 138 pp.
[2] J.A. ROPER and R.H. PRITCHARD, Nature 175 (1955) 639.
[3] S. BENZER, The chemical basis of heredity, Johns Hopkins Press, Baltimore (1958) 70
[4] N. NASHED, Molec. Gen. Genetics 102 (1968) 285.
[5] M.E. CASE and N.H. GILES, Proc. Nat. Acad. Sci., 46 (1960) 659.

[6] O.J. GILLIE, Genetics 58 (1968) 543.

[7] R. LOPPES, R. MATAGNE and P.J. STRIJKERT, Heredity 28 (1972)
    239.

[8] R. LOPPES and R. MATAGNE, Genetica 43 (1972) 422.

[9] J.R.S. FINCHAM and A. CODDINGTON, Cold Spring Harb. Symp.
    Quant. Biol. 28 (1963) 517.

[10] C. YANOFSKY, Bact. Rev. 24 (1960) 221.

[11] F. ROTHMAN and R. BYRNE, J. Mol. Biol. 6 (1963) 330.

[12] J.C. WOOTTON, G.K. CHAMBERS, J.G. TAYLOR and J.R.S. FINCHAM,
     Nature New Biol. 241 (1973) 42.

[13] D.G. CATCHESIDE, Cold Spring Harb. Symp. Quant. Biol. 23
     (1958) 137.

[14] J.R.S. FINCHAM, J. Gen. Microbiol. 21 (1959) 600.

[15] S. BRENNER, Biochemistry of human genetics, Ciba Found. Symp.,
     Churchill London (1959) 304.

[16] I.M. KLOTZ, N.R. LANGERMAN and D.W. DARNELL, Ann. Rev. Biochem.
     39 (1970) 25.

[17] F.H.C. CRICK and L.E. ORGEL, J. Mol. Biol. 8 (1964) 162.

[18] O.J. GILLIE, Genet. Res. 8 (1966) 9.

[19] C.T. KORCH, Genetics 74 (1973) 307.

[20] D. PERRIN, Cold Spring Harb. Symp. Quant. Biol. 28 (1963)
     529.

[21] A. ULLMANN, D. PERRIN, F. JACOB and J. MONOD, J. Mol. Biol.
     12 (1965) 918.

[22] M.J. SCHLESINGER and C. LEVINTHAL, J. Mol. Biol. 7 (1963) 1.

[23] A. GAREN and J. GAREN, J. Mol. Biol. 7 (1963) 13.

[24] A. CODDINGTON and J.R.S. FINCHAM, J. Mol. Biol. 12 (1965) 152.

[25] A.S. ISSALY and J.L. REISSIG, Arch. Biochem. Biophys. 116
     (1966) 44.

[26] D. ZIPSER and D. PERRIN, Cold Spring Harb. Symp. Quant. Biol.
     28 (1963) 533.

[27] A.S. ISSALY, S.A. CATALDI, I.M. ISSALY and J.L. REISIG, Bio-
     chem. Biophys. Acta 209 (1970) 501.

[28] F.K. ZIMMERMAN and E. GUNDERLACH, Molec. Gen. Genetics 103
     (1969) 348.

[29] F.K. ZIMMERMAN, I. SCHMIEDT, A.M.A. TEN BERGE, Molec. Gen.
     Genetics 104 (1969) 321.

[30] J.L. LI and G.P. REDEI, Theoret. Appl. Genet. 39 (1969) 68.

[31] D. SCHWARTZ, Proc. Nat. Acad. Sci. 68 (1971) 145.

[32] D. SCHWARTZ, Proc. Nat. Acad. Sci. 46 (1960) 210.

[33] D. SCHWARTZ, Proc. Nat. Acad. Sci. 48 (1962) 750.

[34] D. SCHWARTZ, Proc. Nat. Acad. Sci. 51 (1962) 681.

PRINCIPLES OF GENETIC REGULATION IN LOWER AND HIGHER PLANTS

R. LOPPES [*] and R.F. MATAGNE

Laboratory of Molecular Genetics, Department of Botany
University of Liège, Sart Tilman, B-4000 Liège, Belgium

Living organisms are generally able to adapt themselves to relatively wide and sudden variations of the environmental conditions. As a result of a change in their surroundings, they may produce one or several additional enzymes specifically related to the new external conditions. This property of adaptation may be easily demonstrated with unicellular organisms the metabolism of which is strongly dependent on the growth medium. If a yeast cell is transferred from its normal medium containing mineral nitrogen to a medium containing arginine as the sole nitrogen source, it will rapidly synthesize two enzymes (arginase and ornithine transaminase) which are needed for degrading arginine into NH_4^+ and glutamate [1]. The production of great amounts of these two enzymes will allow the cell to make all its nitrogenous compounds from arginine. Hence, the induction of arginine breakdown enzymes is a prerequisite for survival of the yeast in these particular conditions. That the repression of enzyme synthesis is a prerequisite for survival is also obvious. Certain species of *Pseudomonas* are able to grow on more than 100 different organic substrates [2]. The enzymes necessary for degrading a specific compound are generally not produced when this compound is not present in the culture medium. Mutants have been obtained in which the enzymes catalyzing the breakdown of a given compound may constitute, in non-inducible conditions, up to 10 % of the total protein. It is clear that the cell could not bear too many mutations of this kind which would result in an accumulation of useless proteins.

[*] Chercheur qualifié du Fonds National Belge de la Recherche Scientifique.

In higher organisms, cell differentiation results in a variety of tissues which differ in their gene activities although their chromosomes carry identical basic information. It is evident that such a repartition of the biochemical work which has developed in animals and higher plants can only last thanks to a tight control of gene transcription.

We would like to illustrate here how mutants impaired in regulatory functions can be used as tools for studying the regulation of gene expression. We shall mainly deal with microeucaryotes like fungi and yeast. The few data obtained up to now on the genetic regulatory mechanisms in higher photosynthetic organisms will be discussed in relation to the patterns of regulation now apparent in bacteria and fungi.

THE USEFULNESS OF SPECIFIC MUTANTS IN REGULATION STUDIES.

Before investigating how a given metabolic pathway is regulated, it is necessary to first know the different enzymatic steps involved in this pathway. Some knowledge about these reactions can be gained from biochemical studies, but mutants specifically blocked in one enzymatic reaction are the essential tools to relate gene and specified protein coded by that gene. When this is done, one must determine which culture conditions modify one or several enzyme activities. The terms "induction" and "derepression" will be used respectively to mean that the enzyme is produced in response to adding a compound to the growth medium or to depriving it from some metabolite [3]. That the increase of the enzyme activity is the result of specific transcription of the related gene and is not due to "activation" of a preexisting protein can be established easily with radioisotopic precursors of proteins [4].

A careful genetic analysis of the various types of mutants allows to determine whether certain (or all) genes are closely linked or not and are candidates for being part of an operon. In *E. coli*, for example, the synthesis of arginine from glutamic acid is catalysed by 8 enzymes; the structural genes have been mapped : 4 genes (ECBH) are clustered and 4 genes are scattered on the chromosome. The genetic background is very different here from that observed in the lactose operon of *E. coli* or in the histidine operon of *S. typhimurium* where all the structural genes are clustered. Nevertheless, all the enzymes of the arginine biosynthesis in *E. coli* are repressed by arginine, which suggests that part of the mechanism leading to repression is common for all the enzymes of the pathway, even when these are coded by unlinked genes.

To better understand the matter, it is necessary to isolate

and to investigate mutants disturbed in their regulatory system. A widely used method consists in selecting strains which are resistant to an analog of the co-repressor. In *E. coli* [5] and in *S. cerevisiae* [6], mutants impaired in their ability to repress the arginine biosynthetic enzymes have been isolated as resistant to canavanine. This compound is incorporated into protein, which results in lethal damage for the cell. Owing to the fact that canavanine acts as a false co-repressor, little arginine is produced in wild-type cells grown in the presence of the analog. If, by mutation, the arginine biosynthetic enzymes are strongly derepressed in the presence of canavanine, the intracellular concentration of arginine will reach such a level that it will successfully compete with canavanine for incorporation into protein.

In a few enzymatic systems (phosphatases, for example) it is possible to test the enzyme activity on the whole colonies. In this case, no "selection" procedure has to be used and the regulation mutants can be directly visualized as producing the enzyme constitutively in repression conditions or producing little enzyme in derepression conditions [7].

CONSEQUENCES OF MUTATIONS IN REGULATOR GENES. NEGATIVE OR POSITIVE CONTROL

The control of gene transcription is negative or positive according as the active product of the regulator gene prevents or allows transcription. Hence, the study of regulation mutants makes it possible to discriminate between the two types of control susceptible to operate in a given system.

Let us consider a cluster of 3 genes (A, B, C) governing the synthesis of 3 related enzymes (a, b, c) whose activity decreases when the organism is grown in the presence of a given metabolite (M). As shown in fig. 1 nonsense mutations in the regulator (R) gene lead to de-repressed enzyme production when the control is negative and to super-repressed enzyme production when the control is positive. In other words, if the control is negative, nonsense mutants of R will be found which produce great amounts of the enzymes a, b and c in the absence and in the presence of M; conversely, if the control is positive, nonsense mutants of R will be found which produce no enzyme in the absence or in the presence of M.

It must be pointed out that certain missense mutations of R can lead to super-repression in a negatively controlled system and to "constitutivity" (i.e. a permanent synthesis) in a positively controlled system. But the important feature is that "de-repressed" is always dominant over "super-repressed" when the control is positive but recessive when the control is negative.

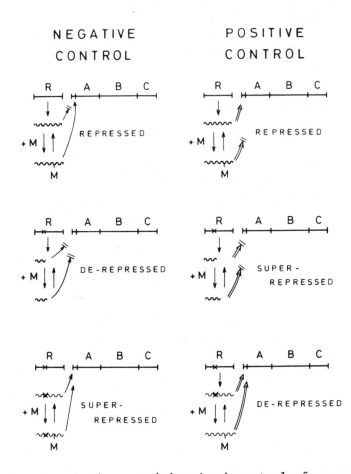

Fig. 1. Negative (⟶) or positive (⟹) control of repression.
The regulator protein coded by gene R can exist in two
conformations according as co-repressor (M) is present
or not. In a negatively controlled system, M activates
the product of R which becomes effective in switching
the operon off. In a positively controlled system, M
inactivates the product of R which becomes ineffective
in switching the operon on. The effects of mutations in
R gene are explained in the text.

Let us assume the control of (A B C) to be found negative. A, B and C being genetically clustered, they can be postulated being parts of an operon. To prove this unequivocally, it is necessary :

1) to show that the derepression of the enzymes a, b and c is coordinate, i.e. that equimolar amounts of enzymes are produced in all cases. The gene cluster *arg* ECBH of *E. coli*, for example, has first been thought to behave as one operon. However it has been shown afterwards [8] that C, B and H were coordinately repressed, whereas E was repressed to a lesser extent.

2) to show the existence of typical operator mutations. Mutations must theoretically occur at one end of the group of structural genes, in the operator-promotor region, where RNA synthesis is initiated along one of the DNA strands and where regulator proteins interact for inhibiting or switching on RNA synthesis.

How is it possible to distinguish a mutation in a regulator gene from a mutation of the operator ?

1) The regulator genes are generally not linked to the structural genes they control.

2) Like mutations in the regulator gene(s), mutations in the operator region have a pleiotropic effect in that they can affect the expression of several structural genes but, unlike mutations in the regulator genes, they affect only those genes which are coordinately transcribed.

3) Deletions in the operator may have the same phenotypical effect as deletions in a regulator gene but these two kinds of mutations can be distinguished on the basis of their genetical behaviour. As can be seen in fig. 2, the mutations of O^c (operator-constitutive) and R^c (regulator gene constitutive) both result in derepression of protein synthesis. Yet when R^c is coupled to its wild-type allele in a cis-trans test, the active regulator gene is dominant in the trans configuration. On the contrary, the operator mutations do not affect the transcription in the trans position and O^c is then dominant over O. Because the constitutive allele is dominant over the wild-type, O^c mutants (but not R^c mutants) can be selected directly for constitutivity from a population of diploid cells.

To conclude this chapter devoted to the different types of mutants which can be detected and which are needed to characterize a regulation system, one should point out the difficulty sometimes encountered to decide whether one is dealing with a regulation mutant or a structural one.

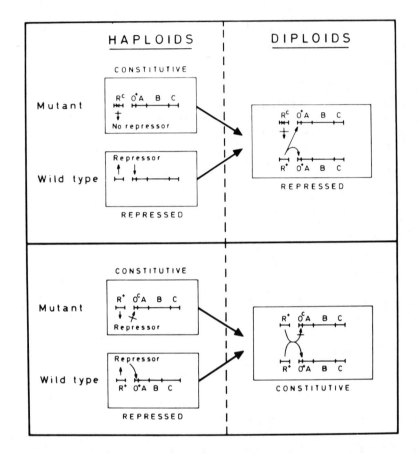

Fig. 2. Genetic behaviour of deletions in regulator gene (R^c) and operator (0^c) in a negatively controlled system. The two types of mutations can be distinguished according to their effect in trans configuration.

In a system including several functionally related enzymatic reactions, mutations will usually be found which are not linked to structural genes (whether these are clustered in an operon or scattered within the genome) and modify the rate of synthesis of several enzymes.

In a system where only one enzyme is susceptible to be regulated by a given factor, a mutation taking place in a regulator gene or in a structural gene may equally result in a lack of enzymatic activity. If two mutations are found in which this enzyme activity is lacking and do not map at closely linked sites, it can be postulated that one occurs in a structural gene and the other one in a regulator gene. Deciding between these two alternatives may require a lot of experimental work as can be realized by examining, for example, the problem of maltase mutants in *Saccharomyces*.

Maltase is inducible by maltose in the wild-type strain. Mutants have been obtained which produce maltase constitutively. From one of these strains (*MAL* 4), Kahn *et al.* [9] have isolated a series of mutants unable to ferment maltose. The problem was to determine whether the loss of activity resulted from a mutation in a structural gene or from a mutation in a regulator gene leading to uninducibility.

Such mutants were allelic or closely linked to *MAL* 4 and exhibited a low but detectable enzyme activity. They did not complement each other and were recessive. At least some of them were revertible and the revertants synthesized an enzyme with properties (K_m, substrate specificity, heat sensitivity) similar to those of the *MAL* 4 strain. This suggested that the maltose-negative mutants had arisen from a mutation in a regulator gene, since revertants obtained from structural mutants generally produce enzymes which differ from the wild-type enzyme in some of their properties.

The same conclusion could be drawn from immunological studies. In a strain carrying a missense mutation in a structural gene, it is expected to find a low enzyme activity beside a great amount of "CRM" protein, immunologically related to the maltase of the parent strain (ratio enzymatic activity/immunological reactivity much lower than in *MAL* 4). On the contrary, this ratio is expected to be the same as in *MAL* 4 when a regulator mutation switches off the transcription of the structural gene. All the mutants investigated displayed the same ratio enzyme activity/immunological reactivity, which confirmed the regulatory function of *MAL* 4.

The examples quoted up to now have been indiscriminately taken from the literature dealing with prokaryotic or eukaryotic microorganisms. The general principles of metabolic regulation seem to be similar in bacteria and fungi, in that regulation is

apparently mediated by regulatory proteins which are activated or
inactivated by effectors. However we do not yet know how this type
of regulation works in *Eukaryotes* at the molecular level.

Several bacterial operons (lac, his) have been demonstrated
to actually work *in vitro* [for a review, 10] and to obey the laws
predicted from the behaviour of particular mutants. The current
work now in progress with microeukaryotes is mainly directed
towards the isolation of mutants. Attempts are made to define them
following models derived from a combination of results obtained in
bacteria. Umbarger [11] believes that in some cases, "the estheti-
cally pleasing model developed in studies with bacterial systems
may provide more of hindrance than a guidepost".

In fact, the models obtained with *Prokaryotes* are not applicable as such to *Eukaryotes*. This is not surprising owing to the
complex organisation of *Eukaryotes* with their complex chromosomes
and well defined nuclei with the morphological and functional
compartmentation of the cell and with their multiple independent
transcription and translation systems.

Let us now discuss some problems related to enzyme regulation
in *Eukaryotes*, namely the scarcity of true operons, the apparent
hyper complexity of certain regulatory mechanisms and the existence of proteins combining catalytic and regulatory functions.

OPERONS IN EUKARYOTES ?

In bacteria, the genes corresponding to a given pathway are
generally closely linked. The most typical example is probably
that of the histidine operon in *S. typhimurium*, containing 9 con-
tiguous genes. In *Neurospora*, *Aspergillus* and *Saccharomyces*, most
genes coding for the enzymes of the histidine biosynthesis are
dispersed throughout the genome. There are, in bacteria, exceptions to clustering : the genes of the arginine system in *E. coli*
clearly illustrate this possibility. Nevertheless it can be said
that gene clustering is common in bacteria whilst exceptional in
Eukaryotes. According to Jacob and Monod [12], the scattering of
structural genes must not necessarily be considered as an objec-
tion to the operon theory. In *Eukaryotes*, a given genetic system
may well be constituted of several unlinked operons (each with
one structural gene and one operator) all of them being under the
control of the product of one regulator gene.

In bacteria, evidence for the existence of a given operon
depends on the finding of operator-constitutive (0^c) mutants. Up
to now, very few possible 0^c mutants have been found in *Eukaryotes*.

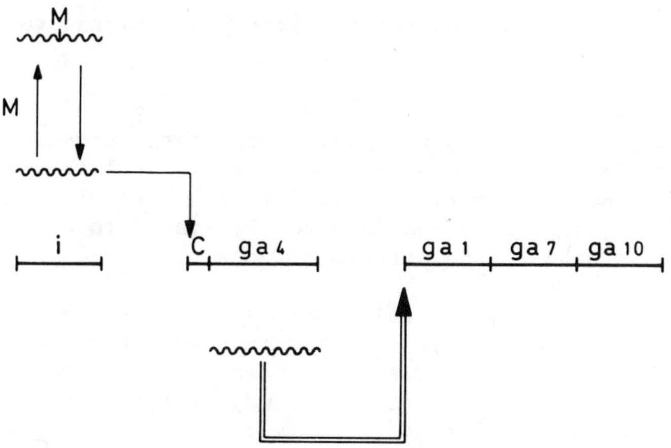

Fig. 3. Control of the galactose cluster in *Saccharomyces* according to Douglas and Hawthorne [37]. In the presence of co-inducer (M) the product of the regulator gene (i) does not act any more on C for switching off the synthesis of the ga_4 gene product. The ga_4 gene product is required for transcription of ga_1, ga_7 and ga_{10}. ⟶ negative control; ⟹ positive control.

In yeast, the utilization of galactose is mediated by 3 enzymes which are inducible by galactose. The corresponding structural genes ga_1, ga_7 and ga_{10} (fig. 3) are clustered. Three types of regulation mutants have been found (review by Hartwell [13])

ga_4 : loss of the three enzyme activities; recessive mutation

i : constitutive synthesis of the 3 enzymes : recessive mutation only expressed in the presence of the wild ga_4 gene

C : constitutive synthesis of the 3 enzymes; dominant mutation expressed only when in cis position to the wild ga_4 gene.

These mutants can be interpreted by assuming that the gene *i* produces a repressor that acts on C (operator site ?) to regulate the synthesis of the ga_4 product which in turn positively controls the synthesis of the 3 enzymes. The peculiarity of this "operator" lies in the fact that it does not directly control the cluster but rather controls a regulator gene the product of which controls the

structural genes. No operator region tightly associated to the
cluster has been found.

Toh - E and co-workers [14, 15] have recently studied the
genetic regulatory system controlling phosphatase formation in
Saccharomyces. They have isolated, among other regulatory mutants,
one which could be an 0^c mutant. Surprisingly, like with the
galactose system, this mutation is strongly linked to a regulator
gene, itself unlinked to the structural gene.

The classical operon not only implies the presence of an
operator but also of a cluster of genes involved in the same
metabolic pathway. Such clusters are present in the chromosomal
map of *Neurospora*. The most detailed study of these possible
operons has been carried out on the *arom* region [for reviews,
see 3 and 16] : this is composed of 5 genes coding for 5 enzymes
catalyzing successive steps in the biosynthetic pathway of
aromatic amino acids. The synthesis of these enzymes is highly
coordinate. Mutations may be induced in this region which abolish
separately each of the enzyme activities. Moreover, certain mutations in the first structural gene have a pleiotropic effect and
can suppress all enzyme activities. In bacterial operons, such
pleiotropic effects have been shown to result from nonsense
mutations leading to an early interruption of mRNA synthesis.

The analogy of the *arom* cluster with a bacterial operon is
however not complete. No evidence has been brought that an
operator region does really exist in this system (it is perhaps
relevant to point out that the synthesis of these 5 enzymes is
constitutive and that the pathway is regulated by feedback inhibition of the first enzyme, this latter being coded by a gene
distant from the cluster). The biochemical analysis has allowed
defining this eukaryotic cluster. Purification of one of the
"enzymes" always resulted in the simultaneous purification of the
other ones. This was due to the fact that the 5 activities determined by the *arom* cluster are actually associated in a protein
complex of molecular weight about 230.000. This complex seems to
be composed of 5 different polypeptides each of which corresponds
to one enzyme.

The clustering of genes in a true operon seems to be advantageous to the economy of the cell. As suggested by Calvo and
Fink [16], the aggregation of related enzymes results in "seques-
tering intermediates and preventing them from entering into
degradative cycles or from diffusing out of the cell". It is not
clear however why enzyme aggregates should be encoded by a gene
cluster.

Another problem arises when surveying the regulation systems
described in *Eukaryotes*. It relates to the number of genes con-

cerned with the production of a given metabolite. We previously quoted the example of the "maltase" mutants in yeast. Up to now, no less than 7 different genes have been detected (structural or regulator genes) which make the cell able to ferment maltose [17]. In the Basidiomycete *Coprinus lagopus*, the synthesis of alkaline phosphatase is under the control of 3 structural and 5 regulator genes [18]. In *Aspergillus*, about 10 genes are concerned with the production of the same enzyme [19]. Recent results on the control of the derepressible phosphatase synthesis in yeast show [14] an extremely complex situation where the single structural gene is controlled by at least 5 different loci, one of them being possibly an operator.

It is far from clear why so many genes are involved in the regulation of the same function, or why they so often interact in such a sophisticated way. Eukaryotic cells contain lots of DNA (many authors say "too much") and it might be assumed that after the setting of a first regulation system, other systems have arisen (maybe by gene duplication) paralleling the first one, or reinforcing it, each additional system progressively refining the overall control

PROTEIN-PROTEIN INTERACTIONS

All regulation mechanisms we have been dealing with up to now were related to the control of transcription. This very efficient system results in a rapid modification of the production of new RNA molecules and, ultimately, of new specific proteins.

This system is expected to be very effective only if mRNA has a short life, otherwise the synthesis of proteins would continue in the absence of transcription. In bacteria, many mRNA species are unstable. On the contrary, the eukaryotic RNA's may have a half life of several hours and the effects of switching off transcription may be much delayed. Of special interest are in this case the systems which operate in the cell to control the activity of the enzymes.

This type of control is often mediated by small molecules which modify the allosteric properties of the enzyme.

We shall not deal here with allosteric modifications but rather discuss the finding that proteins can exhibit a given catalytic function and also play a role in the regulation of another enzyme. The most obvious example is that of arginase in yeast. In this organism, the biosynthesis of arginine proceeds from glutamate as schematically shown in fig. 4. When the wild-type strain is grown in the presence of arginine, several anabolic enzymes are repressed [20] whereas the catabolic enzymes

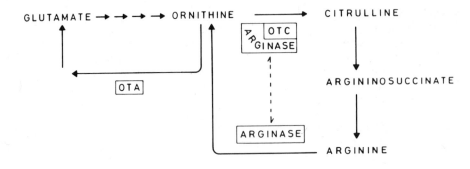

Fig. 4. The control of ornithine transcarbamylase activity by
arginase in *Saccharomyces cerevisiae*.

arginase and ornithine transaminase are induced [1]. Regulation
mutants (*arg*R) were found [21] in which the biosynthetic enzyme
ornithine transcarbamylase (OTC) was no longer repressed by
arginine. These *arg*R mutants were also shown to lack arginase
and ornithine transaminase. Consequently they failed to use arginine as the sole nitrogen source [22]. *In vitro* experiments demonstrated that a protein was produced in the wild-type strain, which
inhibited OTC in the presence of ornithine and arginine. This regulatory protein was missing in *arg*R. As this mutant was impaired in
the anabolism and the catabolism of arginine, the same regulatory
protein was expected to be involved in both functions. The regulatory protein was then identified as being arginase itself. A direct
demonstration of the binding of OTC to arginase was obtained *in
vitro* in the presence of arginine and ornithine. This system
prevents the waste of energy which would result from the urea
cycle operating while arginine is catabolized [23].

   We would like to mention another example of the regulation of
the activity of an enzyme by another enzyme. In 1968, Manney observed that when yeast was grown in certain conditions, the tryptophan synthetase activity (TS) exponentially disappeared in crude
extracts incubated at 37° C. The study of this phenomenon led the
author to conclude that in yeast several macromolecular factors
are present which affect the stability of TS [24]. This "inactivating principle" was further investigated by Holzer and co-workers.
These authors [25] purified two different inactivating enzymes
(inactivases I and II) which had proteolytic properties specifically directed against TS. The inactivases were almost absent in

exponential cultures but accumulated in stationary phase cultures. This feature appears quite logical since high levels of biosynthetic enzymes like TS are no longer required when the stationary phase is reached. Very recently, Holzer's group has found a specific TS inactivase inhibitor of high molecular weight. The properties of this inhibitor are somewhat similar to those of protease inhibitors [26]. More difficult to understand is the reason why the inhibitor of the TS inactivases, like the inactivases themselves, seems to be mainly produced in the stationary phase of growth.

It is well known that nitrate reductase can be induced by nitrate in different organisms. In *Neurospora*, deprivation of nitrate or addition of ammonium salts results in a rapid *in vivo* inactivation of the enzyme [27, 28]. The rate of inactivation is slower in the presence of cycloheximide which inhibits protein synthesis. Contrary to what happens with the yeast tryptophane synthetase, no free "inactivator principle" is found in extracts containing inactivated nitrate reductase. Nitrate seems to be required for protecting the enzyme *in vivo*. To explain the effect of cycloheximide, Subramanian and Sorger suggest that nitrate and ammonium control the stability of the enzyme *in vivo* by modifying its conformation in such a way that it is or not recognized by a rapidly turning-over protease. This view is in agreement with the fact that *nit*-1 and *nit*-3 mutants which have an abnormal nitrate reductase, do not display any enzyme inactivation by NH_4^+. Hence, the integrity of the nitrate reductase molecule seems to be required for the *in vivo* inactivation.

REGULATION MECHANISMS IN HIGHER PLANTS

When surveying the numerous studies devoted to enzyme regulation in higher plants, one can be disappointed by the lack of sound genetic basis. The most commonly used tools are the "specific metabolic inhibitors" of protein (cycloheximide, chloramphenicol), RNA (actinomycin D) and DNA (5-fluorodeoxyuridine) synthesis.

The results obtained with the inhibitors have sometimes led to erroneous interpretations. Pardee and Prestidge [29] had observed in *E. coli* that the synthesis of the *lac* operon repressor was not inhibited by 5-methyltryptophane. As this compound inhibited protein synthesis, it was concluded that the repressor could not be a protein. These results led Jacob and Monod [12] to postulate that the repressor was RNA. In fact, it was found later that 5-methyltryptophan does not inhibit all protein synthesis and that the *lac* repressor can be produced in its presence. With this restriction in mind, it can be said that quite interesting data have been gathered in plants thanks to the use of inhibitors. A good example is the regulation of invertase synthesis in sugar cane tissue by giberellic acid and other hormones [30].

By pretreating the tissue with glucose, the production of mRNA becomes a limiting factor for the production of invertase. The synthesis of invertase is stimulated by abscisic acid (ABA) while RNA synthesis is blocked by 6-methylpurine. On the other hand, ABA does not modify the degradation rate of invertase when the synthesis of this enzyme is blocked by cycloheximide. It can be concluded that ABA acts at a stage posterior to the formation of invertase mRNA and anterior to the degradation of invertase. These results, of course, cannot be interpreted to propose that the hormone acts on an hypothetical "operator" gene switching on transcription. They rather mean that the degradation of certain mRNA can specifically be controlled.

In the example above, the hormonal control seems to be exerted at the post-transcriptional level. Other results however [for a review, see 31] are better interpreted by a model of control intervening at the transcriptional level.

Another type of control operates at the level of transcription in *Eukaryotes* and is presumably of extreme importance in higher plants, i.e. the control by proteins which specify the availability of chromosomal DNA to the action of RNA polymerase. It is well known that the association of DNA with histones greatly prevents DNA to serve as a template for RNA polymerase. Several schemes accounting for the effects of histones have been proposed by Giorgiev [32]. According to this author :

1) all DNA could be combined to histones and, in this case, non histone proteins could recognize specific base sequences in the DNA, interact with them and cancel the inhibitory effect of histones;

2) alternatively, certain histones could recognize specific multiple DNA base sequences which would be promotor sites. No RNA synthesis could take place when histones are linked to the promotor site. The inhibition of transcription could be suppressed by chemical modification of the histones. Non histone proteins would be responsible for the rate of RNA synthesis in these "open" parts of the genome.

The two regulation systems we have just mentioned do not certainly act in a highly specific way on the production of a given enzyme. Another system is operative in higher plants which has something similar to the operator-regulator system working in bacteria. For a number of enzymatic systems indeed, a rapid enzyme synthesis is induced by the substrate. Many investigations concerned with this problem in plants have been made with nitrate

reductase [for a review, see 33]. This is not surprising owing to
the fact that nitrate reductase plays an essential role in the
assimilation of nitrogen. It is well established that nitrate reductase is inducible by nitrate in most plant species. In certain
cases, it was demonstrated that induction was dependent upon RNA
and protein synthesis. Nevertheless, the situation is further
complicated by the fact that the extent of induction is modified
by numerous factors such as oxygen, carbon dioxide, light, drought,
age and genetic background.

Although it was shown in several cases that the level of
nitrate reductase activity is under genetic control, these studies
are in a too primitive state to give any information about the
mechanisms of control. As we have seen, there is no unquestionable
evidence for the existence of operons in *Eukaryotes*. A regulation
of the transcription through low molecular weight effectors certainly exists in higher organisms but one could wonder whether
this type of control is efficient enough and, moreover, whether it
is fast enough. All tissues of a plant taken as a whole are not in
a close contact with the inducer and the effects of this latter can
be greatly delayed. Conversely, a plant may dispose in certain conditions of great amounts of a given enzyme. The external conditions

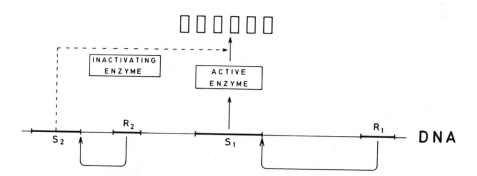

Fig. 5. Two possible levels of control in higher plants. The product of R_1 gene exerts its effect on S_1 at the level of
transcription. Another structural gene S_2 codes for an
enzyme able to inactivate the S_1 product. The synthesis
of the S_2 product itself would be regulated by several
possible mechanisms only one of which is shown here.

can change in such a way that the plant no longer needs this enzyme.
As the cell divisions are not very frequent, a long time will be
necessary before the enzyme be diluted. Since wide fluctuations of
enzyme activities can occur within short periods, it may be inferred that control systems must operate at the level of the stability of the enzyme itself. We previously quoted the case of
yeast tryptophane synthetase which is destroyed during the stationary phase, i.e. when the enzyme is not expected to be diluted
by subsequent cell divisions. Similarly, the nitrate reductase
activity in the leaves of *Hordeum sativum* is lost in the dark, but
rapidly resumes in the light. The disappearance of the nitrate
reductase activity seems to be dependent upon protein synthesis,
which suggests that it might be under the control of an enzymatic
inactivation or degradation system [34]. This type of control is
probably widespread [35] and of paramount importance [36]for
enzyme regulation in higher plants (fig. 5).

REFERENCES

[1] W.J. MIDDELHOVEN, Biochim. Biophys. Acta 93 (1964) 650.
[2] L.N. ORNSTON, Bacteriol. Rev. 35 (1971) 87.
[3] R.L. METZENBERG, Annu. Rev. Genetics 6 (1972) 111.
[4] D.S. HOGNESS, M. COHN and J. MONOD, Biochim. Biophys. Acta 16
        (1955) 99.
[5] W.K. MAAS, Cold Spring Harbor Symp. Quant. Biol. 26 (1961) 183.
[6] J. BECHET, M. GRENSON and J.M. WIAME, Europ. J. Biochem. 12
        (1970) 31.
[7] J.F. LEHMAN, M.K. GLEASON, S.K. AHLGREN and R.L. METZENBERG,
        Genetics 75 (1973) 61.
[8] S. BAUMBERG, D.F. BACON and H.J. VOGEL, Proc. Nat. Acad. Sci.
        U.S. 53 (1965) 1029.
[9] N.A. KHAN, F.K. ZIMMERMANN and N.R. EATON, Molec. Gen. Genetics
        124 (1973) 365.
[10] W.S. REZNIKOFF, Annu. Rev. Genetics 6 (1972) 133.
[11] H.E. UMBARGER, Annu. Rev. Biochem. 38 (1969) 323.
[12] F. JACOBS and J. MONOD, J. Mol. Biol. 3 (1961) 318.
[13] L.H. HARTWELL, Annu. Rev. Genetics 4 (1970) 373.
[14] A. TOH-E, Y. UEDA, S. KAKIMOTO and Y. OSHIMA, J. Bacteriol.
        113 (1973) 727.
[15] A. TOH-E, Y. UEDA and Y. OSHIMA, Genetics, 74 (1973) S 277.
[16] J.M. CALVO and G.R. FINK, Annu. Rev. Biochem. 40 (1971) 943.
[17] N.A. KHAN and N.R. EATON, Molec. Gen. Genetics 112 (1971) 317.
[18] J. NORTH and D. LEWIS, Genet. Res. 18 (1971) 153.
[19] G. DORN, Genetical Res. 6 (1965) 13.
[20] J. BECHET, J.M. WIAME and M. DE DEKEN-GRENSON, Arch. Int.
        Physiol. Bioch. 70 (1962) 564.
[21] J. BECHET and J.M. WIAME, Biochem. Biophys. Res. Comm. 21
        (1965) 266.

[22] P. THURIAUX, F. RAMOS, J.M. WIAME, M. GRENSON et J. BECHET, Arch. Int. Physiol. Biochim. 76 (1968) 955.

[23] F. MESSENGUY and J.M. WIAME, FEBS Letters 3 (1969) 47.

[24] T.R. MANNEY, J. Bacteriol. 96 (1968) 403.

[25] T. KATSUNUMA, H.E. SCHÖTT, S. ELSÄSSER and H. HOLZER, Europ. J. Biochem. 27 (1972) 520.

[26] A.R. FERGUSON, T. KATSUNUMA, H. BETZ and H. HOLZER, Europ. J. Biochem. 32 (1973) 444.

[27] K.N. SUBRAMANIAN and G.J. SORGER, J. Bacteriol. 110 (1972) 538.

[28] K.N. SUBRAMANIAN and G.J. SORGER, J. Bacteriol. 110 (1972) 547.

[29] A.B. PARDEE and L.S. PRESTIDGE, Biochem. Biophys. Acta 36 (1959) 545.

[30] K.R. GAYLER and K.T. GLASZIOU, Planta 84 (1969) 185.

[31] K.T. GLASZIOU, Annu. Rev. Plant Physiol. 20 (1969) 63.

[32] G.P. GIORGIEV, Annu. Rev. Genetics 3 (1969) 155.

[33] L. BEEVERS and R.H. HAGEMAN, Annu. Rev. Plant Physiol. 20 (1969) 495.

[34] R.L. TRAVIS, W.R. JORDAN and R.C. HUFFAKER, Plant Physiol. 44 (1969) 1150.

[35] P. FILNER, J.L. WRAY, J.E. WARNER, Science 165 (1969) 358.

[36] A. MARCUS, Annu. Rev. Plant Physiol. 22 (1971) 313.

[37] H.C. DOUGLAS and D.C. HAWTHORNE, Genetics 54 (1966) 911.

THE ENZYMOLOGY OF NITROGEN FIXATION

John Postgate

Agricultural Research Council, Unit of Nitrogen Fixation
University of Sussex, Brighton, Sussex BN1 9QJ, U.K.

Nitrogen fixation is the name given to the conversion of atmospheric dinitrogen (N_2) into a chemical form which plants and microbes can use for growth. It is the step in the nitrogen cycle which compensates for a loss of fixed nitrogen to the atmosphere caused by microbial reduction of the nitrate ion; the complete nitrogen cycle can be represented in many forms such as that below:

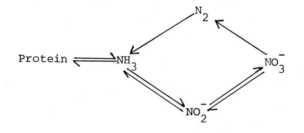

Fig. 1. THE BIOLOGICAL NITROGEN CYCLE

Most parts of the biosphere, except in advanced agricultural communities, are limited in their primary biological productivity by availability of fixed nitrogen, so the fixation of nitrogen is usually a rate-determined step in agriculture as well as natural biological productivity. Fertiliser production by the chemical

industry may account for a few per cent of the total N turnover;
natural or inadvertent conversion of N_2 to oxides of nitrogen
may account for a further few per cent, but nine-tenths of the
global N turnover is due to fixation by microorganisms.

The enzymology, physiology and genetics of nitrogen fixation
is thus an important practical scientific study. The enzymology
has also a fundamental chemical importance because the activation
of the dinitrogen molecule so as to make it chemically reactive
is a difficult chemical process. This chapter is concerned with
recent advances in knowledge of nitrogen fixation at the biochemical
and chemical levels; such advances have been essential prereque-
sites for the developments in understanding of the physiology and
genetics of fixation which form the subject of the following
chapter. The emphasis here will be on the free-living, nitrogen-
fixing bacteria since these have been the major research tools;
symbiotic systems are less amendable owing largely to difficulties
in obtaining regular supplies of material.

The chemistry and biochemistry of nitrogen fixation was the
subject of a monograph (Postgate, 1971) and has also featured in
numerous more recent publications, many of which were reviewed
briefly by Eady & Postgate (1974). These two publications may be
consulted for detailed references to most of the material presented
here.

NITROGENASE

The name nitrogenase was given to the enzyme system responsible
for the fixation of dinitrogen before it was known that two protein
components are involved. The enzyme system has been extracted
from 16 microorganisms, including 4 symbionts with leguminous
plants. Crude extracts containing nitrogenase activity fall into
three main classes.

(1) True solutions, in which no activity sediments over 2 h at
150,000 g. Such extracts are irreversibly destroyed by even brief
exposure to air or oxygen. The first nitrogenase preparation ever
to be obtained (Mortenson et al., 1962) was extracted from Clostridium pasteurianum and was of this class.

(2) Extracts in which activity sediments in such conditions, but
which are irreversibly damaged by oxygen. Crude extracts of Klebsiella pneumoniae, Bacillus polymyxa and Mycobacterium flavum 301
are of this class.

(3) Extracts in which activity sediments in these conditions and
is relatively stable to air or oxygen. Crude extracts from

Azotobacter vinelandii or A.chroococcum are of this class.

Relatively oxygen-tolerant preparations can be obtained from
M.flavum and are associated with membranous material; osmotic
shock can sometimes release an oxygen-sensitive, soluble nitrogenase from A.vinelandii. As will be described shortly, nitrogenase proteins, when purified from any of these sources, prove
to be extremely oxygen-sensitive. These observations indicate
that, in aerobic or facultatively anaerobic bacteria, the nitrogenase proteins can exist in some conformation, probably associated with membranes, in which their oxygen-sensitive sites are
passively protected from damage by oxygen.

Studies with crude nitrogenase preparations demonstrate three
other points of general importance;

(1) ATP is consumed in relatively large amounts. A crude, particulate preparation from A.chroococcum can consume 2.5 molecules
of ATP per electron transferred to the substrate, N_2. The ATP
consumed in vivo is probably large, too.

(2) The reaction is essentially the reduction of dinitrogen to
ammonia, but no intermediate has been detected at the level of
hydrazine or diimine.

(3) A ferredoxin or a flavodoxin seems generally to be the natural
electron donor to nitrogenase, even in aerobic, nitrogen-fixing
systems such as azotobacters or the legume nodule. In the laboratory, a low potential dye such as methylviologen will replace the
'doxin. Sodium dithionite will react directly with the enzyme
system and is much used in research. Magnesium ions are essential
for nitrogenase function.

Nitrogenase proteins have been purified from six sources.
Some properties of five are summarised in Table 1; some of the data
for Kpl are recently revised and unpublished. The enzyme consists
of two proteins: one of molecular weight about 220,000, containing
molybdenum and a considerable amount of non-haem iron and labile
sulphide; a smaller protein of molecular weight around 70,000
containing only non-haem iron and labile sulphide. The Mo-protein
is usually tetrameric and usually heteromeric: with Avl there is
a conflict of published data, some authorities claiming that it is
homomeric. The Fe-protein is dimeric and has some resemblences
to a dimer of a plant ferredoxin. It is notable that both proteins,
when purified, are irreversibly destroyed by exposure to air or
oxygen and the Fe-protein is exceptionally oxygen-sensitive. This
is no doubt why reports of purified Fe-protein are rather few. The
proteins obtained from aerobic systems such as azotobacters and

TABLE 1. SOME PROPERTIES OF NITROGENASE PROTEINS

	Cp1	Kp1	Av1	Rj1	Cv1	Cp2	Kp2
Mol.wt	220 000	218 000	270 000	200 000	...	55 000	66 700
Sub-units	50 700, 59 500	51 300, 59 600	54 000, 60 000	50 000	(2 types)	27 500	34 000
Mo/mol	2	2	2	1.3	1.3	0	0
Fe/mol	22-24	30-36	32-36	29	17	4	4
S^{2-}/mol	22-24		28	26	14	4	3.8
O_2-sensitivity ($t_{\frac{1}{2}}$ in min)	+	10	+	4.5	+	++	0.75

Code: Cp signifies Clostridium pasteurianum; Kp, Klebsiella pneumoniae. Ar, Azotobacter vinelandii; Rj, Rhizobium japonicum bacteroids; Cv, Chromatium vinosum; 1, Mo-protein; 2, Fe-protein.

leguminous root nodules are quite as oxygen-sensitive as those from the anaerobes.

The component proteins of nitrogenase show considerable structural and chemical similarity. This similarity extends to the fact that one can take the Mo-protein from one organism and the Fe-protein from another organism and frequently construct a fully active, hybrid nitrogenase. A table compiling recent data on such cross-reactions was published by Postgate (1974) who mentioned that immunological cross-reactivity is often observed: anti-serum prepared to K.pneumoniae Mo-protein (Kp1) will precipitate analogous proteins from B.polymyxa and A.vinelandii for example. Immunological crosses do not necessarily parallel biochemical crosses. Nitrogenase proteins from a given organism can often accept electrons from ferredoxins from other organisms.

The component proteins of nitrogenase thus seem biologically and chemically very similar no matter what their origin, though minor divergences are being discovered as new proteins are purified and it will probably be possible, in due course, to construct evolutionary hierarchies among these proteins. The similarity of nitrogenase extends to the wide substrate specificity which the enzyme shows. Table 2 lists a number of substrates which are reduced by nitrogenase and gives their reduction products; a more complete list was provided by Postgate (1974).

TABLE 2 - SOME SUBSTRATES REDUCED BY NITROGENASE

Dinitrogen	N_2	$\longrightarrow$	NH_3
Acetylene	C_2H_2	$\longrightarrow$	C_2H_4
Azide	N_3^-	$\longrightarrow$	$NH_3 + N_2$
Cyanide	CN^-	$\longrightarrow$	$CH_4 + NH_3$
Methyl isocyanide	CH_3NC	$\longrightarrow$	$CH_3NH_2 + CH_4 (+ C_2H_4$ etc.$)$
Nitrous oxide	N_2O	$\longrightarrow$	$N_2 + H_2O$
Hydrogen ion	H_3O^+	$\longrightarrow$	$H_2 + H_2O$

The reduction of acetylene to ethylene forms the basis of the now famous acetylene test for nitrogen fixation. This test provides an assay for nitrogen fixation which appears to work both in vitro and in vivo and is approximately 1,000 times as sensitive

as any technique previously available. It has become essential
for research on nitrogen fixation and a brief discussion of the
technique, with references, forms an appendix to the present
chapter. Most of the other substrates are small molecules with
triple bonds which can reasonably be regarded as structural
analogues of the dinitrogen molecule. The analogue carbon monoxide
is not reduced by nitrogenase but is a powerful specific inhibitor
of the reduction of dinitrogen and of other substrates. The enzyme
is also capable of reducing the hydrogen ion, thereby promoting
evolution of hydrogen gas. This reaction obviously does not arise
from structural analogy and it is not inhibited by carbon monoxide.
For all these reactions, a supply of ATP is required and the ATP/
electron stoichiometry is more or less independent of the substrate.

The study of the reduction of these alternative substrates has
given valuable information concerning their interaction with the
enzyme. An early observation made by Dilworth (1966) was that if
acetylene reduction takes place in D_2O, the product, deuteroethylene,
is largely the cis-isomer:

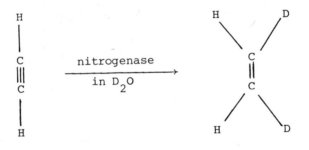

From a chemical viewpoint, this observation suggests that the
substrate is bound sideways-on, a reaction which might well occur
if it is bound to a transition metal. The products of the reduction of vinylcyanide were studied by Hardy, Knight & Jackson
(1967) who observed propylene among the products, which indicated
that, during reduction, a proton migration had taken place of the
sort that normally required catalysis by a transition metal. More
direct evidence that the substrates become bound to a transition
metal arises from the study of the reduction products of methyl
isocyanide. The products of enzymic reduction are methylamine,
methane and certain C_2 by-products. These are only obtained in
chemical environments in which isocyanides are, or become,
complexed to transition metals; the reduction of free methyl

isocyanide yields dimethylamine. Experiments of this kind encourage the view that either the iron or the molybdenum atoms of nitrogenase are directly involved in substrate binding.

Though electron paramagnetic resonance (e.p.r.) can be a valuable probe for studying molybdo-enzymes, it is only useful if the oxidation state of the Mo atom has an unpaired electron (e.g: Mo^V). Both component proteins of nitrogenase can be epr-active, but there is good evidence from isotope substitution experiments with ^{95}Mo or ^{57}Fe that all the signals are assignable to Fe. E.p.r., supplemented by Mössbauer (γ-resonance) spectroscopy, has given considerable insight into the behaviour of the iron in the two nitrogenase proteins and has permitted a reaction sequence to be proposed.

To understand the reasons underlying present views of the mechanism of nitrogenase function it is necessary to bear in mind that the enzyme, to be active, requires the presence of the two protein components, a buffer (which should not be phosphate because this may be inhibitory), magnesium ions, a reductant (usually sodium dithionite in the laboratory, though reduced viologens also donate electrons to nitrogenase) and a supply of ATP. High levels of ATP can inhibit the enzyme, so ATP is usually supplied continuously but at a low concentration by making use of an ATP-regenerating system. A widely used system is a mixture of creatine phosphate, creatine kinase and ATP, which regenerates ATP from the ADP formed by nitrogenase action. A typical reaction mixture for measuring nitrogenase activity contains the following reagents in 1.5 ml of water under argon or nitrogen:

	'HEPES' buffer (pH 7.8)	40 μmol
ATP-regenerating	ATP	8 μmol
system	$MgCl_2$	20 μmol
	Creatine phosphate	15 μmol
	Creatine kinase	200 μg
nitrogenase	Mo-Fe protein	50 μg
	Fe protein	50 μg
	$Na_2S_2O_4$	20 μmol

Evidence bearing on the rôles of the two proteins in such
conditions will be outlined briefly.

Mössbauer spectroscopy.

This technique has indicated changes in the redox state of the
iron in the Mo-protein during enzyme function. Figure 2 shows line
sketches of the Mössbauer spectra at 4.2°K of 57 Fe-labelled Mo-
protein from Klebsiella pneumoniae: they show that the native
protein can exist with its

         oxidized   intermediate   reduced

iron in three oxidation states. The most oxidized, formed with a
dye (Lauth's violet), is probably not involved in enzymic function.
Treatment with $Na_2S_2O_4$ gives the intermediate state; the fully
reduced state only appears when ATP and the Fe-protein are also
present, i.e.: when the enzyme is functioning. Aceteylene alters
this behaviour pattern hardly at all, so Mössbauer spectra supply
no evidence for interaction between Fe and substrate.

Epr spectroscopy

The intermediate redox form of the Mo-Fe protein has a most
unusual epr signal, with resonance at g = 4.32, 3.63 and 2.009 at
pH 7. The signal at g = 3.63 is unique to nitrogenase and has been
used in living bacteria to detect the protein in mutants and to
monitor synthesis of the protein in studies on the regulation of
nitrogenase synthesis. In more alkaline solutions, these signals
change appreciably, with a pK at 0°C at pH 8.7. Acetylene shifts
the pK of these changes to pH 8.2, thus antagonising whatever
symmetry change hydrogen ions cause which affects the epr-active
site. This observation provides oblique evidence that the substrate ions react with the intermediate oxidized forms of the

Mo-protein, at a site which is not epr-active.

The epr signals of the Mo-protein vanish in the functioning enzyme (returning when reductant is exhausted) and are absent from the oxidized form.

The Fe protein shows an epr signal at $g = 1.94$ which resembles that of a plant ferredoxin; it disappears when the protein is carefully oxidized so as to avoid denaturation. Thus this protein can exist with its Fe reduced (and epr-active) or oxidized. ATP, in the presence of Mg^{2+} causes a marked change in the shape of the epr-signal, indicating that a structural change in the molecule has taken place.

Kinetics

Classical steady state kinetics, using dilution and studies on mixtures of the components at different stoichiometries, indicate that the two proteins associate to form a complex during enzyme function (see Eady et al., 1974). ATP interacts with that complex in the form of MgATP; other species such as ATP and Mg_2ATP are inactive or inhibitory (Thorneley & Willison, 1974). Stopped flow kinetics show that MgATP increases the accessibility of the SH groups of the Fe protein to a sulphydryl-specific reagent; concurrently its already considerable sensitivity to O_2 denaturation is enhanced and the chemical removal of the Fe by chelating agents is facilitated. Indications are thus that the MgATP converts the reduced form of the Fe protein into a more powerful reductant, but no data on E'_o values of the two species have been published at the time of writing. (June, 1974).

Equilibrium dialysis

^{14}C-labelled ATP is bound by Fe proteins in both co-chromatography and gel equilibration experiments. Tso & Burris (1973) assigned a stoichiometry of 2 ATP molecules/mole Fe protein with differing binding constants; it does not necessarily follow that both ATP molecules are converted to ADP when the complex is functional. An equilibrium dialysis experiment by Kelly & Lang (1970) indicated that the complete enzyme system was necessary for binding of ^{14}C-labelled HCN, antagonized by CO.

Sedimentation

Evidence for chemical interaction of MgATP and the Fe protein is supported by the observation that the sedimentation coefficient

is increased in the presence of ATP. This effect has been interpreted as an ATP-induced monomerization followed by formation of
tri- and/or tetramers; ADP has a similar effect and the phenomenon
is only observed in the absence of dithionite, so the significance
of these observations is not clear. Sedimentation of mixtures of
Mo-protein and Fe-protein in the absence of dithionite shows that
a sedimentable 1:1 molar complex is formed. ATP does not alter
this effect, but the species is not observed if dithionite is
present.

These are the main physico-chemical approaches which are converging to provide evidence that the Mo-protein is the substrate-
binding component of nitrogenase and the Fe protein, after interaction with MgATP, is the primary electron donor in the active
enzyme complex, though the electron is transferred to substrate
via the Mo-protein. This view leaves open the question how a substrate such as the N_2 molecule is bound to the Mo-protein, a question
on which no biochemical evidence is available beyond the three
points already mentioned:

(1)   that the stereochemistry of acetylene reduction suggests
that the substrate is bound sideways on,

(2)   that the Mössbauer and epr experiments give no reason
to suggest that Fe is a binding site,

(3)   that the reduction products from certain substrate analogues
suggest that the binding state is nonetheless a transition metal.

Examples of systems in which the dinitrogen molecule can be
bound to a transition metal have arisen as a result of new developments in the chemistry of metal complexes during the past decade.
The relevance of such studies to thinking about biological fixation
was discussed by G.J.Leigh, J.Chatt and R.L.Richards in a monograph
(Postgate, 1971). The best characterized examples are the dinitrogen complexes, which have a triply bonded N_2 molecule bound to a
metal atom. An example whose structure is known completely is the
cobalt complex:

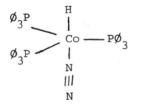

($\emptyset_3$P is
triphenylphosphine)

which was the second to be reported and which is formed by interaction of a complex cobalt hydride with N_2. Most of the dinitrogen
complexes are formed indirectly, the N_2 group being derived from
azide or hydrazine rather than N_2. From the point of view of
biologists, an interesting fact is that binuclear complexes exist
such as the following:

$$[(NH_3)_5Ru-N\equiv N-Ru(NH_3)_5]^{4+}$$

and this compound, in dilute alkali, will exchange normal N_2 for
$^{15}N_2$, thus indicating that metal-N_2 bonds can be broken and re-
formed in water. In these complexes, the stretching frequency of
the $N\equiv N$ triple bond, an indication of its strength, changes. In
the unsymmetrical complex:

$$[(\emptyset Me_2P)_4ClRe-N\equiv N-MoCl_4(Et_2O)]$$

the stretching frequency approaches that of a double bonded $N=N$
group (as in azobenzene). Thus complexing to a transition metal
could overcome the considerable energy barrier involved in splitting
the $N\equiv N$ bond and rendering the N_2 group reducible. So far, however,
no dinitrogen complex has been reduced in protic solution to give
ammonia, but the tungsten complex below has been protonated to give
a partly reduced N_2 group:

$$[(\emptyset_2P-CH_2\cdot CH_2-P\emptyset_2)_2W(N\equiv N)_2] \longrightarrow [(\emptyset_2P-CH_2CH_2-P\emptyset_2)_2ClW=N-NH_2].$$

It is interesting that the N_2 group protonates unsymmetrically.
In theory, a compound which would accept a third proton on the
terminal N atom ought to release NH_3, yielding a nitride (R-W$\equiv$N)
which would hydrolyse to give another molecule of ammonia. Thus
two NH_3 molecules would be derived from dinitrogen, as in biological
fixation.

Such chemical studies will probably lead to a precise knowledge
of the mode of interaction of N_2 with the prosthetic metal atom of
nitrogenase. At a less precise level, a number of chemical systems
have been described which reduce acetylene, isocyanide and even N_2
in aqueous environments at room temperature, as does nitrogenase.
Examples are a system described by Shilov in the U.S.S.R., where

sodium molybdate, magnesium ions, and titanous chloride as reductant, reduce N_2 to hydrazine and traces of NH_3. Schrauzer et al., (1974) found that a molybdenum thiol catalyses reduction of acetylene and isocyanides to the biological products by borohydride; formation of traces of NH_3 from N_2 was claimed. Iron pyridyl complexes catalyse comparable reductions (Newton et al., 1971); a gluta-thione-Mo complex reduces acetylene or hydrazine (Werner et al., 1973). Some of these systems are stimulated by ATP. The precise chemistry of these processes is vague and their relevance as models for nitrogenase action is dubious, but there is no doubt that a more complete understanding of their mode of action, partic-ularly of the possible involvement of transient dinitrogen complexes, will advance our knowledge of the biological process.

Both chemical and biochemical data are converging to the extent that it is now possible to propose mechanisms for the action of nitro-genase. The scheme in Figure 3 is an example. Essentially it proposes a mechanism whereby the oxidized form of the dimeric Fe protein (symbolized as P2) accepts an electron from a natural donor such as a ferredoxin and reacts with MgATP to form a reductant of lowered redox potential and altered conformation. This forms a complex with the intermediate redox form of the tetrameric Mo-protein (P1) which has bound the substrate at a transition metal site. In the complex, electron transfer from P2 to P1 occurs, giving the fully reduced species; the oxidized P2 releases APD + Mg and either becomes re-charged with MgATP or is replaced by a new reduced MgATP-P2 complex. The electron transfer event occurs repeatedly, consuming one ATP/electron, until the stoichiometry for product formation is complete (6 electrons for N_2, 2 for C_2H_2) and only then does the reduced product dissociate from P1 leaving the intermediate form of P1 again. Thus the substrate remains bound to a single molecule of P1 during reduction and no chemical intermediates are detectable. CO can block interaction of the triply bonded substrates with P1, but the hydrogen ion can interact with the prosthetic site even if CO is bound there.

The scheme leaves certain questions unanswered, including the consumption of nearly 2.5 ATP/electron in vitro. It also goes beyond the present experimental evidence in several respect, of which three should be mentioned.

(a) It accepts that the 1:1 P1:P2 complex is the functional enzyme,

(b) It assumes that the prosthetic metal for substrate binding in P1 is molybdenum (for which view there is no substantial evidence),

(c) It proposes a 2-site attachment located sideways with respect to the topography of the protein surface.

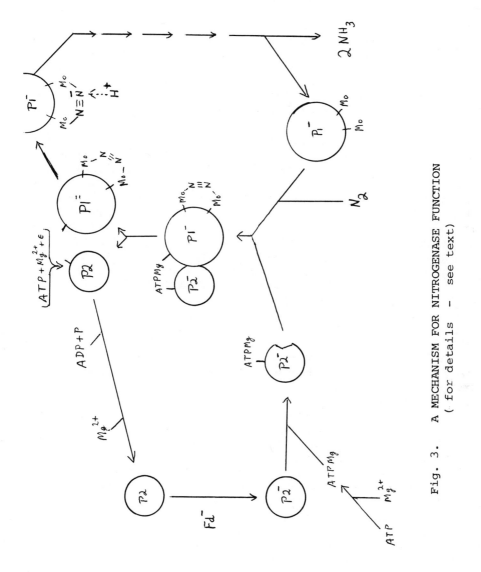

Fig. 3.   A MECHANISM FOR NITROGENASE FUNCTION
(for details — see text)

The principal virtue of the scheme in Figure 3 is that it is
a rationalization of present knowledge which is not inconsistent
with either our present knowledge of the enzymology of nitrogenase
or of the chemistry of dinitrogen. Even two years ago schemes of
this type were much more speculative in character.

APPENDIX: The acetylene test for nitrogen fixation

The discovery in the mid-sixties that nitrogenase reduces
acetylene specifically to ethylene (Dilworth, 1966; Schöllhorn &
Burris, 1967) lead to the development of a technique for detecting
the enzyme, using this reaction together with flame ionization gas
chromatography, which has proved extremely valuable and applicable
in a wide variety of biological contexts. It is effective with
free-living nitrogen-fixing organisms, with enzyme preparations,
with nodulated plants and rhizosphere associations, with soil cores
and water samples. It has been used with living termites (Breznak
et al., 1973; Benemann, 1973) human excrement (Bergersen & Hipsley,
1970) and has been injected into the rumen of a live sheep to seek
nitrogen fixation (Hobson et al., 1973). Hardy et al., (1968) gave
an early account of its use, giving practical details; another description of its practical use was given by Postgate (1972b); the
technique is described in most modern handbooks of microbial ecology
and will not be described in detail here.

Certain principles require emphasis. When new nitrogen-fixing
systems are being investigated, particularly when using material of
plant origin, a control testing for ethylene formation in the
absence of acetylene is mandatory. Certain chemical systems (e.g.:
colloidal palladium) catalyse reduction of acetylene to ethylene
by materials such as hydrogen, so evidence that the reduction process
is biological requires confirmation with $^{15}N_2$; evidence that ammonia
in the medium represses acetylene-reducing activity is valuable
circumstantial evidence in favour of nitrogenase function when studying microbes in the laboratory. Aerobic systems should always be
tested in micro-aerobic conditions (a pO_2 of 0.04 is reasonable)
and blue-green algae should be tested at low illumination levels.
With many strains of aerobic microbes, the nitrogenase is inactive
or damaged at atmospheric oxygen concentrations or, in the case of
blue-green algae, at high illuminations (which lead to high photosynthetic O_2 output). Most anaerobic bacteria can be handled
briefly in air before testing anaerobically, but some (e.g.:
Desulfovibrio) are apparently so sensitive that the enzyme in suspension is damaged even when the living cells are exposed to air.
Techniques for growing anaerobes anaerobically and testing them
without exposure to air have been described.

Enzyme preparations are normally handled in the absence of air and, with very few exceptions, must never be exposed to air even during preparation for the test. Sodium dithionite can be damaging to certain enzyme preparations, particularly rather dilute ones; buffers are sometimes inhibitory to the enzyme system and so may be high concentrations of ATP. The use of an ATP-regenerating system to avoid high ATP concentrations was described in the test. Enzyme preparations will also accept electrons from reduced ferredoxin, a plant chloroplast preparation in which photo-system 2 has been inactivated by heat, or a system such as the en-zyme hydrogenase and an atmosphere of hydrogen which generates a reduced viologen dye such as methyl viologen. These systems may be used in experiments where the presence of sodium dithionite is un-desirable. With simple enzyme preparations and cultures of bacteria, the acetylene reduction rate normally falls between 3 and 4 times the nitrogen fixation rate. It is not safe to use this coefficient on more complex systems such as whole plants or soil cores, because acetylene is more water-soluble and lipophilic than nitrogen and its relatively high diffusion rate may give a false impression of the nitrogen-fixing capacity of the system being studied.

Given appropriate controls and reasonable caution in inter-pretation, the acetylene test is an invaluable tool in the study of nitrogen fixation at all levels ranging from enzymological through ecological to genetical. It should be unnecessary to say that the most rigid precautions concerning the integrity of the system being studied are necessary: contaminant nitrogen-fixing bacteria in puta-tively pure cultures must have been responsible for many false reports of nitrogen fixation among microbial genera; adequate bacteriological examination of plant tissue cultures for contamin-ant nitrogen-fixing bacteria are often missing from published reports of nitrogen-fixing symbioses cultured in vitro.

REFERENCES

Benemann, J. (1973) Science, 181, 164.

Bergersen, F.J. & Hipsley, E.H. (1970) J.gen.Microbiol., 60, 62.

Breznak, J.A., Brill, W.J., Mertins, J.W., & Coppel, J.C. (1973) Nature, Lond., 244, 577.

Dilworth M.J., (1966) Biochim.biophys.Acta, 127, 285.

Eady R.R. & Postgate, J.R. (1974) Nature,Lond., 249, 805.

Eady, R.R., Smith, B.E., Thorneley, R.N.F., Yates, M.G. & Postgate J.R. (1974) in Nitrogen fixation and the biosphere. Ed. Nutman, P.S. & Stewart, W.D.P., International Biological Programme.

Hardy, R.W.F., Burns, R.C. & Holsten, R.D. (1973) Soil Biol.Biochem. 5, 47.

Hardy, R.W.F., Knight, E. & Jackson, E.K. (1967) Bact.Proc., p.112.

Hardy, R.W.F., Holsten, R.D., Jackson, E.K. & Burns, R.C. (1968) Plant Physiol., 43, 1185.

Hobson, P.N., Summers, R., Postgate, J.R. & Ware, D.A. (1973) J.gen.Microbiol., 77, 225.

Kelly, M. & Lang, G. (1970) Biochem.biophys.Acta, 223, 86.

Mortenson, L.E., Mower, H.F. & Carnahan, J.E., (1962) Bacteriol.Rev., 26, 42.

Newton, W.E., Corbin, J.L., Schneider, P.W., and Bulen, W.A. (1971) J.Amer.Chem.Soc., 93, 268-9.

Postgate, J.R. (1971) The Chemistry and biochemistry of nitrogen fixation. London: Plenum Press.

Postgate, J.R. (1972) in Methods in Microbiology. Ed: Norris, J.R. & Ribbons, D.W., 6b, 343. London: Academic Press.

Postgate, J.R. (1974) in Evolution in the Microbial World. Ed: Carlile, M.J. & Skehel, J.J. Symp.Soc.gen.Microbiol., 24, 263. Cambridge U.Press.

Schollhorn, R. & Burris, R.H. (1967) Proc.nat.Acad.Sci., U.S.A., 57, 213.

Schrauzer, G.N., Doemeny, P.A., Kiefer, G.W., Kisch, H. & Tano,K. (1974) International Conference on the chemistry and uses of molybdenum, Reading, 1973.

Thorneley, R.N.F. & Willison, K.R. (1974) Biochem.J., 134, 211.

Werner, D., Russell, S. & Evans, H.J. (1973) Proc.nat.Acad.Sci., U.S.A., 70, 339.

THE PHYSIOLOGY AND GENETICS OF NITROGEN FIXATION

John Postgate

Agricultural Research Council, Unit of Nitrogen
Fixation
University of Sussex, Brighton, Sussex BN1 9QJ, U.K.

The enzymological studies of nitrogenase outlined in the previous chapter have led to important reassessments of nitrogen fixation in the biosphere, and have permitted rapid advances in the study of the genetics of nitrogen fixation. These developments have stemmed partly from the practical value of the acetylene test and partly from the recognition of the metalloenzyme character of nitrogenase, its extreme oxygen sensitivity and its apparent waste of ATP. In this chapter, certain physiological, ecological and genetical consequences of recent biochemical knowledge will be discussed.

THE PHYSIOLOGY OF NITROGEN FIXATION

The manifest oxygen sensitivity of purified nitrogenase proteins, particularly the Fe-protein, immediately raises the simple physiological question of how do aerobic nitrogen-fixing microbes, or symbiotic systems, protect the functioning enzyme from oxygen damage ? At a physiological level, at least four expedients have been developed by such organisms to avoid oxygen damage.

Respiratory protection.

The best known aerobic nitrogen-fixing bacteria belong to the family Azotobacteracae which includes the genera Azotobacter, Beijerinckia and Derxia. The azotobacters have the highest respiratory activity of living organisms, and in recent years evidence has accumulated that this respiratory activity not only has the normal function of ATP generation, but also serves to protect functioning nitrogenase from damage by oxygen (see a review by Postgate 1974a,

who cited references). The evidence for respiratory protection
of nitrogenase can be summarised as follows.

1.   Ordinary cultures of either Azotobacter chroococcum or
A.vinelandii are inhibited by vigorous aeration when fixing nitrogen, but not when growing with adequate supplies of an ammonium
salt. This oxygen sensitivity is enhanced when the organisms are
grown with limited supplies of a respirable carbon source.

2.   The amount of nitrogen fixed per gramme of carbon source consumed in continuous cultures of azotobacters is maximum when the
organisms are starved of oxygen and becomes extremely low, implying
a considerable wastage of carbon source, when the oxygen concentration
is high.

3.   Continuous cultures can be acclimatised to high concentrations
of oxygen in the atmosphere. The respiratory activity and the
content of terminal oxidase are then discovered to have increased
3 to 5-fold but the nitrogenase activity is little changed.

4.   An oxygen stress to an oxygen-limited continuous culture of
azotobacter results in immediate cessation of nitrogen fixation
followed by an increase in respiratory activity so that the dissolved oxygen concentration returns to a low value and nitrogen
fixation starts again.

5.   Aerobic nitrogen-fixing bacteria of low intrinsic respiratory
activity (such as Mycobacterium flavum 301) show high natural oxygen
sensitivity and only grow well in microaerobic conditions.

     Consistent with the concept of respiratory protection is the
evidence reviewed by Yates and Jones (1974) that azotobacters
possess a branched electron transport chain. One of these has a
relatively high capacity to generate ATP and the other a relatively
low capacity; the latter is the one that normally functions when the
oxygenation of the culture is high. A corollary of these observations
is that respiration is, even when serving its protective function,
always coupled to ATP generation to some extent. Thus respiratory
protection must involve some wastage of ATP and, conversely, in
conditions where ATP supplies are limited, a conflict between respiratory protection and respiratory chain phosphorylation may develop.
Evidence that phosphate-limited populations of azotobacter are hyper-
sensitive to oxygen inhibition, when fixing nitrogen, has been interpreted along the lines of a conflict between respiratory protection
and respiratory control.

Conformational protection

In the previous chapter, evidence was mentioned that one can obtain a crude nitrogenase preparation from azotobacters which is not sensitive to oxygen, though when the proteins are purified from it they show the usual oxygen sensitivity. In such preparations, the nitrogenase proteins appear to be in some conformation in which they are passively protected from oxygen damage, and this protection appears to involve association with membranes. Comparable particulate preparations from Mycobacterium flavum 301 are oxygen-sensitive, but membrane-associated preparations can be obtained from this organism which also passively tolerate oxygen. Early studies of continuous cultures of A.chroococcum, discussed by Postgate (1974a), provided evidence that the organisms regulated their nitrogenase activity in response to their mean residence time in the culture vessel: effectively in response to the length of time each individual cell was exposed to oxygen. The hypothesis has therefore been proposed that the membrane-associated, oxygen-sensitive form of nitrogenase represents a conformation of the two proteins which the enzyme can assume in the living cell when the organisms are subject to an oxygen stress greater than respiratory protection can cope with. Supporting evidence for this view is provided by the evidence that populations of A.chroococcum, when subject to an abrupt oxygen stress (increased shaking rate in air, or increased pO_2) abruptly 'switch off' their nitrogenase activity. They can 'switch on' the activity again with varying degrees of rapidity when the previous conditions are restored. Conformational protection probably implies some form of sub-cellular compartmentation in which membranes are involved; it still has the status of a working hypothesis rather than an established physiological protection mechanism because the evidence for it is oblique. The oxygen-sensitivity of the oxygen-tolerant subcellular particulate nitrogenase, extractable from azotobacters, can be enhanced by adding ATP or chelating agents, suggesting that metals are perhaps involved in conformational protection.

Heterocyst formation

The nitrogen-fixing blue green algae, of which there are many representatives, have a particular problem with oxygen because their photosynthesis leads to oxygen evolution. In the heterocystous blue green algae there is now good evidence that the heterocysts represent a specialised compartment to which nitrogen fixation is usually restricted. Heterocysts have the distinguishing feature

that they lack photosystem 2, the oxygen-evolving component of
photosynthesis, and therefore may reasonably be regarded as
specialised compartments to which access of oxygen is minimised.
The view that the heterocysts represent oxygen-restricting compartments for nitrogenase function, though not universally accepted, is
very compelling (see Stewart, 1973). Nevertheless, there exist
blue-green algae which do not possess heterocysts and which can
fix nitrogen; consistent with this view of the function of heterocysts is the fact that the majority of non-heterocystous blue green
algae only fix at low oxygen tensions or low illuminations. Some
evidence for respiratory protection in blue green algae also exists.

The root nodule as a compartment

Many leguminous plants form the classical nitrogen-fixing
symbiosis: nodules appear among their roots in response to invasion
by the bacterium Rhizobium and, within these nodules, the rhizobia
become near-dormant 'bacteroids' which acquire the ability to fix
nitrogen. The free-living bacteria have never been shown to fix
nitrogen in the absence of the plant. From a physiological viewpoint,
an important recent development has been the recognition of the
function of leghaemoglobin, a haemoprotein characteristic of the
legume symbiosis and not normally found in the separate plant or
free-living bacteria. Nitrogen fixation by isolated bacteroids,
and presumably by the complete symbiotic system, requires oxygen
and therefore, presumably, presents problems of oxygen restriction
comparable to those found in azotobacter or the blue-green algae.
Wittenberg et al (1974) have shown that leghaemoglobin, which has
a high affinity for oxygen, very probably serves as an oxygen-
transport protein with the special property of delivering oxygen to
the bacteroids at what is effectively a very low pO_2. The presence
of leghaemoglobin is essential for effective nitrogen fixation; it
seems that the nodule, with its attendant leghaemoglobin, represents
another example of an oxygen-restricting compartment in which nitrogen
fixation can occur in nature. Presumably comparable oxygen-restricting
stratagems will be discovered in the non-leguminous symbiotic systems,
but physiological and biochemical studies of these are much less advanced.

Thus, from a physiological point of view, we now recognise four
plausible oxygen-restricting mechanisms which enable aerobic organisms
to fix nitrogen in air. Other mechanisms probably exist: the gum
characteristic of many nitrogen-fixing bacteria probably serves to
restrict diffusion of oxygen to the cells; anaerobes such as Clostridium pasteurianum or the facultative organism Klebsiella pneumoniae
(the latter only fixes nitrogen when growing anaerobically) can be

harvested in air and the nitrogenase enzyme can be extracted, so
there is probably some passive protection mechanism in these organisms. Unpublished work in the writer's laboratory by Dr. T.H. Black-
burn suggests that, in the anaerobe Desulfovibrio desulfuricans, such
passive protection scarcely exists: even taking a sample of a growing,
nitrogen-fixing culture in air can lead to damage to the organism's
nitrogenase.

THE ECOLOGY OF NITROGEN-FIXING SYSTEMS

    The application of the acetylene test and the recognition of
the oxygen-sensitivity of nitrogenase have led to extensive revisions
of the accepted list of free-living nitrogen-fixing bacteria. This
topic has been reviewed comprehensively by Dalton (1974) and will not
be discussed here except to make one point of general importance.
There now exist no authenticated instances in which nitrogen is fixed
by a eukaryote: the property seems to be exclusive to prokaryotic
microbes - the bacteria and blue-green algae.

    Considerable reassessment of the relative agronomic effectiveness
of various nitrogen-fixing associations has taken place in the light
of our newer knowledge. Table 1 gives the relative agronomic effic-
iencies of a number of nitrogen-fixing systems as they stood about 4
years ago.

Table 1. ESTIMATED AMOUNTS OF NITROGEN BROUGHT TO
          SOIL (Kg/Hectare/year) BY VARIOUS NITROGEN-
          FIXING SYSTEMS

Legumes	Lucerne	300 - 600
	Clover	150 - 300
	Lupin	150
	Pulse	50 - 60
	Alder	100 (leaf fall alone)
	Blue-green algae	25
	Azotobacter	0.3
	Clostridia	0.1 - 0.5

Continuous culture experiments enable us to up-grade the
efficiency of azotobacter about 3-fold but otherwise the free-
living bacteria remain relatively trivial in agronomic terms.
The blue-green algae are still the most important nitrogen-fixing
systems in Arctic and certain arid environments; they are also the
primary colonisers of volcanic or devastated soils. They are probably the primary nitrogen-fixing organisms in the pelagic zone
of the sea. In association with fungi they are important symbiotic
fixers as lichens; they form associations with plants ranging from
liverworts through mosses and cycads to the angiosperm Gunnera.
Their agronomic importance can be considerably greater than given in
the table: Dr. Y.Dommergues (personal communication) has deduced
from acetylene reduction tests that, in the rice paddies in the warm
season, they can fix at a rate of 240 Kg N/Hc/year.

The non-leguminous associations represented by alder in the table
are very important over many parts of the planet and are often pioneer
plants. Their quantitative contribution has yet to be evaluated. The
symbiotic microbe, thought to be a streptomycete, has not yet been
isolated unequivocally.

The leaf nodule association is now discounted. Certain plants
such as Psychotria have nodules in their leaves which contain bacteria,
some of which may fix nitrogen. There is little doubt that the microbe
has a favourable effect on the growth of the plant, but the effect is
probably due to gibberellin-like materials because non-nitrogen-
fixing bacteria appear to be equally beneficial and no acetylene
reduction can be detected in nodules, even when deliberately infected
by nitrogen-fixing strains of symbiotic bacteria (Bettleheim, Gordon
and Taylor, 1968; Becking, 1971). More casual association between
free-living nitrogen-fixing bacteria and the phyllosphere of plants
such as sugar cane (Ruinen, 1956) is still not in doubt: the associated nitrogen-fixing organism becomes washed into the soil by rain
and improves its nitrogen status.

Another association which must now be discounted is that between
mycorrhiza and the conifer Podocarpus. Earlier evidence for fixation
by the endotrophic mycorrhiza of this plant has more recently been
attributed to free-living nitrogen-fixing bacteria casually associated with the rhizosphere (Silvester and Bennett, 1973).

Potentially one of the most important consequences of newer
knowledge has been the recognition of relatively casual associations
between free-living nitrogen-fixing bacteria and the roots of plants.
These have been called 'associative symbioses'. The first to be
established was an association between the sand grass Paspalum
notatum and a species of azotobacter: Azotobacter paspali (see
Dobereiner, Day and Dart, 1972). The acetylene test indicates that
this association is capable of bringing nearly 100 Kg N/Hc/year to

a tropical soil (cf. table 1). A degree of host specificity exists: cultivars of the sand grass incapable of forming the association exist and the azotobacter is only found in the rhizosphere; the dominant free-living nitrogen-fixing organism in the surrounding soil being generally either Derxia or Beijerinckia. A.paspali forms a sheath-like structure round the root, and, once established there, becomes relatively dormant but continues to fix nitrogen. Paspalum species are widely distributed in tropical and sub-tropical areas; they could become an important forage crop for tropical and sub-tropical agriculture and the development and use of appropriate cultivars and bacteria is an important current topic in agricultural research. At a conference on nitrogen fixation in Pullman, Washington, U.S.A.,this year, Dr. Johanna Dobereiner announced the discovery of another associative symbiosis, seemingly equally important, between the grass Digitaria decumbens and a nitrogen fixing bacterium Spirillum lipoferum. Associations between the roots of rice and Beijerinckia, corn and various nitrogen-fixing enterobacteria, temperate weeds and water plants with unspecified nitrogen-fixing organisms, have also been reported and were briefly mentioned by Postgate (1974b). It seems that such associative symbioses arise wherever selective pressure favours them.

The reassessment of nitrogen fixation in the biosphere, consequent upon our newer knowldege of the enzymology of the process, is still in progress and is an exciting aspect of research in this area.

THE GENETICS OF NITROGEN FIXATION

Recognition of oxygen-sensitivity and the binary nature of the enzyme, together with use of the acetylene test, has permitted considerable advances in the study of the genetics of nitrogen fixation. The structural and regulatory genes determining nitrogen fixation are referred to as nif; the subject is relatively new and no comprehensive reviews are yet available. The following is a brief summary of the situation at present.

1. The nif genes exist as a cluster on the chromosome of Klebsiella pneumoniae corresponding to 38 to 40 minutes of the Escherichia coli chromosome. An important neighbour is his: a gene determining the biosynthesis of the histidine.

2. The nif gene cluster has been mobilised by transduction using the bacteriophage P1 (see Streicher, Gurney and Valentine, 1972) or by a drug resistant transfer factor R144drd3. This R factor was used to transfer nif from K.pneumoniae to E.coli (Dixon and Postgate, 1972). Dunican and Tierney (1974) have reported mobilisation of nif genes from Rhizobium by a different R factor.

3.   The expression of nif is subject to regulation by NH_3 even
when transferred to a new organism.   Hence at least some part
of the regulatory apparatus forms part of the transferable nif
cluster.   Evidence from laboratories at M.I.T., Madison,(U.S.A.)
and Sussex (U.K.) shows that the regulatory system has much
in common with that regulating the use of histidine (hut) and,
in particular, the enzyme glutamine synthetase is a positive
effector of nif expression.

4.   Hybrids of K.pneumoniae and E.coli have been obtained in
which nif is either integrated into the chromosome or conserved
as a plasmid (Cannon et al., 1974a,b).   A hybrid has been constructed in which nif has been associated with the sex factor F
(Dixon, 1974).   This F'nif plasmid has been used to prepare
nitrogen-fixing Salmonella typhimurium and K.aerogenes in the
writer's laboratory.

5.   Mutants have been obtained of various nitrogen-fixing bacteria
which are unable to fix nitrogen and have been characterized as
unable to synthesise either of the two component proteins, both
of the two component proteins, or electron transport factors
donating to the two component proteins.   Regulatory mutants have
now been constructed which are immune or partially immune to
ammonia repression.

     Virtually all the manipulative genetics has been performed
with nif genes obtained from K.pneumoniae.   Figure 1 indicates
some of the gene transfers which have been performed with these
particular nif genes.   An importance of the transfer of these
genes to E.coli strain K12 is that the whole repertory of mutants
produced by molecular biology over the last two decades is now
available for use with nif genes.   The value of the F'nif plasmid
is already becoming obvious from the ability to prepare other
enterobacteria capable of fixing nitrogen;   association of nif
with a more promiscuous R factor has not yet been successfully
performed, nor has the preparation of a bacteriophage such
as λ carrying nif genes.

THE POSSIBILITIES OF PREPARING NITROGEN-FIXING EUKARYOTES

     Successful intergeneric transfer of nif between prokaryotes
has provoked widespread speculation on the possibility of deliberately
constructing nitrogen-fixing eukaryotes.   Evidence discussed elsewhere in this volume suggests strongly that bacterial DNA can be conserved in plants and, in special circumstances, expressed.   Therefore

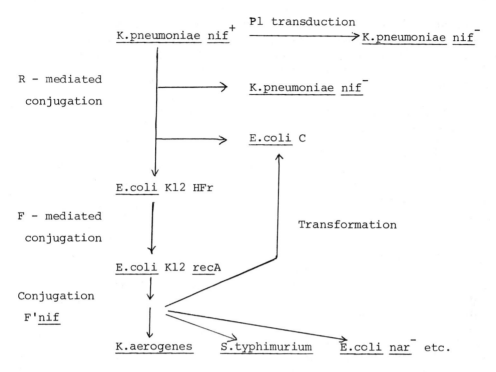

FIGURE 1 - SOME GENETIC MANIPULATIONS UNDERGONE BY nif FROM
                    KLEBSIELLA PNEUMONIAE M5a1

plants themselves become particularly attractive subjects for such
speculation. It must be obvious from the foregoing discussion,
however, that much more is needed than the simple transfer of nif
genes to plants. Indeed, during the evolutionary history of the
nitrogen-fixing symbioses, such gene transfer must have occurred
frequently - yet no nitrogen-fixing plants exist at present.

An important question is whether bacterial nif genes can be
conserved, without expression, in plants. If the answer is affirma-
tive, supporting genes will need to be introduced concerned with a
number of other essential characteristics of nitrogenase: for
example, the regulation of nif gene expression, the uptake and

incorporation of Mo and Fe, the protection of the nif gene product
from oxygen, the synthesis of appropriate electron donor (such as
ferredoxin or flavodoxin), the generation of ATP at an appropriate
site and so on. Though discussion of such possibilities generally
centres on crop plants, the apparent pre-requisites for expression
of nif also apply to other eukaryotes, including fungi which might
be considered as candidates to become nitrogen-fixing symbionts.

The deliberate construction of nitrogen-fixing rhizosphere
commensals seemed a promising approach a few years ago; recognition
of the associative symbioses in recent years suggests that where
selection pressure for such organisms exists, they seem to be present
already. Undoubtedly much scope exists for genetical and physiological
work directed towards maximisation of the host-bacterial interaction
in these symbioses.

The possibility of deliberately constructing a plant organelle,
analagous to a mitochondrion or chloroplast, which would fix nitrogen
has also been discussed. A step in this direction would be the preparation of a benign bacterial endophyte carrying nif genes and the
establishment of this, at a later stage, as an independent replicon
in the plant. The ability of plant protoplasts to take up small
particles suggests that projects along these lines are not mechanically
impossible, but clearly a lot needs to be known about the establishment of independent replication by such a system. Moreover, the
existence of widespread associations between blue-green algae and
plants suggests that, if the formation of a nitrogen-fixing organelle
were easy, it ought to have emerged already during evolutionary time.

A somewhat different approach is that of constructing 'conventional'
hybrids of desirable agricultural crop plants with other plants which
already form the nitrogen-fixing symbiosis. The recent discovery of
a system in which Rhizobium forms an association with a non-leguminous
plant (Trema aspera; Trinick, 1973) is encouraging in this context.

At a more modest level, much can be done to study the genetics
of effectiveness in Rhizobium, analysing the numerous determinants
whose concatenation must be necessary for optimal nitrogen-fixing
capacity. In this context, the claim to have obtained expressable
nif genes from Rhizobium after transfer to K.aerogenes (Dunican and
Tierney, 1974) is most exciting. At present the genetics of Rhizobium
is in its infancy.

Constitutive mutants, not only of rhizobia, which would fix nitrogen
no matter what the nitrogen status of the soil might be, could be of
great value in agriculture, provided ammonia toxicity were avoided
(their use has been suggested, half humourously, to produce nitrogen-
fixing ruminant animals - Postgate, 1974b).

Above all, it is important not to confuse speculation with fact. The sort of gene transfer experiments envisaged in this section require a great deal more knowledge about the genetic determination, regulation, and physiological expression of nif genes in a very wide variety of microorganisms, as well as a great deal of new knowledge of plant physiology and genetics. Perhaps a major advance of the last two years has been that one can now see clearly some of the grave obstacles presented by the prospect of manipulating nif genes into crop plants.

REFERENCES

Becking, J.H. (1971) in Biological nitrogen fixation in natural and agricultural habitats, ed. T.A. Lie & G.C. Mulder, Pl. Soil (Special vol.), 361.

Bettleheim, K.A., Gordon, J.F. & Taylor, J. (1968) J.gen.Microbiol., 54, 177.

Cannon, F.C., Dixon, R.A., Postgate, J.R. & Primrose, S.B., (1974a) J.gen.Microbiol., 80, 227.

Cannon, F.C., Dixon, R.A., Postgate, J.R. & Primrose, S.B., (1974b) J.gen.Microbiol., 80, 241.

Dalton, H. (1974) Critical Rev.Microbiol., 3, 183.

Dixon, R.A. (1974) Genetical Research (in press)

Dixon, R.A. & Postgate, J.R. (1972) Nature, Lond., 237, 102.

Dobereiner, J., Day, J. & Dart, P.J. (1972) J.gen.Microbiol., 71, 103.

Dunican, L.K. & Tierney, P.B. (1974) Biochem.biophys.res.Commun., 57, 62.

Postgate, J.R. (1974a) in Biological nitrogen fixation, ed. A.Quispel. Amsterdam: North Holland.

Postgate, J.R. (1974b) J.applied Bact., 37, 180.

Ruinen, J. (1956) Pl.Soil, 22, 375.

Silvester, W.B. & Bennett, K.J. (1973) Soil.Biol.Biochem., 5, 171.

Stewart, W.D.P. (1973) Annu. Rev.Microbiol., 27, 283.

Streicher, S.L., Gurney, E. & Valentine, R.C. (1972) Nature,Lond., 239, 495.

Trinick,H.J. (1973) Nature,Lond., 244, 459.

Wittenberg, J.B., Bergersen, F.J., Appleby, C.A. & Turner, G.C., (1974) J.biol.Chem. (in press).

Yates,M.G. & Jones, C.W. (1974) Adv.Microbial Physiol., (in press).

Molecular Biology of the Genus *Agrobacterium*

J. DE LEY

Laboratory of Microbiology and microbial Gene-

tics - State University - 9000 Gent - Belgium

We started this study several years ago, because knowledge of molecular biology of a bacterial genus was very fragmentary. A number of questions needed an answer such as : What are the relationships (homology) between the genomes of the individual strains in a genus ? how homogeneous or heterogeneous are the molecular weights and base compositions of the genome DNA ? is a bacteriological species a genetically homogeneous group of strains ? what are the correlations between the genotypic and the phenotypic properties of the strains ? etc.

We selected the genus *Agrobacterium* for several reasons. Firstly, the number of strains known, about 300, is not too large. They have been isolated all over the world. We have most of them in our collection. Secondly, the number of species is rather small : it contains the crown gall bacteria *A. tumefaciens*, the cane gall bacteria *A. rubi*, the hairy root disease bacteria *A. rhizogenes*, and non-pathogenic strains called *A. radiobacter*. About eleven other species such as *A. gypsophilae*, etc. are taxonomic mistakes. Thirdly, many strains cause crown gall, a plant tumor disease, reminescent of some animal tumors. Excessive root formation is another type of abnormal outgrowth. A better knowledge of these bacteria is required for the elucidation of the pathogenic mechanisms.

We used a variety of methods.
1. DNA:DNA hybridizations.
2. Determination of mismatching in the DNA hybrids from thermal stability.

3. Determination of DNA base composition.
4. Determination of DNA genome size.
5. Numerical analysis of phenotypic features.
6. Numerical analysis of protein profiles.
7. Comparison of physical properties and amino acid
   sequence of soluble cytochrome c.
8. Detection of intergeneric relationship by DNA:rRNA
   hybridization.

   Agrobacterium consists genotypically and phenotypically of 11 races. Three are large and contain each
about 70 strains. We call them the B6, the TT111 and
the rhizogenes race. The remaining 8 races contain between 1 and 10 strains. Within each race the strains
are at least 80 % DNA-homologous. The B6, the TT111
and five small races hybridize at ca 50 % homology. We
call it the tumefaciens-radiobacter cluster. This cluster, the rhizogenes race, the rubi race and two individual strains 1650 and 1771 hybridize at about 15 % DNA
homology.

   The thermal stability of the DNA hybrids within
each race is about the same as for the homoduplex. Between two races of 50 % homology the duplexes are about
6° C less stable. Between races of 15 % homology the
stability is at least 13° C lower. The less two races
are evolutionary related, the more mutations occurred
within the common DNA parts.

   The % GC of all agrobacteria is in the narrow
range of 58-61. The races rubi, 1650 and 1771 are at
the low side with 58-59 % GC. All the other strains have
a % GC in the range 59-61.

   The overall average molecular weight of the *Agrobacterium* genome DNA is 3.4 x 10^9, which is rather large
for a bacterial genome. The range is 3.1-3.6 x 10^9.
Only strain 0363 has a significantly smaller genome of
2.7 x 10^9. The genotypic heterogeneity of the genus is
not reflected either in its % GC or in its genome size.

   Numerical analysis of over a hundred phenotypic
features revealed essentially the same races, but the
differences are smaller than from DNA hybridization.
Organisms within each genetic race show no significant
phenotypic differences. Genetic races at the 50 % homology level differ by at most 5 features. The rhizogenes
race differs by some 20 features from the tumefaciens-
radiobacter cluster. The three other races at 15 % homology differ more phenotypically. The relationships
between races, obtained from DNA:DNA hybridization in
stringent conditions, are lower than the phenotypic
relationships. This apparent paradox can be explained

by mutations, located mainly outside the active center
of the enzymes.

The nature and number of protein molecules in a
cell are a kind of crude copy of the genome DNA. Numerical analysis of PAGE protein patterns yield again the
same eleven races. The above hypothesis is thus confirmed. PAGE in our modification with the computerized
clustering, is extremely well suited as a simple and
quick identification method.

Differences in PAGE protein patterns are obviously due to differences in the primary structure of the
homologous proteins. Therefore we prepared cytochrome
c--556 from the races B6, TT111 and rhizogenes in the
pure state. The cytochromes c-556 of two strains from
the B6 race are physically identical, and so is the
sequence of 8 N-terminal amino acids. Cyt c-556 from a
strain of the TT111 race is distinctly different in isoelectric point and electrophoretic mobility. The same
is true for a strain from the rhizogenes race and here
are some clearcut differences in the N-terminal amino
acid sequence.

The rRNA cistrons in the tumefaciens-radiobacter
cluster are almost undistinguishably the same. There
are but small differences with the rubi, rhizogenes,
1650 and 1771 races. We also looked for the closest ge-
neric relatives of *Agrobacterium* by DNA:rRNA hybridization. There are considerable similarities between *Agrobacterium* rRNA cistrons with these of *Rhizobium*, *Myco-
plana*, *Azotomonas*, *Phyllobacterium* and the blue bacteria from *Ardisia*. These genera might well be related
at the family-level. The numerous other genera of both
Gram-positive and Gram-negative organisms which we investigated, have less similarity in their rRNA-cistrons
with *Agrobacterium*.

In the above results the crown gall strains, the
rhizogenic strains and the non-pathogenic strains do
not cluster according to their phytopathogenicity. DNA
of pathogenic strains quite often hybridizes for almost 100 % with DNA of non-pathogenic strains, and DNA
of several crown gall strains hybridizes for almost 100
% with DNA of the rhizogenes strains. If the cause of
both diseases resides in DNA, it constitutes at most
a few per cent of the bacterial genome. The present
species names, species concept and species differentiation in *Agrobacterium* is not justified.

Agrobacterium is now probably one of the most thoroughly known genera in bacteriology.

REFERENCES

M. BERNAERTS, J. DE LEY
3-Ketoglycosides, new intermediates in the metabolism of dissacharides by bacteria.
Biochim. Biophys. Acta, 30, 661-662 (1958).

M. BERNAERTS, J. DE LEY
Une nouvelle voie de décomposition des disaccharides.
Abstr. Comm. Intern. Congr. Microbiol. Stockholm
(1958).

M. BERNAERTS, J. DE LEY
3-Ketoglycosides, nieuwe stofwisselingsprodukten ge-
vormd door bacteriën uit disacchariden.
Arch. Int. Physiol. Biochim. 68, 209-210 (1960).

M. BERNAERTS, J. DE LEY
Microbiological formation and preparation of 3-keto-
glycosides from disaccharides.
J. gen. Microbiol. 22, 129-136 (1960).

M. BERNAERTS, J. DE LEY
The structure of 3-ketoglycosides formed from dis-
accharides by certain bacteria.
J. gen. Microbiol. 22, 137-146 (1960).

M. BERNAERTS, J. DE LEY
An improved method for the preparation of 3-keto-
glycosides.
Ant. v. Leeuwenhoek J. Microbiol. 27, 247-256 (1961).

M. BERNAERTS, J. DE LEY
A biochemical test for crown gall bacteria.
Nature (London), 197, 406-407 (1963).

M. BERNAERTS, J. FURNELLE, J. DE LEY
The preparation of some new disaccharides and D-al-
lose from 3-ketoglycosides.
Biochim. Biophys. Acta, 69, 322-330 (1963).

J. VAN BEEUMEN
The enzymatic formation of 3-ketolactose by *Agrobac-
terium tumefaciens*.
Ant. v. Leeuwenhoek J. Microbiol. 31, 469 (1965).

J. DE LEY, A. RASSEL
DNA base composition, flagellation and taxonomy of
the genus *Rhizobium*.
J. gen. Microbiol. 41, 85-91 (1965).

J. DE LEY, M. BERNAERTS, A. RASSEL, J. GUILMOT
Approach to an improved taxonomy of the genus *Agro-
bacterium*.
J. gen. Microbiol. 43, 7-17 (1966).

J. DE LEY, J. VAN BEEUMEN
Aldo-hexose dehydrogenase, a new enzyme from *Agro-
bacterium*.
IX° Intern. Congress Microbiol., Moscow, Proc. (1966).

M. BERNAERTS, J. DE LEY
Mechanism of the 3-ketolactose test for *Agrobacterium*.
Arch. f. Mikrobiol. 56, 81-90 (1967).

G. HEBERLEIN, J. DE LEY, R. TYTGAT
Deoxyribonucleic acid homology and taxonomy of *Agrobacterium*, *Rhizobium* and *Chromobacterium*.
J. Bacteriol. 94, 116-124 (1967).

J. VAN BEEUMEN, J. DE LEY
Hexopyranoside : Cytochrome c oxidoreductase from *Agrobacterium tumefaciens*.
Eur. J. Biochem. 6, 331-343 (1968).

J. DE LEY
DNA base composition and hybridization in the taxonomy of phytopathogenic bacteria.
Ann. Rev. Phytopathol. 6, 63-90 (1968).

M. ANTEUNIS, J. VAN BEEUMEN, A. DE BRUYN, J. DE LEY
NMR Experiments on acetals. XIX. The NMR analysis and structure of 3-keto-lactose and β-D-galactose.
Bull. Soc. Chim. Belges, 78, 651-658 (1969).

J.B. VAN DER PLAAT, L.N. VERNIE, J. DE LEY
Suspected mutant of *Agrobacterium tumefaciens* with an altered DNA.
Mutation Research, 7, 466-468 (1969).

J. VAN BEEUMEN, J. DE LEY
Polarographic method for determination of 3-keto sugars.
Anal. Biochem. 44, 254-261 (1971).

J. VAN BEEUMEN, J. DE LEY
Polarography of 3-keto-sugars.
Bull. Soc. Chim. Belges, 80, 683-699 (1971).

J. DE LEY
Agrobacterium : intrageneric relationships and evolution.
Proc. Third International Conference on Plant Pathogenic Bacteria, April 1971 - Pudoc, Wageningen, 1972.

J. DE LEY, M. GILLIS, C.F. POOTJES, K. KERSTERS, R. TYTGAT, M. VAN BRAKEL
Relationship among temperate *Agrobacterium* phage genomes and coat proteins.
J. gen. Virol. 16, 199-214 (1972).

J. DE LEY AND COLLABORATORS
Verwantschap en evolutie van plantenkankerbakteriën.
Biol. Jb. Dodonaea, 40, 32-39 (1972).

M. DE CLEENE, K. OTTEN
Het voorkomen van *Agrobacterium*-kanker (crown gall) bij economisch belangrijke plantengeslachten.
De Belgische Tuinbouw, 12, 196-197 (1973).

K. KERSTERS, J. DE LEY, P.H.A. SNEATH, M. SACKIN
Numerical taxonomic analysis of *Agrobacterium*.
J. gen. Microbiol. <u>78</u>, 227-239 (1973).

J. DE LEY, R. TYTGAT, J. DE SMEDT, M. MICHIELS
Thermal stability of DNA:DNA hybrids within the ge-
nus *Agrobacterium*.
J. gen. Microbiol. <u>78</u>, 241-252 (1973).

J. DE LEY
Biologie moléculaire, phylogénie et taxonomie du
genre *Agrobacterium*.
Ann. Phytopath. <u>5</u>, 102 (1973).

J. DE LEY
Phylogeny of procaryotes.
Taxon, <u>23</u>, 291-300 (1974).

CROWN GALL : A MODEL FOR TUMOR RESEARCH AND GENETIC ENGINEERING

R.A. Schilperoort and G.H. Bomhoff

Laboratory of Biochemistry, State University

Wassenaarseweg 64, Leiden

PART I. GENERAL CONSIDERATIONS ABOUT THE CROWN GALL DISEASE

Introduction

The purpose of this section is not to give a complete review of all what is known today about Crown gall but to recapitulate some of its principal features. This will be done especially in relation to its possible usefulness as a model for tumor research and to find ways for well defined genetic modification of plant cells (Genetic Engineering). Presumably genetic modification of plant cells is not directly relevant in near future for the improvement of plant species in aid of agriculture but might be an important tool for the study of the regulatory processes involved in differentiation, morphogenesis and uncontrolled growth (tumor induction). Several excellent reviews on the whole field of Crown gall research have appeared and can be used for more detailed information (1, 2, 3).

More than 65 years ago Smith and Townsend found that the plant tumor Crown gall is caused by a bacterium now called Agrobacterium tumefaciens. In the animal kingdom several so called oncogenic viruses are known to induce tumors. These are DNA as well as RNA viruses and recent developments in this field suggest an important role of RNA viruses in oncogenesis possibly also in human beings. Crown gall, however, is the sole known tumor disease caused by a bacterium. Such an agent in our opinion could also play a role in oncogenesis in animals or human beings. We may be strengthened in this idea if we realise that tumor growth on plants can arise as in the case of animal cells under the influence of a RNA-

virus (the Wound Tumor Virus) and radiation. Also tumors of
probable genetic origin have been known for long time to occur in plants. They are found both within species and in
species hybrids. Especially much is known about the genetically tumor-prone hybrids of Nicotiana. Moreover habituation
i.e. the ability of plant tissues to grow in the absence of
phytohormones after prolonged cultivation in vitro might be
compared to the establishment of animal cell-lines which frequently show a malignant character. The analogy in the etiology of uncontrolled growth for both "green" and "white" cells
suggests fundamentaly comparable principles in oncogenesis in
both systems. Tumors in human beings may develop from cells
long after some agent has left its traces in these cells.
Only under the influence of special environmental changes e.g.
of hormonal nature or chemical carcinogens the cells are
triggered in such a way that a new property of the cell brought
about by the original agent becomes effective. In this light
we might even wonder, although rather speculative, whether
a particular bacterial species exists which is able to infect
animal or human cells with an oncogene. Later in developing
tumors, this oncogene becomes manifest as e.g. a RNA virus
(c-type particle).

The Crown gall disease offers us an unique possibility to
investigate at the molecular level how a bacterium is able to
convert a normal cell into a tumor cell. If we know the Tumor
Inducing Principle(TIP) of this bacterium we seriously can
look for similar bacterial species in human oncogenesis.

The plant system has another important advantage i.e. the
totipotency of the plant cells. From single plant cells complete plants can be regenerated. By this the tumor problem can
directly be investigated in relation to cell differentiation.
This possibility is largely extended by recent developments
in the isolation of plant protoplasts, fusion of protoplasts
for somatic cell hybridization and the availability of diploid
and haploid plants from the same species. Now in principle
biochemical work can be combined with genetic work formerly
only possible with micro-organisms. Due to these developments
and the use that can be made of bacterial enzymes operating in
DNA-synthesis and restriction, Genetic Engineering will soon
be reality (4). Inevitably this kind of research will raise
questions about its ethical implications. Indeed, manipulating
members of the animal kingdom certainly will lead to serious
conscientious objections. The absence of a nervous system at
least spares us the creating of monsters when using members
of the Plant Kingdom. In this field too Crown gall might be
used as a model, since several data suggest that this tumor
disease represents a naturally occurring case of genetic
information transfer from the inciting bacteria into the plant
cell. If a bacterial plasmid is transferred into the plant
cells, as supposed recently (5), then in principle all kinds

of genetic information can be intentionally introduced into plant genomes. A. tumefaciens cells, provided with the desired genetic information in its plasmid, might possibly be used in future to acieve a reproducible and efficient transfer of genes. If part or the complete plasmid DNA escapes restriction mechanisms which possibly act in plant cells too, then this type of DNA is preferred over arbitrary chosen other DNAs, in experiments intended to modify plant cells in vitro genetically with DNA.

The Crown gall disease

Crown gall is a nonself-limiting disease that affects not only a few sensitive plant species, but a great number of species and families, most of them being dicotyledones. Once the tumor induction by A. tumefaciens has taken place, the continued abnormal and autonomous proliferation of the tumor cell becomes entirely independent of the inciting bacterium. It is generally believed that Crown gall is a real plant cancer having several characteristics in common with animal tumors. It displays, contrary to normal tissue, autonomous, phytohormone independent growth when brought into tissue culture as well as after transplantation on healthy plants.

The following sequence of events in tumor formation is tentatively suggested from data of experiments with Kalanchoë. The diagrammatic representation as shown in fig.1 is based on the one proposed earlier by Klein (6). This may hold also for other plant species. In the case of Kalanchoë the tumors originate mainly in the cortex.

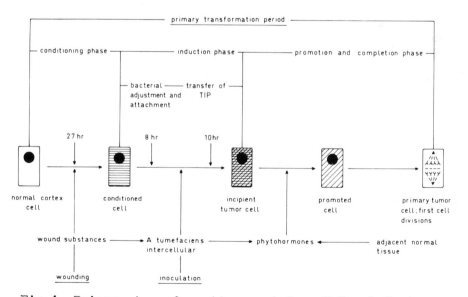

Fig.1. Primary transformation period on Kalanchoë stems.

Conditioning phase

        Wounding is an essential requirement for tumor formation
with a virulent strain of A. tumefaciens. The wound sites
show a progressively increasing followed by a decreasing ability to react to the bacterial stimulus. The process by which
these uninfected sites become first sensitive and then refractory to the tumorogenic stimulus is referred to as conditioning.
It represents all of the metabolic events that must take place
before the bacteria can induce a transformation.

        Although conditioning can occur at both 25ºC and 32ºC,
the process is accelerated at 32ºC. Maximum conditioning at
25, 32 and 36ºC has been shown to occur prior to the first
observed wound-stimulated cell divisions (7). The optimum in
conditioning at 25ºC is reached after about 27 h. It is suggested that there exists a particular cellular stage, between
quiescence and division, during which the cell can respond to
the tumorogenic stimulus. Only during this sensitive stage,
which is finite in duration, a cell can be diverted from its
morphogenetic path to form a tumor. The experiments using anti-
metabolites to see whether tumor formation could be inhibited
(8) provide support in favor of the DNA-synthesis period "S"
of the mitotic cycle as the sensitive stage involved in tumor-
initiation.

Induction phase

        The time found to be required to convert a conditioned
cell to a tumor cell is at least 8 h at 25ºC, after a bacterial adjustment period of another 8 to 10 h. Thus if the
length of the sensitive phase of the host cells is less than
8 h no tumors will form. If this hypothesis is correct then
it might account for the failure to form tumors at 32ºC and
for the failure of certain cells, which do divide as a result
of wounding, to form tumors in the presence of bacteria (7).
A. tumefaciens cells penetrate into the intercellular spaces
and into the injured cells which are filled with woundsap. In
these places the bateria replicate and interact with the
adjacent plant cells. They never penetrate into undamaged
cells. A bacterial attachment to a limiting number of specific
sites in the conditioned wounds seems to be an essential stage
in tumor initiation(9,10,11). The association of the bacterial
cells to the cell wall as shown by electron microscopic observations (fig.2) presumably demonstrate such an attachment.
If the bacterial attachment is considered as an initial stage
of tumor induction this could explain the existence of the
essential phase of bacterial adjustment. It was found that
avirulent Agrobacterium cells were able to compete with virulent cells for the attachment sites. However, only viable
avirulent cells were able to do so. They failed to show this

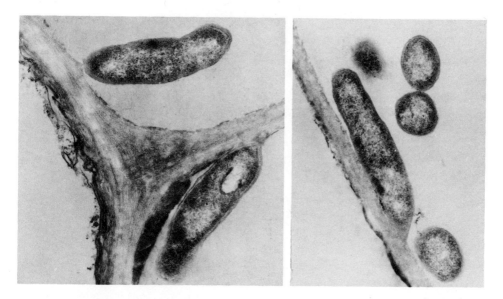

Fig. 2. Association of Agrobacterium cells to the cell wall.

phenomenon when killed at 60°C. This might indicate that under conditions of bacterial adjustment the bacteria undergo a change in their surface properties essential for the bacterial attachment to occur. The attachment is postulated to be a preliminary step to the injection of bacterial DNA into intact cells (10). In that case DNA is the TIP, which will be discussed later.

Promotion and completion phase

The processes that occur in the promotion and completion phase are not well known. The conversion of normal cells in Crown gall cells most likely is not an "all-or-none" phenomenon, but rather a progressive process. As in differentiation the basis of progression is thought to be a change in gene expression and thus of epigenetic nature, leading to a phenotypically different cell. In the case of induced uncontrolled growth like e.g. Crown gall in our opinion changes of gene expression of the host cell might be triggered by a genetic modification of the cell genome. Others believe that the nuclei of normal and tumor cells are genetically equivalent (12).

The incipient tumor cell may be considered to have acquired TIP from the bacteria and by this the cell is fated to become a tumor cell. However, stable transformation and phenotype of the resulting tumor are determined by environmental factors. The local concentration of phytohormones synthesized

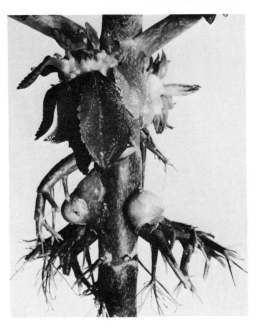

Fig. 3. Tumors on Kalanchoë stem induced by weakly virulent
   Agrobacterium tumefaciens strain (E III 9.6.1.)

by the bacteria and derived from adjacent normal tissue seems
to be of great influence on the final outcome of the transformation process. The variation encountered in the reaction of
different host species in response to infection with A. tumefaciens are attributed to variations in the internal hormonal environment provided by the host (13). Cells of plant species
such as sunflower, possessing low competence for regeneration,
develop into typically unorganized tumors irrespective whether
strongly or weakly virulent strains are used. However, tumors
bearing abnormal supernumerary organs which are called teratomata are produced in the upper half of stems of highly regenerative plants like Tobacco and Kalanchoë infected with moderately virulent strains. In the lower half only unorganized tumors
are formed by such strains. An example of both types of tumors
is shown in fig. 3. When pluripotent cells of e.g. Kalanchoë
are transformed to tumor cells by a highly virulent strain,
they lose permanently the capacity to organize morphologically more or less normal structures (teratomata), indicating that
the cellular factors concerned with differentiation and organ-

ization are completely overwhelmed by the tumorogenic stimulus
of the bacteria.

From experiments showing an increase in the size of tumors that develop on Kalanchoë stems at 32°C with increasing
duration of the induction period at a lower temperature it was
stated that progression in Crown gall is due to a cumulative
action of TIP, and that TIP is inactivated at 32°C. The viability of the bacteria and their capability to induce tumors
is not influenced by the heat treatment. Normal wound healing
was said to run its ordinary course. More detailed studies on
the influence of temperature have shown that cell division
induced by wounding as well as the competence of the host cells
(conditioning) actually is strongly affected by temperature(7).
A comparison of the results of the former experiments with
Kalanchoë plants(14) with those obtained on the influence of
temperature performed with the same plant species show that the
results can be explained by a decline in competence that occurs
after an optimal conditioning period. The results are even inconsistent with the thermal-inactivation hypothesis(15). Thus,
what was thought to be progression in fact is a reflection of
a difference in the number of converted cells. The original
concept of progression in Crown gall tumorogenesis came from
experiments with periwinkle (Vinca rosea L.) taking advantage
of the fact that A. tumefaciens cells can be eliminated when
infected plants are held at 46-47°C for 3 or more days. This
treatment does not affect the tumor development at normal temperature afterwards. Tumor size and growth rate were found
to be dependent on the duration of the induction period at
normal temperature before eliminating the bacteria. The tumors
have a maximum size and growth rate when the induction period
is 4 days or longer. Interestingly tumors put into tissue
culture displayed a decrease in requirement of growth substances with increasing duration of the induction period at normal
temperature (16). This phenomenon is taken as a demonstration
of progression leading to partially or completely converted
cells depending on the duration of the presence of viable bacteria within the susceptible host tissue. In fact then only the
bacteria determine through continued presence the final outcome of epigenetic changes in the incipient tumor cell during
the promotion phase. We, however, wonder whether the results
with periwinkle could also be explained by a different ratio
of fully converted cells to non Crown gall cells in the tumors
depending on the duration of the induction period before the
bacteria are killed. Moreover, what looks to be a cumulative
bacterial action could also be caused by the heat treatment at
46-47°C. It is not known whether heat treatment which does not
kill the plant cells, might stop further progression in incipient tumor cells, which otherwise would have become fully
converted cells even without the help of bacteria present.

We in fact question whether there is any evidence showing
that the bacteria, through a more or less lasting presence
after initiation of the incipient tumor cell, which in itself
is accomplished in a rather short time (fig.1) determine
whether partly or fully converted cells will develop. We do not
deny the existence of different degrees of conversion but in
our opinion the degree of conversion is largely dependent on
the course of processes that occur in the incipient tumor cell
after acquisition of TIP, from the bacteria. The bacteria then
do not influence so much the processes once started. The course
of the processes is presumably only determined by the genetic
constitution of the host cells and by gradients of growth
regulators in the plant (position effect). The role of these
different determinants is clearly demonstrated in experiments
using crosses of different species of Kalanchoë (17). Different
kinds of tissue of Kalanchoë reacted independently (position
effect). Similar types of tissue of these various species did
not react in the same way (difference in gradients of growth
regulators in plants with other genetic constitution). However, the reaction of different cell types of the F-hybrids
had its own character, sometimes clearly influenced by one of
the parents. This means that the outcome of cell conversion was
influenced by a genetic factor in the cells. It was found too
that, when one of the parents of the hybrid is unable to form
tumors on the leaves, in the F_1 hybrids, this ability also can
be lacking. In plants as well as in animals growth can be the
result of two types of processes i.e. cell enlargement or cell
enlargement combined with cell division. The basic cellular
mechanisms underlying these growth processes are regulated
by hormones. In plant cells the auxins are involved in cell
enlargement while cytokinins and auxins in a synergistic way
promote growth by cell division. The autonomous growth of
plant cells might be directly related to a very early activation of the two intracellular hormone-synthesizing systems
(auxins and cytokinins). The resulting deviation of the phytohormone balance from normal consequently leads to a progressive
activation of several biosynthetic systems in the tumor cells,
which becomes hereditary stable.

A changed ion-permeability of the cell membrane may play
an important part in the autonomy of the tumor cells (18) and
may underly the changed phytohormone balance. It was found
that particular ions, which are well-known activators of metabolic processes, could penetrate to the proper locus in tumor
cells much more efficiently than in normal cells. The changed
ion-permeability of the tumor cells can not be the only explanation for autonomy, however, as unlike the auxin requirement
of the normal cells, the cytokinin requirement cannot be met

by addition of ions. Nevertheless the changed permeability of
the tumor cells might be one of the most important results of
transformation. Changes in the cell surface of animal cells
have also been recognized as an important phenomenon in tumorous conversion. Membrane alterations have indeed been postulated to be the basis of malignancy (19).

Part II. THE NATURE OF THE TUMOR-INDUCING-PRINCIPLE
         ELABORATED BY A. TUMEFACIENS

Introduction

     The tumorous character is inherited in a dividing populat-
ion of cells and is highly stable. The fundamental question
arises whether this can be achieved in the absence of any change
in the integrity of the genetic information normally present in
a cell (12) or that some somatic cell mutation is an essential
prerequisite for either the establishment or maintenance of the
tumorous state.
     Without any change in the genetic information content of
the cells the tumorous state is evoked only by a change in gene
expression which in some way is heritably stabilized. In that
case neither nucleic acids from A. tumefaciens nor a DNA- or
RNA-virus elaborated by the inciting bacterium can be involved,
since these agents when penetrated into the cell would change
the genetic information content of the cell. A. tumefaciens
then must synthesize a particular metabolite that is able to
change gene expression persistently in the relatively short
time that the bacterium is needed for tumorous conversion
(about 10 h in Kalanchoë plants).
     The concept that a change in the integrity of the genetic
information of the cell is not an essential prerequisite in
establishing and maintenance of the tumorous state came from
experiments which show that starting from a graft of teratoma
tissue of single cell origin on the cut stem-tips of tobacco
plants finally normal plants could be obtained (20). Although
for these experiments it was stated that the first shoots developed from the graft and not from surrounding normal tissue,
others repeating these experiments could establish that only
shoots developed from cells of the host plant (21). Tobacco
plants could also be regenerated from unorganized tumor tissue
grown in vitro (21). However, the plants were sterile and did
not resemble the tobacco variety from which they were originally derived. A severe loss of chromosomes occurred during the

regeneration process. If the plants actually developed from
real Crown gall cells in the tumor tissues used, the loss of
chromosomes might have eliminated genetic modifications when
these had been introduced by A.tumefaciens. Furthermore, it
is very difficult to be sure that the plants regenerate from
Crown gall cells in tumor callus tissue that might consist of
different types of cells. Starting from single cells up to now
no regenerates could be obtained (21).

In our opinion the reversion of the tumorous state into
normal has still not been firmly established in the case of
Crown gall. Like in oncogenesis by DNA- and RNA-virusses in
animals A.tumefaciens might have modified the genetic information content of the incipient tumor cell. It might do so by
introducing some type of its own DNA or RNA into the plant
cell or by producing a DNA- or RNA-virus that is able to convert the cell. The participation of bacterial RNA in Crown gall
induction has been postulated from data obtained by different
types of experiments (22,23,24,25). An undisturbed RNA synthesis in both the inciting bacteria and the host cells during
the first stages of Crown gall induction has also been found
to be important (26,27).

A lysogenic phage of A.tumefaciens cells has frequently
been brought in relation with the tumor inducing capacity of
A.tumefaciens. Several A.tumefaciens strains are lysogenic
indeed. Especially much attention has been paid to a phage
called PS8. This phage has been isolated from one of the
plaques that arose when homogenates of sunflower Crown gall
callus culture (originally induced by strain B6) were tested
for phage activity against A.tumefaciens strain B6-806 (28).
Phages of the same type were isolated from single plaques on
B6-806 when homogenates of many different kinds of Crown gall
cultures of Tobacco including those induced by strain A6 were
tested (29). This, however, needs not to be a general phenomenon, since another A6-induced sterile Crown gall callus
tissue of Tobacco did not contain detectable phage activity
(30). Moreover, preliminary evidence shows that the B6-806
strain most probably carries a defective prophage but is not
immune to superinfection with phage PS8 (30).The morphology
of this phage resembles that of PS8. Nucleic acid hybridization experiments, should show whether the defective phage
from B6-806 is genetically equivalent to PS8. Although phage
particles were ineffective, conflicting data have been presented on the tumor inducing capacity of PS8-DNA itself (31,
32). Anyhow, the induction of PS8 is not likely to be an essential prerequisite for tumor induction since non-phage producing strains were found to be as pathogenic as their PS8-
lysogenic derivatives showing a high frequency of spontaneous induction (33).

Several lines of evidence tentatively suggest that Crown gall cells contain genetic information obtained from A. tumefaciens cells. A. tumefaciens cross-reacting antigens have been detected in sterile Crown gall tissues (34,35,36). Moreover nucleic acid hybridization experiments have been reported showing A. tumefaciens like RNA to be present in tumor cells (37,38) while also complementarity between A. tumefaciens DNA and DNA isolated from sterile Crown gall tissue seems to exist (10,39,40).

Recently base-sequence homology has also been detected between PS8 cRNA (complementary RNA) and the DNA from sterile Crown gall tissue induced by strain A6 (30). Phage activity could not be detected in homogenates of this tissue. The interpretation of the results is complicated by the fact that no PS8 can be induced from the PS8-insensitive A6 cells. Moreover, no PS8-DNA can be detected in DNA isolated from these A6 cells with a routine isolation method. It has been postulated that the PS8-like DNA sequences detected in Crown gall DNA preparations are part of a large plasmid which has been found in A6 cells. The plasmid is lost, however, with the common DNA isolation procedure.

To know more about the significance of the results obtained, different features of the hybridization reaction between Crown gall DNA and cRNA transcribed from PS8-DNA and A6-DNA have been investigated. Furthermore, the hybrids formed have been characterized with regard to RNAase and DNAase resistance, melting temperature, S-value of the cRNA melted from RNAase treated hybrids and buoyant density in Cs_2SO_4 gradients (41). All the data indicate that the cRNA molecules not simply anneal to homologous DNA present in the Crown gall DNA preparation. This analysis of the Crown gall -(PS8-cRNA) hybrid shows that the amplification of PS8 genomes in Crown gall DNA, as supposed earlier, actually does not exist. Preliminary renaturation (Cot) experiments even indicate that one complete genome of PS8 might not be present in Crown gall DNA.

Recent data support the idea that a plasmid in A. tumefaciens cells is directly involved in tumor induction, since it was found that plasmid is only present in cells of virulent strains and not in those of wildtype avirulent strains (5). Because experiments with plasmid DNA and cRNA have still to be done, we actually do not know if plasmid DNA or part of it is integrated in the host genome.

Specific markers for Crown gall cells ?

Various reports have shown the presence of the unusual amino acid derivatives octopine N^2-(D-1-carboxyethyl)-L-arginine (42,43), octopinic acid N^2-(D-1-carboxyethyl)-L-ornithine (44) nopaline N^2-(1,3-dicarboxypropyl)-L-arginine (45), and

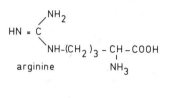

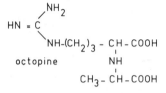

HN = C
NH₂
NH-(CH₂)₃ - CH - COOH
nopaline   NH
HOOC-(CH₂)-CH-COOH

Fig. 4.

lysopine N²-(D-l-carboxyethyl)-L-lysine (46,47)in Crown galls
on various plants and in tissue culture. In these tumors the
presence of one of these derivatives seems to be independent of
the plant species, but only determined by the type of bacterium
used for inoculation. Moreover strains of Agrobacterium tumefaciens which induce tumors containing octopine (nopaline) are
capable of catabolizing octopine (nopaline) in a synthetic
medium (48). This correlation has led to the hypothesis that
the information for the synthesis of these compounds is located on bacterial genes which are transferred during tumor formation (49). If so the presence of these amino acid derivatives
would be a very useful marker for tumor cells transformed by
Agrobacterium tumefaciens. Moreover compared to the detection
of bacterial DNA through complicated hybridization experiments
or to the immunological methods for demonstrating cross-reacting
antigens, experiments to detect these amino acid derivatives
are much easier to accomplish. Experiments by Seitz and Hochster
(50),but not confirmed by others(51,52),however, suggest that
lysopine is a normal plant metabolite, though present in a
much lower concentration than in tumor tissue. In that case
the production is only stimulated in transformed cells.

In order to confirm the specificity of the presence of
these compounds in tumor tissue, we analyzed various plant
tissues for the presence of octopine and nopaline.

Methods

All tissues were frozen in liquid air and lyophilized immediately after harvest. Samples were ground to a fine powder and extracted with distilled water. The resulting slurry was centrifuged for 10 min at 3000xg and the supernatant was directly used for high-voltage electrophoresis. Using a formic acid-acetic acid-water mixture (11:30:159 ^{V}/v) we obtained a clear separation of the different guanidine compounds in only 20 min. The papers were thoroughly air-dried before colouring with a specific fluorescent reagent (53). The identification of octopine, arginine and γ-guanidobutyric-acid in all tissues was confirmed by co-electrophoresis of a standard mixture of these compounds (fig.5). The results are summarized in fig.6.

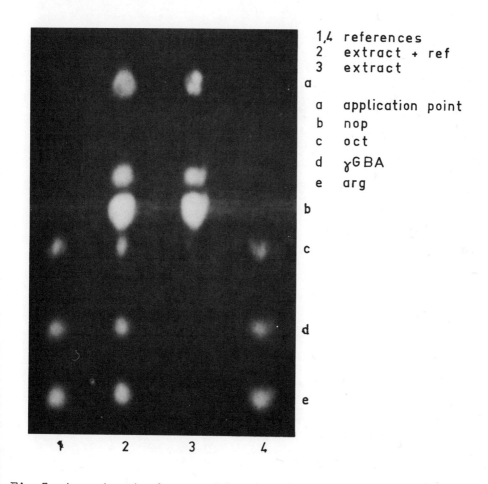

1,4 references
2   extract + ref
3   extract
a

a   application point
b   nop
c   oct
d   γGBA
e   arg

Fig.5. An extract of a nopaline-tumor after high-voltage electrophoresis.

Plant tissues analyzed for the presence of octopine and nopaline (1).

Kalanchoë daigremontiana.

healthy stem		-
young leaves		-
plantlets produced in leaf notches		-
adventitious roots formed on the stem		-
stem tumors	(A6, B6)	Oct.
	(E III 9.6.1, C-58, T37)	**Nop.**

Nicotiana tabacum.
var. White Burley (WB)
var. Xanthi (X)
var. Wisconsin (W)

(WB,X) healthy stem		-
(WB,X) young leaves		-
(WB) leaf tumors	(B6S3)	Oct.
(WB) stem tumors	(A6, B6)	Oct.
(X) stem tumors	(B6, B6-806, 15955)	Oct.
(WB) stem tumors	(C-58)	Nop.
(WB,W) normal tissue		-

tissue culture material

(WB) Crown gall	(A6)	Oct.
	(E III 9.6.1.)	Nop.

Helianthus annuus.
var. giganteus

healthy stem		-
stem tumors	(A6, B6)	Oct.
	(C-58)	Nop.

(1) In brackets, the strain of Agrobacterium tumefaciens used for tumor induction.

Fig. 6

Results

These data show a strict correlation between Agrobac-terium transformed tumor tissue and the presence of octopine or nopaline, depending on the bacterial strain used. Though the method we used, enables a detection of the amounts of octopine reported to be present in root tips of bean seedlings, root tips and hypocotyls of pea seedlings (54) and normal tis-sue of tobacco and sunflower (55), we could not confirm their results using the same plant varieties and corresponding cul-ture conditions. In the pea and bean tissue extracts we found besides arginine more than four different guanidine-compounds which were, however, clearly separated from a reference octo-pine spot, added to the sample. The Leguminosae are indeed notorious for the presence of guanidine compounds (56). Re-covery of octopine added to the tissue material before ex-traction was in all cases more than 90%.

Recently three different habituated White Burley tissues were initiated in our laboratory. All habituated tissues show-ed a higher nuclear DNA content compared to the original normal callus tissue, while one of them acquired a DNA content not significantly different from that of Crown gall tissue (57). In none of these tissues octopine or nopaline was found. A habituated tissue of Scorsonera hispanica was also negative. This too is in straight contrast with earlier results (54), where it was stated that a habituated White Burley tissue, in-itiated about 27 years ago in the laboratory of Gautheret con-tained octopine. Though we could confirm their results, using this old tissue line, we have up to now no explanation for the conflicting data obtained with habituated tissue.

In order to study several aspects of tumor induction more precisely, a model system was developed in our laboratory by Dr. Newell using sterile cortex segments of young Kalanchoë stems. These tissue slices were inoculated with virulent bac-teria and placed on a nutrient agar medium. Seven days later a ridge of light-coloured tissue could be seen at the top of the segment, which was morphologically distinct from normal wound cambium. Using avirulent Agrobacteria only wound healing was observed. To substantiate the tumorous character of these cells we analyzed the light-coloured tissue, the rest of the segment below this ridge and also the same parts from segments inoculated with avirulent strains. Only in the tumorous tissue octopine or nopaline could be found. This result clearly demon-strates the usefulness of these guanidine-compounds as markers for tumor tissue where other techniques are not feasible.

In part I we already mentioned the occurrence of complex tumors so called teratomata. Work by Braun (58,59) on Kalan-choë strongly suggest on histological and morphological grounds that the teratomata shoots are of tumorous origin.

In shoots and roots protruding from these complex tumors, we
found high amounts of nopaline, while plantlets on the edges
of normal leaves and adventitious roots on healthy stems were
always negative. This result could be an indication for the
presence of bacterial genes in these tumor cells, which are
capable of some form of differentiation. Even under these
circumstances the information for the synthesis of nopaline
cannot come under repression in the plant cell. Comparable
results were found in tissue culture material of these tumors
which, under certain conditions, also showed shoot and bud
formation.

Bacterial catabolism

Another interesting aspect of these guanidine-compounds
concerns their utilization by different Agrobacterium strains.
In the introduction we mentioned the correlation between the
induction of octopine (nopaline)forming-tumors and the ability
to degrade these compounds by the virulent bacteria. Reports by
Petit and Tourneur (60) and Lippincott et al.(61), in which
the authors show that the loss of virulence is, with only a few
exceptions, accompanied by loss of the capability to catabolize
octopine, nopaline or both, further emphasize the importance
of further research in this direction.

An important extention was the discovery of the presence
of a large plasmid in all virulent Agrobacterium tumefaciens
strains tested, belonging to different taxonomical groups (5).
Especially interesting was the absence of this plasmid in the
avirulent strain C-58(C-9) which was simply obtained by incubating the strain C-58 at 37°C in analogy with the experiments of Hamilton and Fall (62). Also in the "spontaneous"
avirulent derivative IIBNV6, obtained by Braun, no plasmid
could be found (63).

By growing these avirulent strains and the parent virulent strains (C-58 and IIB) in a synthetic medium, we found
that only the virulent Agrobacteria were capable to degrade
nopaline while the derivative avirulent strains could not catabolize it (64). Though we do not know if the plasmid codes
for an octopine (nopaline) degrading enzyme system, or if it
effects a membrane alteration necessary for the uptake of octopine (nopaline) these results suggest an important function of
the plasmid in both virulence and the degradation of octopine
and nopaline.

Discussion

One of the main reasons for contradictory or badly reproducible results in Crown gall research at the molecular
level in our opinion is based on the fact that we are unaware
of unique properties of the Crown gall cell. Phytohormone in-
dependency only is not a good criterion, since habituated cells

show the same property without ever being in contact with <u>A.</u> <u>tumefaciens</u>. The same seems to hold for transplantation experiments although this might largely depend on the host plant selected for grafting. On <u>Xanthi</u> e.g. both phytohormone dependent <u>Xanthi</u> normal callus tissue and phytohormone independent <u>Xanthi</u> callus tissue derived from tumors give rise to outgrowth, while on <u>White Burley</u> only <u>White Burley</u>-Crown gall tissue is transplantable. On account of this for Crown gall research one has to be careful in selecting plants for tumor induction and further experiments.

In our opinion octopine or nopaline, depending on the strain to be used, at this moment should be taken as the best marker for Crown gall cells. It has the advantage that it can be detected at very low concentrations with rather simple techniques.

ACKNOWLEDGEMENT:

The assistance of Dr. E. Newell in various parts of the experimental work is highly appreciated.

REFERENCES

1. Progress in experimental tumor research.vol.15.Plant Tumor Research.(1972) vol.ed.A.C.Braun.(ed.Karger,Basel).

2. Bopp,M.(1973). Entwicklungsphysiologie. in:Fortschritte der Botanik.Band 35.H.Ellenberg et al.(ed.Springer-Verlag, Berlin)p147.

3. Butcher, D.N.(1973).The origins, characteristics and culture of plant tumour cells. in: Plant tissue and cell culture.H.E.Street.(ed.Blackwell Sc.Publ.,Oxford)p356.

4. Heyn,R.F.,A.Rörsch,R.A.Schilperoort(1974).Prospects in genetic engineering of plants. Quarterly Review of Biophysics $\underline{7}$,35.

5. Zaenen, I.,M.van Larebeke, H.Teuchy,J.Schell,(1974). Supercoiled circular DNA in Crown gall inducing <u>Agrobacterium</u> strains. J.Mol.Biol.(in press).

6. Klein, R.M.,G.K.K.Link (1955).The etiology of Crown gall. Quarterly Review Biology $\underline{30}$,207.

7. Lipetz, J.(1966).Crown gall tumorigenesis II.Relations between wound healing and the tumorigenic response. Cancer.Res.$\underline{26}$,1597.

8. Bopp,M.(1966).Die Wirkung von Nukleinsäurehemmstoffen auf die Morphogenese von Pflanzen.Biol.Rundschau $\underline{4}$,25.

9. Lippincott, B.B.,J.A.Lippincott(1969).Bacterial attach-
    ment to a specific wound site as an essential stage
    in tumor initiation by Agrobacterium tumefaciens.
    J.Bact.97,620.

10. Schilperoort, R.A.(1969) Investigations on plant tumors-
    Crown gall.On the biochemistry of tumor induction by
    Agrobacterium tumefaciens. Thesis,Leiden (ed.Demmenie,
    Leiden).

11. Bogers, R.J.(1972).On the interaction of Agrobacterium
    tumefaciens with cells of Kalanchoë daigremontiana.
    Proc.3rd Int.Conf.Plant Pathogenic Bacteria.
    Wageningen (ed.Pudoc,Wageningen) p239.

12. Braun, A.C.(1970).On the origin of the cancer cell.
    Amer.Scientist 58,307

13. Stonier,T.(1962).Normal, abnormal and pathological rege-
    neration in Nicotiana. in: Regeneration. D.Rudnick.
    (ed. Ronald Press, New York)p85.

14. Braun, A.C., R.J.Mandle(1948).Studies on the inactivation
    of the tumor-inducing-principle in Crown gall. Growth
    12, 255.

15. Beardsley, R.E.(1972).The inception phase in the Crown
    gall disease. in:Progress in experimental tumor re-
    search vol.15.Plant Tumor Research.vol.ed.A.C.Braun
    (ed.Karger, Basel)p1.

16. Braun, A.C.(1958).A physiological basis for autonomous
    growth of the Crown gall tumor cell.P.N.A.S.(USA)
    44,344.

17. Bopp, M.,F.Resende.(1966).Crown gall Tumoren bei verschie-
    denen Arten und Bastarden der Kalanchoidedae. Portu-
    galiae Acta Biologica 9,327.

18. Wood, H.N., A.C.Braun (1965).Studies on the net uptake of
    solutes by normal and Crown gall tumor cells. P.N.A.S.
    (USA) 54,1532.

19. Holley, R.W.(1972).A unifying hypothesis concerning the
    nature of malignant growth.P.N.A.S.(USA) 69,2840.

20. Braun, A.C.(1959). A demonstration of the recovery of the
    Crown gall tumor cell with the use of complex tumors
    of single-cell origin. P.N.A.S.(USA) 45,932.

21. Melchers, G.(1971).Tumoren als Folge von Mutation, Infek-
    tion oder Modifikation der Entwicklung. Mitteilungen
    aus der Max-Planck-Gesellschaft Heft 2,72.

22. Braun, A.C., H.M.Wood (1966). On the inhibition of tumor
    inception in the Crown gall disease with the use of
    ribonuclease A. P.N.A.S.(USA) 56,1417.

23. Beljanski, M.,A.Kurkjian, P.Manigault (1972). Transform-
    ation of Agrobacterium tumefaciens into a non-onco-
    genic species by an Escherichia coli RNA. P.N.A.S.
    (USA) 69,191.

24. Swain, L.W., J.P.Rier (1972). Cellular transformation in
    plant tissue by RNA from Agrobacterium tumefaciens.
    Bot.Gaz. 133,318.

25. Beljanski, M., M.I.Aaron-Da Cunha, M.S.Beljanski, P.
    Manigault, P.Bourgarel (1974).Isolation of the tumor-
    inducing RNA from oncogenic and nononcogenic
    Agrobacterium tumefaciens. P.N.A.S. 71,1585.

26. Beiderbeck, R.(1972).Rifampicin und der Phage PS8 von
    Agrobacterium tumefaciens. Z.Naturforsch.27b,584.

27. Beiderbeck,R.(1972). α-Amanitin hemmt die Tumorindukti on
    durch Agrobacterium tumefaciens.Z.Naturforsch.27b,
    1393.

28. Parsons, C.L., R.E.Beardsley(1968). Bacteriophage activity
    in homogenates of Crown gall tissue.J.Virology 2,651.

29. Tourneur, J.,G.Morel (1970).Sur la présence de phages
    dans les tissus de "Crown gall" cultivés in vitro.
    C.R. Acad.Sc.série D(Paris) 270,2810.

30. Schilperoort, R.A., N.J.van Sittert, J.Schell (1973).
    The presence of both phage PS8 and Agrobacterium
    tumefaciens A6 DNA base sequences in A6-induced
    sterile Crown gall tissue cultured in vitro. Eur.J.
    Biochem. 33,1.

31. Leff, J.,R.E. Beardsley (1970).Action tumorogène de l'acide
    nucléique d'un bactériophage présent dans les cultures
    de tissus tumoral de tournesol (Helianthus annuus).
    C.R.Acad.Sc. série D(Paris) 270,2505.

32. Beiderbeck,R.,G.T.Heberlein, J.A.Lippincott(1973). On the
    question of Crown gall tumor initiation by DNA of
    bacteriophage PS8. J.Virol.11,345.

33. Brunner, M.,C.F. Pootjens(1969).Bacteriophage release in
    a lysogenic strain of Agrobacterium tumefaciens.
    J.Virol.3,181.

34. Schilperoort, R.A., W.H. Meys, G.M.W. Pippel, H.Veldstra
    (1969). Agrobacterium tumefaciens cross-reacting
    antigens in sterile Crown gall tumors. FEBS Letters
    3,173.

35. Torok, D.de, R.A. Cornesky(1970). Antigenic and immuno-
       logical determinants of oncogenesis in plants in-
       fected with Agrobacterium tumefaciens in: Les cul-
       tures de tissus de plantes. Coll.Int.C.N.R.S. no.
       193, Strasbourg (éd.C.N.R.S.,Paris)p443.

36. Chadha, K.C.,B.I.S.Srivastava(1971). Evidence for the pre-
       sence of bacteria-specific proteins in sterile Crown
       gall tissue. Plant Physiol.48,125.

37. Milo, G.E.,B.I.S.Srivastava (1969).RNA-DNA hybridization
       studies with Crown gall bacteria and the tobacco tu-
       mor tissue. Biochem.Biophys.Res.Comm.34,196.

38. Sittert, N.J.van (1972). Onderzoekingen over Crown gall.
       Analyse van DNA en RNA in de tumor cel. Thesis,Leiden.
       (ed.Pasmans, The Hague).

39. Quétier, F.,T.Huguet,E.Guillé (1969). Induction of Crown
       gall:partial homology between tumor cell DNA, bacteri-
       al DNA and the G+C rich DNA of stressed normal cells.
       Biochem.Biophys.Res.Comm.34,128.

40. Srivastava, B.I.S.(1970). DNA-DNA hybridization studies
       between bacterial DNA, Crown gall-tumor cell DNA and
       the normal cell DNA. Life Science 9,889.

41. Schilperoort, R.A., J.J.M. Dons, H.Ras(1974).Characteri-
       zation of the complex formed between PS8 cRNA and
       DNA isolated from A6-induced sterile Crown gall
       tissue. 2nd John Innes Symposium. Modification of the
       information content of plant cells. July 1974,Norwich,
       England.

42. Ménagé, A., G. Morel(1964). Sur la présence d'octopine dans
       les tissus de Crown gall. C.R.Acad.Sc. série D (Paris)
       259,4795.

43. Goldmann-Ménagé, A. (1970). Recherches sur le métabolisme
       azoté des tissues de Crown gall cultivés in vitro.
       Thèse(Paris) Ann.Sc.Nat., Bot.,Paris 12e série 11,
       223.

44. Ménagé, A.,G.Morel(1965).Sur la présence d'un acide aminé
       nouveau dans les tissus de Crown gall. C.R.Acad.Sc.
       série D (Paris) 261,2001.

45. Goldman, A., D.W. Thomas, G.Morel (1969).Sur la structure
       de la nopaline, métabolite anormale de certaines
       tumeurs de Crown gall. C.R.Acad.Sc.série D (Paris)
       268,852.

46. Lioret,C.(1956).Sur la mise en évidence d'un acide aminé non identifié particulier aux tissus de Crown gall. Bull.Soc.fr.Physiol.vég. 2,76.

47. Biemann, K., C.Lioret, K. Asselineau, E.Lederer, I.Polonski(1960). Sur la structure chimique de la lysopine, nouvel acide aminé isolé du tissu de Crown gall. Bull.Soc.Chim.biol. 42,979.

48. Petit, A., S.Delhaye, J.Tempé, G. Morel(1970).Recherches sur les guanidines des tissus de Crown gall. Mise en évidence d'une relation biochimique spécifique entre les souches d'Agrobacterium tumefaciens et les tumeurs qu'elles induisent. Physiol.Vég.8,205.

49. Morel,G. (1970).Déviations du métabolisme azoté des tissus de Crown gall. in: Les cultures de tissus de plantes. Coll.Int.C.N.R.S. no.193 Strasbourg. (éd. C.N.R.S., Paris)p463.

50. Seitz, E.W., R.M.Hochster(1964). Lysopine in normal and in Crown gall tumor tissue of tomato and tobacco. Canad.J.Bot.42,999.

51. Lejeune,B.(1967).Etude de la synthèse de lysopine in vitro par des extraits de tissus de Crown gall. C.R. Acad.Sc.série D (Paris) 265,1753.

52. Lejeune,B.(1972).Recherches sur le métabolisme de la lysopine dans les tissus de Crown gall de Scorsonère cultivés in vitro. Thèse,Paris.

53. Yamada, S., H.A.Itano(1966).Phenanthrenequinone as an analytical reagent for arginine and other mono-substituted guanidines. B.B.A. 130,538.

54. Wendt-Gallitelli, M.F., I.Dobrigkeit(1973). Investigations implying the invalidity of octopine as a marker for transformation by Agrobacterium tumefaciens. Z.Naturforsch. 28c,768.

55. Johnson, R., R.H. Guderian, F.Eden, M.D.Chilton, M.P. Gordon, E.W.Nester(1974). Detection and quantitation of octopine in normal plant tissue and Crown gall tumor tissue. P.N.A.S. (USA) 71,536.

56. Comparative biochemistry of arginine and derivatives (1965). G.E.W. Wolstenholme, M.P.Cameron. CIBA foundation (ed.Churchill Ltd. London).

57. Dons, J.J.M., M. Valentijn, R.A.Schilperoort,P.van Duijn (1974). Nuclear DNA content and phytohormone requirements of normal, Crown gall and habituated tissues of Nicotiana var. White Burley. Exptl.Cell Res.(to be published).

58. Braun, A.C.(1948).Studies on the origin and development
     of plant teratomas incited by the Crown gall bac-
     terium. Amer.J.Bot.35,511.

59. Braun,A.C.(1951).Recovery of tumor cells from effects of
     the tumor-inducing principle in Crown gall.
     Science 113,651.

60. Petit, A., J.Tourneur(1972) Perte de virulence associée
     à la perte d'une activité enzymatique chez Agrobac-
     terium tumefaciens. C.R. Acad.Sc.série D(Paris)
     275,137.

61. Lippincott, J.A.,R.Beiderbeck, B.B. Lippincott(1973)
     Utilization of octopine and nopaline by Agrobacterium.
     J.Bact. 116,378.

62. Hamilton, R.H., M.Z.Fall(1971). The loss of tumor-initiat-
     ing ability in Agrobacterium tumefaciens by incubation
     at high temperature. Experientia 27,229.

63. Larebeke, N.van, G.Engler, M.Holster, S.v.d.Elsacker,
     I.Zaenen, R.A.Schilperoort, J.Schell. Direct evidence
     indicating that the presence of a large plasmid in
     Agrobacterium tumefaciens strains is essential to the
     Crown gall inducing ability of such strains. Nature
     (to be published).

64. Bomhoff, G.H. (manuscript in preparation).

THE ROLE OF PLASMIDS IN CROWN-GALL FORMATION BY

A.TUMEFACIENS

J. Schell

Laboratorium voor Genetika - R.U.G.

Ledeganckstraat, 35 - GENT - Belgium

I. INTRODUCTION

The gram-negative bacterium <u>Agrobacterium</u> <u>tumefa-</u>
<u>ciens</u> induces crown-gall tumours in many, mostly dico-
tyledonous, plants. Once the tumour induction has taken
place, the autonomous proliferation of the tumour cells
becomes independent of the bacteria since no bacteria
can be detected intracellularly in plant cells that are
being transformed or in the cells of sterile crown-gall
tumours grown in vitro (1). These facts led Braun (2)
to introduce the concept of a Tumor Inducing Principle
(TIP) that would be transferred from the bacteria to
the plant cell thus producing the neoplasmic transformation.
There can be little doubt that the chemical nature of
the TIP is a nucleic acid and probably DNA since one
has demonstrated base sequence similarities between DNA
from <u>A.tumefaciens</u> and crown-gall DNA (3). Recently
however (4) one has observed crown-gall formation induced by RNA fractions. The difficulty in accepting that
these RNA fractions are indeed the TIP resides in the
fact that they can be extracted both from tumor-forming
(oncogenic) and non-oncogenic strains! Certainly more
work will be required to make sure that no artefacts
are involved in these observations.
The main aim of the work to be reported here was
to investigate the real nature of the TIP present in
<u>A.tumefaciens</u>.In our opinion the best way to solve this
problem is to look for a DNA fraction that is present in

oncogenic strains and absent in non-oncogenic strains.
In a very general way one can think of three different
DNA fractions that can be present in any bacterium and
that could carry the TIP in A.tumefaciens : 1° Chromosomal DNA, 2° prophage DNA and 3° plasmid DNA. Since it
should, in theory, be possible to cure A.tumefaciens
strains of possible prophages and, or plasmids, we decided to use the following approach. If either prophage
DNA or plasmid DNA carries the genetic information for
the TIP it should be possible to obtain stable avirulent derivates from oncogenic strains by eliminating
these extrachromosomal elements and subsequently it
should be possible to restore the tumor-inducing capacity of such avirulent derivates merely by reintrodu-
cing either the prophage or the plasmid DNA in their
cells.

II. THE POSSIBLE ROLE OF TEMPERATE PHAGES

        Already in 1927, (5) and with renewed interest
since the discovery of temperate phages in A.tumefaciens
(6), phages have been implicated in crown-gall induction.
Especially the observation that phages can be isolated
from sterile crown-gall tissue (7)(8) and the claim that
free DNA from phage PS8 (a phage reportedly isolated from
crown-gall tissue) induces tumour formation after wounding (9) formed the basis for the hypothesis that an inducible prophage, present in A.tumefaciens strains, would
be the carrier of the TIP.
        In order to investigate this possibility we (10)
set out to make a survey of lysogeny in Agrobacterium.
This work confirmed and extended previous work (11)(12)
(13) suggesting that lysogeny is indeed widespread in
Agrobacterium both in virulent and avirulent strains.
Moreover this work showed that different types of prophages could be detected in these strains.
1° Inducible plaque-forming phages : PB6, PB2A, PV-1
    (LV-1) and PS8 were found to have an identical host-
    range, morphology, anti-serum sensitivity and genome
    size. Moreover hybridization experiments by the he-
    teroduplex method and electron microscopy showed a
    100 % homology between these four phage genomes.
    These results are in agreement with those obtained
    independently by De Ley et al. (14) by DNA : DNA
    hybridisation studies. All these phages are there-
    fore very closely related with the original Ω phage
    described by Beardsley (6) and it is important to
    state that up to now no unrelated plaque-forming
    phages have been discovered in Agrobacterium. However

this could very well be due to the absence of suitable
indicator strains for such phages.

2° Inducible non-plaque forming phages with biological
   activity

With biological activity we mean in this case that
induction lysates are able to kill but not to replicate extensively on a number of indicator strains.
Such activities were found in the A.tumefaciens
strain 396 and in the A.radiobacter strains 8149 and
0362. By the electron microscope negative staining
technique this biological activity was found to be
due to phage like particles.

Based on particle morphology, genome size and the
absence of the formation of heteroduplex molecules it
can be concluded that these phage particles are unrelated and are different from the PB6 (Ω) type phages.

3° Inducible phage-like particles with no measurable
   biological activity were shown to occur in quite a
large number of strains. These could be grouped into
different classes, none of which showed any ressem-
blance to the PB6 type phages.

It is especially important here to note that none of
the phage types discovered thus far can be found in
all the oncogenic A.tumefaciens strains.

     The next step in our study of the possible role of
PB6 (Ω) like prophages in crown-gall formation consisted in attemps to eliminate the prophage from oncogenic
strains. We used two different strains : 1° the weak
oncogenic strain B2A and the highly oncogenic strain B6.
Both contain very similar, inducible, plaque-forming
phages (PB6 and PB2A). Using successive treatments with
U.V. and mitomycin C we (15) succeeded in both cases to
isolate 50 independent derivates that were now sensitive to all the known Ω like phages (PB6 - PB2A - LV-1
and PS8) and that did not produce any Ω-like phage particles upon induction. We can therefore assume that
these phage-sensitive derivates (called B6S and B2AS)
are effectively cured of their Ω-like prophage. Genetic
markers were used to make sure that the B6S and B2AS
strains were isogenic with the parent B6 and B2A strains
and the possibility of contaminants could thus be excluded.

Just as for the previously described phage sensitive
derivates of strain B6, namely B6-806 (6) and V1-C(16)
it turned out that all the B6S and B2AS strains were
exactly as oncogenic as their parent strains. Moreover
lysogenisation of strain B6S with phage PB2A and strain
B2AS with phage PB6 or PS8 (remember that B6 is highly
oncogenic and B2A very weakly oncogenic) did not alter

the oncogenicity of these strains. All these observations
together definitely exclude any possible role of active
phage particles in the tumorigenic process. However the
possibility still existed that the so-called cured
strains B6-806, V1-C, B6S and B2AS were not really completely cured of their Ω-like prophage but now in fact
contained a defective Ω-like prophage. Several indirect
lines of observations pointed to that possibility, the
most convincing one being our discovery (10) that all
of these Ω-phage sensitive derivates of strain B6 will
yield phage-like particles upon prolonged incubation
with mitomycin C. These phage particles are completely
defective in the sense that no biological activity what-
soever can be associated with them. One can only observe
them in lysates by electron microscopy after negative
staining. These defective particles were purified by den-
sity-gradient centrifugation and their DNA was characterized. It turned out that all the defective phages from the
various sensitive strains called PB6-806, PB2AS, PB6S,
PV1-C had an identical particle morphology. The genome
size of PB6-806 was found to be 12.2 mµ as compared with
22.4 mµ for PB6. Furthermore no heteroduplex molecules
could be detected between DNA from a deletion mutant of
PB6 and DNA from PB6-806 indicating that there is no homology between these phages. The conclusion therefore is
that strain B6 is in fact bilysogenic in that it carries
two unrelated prophages : PB6 (or Ω) and PB6S (the defective prophage). The PB6 sensitive strains such as B6S
only carry one (the defective) prophage and hence it can
safely be concluded that the Ω-like phages such as PB6-
PB2A - PS8 and LV-1 are not involved in crown-gall formation.

       Experiments are in progress to try to cure strain
B6S of its defective prophage. However the fact that a
phage particle cannot be detected in many A.tumefaciens
strains would tend to rule out the possibility that this
prophage is involved in tumor formation. Possibly the
most direct evidence for the role of phage PS8 in crown-
gall formation came from the work of Schilperoort et al.
(17) who found PS8 DNA sequences in sterile crown-gall
tissue. Recently however this group of investigators have
discovered (18) that although the reaction between PS8
cRNA and crown-gall DNA appeared to be quite specific,
it was in fact due to some sort of artefact since the
hybrid molecules appear to be the result of an hybridisation between PS8 cRNA and RNA molecules present in
crown-gall DNA preparations. Taking into account all of
this evidence and also the fact that Beiderbeck et al.
(19) were unable to confirm Leff and Beardsley's (9)
observations claiming crown-gall formation by purified

PS8 DNA, it can be stated that there is no evidence indicating that Ω-like phages such as PS8 are involved in
crown-gall formation and that there is good evidence
that this is definitely not the case.

III. THE ROLE OF A LARGE PLASMID

III.A. Detection and isolation of a large plasmid in
    A.tumefaciens strains

The presence of supercoiled circular DNA plasmids
in A.tumefaciens strains could be demonstrated in a
variety of ways (20).

1°) Alkaline sucrose gradient centrifugation

Cells with (^{3}H) labelled DNA were lysed in 0.8 M
NaOH and 1 % sodium dodecyl sulphate. The crude lysate was sheared to reduce the chromosomal DNA to
small fragments and was subjected to zone centrifugation in an alkaline sucrose gradient (5 % to 20 %
linear sucrose gradients with 0.5 M NaCl, 0.02 M
EDTA and 0.3 M NaOH were used).
It is known that under these conditions closed circular DNA molecules sediment three to four times
faster than linear DNA. As can be seen from fig. I
a rapidly sedimenting peak was obtained when B6S
cells were extracted but no such peak could be observed in A.radiobacter S1005 cells.

2°) Dye-buoyant density centrifugation

In order to confirm these results and also to be
able to isolate the plasmid DNA for electron microscopic examination dye-buoyant density equilibrium
centrifugation was used. A neutral lysis procedure
had to be used (see (20)) and again shearing resulting in a selective fragmentation of the chromosomal DNA, had to be used in order to obtain reproducible results.
Fig. 2 shows that both ethidium bromide and propidium iodide could be used to separate the fast
sedimenting supercoiled plasmid DNA from the chromosomal DNA; The best resolution was obtained using
propidium iodide. The fractions under the heavy
peak were pooled, dialyzed against 1 M-ammonium
acetate and examined under the electron microscope.
As was expected double-stranded DNA molecules were
seen, mostly as supercoils. By freezing and thawing
the supercoiled circles could be transformed to
open-circles (plate 1) as a result of single strand
breaks.

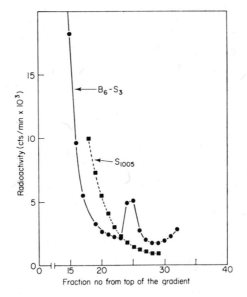

Fig. 1 : Alkaline sucrose sedimentation profile of the
         DNA from a crude lysates of Agrobacterium
         strains
              ● - ● : strain B6S (A.tumefaciens)
              ■ --■ : strain S1005 (A.radiobacter)

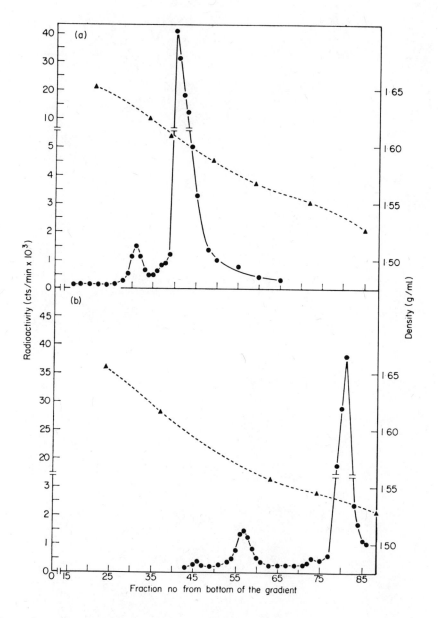

<u>Fig. 2</u> : Dye-buoyant density profiles of the DNA from
crude lysates of strain B6S
a) Caesium chloride/ethidium bromide
b) Caesium chloride/propidium iodide

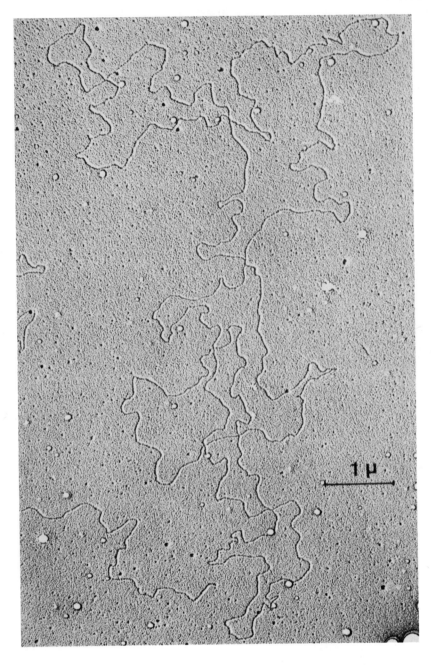

<u>Plate I</u> : Electron micrograph of a plasmid molecule in
the open circular form isolated by CsCl/ethi-
dium bromide from strain B6S.

3°) Neutral sucrose gradient centrifugation

        Since the observed plasmid turned out to be very
large it could be expected that one would be able
to separate them from sheared chromosomal DNA simply
by centrifugation of the crude lysate through a
neutral sucrose gradient. Fig. 3 shows that this
indeed was the case. Since these neutral sucrose
gradients yielded more reproducible results than the
alkaline gradients, this method was used for screening
other bacterial strains for the presence of large plasmids.

III.B. Arguments in favour of the hypothesis that plasmid
        DNA is involved in the tumor-inducing capacity of
        A.tumefaciens strains

     III.B.1. Comparison of oncogenic and non-oncogenic
               Agrobacterium strains
        Based on extensive studies performed by De Ley's
group (see the contribution of Prof. Dr. J. De Ley in
this book) it is known that all A.tumefaciens (oncogenic) and A.radiobacter (non-oncogenic) strains belong
to two large groups and a few minor ones. Each of this
groups contain closely related oncogenic and non-oncogenic strains. Furthermore all A.rhizogenes strains fall
into a third large group.
Both oncogenic and non-oncogenic strains from each of
these groups were tested for the presence of a large
plasmid. As can be seen from the results summarized in
table I, all of the crown-gall inducing strains did contain a large plasmid whereas none of the avirulent
strains did. Furthermore it can be seen from table II
that the mean contour length of the plasmid in various
strains varied from 46.3 mµ to 75.4 mµ and that in some
instances a given strain contained two plasmid populations with a different mean length (strain 925).
     III.B.2. Curing of the plasmid
        Direct evidence indicating that the presence of the
large plasmid in A.tumefaciens strains is essential to
the crown-gall inducing ability of such strains were obtained by showing that there was a 100 % correlation
between curing of the plasmid and loss of tumour inducing capacity.
        From Dr. A.C. Braun we obtained the crown-gall in-
ducing A.tumefaciens strain IIB and its derivative
IIBNV6 which is a stable, non reverting non tumorigenic
strain isolated from strain IIB as a single colony. It
turned out that strain IIB contained a large plasmid

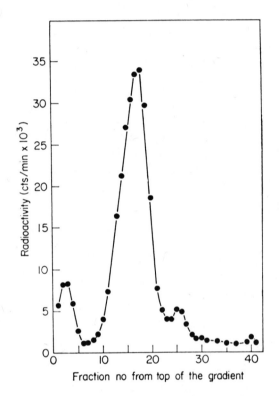

<u>Fig. 3</u> : Neutral sucrose sedimentation profile of the
          DNA of a lysate from a B6S culture.

TABLE I
SOURCE AND PROPERTIES OF THE W.T. BACTERIAL STRAINS USED

SPECIES	STRAIN	CLUSTER (De Ley, 1971)	LYSOGENIC for		Phage detected by E.M.	Pathogenicity	Presence of plasmid
			Ω-type prophage	other			
A tumefaciens	B6	B6	+	-	+	+	+
" "	B2A	B6	+	-	+	+	+
"	11158	B6	-	-	+	+	+
A radiobacter	S 1005	B6	-	-	(•)	-	-
"	TR 1	B6	-	-	+	-	-
"	4718	B6	-	-	-	-	-
A tumefaciens	TT 111	TT 111	-	-	(•)	+	+
" "	A6	TT111	-	-	(•)	+	+
" "	396	TT111	-	+	+	+	+
A radiobacter	8149	TT111	-	+	+	-	-
" "	417	TT111	(•)	(•)	(•)	-	-
A species	0362	0362	-	+	+	+	+
" "	0363	0362	-	-	(•)	-	-
A radiobacter	M2/1	M2/1	-	-	(•)	-	-
A rubi	TR-2	TR-2	-	-	(•)	+	+
A rhizogenes	Kerr 38	rhizogenes	-	-	(•)	+	+
A tumefaciens	3/1	3/1	(•)	(•)	(•)	+	+
" "	RV3	3/1	-	-	(•)	-	-
" "	925	925	-	-	+	+	+
(•) not examined							

For the origin and classification of the
strains used see De Ley et al. (1973)
J. Gen. Microbiol. 78, 241-252.

TABLE II
CONTOUR LENGTHS OF PLASMID DNA IN
A.tumefaciens STRAINS

STRAIN	N° of molecules		mean length (μ) ± S.D.	M.W. ± S.D. (megadalton)
B$_6$-S$_3$	36		54.1 ± 3.1	112.0 ± 6.4
B$_2$A	55		59.1 ± 3.6	122.3 ± 7.5
B$_2$A-S	31		57.0 ± 3.3	118.0 ± 6.8
TT111	35		57.6 ± 2.2	119.2 ± 4.6
Kerr 38	6		71.0 ± 1.2	147.0 ± 2.5
3/1	12		65.0 ± 1.0	134.6 ± 2.1
925	Plasmid I	6	64.3 ± 1.6	133.1 ± 3.3
	Plasmid II	7	46.3 ± 0.9	95.8 ± 1.9
396	5		75.4 ± 2.9	156.1 ± 6.0
ID 135 AO	9		63.0 ± 1.1	130.4 ± 2.3

The plasmid DNA molecules were isolated by
neutral sucrose gradient centrifugation.
The molecular weight estimate given in the
last column was calculated assuming that a
double-stranded DNA molecule has a M.W. of
207×10^4 per mμ length.

whereas no such plasmid could be demonstrated in strain
IIBNV6. Furthermore it had been reported (21) that two
A.tumefaciens strains C58 and ACH-5 could be made to
irreversibly loose their tumour-initiating ability by
incubation at high temperature. An extensive study
showed that in our hands most strains and in particular
B6 strains do not loose their tumour-initiating ability
by growth at 37°C, however we were able to confirm that
indeed the C58 and ACH-5 strains were exceptional and
very readily irreversibly lost their tumour-initiating
ability by growth at 37°C (22). Both strain C58 and
strain ACH-5 were shown to harbor a large plasmid (22).
In order to obtain independently isolated avirulent derivatives and to check the reproducibility of the conversion to avirulence, strains C58 and ACH-5 were stre-
aked out for single colonies and incubated for 5 days
at 37°C. In total 150 colonies were tested for tumour
induction on wounded seeds of Pisum sativum and all
proved to be avirulent ! A total of 12 avirulent colonies were cultured at 28°C and their DNA analysed on
neutral sucrose gradients. All 12 were found to have
lost the large plasmid present in the parental strains!
It is important to note here that with strains B6 and
B6S the same experiments yielded neither avirulent
strains nor curing of the plasmid. One could of course
argue that loss of tumor initiating ability and loss of
the plasmid are two unrelated events both brought about
by growth at 37°C. If this were the case one would expect that under conditions where neither the curing of
the plasmid nor the conversion to avirulence would
have occurred for the totality of the population, one
would find some bacteria for which only one of these
events would have taken place.

   In order to realize these conditions we studied separately the kinetics of appearance of avirulence and
of plasmid free C58 bacteria in a culture grown at 37°C.
The cells were cultured for a total of 38 generations
at 37°C by repeated dilutions into fresh broth. At
various intervals the cells were plated out for single
colonies and these were tested on pea-seedlings for
crown-gall formation. Both virulent and avirulent colonies were thus found. In all cases the virulent strains
turned out to contain the plasmid whereas all the avirulent derivatives had lost the plasmid. From all these
experiments it can safely be concluded that both the
loss of virulence and the loss of the plasmid are 100 %
correlated and hence that the presence of the plasmid
is essential to the cell's ability to initiate tumor
formation.

III.B.3.Other phenotypes determined by the plasmid

III.B.3.a. Sensitivity to agrocins

Recently (23)(24) one has observed that some avirulent A.radiobacter strains can effectively kill a number
of oncogenic strains by the production of bacteriocins.
Not all A.radiobacter strains produce agrocins and not
all A.tumefaciens strains are sensitive to such bacteriocins. We have studied two particular strains : strain
84 (23) and strain S1005 (24). Kerr and Htay (23) have
made the very interesting observation that when a bacte-
riocin-sensitive oncogenic strain is exposed to the
bacteriocin of strain 84, mutant colonies can be selected
that are resistant to the action of the bacteriocin.
These agrocin 84 resistant colonies however turned out
to have irreversibly lost their tumor-initiating ability.
We have repeated and confirmed these author's observations for a number of sensitive A.tumefaciens strains
such as C58 and Kerr 14. It occured to us (25) that a
possible explanation for this phenomenon could be as
follows : if both the tumour-initiating ability and the
factor(s) determining agrocin 84 sensitivity of A.tume-
faciens strains were controlled by genes located on the
large plasmid present in these strains, curing of the
plasmid would result both in irreversible avirulence
and bacteriocin 84 resistance. That this was indeed the
case for strain C58 was demonstrated in different ways :
1°) Curing of the plasmid of stain C58 by growth at 37°C
    resulted in all cases in the simultaneous loss of
    oncogenicity and bacteriocin 84 sensitivity. The
    plasmid free strains thus obtained were all resis-
    tant to the agrocin 84 although they had never been
    in contact with this bacteriocin.
2°) Eight independently isolated bacteriocin resistant
    colonies of strain C58 were obtained by picking a
    surviving colony from each of 8 independent cultures
    of C58 plated on a minimal medium agar plate seeded
    with agrocin 84. Each of these colonies was tested
    for oncogenicity on pea seedlings and its DNA was
    analysed on neutral sucrose gradients and on caesium
    chloride ethidium bromide dye-buoyant density gra-
    dients.
    All eight of these agrocin 84 resistant colonies
    turned out to be non-oncogenic and to be devoid of
    a large plasmid. Analogous experiments were also
    performed using A.radiobacter S1005 strain as the
    bacteriocinogenic strain and A.tumefaciens B6 and
    B6S3 as the bacteriocin-sensitive strains. In this
    case the bacteriocin S1005 resistant colonies of
    strain B6 and B6S3 were neither avirulent (in fact
    they were as highly oncogenic as the parent bacte-

riocin-sensitive strains) nor had they lost the
large plasmid.

It is therefore obvious that the sensitivity to
the agrocins 84 and S1005 is not due to an identical mechanism and that only the sensitivity to
the agrocin 84 is closely associated with the tumor-
initiating properties of the A.tumefaciens plasmids.

III.B.3.b. Exclusion of phage AP-1

It is known that in E.coli certain plasmids can prevent the development of certain phages either by causing
cell surface changes that prevent phage adsorbtion or
by inhibiting phage growth (exclusion) or by inducing
specific restriction endonucleases that break down the
unmodified phage DNA.

It was therefore conceivable that the plasmid present in
A.tumefaciens strains would have a similar effect. Thus
one could hope to find a phage that would grow normally
on plasmid free Agrobacterium strains but not on plasmid
containing strains. Such a phage would be extremely useful since it would provide a selective advantage for
plasmid containing strains. In order to find such a phage
it was decided to enrich phages present in soil water on
a C58 strain cured of its plasmid (this strain will be
calles C58.C9). Several different plaque-types were thus
found, plaque purified on C58.C9 and subsequently plated
on the isogenic plasmid containing C58 strain.

One phage, called AP-1, was found to be unable to form
plaques on the C58 indicator (26). At high multiplicities
of infection the AP-1 phage lyses both C58 and C58.C9
indicator lawns, but plaques are only found on the plasmid free C58.C9 strains.

A preliminary survey indicated that this AP-1 phage can
adsorb to most Agrobacterium strains but will only form
plaques on strains devoid of a plasmid (e.g. A.radio-
bacter S1005).

A further strong indication that phage AP-1 is excluded
by plasmid specific functions can be found in the fact
that the phage does not form plaques on Agrocin 84
sensitive strains but will form plaques on the agrocin
84 resistant mutants derived from such strains.

III.B.3.c. Catabolism of nopaline

It has been observed that the arginine derivatives
octopine and nopaline are present in crown-gall cells
only (for a discussion see R. Schilperoort's contribution in this book "The nature of the tumor inducing
principle elaborated by A.tumefaciens").

The presence in the crown-gall tissue of one of the
other amino acid derivative was found to be independent
of the plants species in which crown-gall was induced.

It would appear that whether octopine or nopaline will
be present in crown-gall tissue depends on the A.tume-
faciens strains used to induce the tumor. The striking
fact is that when a given A.tumefaciens strain induces
the formation of octopine but not nopaline in crown-gall
tissue, that bacterial strain will be able to use octopine but not nopaline as sole source of nitrogen. The
reverse is also true for nopaline inducing A.tumefaciens
strains. C58 is a nopaline inducing strain and it can
grow on nopaline as a sole source of nitrogen. Schilperoort (personal communication) has found that plasmid
cured strains such as C58.C9 are no longer able to catabolize nopaline.

IV. GENERAL DISCUSSION

We have presented evidence indicating that the tumour-
initiating ability of A.tumefaciens strains is not correlated with the presence in these bacteria of Ω (PS8) like
prophages but does very definitely depend on whether or
not these bacteria harbor a large plasmid. A logical
explanation for this observation would be that the plasmid DNA carries Tumour inducing genes and that these
genes can be transferred from the bacteria to the plant
genome, thus causing a neoplasmic transformation. Our
observations do not, at this point, allow any definite
conclusion since it is quite possible that the role of
the plasmid would only be a secondary one, e.g. that the
plasmid would play an essential role in promoting the
transfer of the TIP from the bacteria to the plant cells.
Further experiments are in progress to explain the role
of plasmid DNA in crown-gall formation, such as
1°) Hybridisations between crown-gall DNA ans plasmid
    DNA, to test whether plasmid DNA sequences are in-
    corporated and replicated in transformed plant cells
    (In collaboration with R. Schilperoort)
2°) Transfer of the plasmid DNA from virulent to aviru-
    lent bacterial strains, to test whether non-plasmid
    functions play a role in the tumor-initiating
    mechanism
3°) Isolation of plasmid mutants that can no longer pro-
    mote tumor initiation. A study of such mutants can
    indicate which gene(s) of the plasmid are essential
    for its tumor-initiating ability.
There is however already one observation that suggest
that plasmid DNA is indeed transferred to the plant
cells and is expressed in crown-gall cells. Since the
genes controlling the catabolism (and possibly also

the synthesis) of the typical arginine derivative present in crown-gall tissues : nopaline (and possibly
also octopine) have been shown to be located on the
plasmid DNA, it is conceivable that the synthesis in
the crown-gall cells of these guanidine derivatives is
in fact controlled by plasmid genes. It is this possibility which, in our opinion, offers the main interest
of our work. Indeed this would be the first documented
case whereby an extrachromosomal element belonging to
one type of cellular organisation as an autonomous
plasmid (the bacterium) can be taken up by another
cellular system (the plant cell) and cause the transformation of the latter.

The possibilities for genetic manipulations with
plant materials should be obvious. In particular we can
think of isolating a mutant plasmid that can be transferred to plant cells without causing a neoplasmic
transformation. Various genes of interest could be introduced in this plasmid and thus possibly be stably
transferred to the plant cells.

REFERENCES

1. Stonier, T. (1956). Radioautographic evidence for
        the inter cellular location of crown-gall bac-
        teria. Amer. J. Botany 43, 647.
2. Braun, A.C. (1947). Thermal studies on the factors
        responsible for tumor initiation in crown-gall.
        Amer. J. Botany 34, 234.
3. Schilperoort, R.A., Veldstra, H., Warnaar, S.O.,
        Mulder, G. and Cohen, J.A. (1967). Formation
        of complexes between DNA isolated from tobacco
        crown-gall tumors and RNA complementary to Agro-
        bacterium tumefaciens DNA. Biochim. Biophys.
        Acta 145, 523.
4. Beljanski, M., Aaron-Da Cunha, M.I., Beljanski, M.S.,
        Manigault, P. and Bourgarel, P. (1974). Isola-
        tion of the Tumor Inducing RNA from Oncogenic
        and non-oncogenic A.tumefaciens. Proc. Nat.
        Acad. Sci. U.S.A. 71, 1585.
5. Israilsky, W.P. (1927). Bacteriophagie und Pflanzen
        krebs. II. Zentrallblatt für Bakteriologie, Pa-
        rasitenkunde und Infektionskrankheiten, Jena,
        Abt. II 71, 302.
6. Bearsley, R.E. (1955). Phage production by crown-gall
        bacteria and the formation of plant tumors.
        American Naturalist 89, 175.
7. Parsons, C.L. and Beardsley, R.E. (1968). Bacterio-
        phage activity in homogenate of crown-gall tissue.
        J. Virol. 2, 651.

8. Tourneur, J. and Morel, G. (1970). Sur la présence de phages dans les tissus de crown-gall cultivés in vitro. Comptes rendus de l'Académie des Sciences, Paris, _270_, 2810.

9. Leff, J. and Beardley, R.E. (1970). Action tumorigène de l'acide nucléique d'un bacteriophage dans les cultures de tissus tumoral de tournesol. Comptes rendus de l'Académie des Sciences, Paris, _270_, 2505.

10. Vervliet, G., Holsters, M., Teuchy, H., Van Montagu, M. and Schell, J. (1974). Characterisation of different plaque-forming and defective temperate phages in Agrobacterium strains. J. Gen. Virology : submitted.

11. Stonier, T. (1960). _Agrobacterium tumefaciens_ Conn. I. Release of P^{32} and S^{35} by labeled bacteria in vitro. J. Bacteriol., _79_, 880.

12. Zimmerer, R.P., Hamilton, R.H. and Pootjes, C.F. (1966). Isolation and morphology of temperate _A.tumefaciens_ phages. J. Bacteriol., _92_, 746.

13. Holsters, M. (1970). Een onderzoek over getemperde bakteriofagen bij Agrobacterium. Thesis, Universiteit Gent, Belgium.

14. De Ley, J., Gillis, M., Pootjes, C.F., Kersters, K., Tijtgat, R. and Van Brakel, M. (1972). Relationship among temperate _Agrobacterium_ phage genomes and coat proteins. J. Gen. Virol. _16_, 199.

15. Holsters, M., Van den Elsacker, S., Engler, G. and Schell, J., Unpublished results.

16. Brunner, M. and Pootjes, C.F. (1969). Bacteriophage release in a lysogenic strain of _A.tumefaciens_. J. Virol. _3_, 181.

17. Schilperoort, R.A., Van Sittert, H.J. and Schell, J. (1973). The presence of both phage PS8 and _A. tumefaciens_ A6 DNA base sequences in A6-induced sterile crown-gall tissue cultured in vitro. Eur. J. Biochem. _33_, 1.

18. Schilperoort, R.A., Dons, J.J. and Ras, H. (1974). Characterization of the complex formed between PS8 cRNA and DNA isolated from A6-induced sterile crown-gall tissue. In press.

19. Beiderbeck, R., Heberlein, G.T. and Lippincott, J.A. (1973). On the question of crown-gall tumor initiation by DNA of bacteriophage PS8. J. Virol. _11_, 345.

20. Zaenen, I., Van Larebeke, N.,Teuchy, H., Van Montagu, M. and Schell, J. (1974). Supercoiled Circular DNA in crown-gall inducing Agrobacterium strains. J. Mol. Biol. _86_, 109.

21. Hamilton, R.H. and Fall, M.Z. (1971). The loss of
    tumor-initiating ability in A.tumefaciens by
    incubation at high temperature. Experientia 27,
    229.
22. Van Larebeke, N., Engler, G., Holsters, M., Van den
    Elsacker, S., Zaenen, I., Schilperoort, R.A. and
    Schell, J. (1974). Direct evidence indicating
    that the presence of a large plasmid in A.tume-
    faciens strains is essential to the crown-gall
    inducing ability of such strains. Nature, sub-
    mitted.
23. Kerr, A. and Htay, K. (1974). Biological control of
    crown-gall through bacteriocin production.
    Physiol. Plant Pathol. 4, 37.
24. Holsters, M. (1974). Unpublished results.
25. Engler, G., Holsters, M., Hernalsteens, J.P., Zaenen,
    I., Van Larebeke, N., Van Montagu, M. and Schell,
    J. (1974). Bacteriocin 84 sensitivity : a proper-
    ty of A.tumefaciens strains determined by the
    presence of a large plasmid. To be published.
26. Hernalsteens, J.P., Van Montagu, M. and Schell, J.
    (1974). Phage AP-1, a virulent phage for Agro-
    bacterium strains that is excluded by the TI
    plasmid. To be published.

GENETIC MECHANISMS IN DIFFERENTIATION

AND DEVELOPMENT

G. P. RÉDEI

Department of Agronomy, University of Missouri

117 Curtis Hall, Columbia, Mo. 65201 USA

INTRODUCTION

"In the study of most biological, biochemical, and molecular-genetic problems, just as in the study of many other scientific problems, a full analysis of the facts obtained by experimental investigation of actual phenomena can usually elucidate the mechanisms of the phenomenon, thereby eliminating the need for theoretical hypotheses." (MEDVEDEV 1970). Yet the speculations are rarely saved when genetic mechanisms of differentiation and development are considered.

Developmental genetics, after the spectacular advances in molecular biology, has become increasingly attractive. Unfortunately, this area not only lacks appropriate, versatile and unique tools of operation, there are difficulties even in defining the boundaries of the discipline.

Certainly, we would like to interpret developmental phenomena in biochemical terms. This can be easily done for simple metabolic functions. Morphogenesis is, however, the result of interacting biochemical pathways and the outcome is determined by a balance among several systems, rather by single all-or-none biochemical events. The potentiation is exercised at the chromosomal, chloroplastic or mitochondrial levels and the realization is determined by the cooperation of the genetic system and the environmental stimuli. Generally morphogenetic systems are dependent on three types of activities: cell division and growth, various sensoring operations (intelligence gathering) and determination (BONNER 1965).

Experimental approaches to these problems will be illustrated by chloroplast differentiation under primarily nuclear and nuclear-plastomic control and by experiments on flower initiation in mutants of Arabidopsis.

CHLOROPLAST DIFFERENTIATION IN THE im MUTANTS

Numerous alleles at the *im* locus are available (REDEI, CHUNG and PLURAD 1974), ROBBELEN 1968). All are characterized by a fancy pattern of white and green sectors on all organs of the plants normally green in the wild type (Figure 1). Certain mutants appear almost like albinas under continuous high intensity illumination (1000-2000 ft. candle), while others display only small white sectors when grown identically. When the duration of the daily periods of illumination is reduced to 8-9 hours and the intensity of the

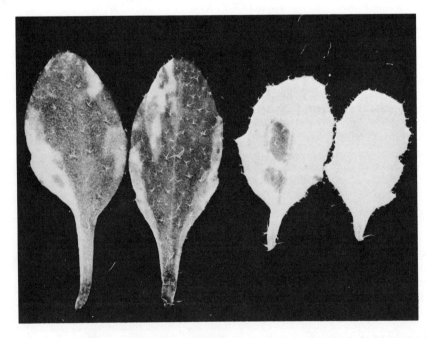

Figure 1.   Characteristic leaves of two different *im* mutants. the mutant on the left has relatively few white sectors while that on the right develops only small patches of green under identical conditions of culture.

light is kept under 500 ft candle both allelic types are difficult
to distinguish from the wild type. The red part of the spectrum
is more conducive to the development of white tissues than the blue
one (RÉDEI 1965, RÖBBELEN 1968).

The phenotype of the plants closely resembles that of various
mutable systems known in many species of plants. The condition is
inherited in a normal mendelian fashion, and the locus responsible
for the variegation was assigned to linkage group 4 by trisomic
analysis. The involvement of mutability of a chromosomal gene locus in the different expressions of a certain allele was easily
ruled out when seeds planted from green and white fruits produced
identical progenies.

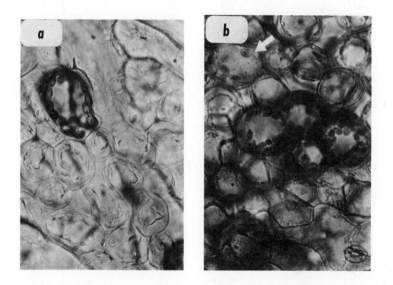

Figure 2.   Comparison of the light microscopic picture of an
            im tissue (a) with that of a plant displaying plas-
            tome segregation (b). Plastid differentiation within
            cells of *im* (a) is all-or-none in contrast to that of
            chm (b), which is functioning as a plastome mutator.
            Note the cells with mixed types of plastids (→).
            Whole leaves or smaller pieces were evacuated with
            an aspirator in water containing 20% glycerol and 4%
            formalin, then they were left for a day or more in
            the refrigerator and before mounting, the tissues were
            torn with forceps and examined under a high-dry ob-
            jective.

Light microscopic examination has shown no sorting out of altered chloroplasts. In all cells, all the plastids were either normal or abnormal (Figure 2A). In the white *im* cells the plastids
appeared shrunken and free of content.

When the plants were cultured on mineral-sugar-agar medium
under conditions unfavorable for plastid differentiation, the leaf
pigment content in the mutant was less than 10% of that of the wild
type. If the medium was made 1-2 x 10^{-5} M for 6-azauracil, pigment
production in the mutant increased 6-8 fold, approaching that of
the wild type. Azauracil feeding has practically no effect on chlorophyll and carotenoid content of the wild type (RÉDEI 1965, 1967).

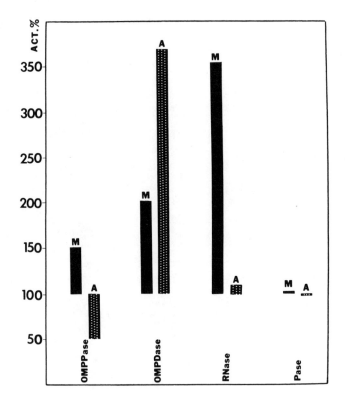

Figure 3.   Altered levels of orotidine-5'-monophosphate pyrophos-
             phorylase (OMPPase), orotidine-5'-monophosphate decar-
             boxylase (OMPDase), acidic ribonuclease (RNase), phos-
             phatase (Pase) in the mutant tissues compared to the
             wild type grown on two media; M: minimal (=100), A: aza-
             uracil medium.

The normalization of the phenotype on this antimetabolite medium indicated that the mutation is involved in a regulatory pro-

cess of RNA or pyrimidine metabolism. Direct evidence was then obtained that the RNA content, was significantly less in the mutant compared to the wild type. Furthermore, the base composition of the RNA was slightly shifted in favor of the pyrimidines.

These analytical data would be understandable if the mutant would overproduce pyrimidines and the same time would break down RNA at an accelerated rate. Overproduction of enzymes is not an uncommon phenomenon in microorganisms (DEMAIN 1971). Indeed, we found that on minimal media three enzymes are present in higher than normal amount in the mutant (CHUNG and RÉDEI 1974, RÉDEI 1967). For the sake of easy comparison enzyme activities are represented in percent of the wild type's grown on minimal media and tested simultaneously (Figure 3).

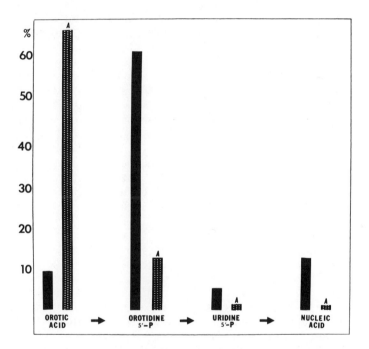

Figure 4.   Changes in substrates and products of pyrimidine synthetic enzymes and RNA in the *im* mutant as a consequence of azauracil feeding. Data are representing percent of radioactivity detectable in compounds indicated below the columns after ^{14}C-orotic acid administration to tissues produced on minimal and azauracil media (A), respectively.

Azauracil feeding reduced the level of OMPPase to almost half of that of the wild type, grown on minimal medium, in the *im* mutant. In contrast, OMPDase appeared in much larger quantities in the plants harvested from the analog medium. The synthesis of a cytoplasmic acid ribonuclease returned to approximately normal level in the azapyrimidine fed plants. Several control enzymes tested, acid phosphatase (Pase), phosphodiesterase, various nucleotidases exhibited approximately identical activities in the mutant and wild type extracts and azauracil had no appreciable effect on their activities.

Thus, azauracil feeding had some selective regulatory effect on the metabolism. The analog itself was effectively metabolized in the cells of the plants. Significant amounts were converted to azauridine-5'-monophosphate and also detectable amounts appeared in RNA as ascertained by measurement the labeling of the appropriate fractions upon ^{14}-C-azauridine administration.

Azauridylic acid is an effective inhibitor of the activity of orotidine-5'-phosphate decarboxylase (CHUNG and RÉDEI 1974), and because of the elimination of feedback inhibition the level of this enzyme can raise (Figure 3). Azauracil feeding results also in the repression of orotidine-5'-phosphate pyrophosphorylase. Thus, one would expect an accumulation of orotic acid in the plants under the conditions of azauracil feeding. We have shown, that this actually happens (Figure 4). When plant tissues were incubated with radioactive orotic acid, this compound was readily converted into orotidine-5'-P (catalyzed by OMPPase) and to uridine-5'-P (mediated by OMPDase) and within four hours even RNA became labeled. When the tissues were grown on azauracil before incubation with orotic acid, over two third of the radioactivity remained associated with the latter compound, indicating the effective block in this biosynthetic pathway.

We have mentioned earlier that due to the metabolic conditions potentiated by the *im* mutation, in the tissues of *im* plants there is an excessive amount of pyrimidines. Apparently, the feeding of azauracil hampers the overproduction of pyrimidines and thus restores the normal pyrimidine:purine ratio. One may expect that an RNA with undesirable base composition could affect adversely plastid differentiation and other functions. The presence of such an RNA has not been shown yet, however. It is also conceivable that substantial amount of a faulty RNA cannot accumulate in the cell because ribonuclease breaks it down as soon as it is formed. The high levels of RNase could be actually detected (Figure 3). There is another possibility for neutralization of the adverse effect of *im* activity by azauracil through the incorporation of the analog into RNA and making it unavailable or less suitable for certain functions. It has been shown that the cyclic phosphates of azauridine or azacytidine are inferior substrates for RNase (RÉDEI 1967a). Most likely several other enzymes are discriminating against analog-containing substrates.

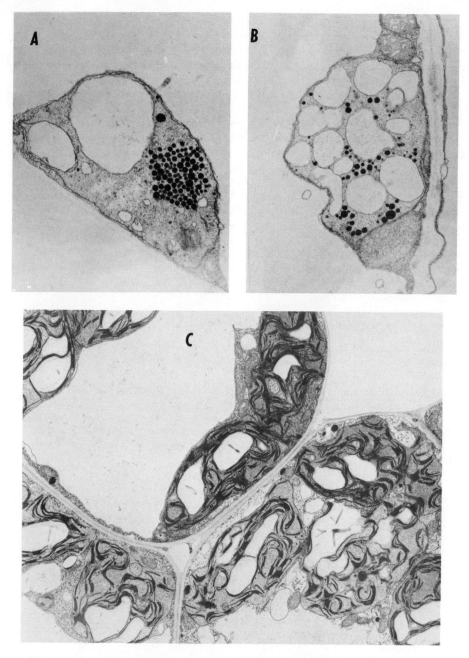

Figure 5.   Electronmicrographs of plastids in the cells
of mature leaves. The two plastids (A, B)
are typical for the white cells of *im* mutants.
Upon azauracil feeding chloroplast differentiation takes place as shown (C).

Feeding of azauracil not only brings about complex changes in the metabolism, it has a dramatic effect on the differentiation of the plastids (Figure 5). In the white cells plastid development is arrested at an early stage. The outer membrane is normal but no signs of tubuli or lamellae within this organelle. Due to the block in normal membrane development, substantial amounts of lipids accumulate as osmiophilic globuli. Characteristic is also the excessive vacuolization. Essentially all the plastids display the same phenotype and no gradations of differentiation are visible within a particular cell. In the plants fed with azauracil at a high concentration (1-2 x 10^{-5} M), two third of the cells become green after a lag period. In the green cells thus formed, the size of individual chloroplasts is larger than normal. Thylakoid structure is well developed but in contrast to the lamellae observed in the wild type (even after azauracil feeding), the internal membranes are curly, forming unusual loops and circles (Figure 5C). In spite of this structural anomaly, the chloroplasts appear to be functional. Large amounts of starch is well visible everywhere (CHUNG, RÉDEI and WHITE 1974, RÉDEI, CHUNG and PLURAD 1974).

SUMMARY

Due to mutation at a single chromosomal locus the activity of at least three enzymes is modified. The mutation thus reveals the existence of a superregulatory function, concerned with the differentiation of the internal structure of a single organelle. Azauracil by repressing the synthesis of OMPPase and RNase and inhibiting the activity and derepressing the synthesis of OMPDase restores the differentiation of the chloroplast lamellae.

CONTROL OF DIFFERENTIATION BY THE PLASTOME

Phenotypic similarity indicates very little concerning the underlying genetic mechanisms. Mutations at a chromosomal gene *chm* (linkage group 3) cause a somewhat similar variegation in the plants as induced by the *im* alleles just described.

Macroscopically the pattern on the leaves appears more intricate, and besides the white and green sectors, yellow mosaicism is also apparent. The patches frequently show gradual transitions in these mutants (Figure 6). In contrast to *im*, the *chm* mutants display cells with more than one type of plastids (Figure 2B).

Upon outcrossing the variegation was transmitted to all the progeny of the female but the reciprocal hybrids were perfectly free of the variegation in the F_1 though it reappeared in ¼ of the F_2. This pattern of transmission along with observations on cells with mixed typed of plastids indicated that the chromosomal mutation functions as a very efficient mutator of the plastome.

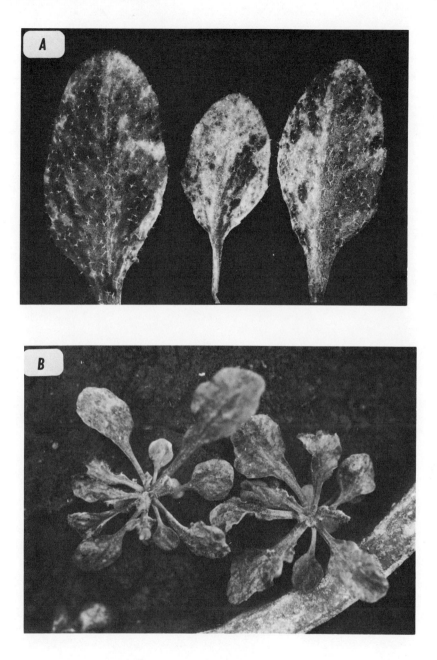

Figure 6. Leaf variegation typical for the *chm* mutants (A).
Leaf shape alterations brought about by the activity
of the *chm* mutator factor (B).

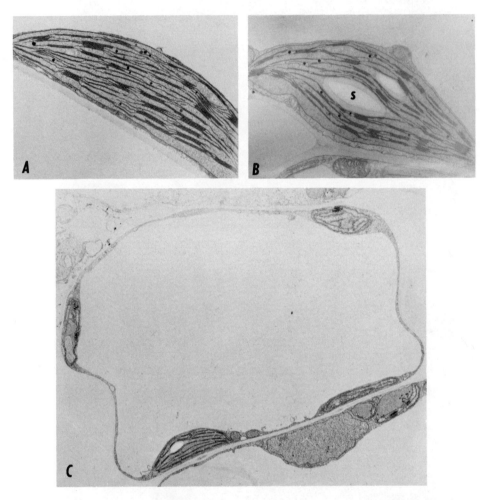

Figure 7.   Electronmicgrograph of a palisade cell with normal and
             abnormal plastids (A).   Normal chloroplasts in higher
             magnification showing some differences in the thylakoid
             arrangement depending on the presence (B) or absence (C)
             of starch (s).

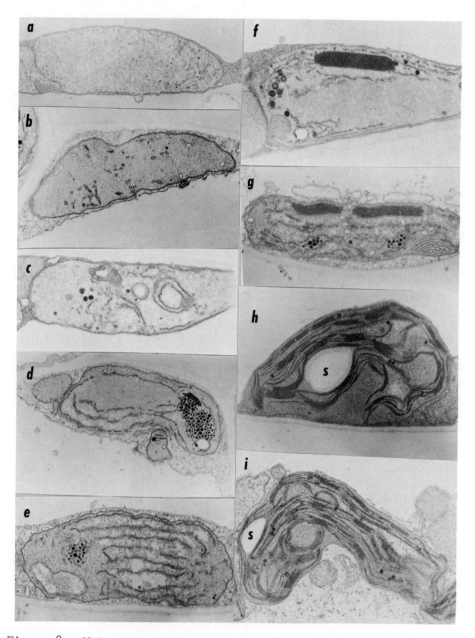

Figure 8. Mutant plastids induced by the activity of the *chm* nuclear factor on the pastome.

Electronmicroscopic examination of the mature leaves of the plants revealed a variety of different types of plastids within single cells (Figure 7a). The use of fully grown leaves for this purpose is advisable to avoid confusion of common developmental differences with genetic changes within the cells. It is not safe to say, even in these cases, that all the morphological changes observed in the plastids are due to different mutations at independent sites of the plastome. A much more reliable information on the nature of the various alterations can be obtained if the mutator is removed from the genome and through sorting out of the cytoplasmic genetic elements, homoplastidic mutant forms are isolated (RÉDEI 1973, RÉDEI and PLURAD 1973).

Due to mutations in the plastome, an almost continuous series of morphological changes are produced (Figure 8). In some plastids only the external membrane and the stroma is formed but there is no evidence for any internal structural elements (Figure 8a). In others, membrane fragments are visible (8b). There are some organelles with abnormal organization of the lamellae; rather than long straight sheets, we observe circular single or double structures (8c). In many chloroplasts the synthesis of the lamellar building blocks is apparently taking place as indicated by the darkly stained drops visible in close association (8d) yet the organization of the raw material into continuous thylakoids is interfered with. Occasionally fairly good thylakoids are formed but they fail to stack up into grana (8e) yet sometimes small starch granules are present in these structurally defective plastids. In other plastids, the few lamellae are immediately piled up into giant grana, fused into unstructured bodies (8f, g). Other mutant plastids are apparently capable of several functions as the presence of large starch (s) granules indicate (8h, i) yet the curly, sometimes circular thylakoids are certainly abnormal. There are some functional disturbances involved because in the plants with the latter types of plastids both male and female fertility is much reduced.

By repeated backcrossing females, carrying these types of abnormal yet photosynthetically functional plastids, we obtained homoplastidic mutant types, free from the mutator gene. In these plants not only the chloroplast structure was altered but there was a conspicuous morphological change of the leaves (Figure 6 B). Though the plants with the altered leaves possessed good vegetative vigor, they produced seeds only occasionally. The plants with variegated leaves frequently produce fruits even on almost white branches, and one can obtain an almost entirely pigment-free progeny which, however, cannot be maintained.

The rate of mutation induced by the mutator gene is extremely high. By the end of the their life cycle all plants produce some evidence of cytoplasmic alterations.

SUMMARY

A variety of plastid alterations can be produced by mutations in the plastome induced by a nuclear gene locus. The mutator is entirely specific for the genetic elements in this particular organelle. It seems as if the nuclear gene would be responsible for the production of a DNA polymerase requiring plastid DNA as template. This hypothetical mechanism may explain the specificity of the mutator, the variety of changes induced in the plastids and the autonomous transmission of the condition even in the absence of chm mutation (mutant template - altered chromosomal DNA - is expected to produce identical copies even in the presence of a normal polymerase, coded by chm+).

From the viewpoint of differentiation the affect of the plastome on the differentiation of leaf shape is a good indication of an integrated circuitry within the cell.

GENETIC CONTROL OF FLOWER INITIATION

Floral initiation has been for many years one of the most active area of research in plant physiology. Annually approximately 200 papers are being published (EVANS 1971), and a vast amount of information has been accumulated (LANG 1965, SCHWABE 1971). Yet the general theory of photoperiodism - if one really exists - faces multiple difficulties. Several details are well worked out but the pieces do not appear to fit together. The hypothetical flowering hormones are refractory to biochemical methods of analysis. The majority of plants used for investigations on photoperiodism are genetically unknown or even unsuitable for this type of analysis.

FLOWERING MUTANTS IN ARABIDOPSIS

Arabidopsis is a photoperiodically very sensitive facultative long-day plant. In several laboratories mutants have been obtained with qualitatively different flowering responses (REINHOLZ 1947, McKELVIE 1962, RÉDEI 1962, RÉDEI, ACEDO and GAVAZZI 1974). Obviously these monogenic mutants lend themselves better for investigations on basic mechanisms than the miscellaneous species with unknown genetic background, widely used.

Our studies have been focused primarily on three loci. Mutants at the *gi* locus require several times as long periods as the wild type for flower initiation under continuous illumination. Under such a light regime, these mutants appear as giant types (Figure 9). Under 8-9 hours daily illumination the differences between mutants and the wild type is much reduced, however. The

two alleles gi^1 and gi^2 are distinctly different. Allele gi^2 is
temperature-sensitive; it flowers much faster at 28 C^o than at 22
(Figure 10).

Mutants at the *1d* locus are not so late as gi^2 under long days
but they are unable to flower under 8-9 hours daily light periods.

The *co* mutants are distinctly later than the wild type in long
days and definitely earlier than the latter under short days. They
display dominance reversal: they are recessive under long days and
dominant under short days. The other mutants are recessive under
both short and long days.

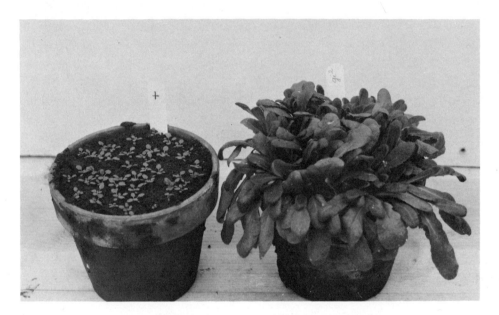

Figure 9.   Columbia wild type (left) and the gi^2 mutant (right)
            grown under continuous illumination at the beginning of
            the appearance of the visible flower buds. The gi^2
            plants are older in days but they are in the same de-
            velopmental stage as the wild type.

The generally accepted view of plant physiologists is that in
photoperiodically sensitive plants light is necessary for flower
initiation in both long- and short-day species (LANG 1965). In
general, Arabidopsis does not have a 'critical daylength', i.e. the
majority of the ecotypes can flower eventually even under 4-5 hours
daily light periods (LAIBACH 1951). Mutations at the *1d* locus are
exceptional, however, since they definitely require long-days if
they are grown under illumination.

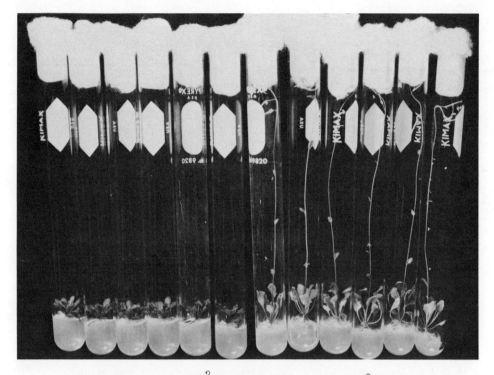

Figure 10.   Flowering in gi^2 at 22 (left) and 28 C^o under long days.

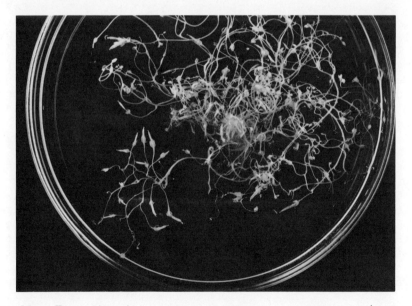

Figure 11.   Flowering in continuous complete darkness in 45 days.

Interestingly, in liquid culture, containing a suitable sugar, all genotypes, including ld, readily flower in the absence of light. The flowering takes place in approximately the same span of time in darkness as required for the wild type under continuous light. If the speed of flower initiation is measured by the commonly used criteria of number of nodes formed before the development of flowers, for flowering complete darkness is more favorable than long days (RÉDEI, ACEDO and GAVAZZI 1974). Not only flower initiation but fruit and seed development can take place in the absence of light (Figure 11).

Thus, the role of light in photoperiodism is an apparent need of revision. Actually, several other short- and long-day plants are capable of flowering in the absence of light (RÉDEI, ACEDO and GAVAZZI 1974. It is obvious from the experiments with mutants of Arabidopsis that the short daily light cycles interfere with flower initiation and long cycles do not have an indispensable effect.

If we wish to use the terminology of microbial genetics, we may say that flowering is derepressed in the dark and it is under negative control in light.

FLOWER INITIATION ON BROMODEOXYURIDINE

There is an additional clue to the mechanism of the genetic control of flowering. On nutrient media containing 5-bromodeoxyuridine, 5-iododeoxyuridine or 5-bromodeoxycytidine (10^{-6} to 10^{-5} M) flowering is accelerated in several genotypes of Arabidopsis (BROWN 1962, 1968, HIRONO and RÉDEI 1966, RÉDEI, ACEDO and GAVAZZI 1974). The nucleoside analogs may reduce the time required for flowering to half or a third of the control and eliminate most of the differences between the genotypes. The ld mutants respond to the analog only under long day conditions, however. In continuous darkness the bromodeoxyuridine treatment has no appreciable effect on any genotype.

Bromodeoxyuridine is a competitive analog of thymidine. At the concentrations used, it does not have much adverse effect on the growth of the plants though root elongation is considerably less on the analog media. Since bromodeoxyuridine is an antimetabolite, its effect is expected to be based on selective interference with certain functions. The logical assumption is that bromodeoxyuridine is working against some type of flowering inhibitor. The genetic and physiological data indicate, furthermore, that there must be at least two types of regulatory compounds in the plants, involved in the repression of flowering. Mutations at the gi^2 and co loci control the synthesis of the precursors of one inhibitor or two different inhibitors. Both of these loci are receptive to bromodeoxyuridine under both short and long day conditions.

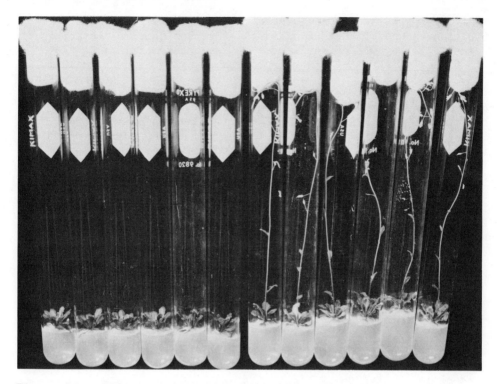

Figure 12.   Effect of bromodeoxyuridine on the flowering of the gi^2 mutant at 22 C°.   Left minimal medium, right 10^{-6} M BrdU.   Compare with figure 10.

Mutations at the ld locus make possible a response under long days but not under short days.   Thus, these mutants seem to carry a genetic defect in disposing of the inhibitor produced under short day conditions.   It should be recalled that these mutants flower early in complete darkness, thus light is not required for flowering *per se*, rather short daily light periods are conducive to inhibition of flowering.   Apparently, under prolonged illumination the inhibitor formed in light may eventually decay.   The ld locus seems to be involved in a step of the control where bromodeoxyuridine cannot release the short day inhibition.

Experiments with radioactive bromodeoxyuridine have shown that all mutants, including ld can take up the analog.   Bromodeoxyuridine may act as a light sensitizer for the compounds associated with. The analog is sensitive to short and long wave length ultraviolet and can destroy other molecules by extraction of hydrogen atoms through its decomposition products (HUTCHINSON 1973).

DNA extracted from the mutants showed that approximately 70-90 million thymine residues may be replaced by bromouracil in an

average nucleus. This constitutes at 20-30% substitution. In spite
of the high amount of the analog in the DNA, the observed effect is
non-genetic; mutagenic effectiveness of nucleoside analogs is very
low in higher plants, including Arabidopsis (HIRONO and SMITH 1969).

The most likely mechanism of action of bromodeoxyuridine is
through DNA, however, since bromouracil or bromouridine are both
ineffective in flowering. BROWN (1968, 1972) has suggested that
bromo- or iododeoxyuridine applied to the apical meristem preferentially inhibit DNA synthesis in the mitotically active cells of
the vegetative apex, forming the flank meristem (anneau initial).
Subsequently, the central initiation zone (méristème d'attente) is
activated, signaling the conversion of the vegetative apex into a
prefloral apex. Upon elimination of the analog from the cells, mitotic activity may be resumed and floral development may take thus
place. This hypothesis is supported by histoautoradiographical
observations. It seems, however, that the histological picture
reflects the consequence rather than the cause of the analog effect
(RÉDEI, ACEDO and GAVAZZI 1974).

It has been observed several years ago (SMITH 1964, OPARA-
KUBINSKA, KURYLO-BOROWSKA and SZYBALSKI 1963) that substituted DNA
has higher affinity for proteins when irradiated by UV. LIN and
RIGGS (1972) noted that the operator site of the *lac* system, containing BrdU, has much tighter binding for the repressor, especially when it is exposed to UV light (LIN and RIGGS 1974). - We have
grown Arabidopsis on ^{14}C-amino acid and ^{14}C-amino acid plus bromodeoxyuridine media. We then extracted DNA with saline-EDTA-SLS
solution and without using any protease or phenol treatment. The
'chromatin' was then precipitated with alcohol and trapped on a dacron web. The filter retained the fibrous material (DNA) but did
not bind any protein, except that bound to DNA. Actually, very
little protein remains associated with DNA under the conditions of
the extraction. Sodium lauryl sulfate splits away histones from
the nucleic acids, and really 0.4 N sulfuric acid extraction removed
practically no radioactivity from the filter, indicating that histones were not present on the dacron web. An incubation of the
extract with protease almost completely prevented the binding of
radioactivity to the filter. Thus, there could be no doubt that
the filter-bound radioactivity was in a protein associated with the
DNA.

A comparison of the BrdU and the normal chromatin revealed
a significant difference in the extent of labeling through amino
acids. Altogether about 30 determinations were made and a higher
amount of protein was invariably present in the BrdU-chromatin
(Table 1). Just as all genotypes incorporated comparable quantities of BrdU into the DNA, all exhibited higher amounts of protein
associated with the DNA when grown on the analog medium. It appeared as if younger plants would have contained somewhat more than

older ones but there was considerable variation from experiment to experiment thus this observation requires confirmation.

Table 1.   Labeling of non-histone protein(s) in normal and BrdU-
           chromatin (cpm/mg fresh weight of plants).

DNA	Source of the label	
	^{14}C- arginine	^{14}C- valine
normal	749 (100%)	815 (100%)
BrdU	1045 (140%)	1399 (172%)

Though in Arabidopsis we do not have direct evidence concerning the role of the tightly bound protein, in mouse fibroblasts BrdU-chromatin has a much reduced template activity (HILL, TSUBOI and BASERGA 1974). This piece of information, together with the reports that in the presence of BrdU several enzymes are synthesized at a lower level (STELLWAGEN and TOMKINS 1971, PRASAD, MANDAL and KUMAR 1973, TOMIDA, KOYAMA and ONO 1974, WALTHER et al. 1974), gives useful clues to the mechanism of action of bromodeoxyuridine on flowering. It seems that a non-histone protein has a tighter than normal binding to BrdU-DNA and thus selectively prevents the transcription of part of the genome. On the basis of experiments discussed above, the conclusion was made that flowering is under negative control in light. Thus it seems that in the presence of BrdU in the DNA the transcription of the flowering repressor may be hampered.

SUMMARY

   Flower differentiation in Arabidopsis is mediated through a series of gene loci. Though this is a long-day plant by the definition of classical plant physiology, light is not required for flowering in any of the genotypes studied. Short periods of daily illumination generate some unidentified flowering suppressor(s) which may, however, decay upon prolonged exposure to light. In light, the DNA nucleoside analog may interfere with the production of the flowering inhibitors(s), possibly through the prevention of transcription of the genome containing the analog. A non-histone type of protein has been shown to accumulate on BrdU-DNA of Arabidopsis.

CONCLUSIONS

   Differentiation and development can be potentiated by nuclear and organelle genetic systems. In the determination and the re-

gulation of morphogenesis and development genetic and epigenetic mechanisms seem to cooperate. The realization of differentiation seems to require selective synthesis or activation of proteins. At the moment no single detailed theory can account for the variety of mechanisms involved in these processes.

ACKNOWLEDGEMENT - Contribution from the Missouri Agricultural Experiment Station. Journal Series Number 7061. Approved by the Director.

TECHNIQUES

CULTURE OF PLANTS

Seeds were planted on the surface of soil of sufficient drainage and watered with a fine mist with the aid of superfine nozzles (Fogg-It Nozzle Co., Box 1752, Oakland 4, Calif. 94604). Arabidopsis seed requires at least 15 min. red light for germination. - Alternatively aseptic cultures were established on mineral media (mgs/l double dist. water: NH_4NO_3 40, $M_gSO_4.7H_2O$ 20, $CaH_4(PO_4)_2 H_2O$ 20, KH_2PO_4 20, K_2HPO_4 10, $FeC_6H_5O_7.3H_2O$ 0.5) supplemented with 2% glucose or sucrose and solidified with agar, in minimal amount to prevent submersion of the seed. In the dark cultures liquid medium was used with 0.5% sugar; germination was induced with 1 hr exposure of the seed to white light after overnight imbibition. In long day cultures supplementary illumination was provided with ca. 200 ft. candle fluorescent or incandescent light. Optimal temperature for growth is 22-25 C^O.
The seed was surface desinfected for aseptic cultures with a 5% solution of $Ca(OCl)_2$ for 8 min., then rinsed 4-5 times with sterile water. Planting was done in a glove box sterilised with 70% ethanol, sprayed with a window cleaner.

MUTATION INDUCTION

10-12 kR X-rays to 24 hrs presoaked seed or 0.2% ethyl methanesulfonate, 15 hrs, followed by 3-4 hrs washing in running water were used.

LINKAGE

Studied in F_2 coupling phase and calculation by formulas of IMMER (1930), alternatively by trisomic analysis which may provide information on centromere positions (LEE-CHEN and STEINITZ-SEARS 1969) on the basis of double reduction frequency (BURNHAM 1962). Mutator genes, specific for the plastome were identified by alternative reciprocal backcross schemes (RÉDEI 1973, ROBBELEN 1966). Allelism of mutator factors, specific for the plastome was shown as given earlier (RÉDEI 1973)

RNase
*3 mg/ml yeast RNA incubated with an appropriate extract, the re-
action stopped by the addition of 3 vol. acetic acid:tertiary butanol
(1:2 v/v) on ice bath and the acid soluble O.D. was measured spec-
trophotometrically at 260 nm. (RÉDEI 1967b).*

PHOSPHATASE
*was assayed with the splitting of p-nitrophenyl phosphate, disodium
0.875 mg/ml,(fresh)in 0.2 M citrate buffer, pH 5, after 15 min. incubation the reaction was stopped with 2.5 ml 0.2 N NaOH and O.D.
determined at 400 nm (CHUNG and REDEI 1974).*

NUCLEOTIDASES
*were incubated with appropriate substrates (2mg/ml pH 7.5 Tris
buffer) and with enzyme extracts previously heated to 60 C^o for
10 min. to inactivate unspecific phosphatases. The liberated
inorg P was determined by a modified Fiske and SubbaRow method,
using a sample in 3.9 ml, 0.5 ml 5 N H_2SO_4, 0.5 ml 2.5% $(NH_4)_6Mo_7
O_{24}.4H_2O$, 0.1 ml reducer (125 mgs/10 ml water) consisting of a
mixture of ground 1-amino-2-naphtol-4-sulfonic acid (0.2g), $NaHSO_3$
(1.2 g) and Na_2SO_3 (1.2 g), stored in dark, tightly stopped. After
10 min. O.D. was measured at 660 nm and compared with KH_2PO_4 standard (10^{-6} mole/ml).*

OROTIDINE-5'-MONOPHOSPHATE DECARBOXYLASE
*was assayed in the 15,000 g supernatants of tissue extracts (1g/
3 ml,pH 7.2 Tris-HCl, 0.05 N, containing sucrose, 0.25 M). 1 ml
final volume contained Tris (to 20 mM), orotidine-5'-phosphate
(to 0.02 mM and 0.02 µCi of orotidine-carboxyl-^{14}C-5' monophosphate
triammonium salt), KF (to 0.01 M) and an aliquot of the enzyme.
The incubation took place at room temperature for 10 min. in a
small weighing bottle with a shallow vial placed in the center
with 0.3-0.5 ml 3% KOH. The reaction was stopped with 0.4 ml 1 N
$HClO_4$ and after 15 hours the CO_2 absorbed by the alkali in the
center was counted in 0.1 ml aliquots with 75% efficiency in
scintillation spectrometer (CHUNG and RÉDEI 1974).*

OROTIDINE-5'-PHOSPHATE PYROPHOSPHOSPHORYLASE
*was assayed in 1 ml mixture of Tris-HC1 buffer, pH 7.2 (to 20 mM,
orotic acid-6-C^{14} (to 0.1 mM and 1 µCi), phosphoribosylpyrophos-
phate (to 0.1 mM), $MgCl_2$ (to 4 mM), yeast orotidine-5'-phosphate
decarboxylase (0.06 units) and an aliquot of plant extract containing the enzyme.*

PHOSPHODIESTERASE
*was assayed in 1 ml pH 7.2 Tris-HC1 containing 1.2 mg p-nitrophenyl-
thyminephosphate and plant extract, after 1 hour incubation it was
diluted to 6 ml with water and O.D. was measured at 400 or 540 nm
(RÉDEI 1967b).*

*All enzyme activities were expressed on protein basis determined
by the method of Lowry et al. 25-300 µg samples of protein in 1 ml
buffer or 0.01 N NaOH were mixed with 5 ml mixture, containing 100
parts 2% Na₂CO₃ and 1 part each of 1% CuSO₄ and 2.7% NaK-tartrate;
after 10 min. 0.5 ml 1 N commercial Folin-Ciocalteau reagent was
added with instantaneous mixing and after 30 min. O.D. was measured
at 750 nm. Standard was established on the basis of egg or serum
albumin solutions. Note that many buffers interfere with this
method (GREGORY and SAJDERA 1970).*

RNA
*was determined quantitatively by a modified Schmidt and Thannhauser
procedure. An appropriate sample was homogenized and extracted
several times with methanol-acetone-water (4.5:4.5:1) until practically all pigment was removed. Residue was extracted 3 x with cold
0.2 N perchloric acid or 10% trichloro acetic acid, then with etha-
nol-ether (2:1) at 50 C° 30 min. The residue was digested with
0.33 N KOH at 37 C° for 7-16 hours. The soluble supernatant brought
to pH 2-3 with perchloric acid in the cold, than two volumes ethanol added after 2 hours in the cold it was centrifuged at 8,000
rpm. The supernatant, containing RNA nucleotides was adjusted to
pH 7-8 and then purified on Dowex-1x8-200 (The resin was washed
previously 3 times with 1 N HCl and 1 N NH₄OH each and distilled
water in between and after until neutral, finally again with 1 N
HCl and water to keep it the chloride form). After adding the solution to a 4-5 cm long small column, it was washed with a few ml
of water, then the nucleotides were eluted with 0.12 N HCl and their
O. D. Was determined at 260 nm. Alternatively the nucleotides were
individually separated on similar Dowex resin of 400 mesh converted
the formate form by passing through 1 N Na-formate until an 0.1 N
AgNO₃ test showed no more signs of chloride in the eluates (white
precipitate upon adding 2-3 drops), and then at least three bed
volumes of 1 N formic acid. The 15 x 1 cm column was subsequently
washed with distilled water until effluent was the same as the inflow in pH and O.D. The concentrated nucleotide mixture (pH 8-9)
was applied to the column and eluted sequentially with 0.01 M
HCOOH, 0.15 M HCOOH, 0.01 HCOOH containing 0.05 M NaOOCH, 0.1 M
HCOOH containing 0.15 M NaOOCH (MARKHAM 1955). The progress of
elution was monitored in the 5 ml fractions by O.D. measurement at
250, 260, 270 and 280 for the identification of the nucleotides.
The sequence of elution was cytidylic, adenylic, uridylic and
guanylic acids (2'- and 3'-monophosphates partly separated) with
a characteristic absorption ratios as follows 250/260 nm: 0.45,
0.85, 0.80 and 0.90, 280/260: 2.0, 0.23, 0.28 and 0.68, respectively. Their total quantities was determined on the basis of the
molar extinction coefficients at 260 nm being 6.6, 14.5, 9.9 and
12.0, respectively at pH 2. In the combined nucleotides O. D. x
33.16 corresponds to approximately µg/ ml RNA.
Alternatively RNA was extracted by a hot phenol method (GIRARD 1967)
and the labeling was estimated by scintillation counter.*

DNA

*was extracted according to LEDOUX, HUART and JACOBS (1971) and it
was further purified by extraction with an equal volume of 88%
phenol (freshly distilled over aluminum turnings and 0.05% $NaHCO_3$
added in 12 volume of water); after 30 min. gentle shaking 2 vols.
of chloroform was added with an additional minute shake, then the
phases were separated in the centrifuge (8,000 rpm, 15 min.) Upper
phase combined with 2 parts cold ethanol and after 2 hrs in the cold,
DNA fibers were spooled out or sedimented by centrifugation in the
cold. The DNA was washed with 70% ethanol until all traces of
phenol were removed. Fibers taken up in 0.15 M NaCl-0.015 Na-ci-
trate and used for density gradient centrifugation as indicated by
LEDOUX et al. The density of the fractions was determined with the
aid of a Bausch and Lomb Abbe 3L refractometer at 25° C and refractive index was converted into density values with the Table provided by Handbook of Biochemistry. (DNA solutions were transferred
only with blunted pipets). Base composition was estimated with
the formula of De LEY (1970). The density of BrU-A was taken 0.2 g
heavier than T-A DNA as indicated by WAKE and BALDWIN (1962).*

NON-HISTONE PROTEIN

*was extracted as DNA but no protease, RNase or phenol was applied.
Before homogenization the plants were submerged for 10 min. in the
saline-EDTA-SLS at 60 C^o and processed further after cooling. To
the crude extract 750-150 mg slightly sheared salmon sperm or thymus DNA was added and after mixing the chromatin was precipitated
with 2 volumes of -15 C^o ethanol for at least 30 min. then filtered
through two layers of dacron web (Pellon, New York) without suction.
Radioactivity on the disks was measured by scintillation counting.*

6-AZAURACIL-2-C^{14} METABOLITES

*were extracted from plants (grown on media containing 0.125 µCi/ml)
after thorough washing with hot 80% ethanol or -15 C^o methanol:
acetone: water (45:45:5 v/v) mixture and concentrated in a Rotava-
por. The concentrates were co-chromatographed with authentic cold
samples on polyethyleneimine-cellulose thin-layer plates (Brinkman
Instr., Westbury, New York), developed with tetrahydrofurfuryl alcohol: isoamylalcohol: 0.08 M potassium citrate buffer, pH 3.0 (1:
1:1, v/v) mixture (Carpenter 1952). The spots were located under
short wavelength ultraviolet light, eluted with 0.5 ml 1 N HC1 and
counted by liquid scintillation.*

OROTIC ACID METABOLISM

*was followed in extracts of plants (100 mg) grown aseptically for
four weeks, then incubated at 28 C^o in 3 ml 0.01 M sodiumphosphate
buffer pH 5.8, containing 10 µCi of orotic acid-6-C^{14}. The free
nucleotides, nucleosides and bases were extracted with hot 80%
ethanol and 0.2 N percholoric acid and separated on thin-layer
plates. The soluble material was digested with KOH for nucleic
acid determination. In appropriate samples the radioactivity was
measured as described above.*

LEAF PIGMENTS
were analyzed according to RÖBBELEN (1957).

SCINTILLATION COCKTAIL
*consisted of 10 ml mixture o toluene and Triton-X-100 (1000 ml:500
ml) containing 8.25 g 2,5-diphenyloxazole (PPO) and 0.25 g 4-bis-2-
(4-methyl-5-phenyloxazoly1)-benzene (Me₂POPOP). Efficiency was estimated with toluene internal standard.*

ELECTRONMICROGRAPHY
*was done on mature leaves fixed for 3 hrs in 5% glutaraldehyde buf-
fered to pH 7.4 with sodium cacodylate and postfixed in 1% osmium
tetroxide. Dehydration in alcohol series was followed in propylene
oxide. Embedding was in Epon 812. Ultrathin sections were stained
on 300 mesh grids in uranyl acetate and Reynold's lead citrate
(SJØSTRAND 1967).*

LITERATURE CITED

BONNER, J.   1965 The Molecular Biology of Development.   Oxford Univ.
     Press, New York.

BROWN, J. A. M.   1962 Effect of thymidine analogues on reproductive
     morphogenesis in Arabidopsis thaliana (L.) Heynh.   Nature 195:
     51-3.

BROWN, J. A. M.   1968 The role of competitive halogen analogues of
     thymidine in the induction of floral morphogenesis.   Pp. 117-
     38.   Cellular and Molecular Aspects of Floral Induction. Ber-
     nier, G. Ed., Longman's Green and Co. London.

BROWN, J. A. M.   1972 Distribution of ³H-thymidine in Arabidopsis
     vegetative meristems after 5-iododeoxyuridine treatment. Amer.
     J. Bot. 59: 228-32.

BURNHAM, CH.   1962 Discussions in Cytogenetics.   Burgess, Minne-
     apolis.

CARPENTER, D. C.   1952 Paper chromatography of nucleic acid deri-
     vatives Anal. Chem. 24: 1203-4.

CHUNG, S. C. and G. P. RÉDEI 1974 An anomaly of the genetic regula-
     tion of the de novo pyrimidine pathways in the plant Arabidop-
     sis. Biochem. Genet. 11: 441-53.

DeLEY, J. 1970 Reexamination of the association between melting
     point, buoyant density and chemical base composition of deoxy-
     ribonucleic acid. J. Bacteriol. 101: 738-54.

DEMAIN, A. L. 1971 Overproduction of microbial metabolites and enzymes due to alteration of regulation. Adv. Biochem. Engin. Ghose, T. K. and A. Fichter, Eds., 1: 113-42.

EVANS, L. T. 1971 Flower induction and the florigen concept. Ann. Rev. Plant Physiol. 22: 365-94.

GIRARD, M. 1967 Isolation of ribonucleic acids from mammalian cells and animal viruses Pp. 581-96. Methods in Enzymology, Colowick, S. P. and N. O. Kaplan, Eds., Vol. 12A. Acad Press, New York.

GREGORY, J. D. and S. W. SAJDERA 1970 Interference in the Lowry method for protein determination. Science 169: 97-8.

HILL, B. T., A. TSUBOI and R. BASERGA 1974 Effect of 5-bromodeoxy-uridine on chromatin transcription in confluent fibroblasts. Proc. Nat. Acad. Sci. U. S. 71: 455-59.

HIRONO, Y. and G. P. RÉDEI 1966 Early flowering in Arabidopsis induced by DNA base analogs. Planta 71: 107-112.

HIRONO, Y. and H. H. SMITH 1969 Mutation induced in Arabidopsis by DNA nucleoside analogs. Genetics 61: 191-99.

HUTCHINSON, F. 1973 Lesions produced by ultraviolet light in DNA containing 5-bromouracil. Quart. Rev. Biophys. 6: 201 :46.

IMMER, F. R. 1930 Formulae and tables for calculating linkage intensities Genetics 15: 81-98.

LAIBACH, F. 1951 Über sommer- und winterannuelle Rassen von Arabidopsis thaliana (L.) Heynh. Ein Beitrag zur Ätiologie der Blütenbildung. Beitr. Biol. Pflanzen 28: 173-210.

LANG, A. 1965 Physiology of flower initiation Pp. 1380-1563. Encyclopedia of Plant Physiology, Ruhland, W., Ed. Vol. 15/1: Springer Vlg. Berlin.

LEDOUX, L., R. HUART and M. JACOBS 1971 Fate of exogenous DNA in Arabidopsis thaliana. Pp. 159-75. Informative Molecules in Biological Systems, Ledoux, L. Ed., North Holland, Amsterdam.

LEE-CHEN, S. and L. M. STEINITZ-SEARS 1967 The location of linkage groups in Arabidopsis thaliana. Can. J. Genet. Cytol. 9: 381-84.

LIN, S.-Y. and A. D. RIGGS 1972 Lac operator analogues: bromodeoxy-uridine substitution in the lac operator affects the rate of dissociation of the lac repressor. Proc. Nat. Acad. Sci. U.S. 69: 2574-76.

MARKHAM, R.   1955 Nucleic acids, their components and related com-
    pounds. Modern Methods of Plant Analysis, Pp. 264-304, Paech,
    K. and M. V. Tracey, Eds. Vol. 4., Springer Vlg. Berlin.

McKELVIE, A. D.   1962   A list of mutant genes in Arabidopsis tha-
    liana (L.) Heynh.   Radiation Bot. 1: 233-41.

MEDVEDEV, ZH. A.   1970 Molecular-Genetic Mechanisms of Development.
    Plenum, New York.

OPARA-KUBINSKA, Z., Z. KURYLO-BOROWSKA and W. SZYBALSKI   1963   Ge-
    netic transformation studies III. Effect of ultraviolet light
    on the molecular properties of normal and halogenated deoxy-
    ribonucleic acid. Biochim. Biophys. Acta 72: 298-309.

PRASAD, K. N., B. MANDAL and S. KUMAR   1973   Human neuroblastoma
    cell culture. Effect of 5-bromodeoxyuridine on morphological
    differentiation and levels of neural enzymes. Proc. Soc. Exp.
    Biol. Med. 144: 38-42.

RÉDEI, G. P.   1965 Genetic control of subcellular differentiation.
    Arabidopsis Research. Rep. Inst. Symp. Göttingen, Röbbelen,
    G., Ed. University of Göttingen.

RÉDEI, G. P.   1967a Suppression of a genetic variegation by 6-aza-
    pyrimidines. J. Heredity 58: 229-35.

RÉDEI, G. P.   1967b Biochemical aspects of a genetically determined
    variegation in Arabidopsis.   Genetics 56: 431-43.

RÉDEI, G. P.   1973 Extra-chromosomal mutability determined by a
    nuclear gene locus in Arabidopsis.   Mutation Res. 18: 149-62.

RÉDEI, G. P., S. C. CHUNG and S. B. PLURAD   1974 Mutants, antimeta-
    bolites and differentiation.   Brookhaven Symp. Biol. 25: 281-
    96.

RÉDEI, G. P., and G. ACEDO and G. GAVAZZI   1974 Flower differentia-
    tion in Arabidopsis.   Stadler Symp. Columbia 6: (in press).

RÉDEI, G. P. and S. B. PLURAD   1973 Hereditary structural altera-
    tions of plastids induced by a nuclear mutator gene in Ara-
    bidopsis.   Protoplasma 77: 361-80.

REINHOLZ, E.   1947 Auslösung von Röntgenmutationen bei Arabidopsis
    thaliana (L.) Heynh. und ihre Bedeutung fur die Pflanzenzüch-
    tung und Evolutionstheorie. FIAT Rep. 1006: 1-70.

RÖBBELEN, G.   1957 Untersuchungen an Strahleninduzierten Blattfarbmutanten von Arabidopsis thaliana (L.) Heynh. Zeitschr. Ind. Abst. Vererb.-Lehre. 88: 189-252.

RÖBBELEN, G.   1966 Chloroplastendifferenzierung nach geninduzierter Plastommutation bei Arabidopsis thaliana (L.) Heynh. Zeitschr. Pflanzenphysiol. 55: 387-403.

RÖBBELEN, G.   1968 Genbedingte Rotlicht-Empfindlichkeit der Chloro-plastendifferenzierung bei Arabidopsis. Planta 80: 237-54.

SCHWABE, W. W.   1971 Physiology of vegetative reproduction and flowering Pp. 233-441.   Plant Physiology, Steward, F. C., Ed. Vol. 6A. Acad. Press, New York.

SJØSTRAND, F. S.   1967 Electron Microscopy of Cells and Tissues. Vol. 1. Instrumentation and Techniques. Acad Press, New York.

SMITH, K. C.   1964 Photochemistry of nucleic acids. Pp. 329-88. Photophysiology, Giese, A. G., Ed. Vol. 2. Acad Pres, New York.

STELLWAGEN, R. H. and G. M. TOMKINS   1971 Differential effect of 5-bromodeoxyuridine on the concentration of specific enzymes in hepatoma cells in culture. Proc. Nat. Acad. Sci. U. S. 68: 1147-50.

TOMIDA, M., H. KOYAMA and T. ONO   1974 Hyaluronic acid synthetase in cultured mammalian cells producing hyaluronic acid.   Oscil-latory change during the growth phase and suppression by 5-bromodeoxyuridine. Biochim. Biophys. Acta 338: 352-63.

WAKE, R. G. and R. L. BALDWIN   1962 Physical studies on the repli-cation of DNA in vitro. J. Mol. Biol. 5: 201-16.

WALTHER, B. T., R. L. PICTET. J. D. DAVID and W. J. RUTTER   1974 Mechanism of 5-bromodeoxyuridine inhibition of exocrine pancreas differentiation. J. Biol. Chem. 249: 1953-64.

PLANT CELL CULTURES: PRESENT AND PROJECTED APPLICATIONS FOR STUDIES IN CELL METABOLISM

H.E. Street

Botanical Laboratories

University of Leicester, Leicester, LE1 7RH, U.K.

INTRODUCTION

The primary phenotypic expression of genetic information is at the level of cellular metabolism. Sophisticated methods of monitoring qualitative and quantitative changes in cellular metabolism are therefore essential to studies in genetic manipulation. This lecture is therefore concerned to evaluate how far recent advances in plant cell culture now provide us with the necessary capability to monitor metabolism at the level of higher plant cells.

The range of metabolic changes which we may be called upon to characterise is limited only by the finite complexity of cellular metabolism. Clearly therefore one 'limiting' factor is the range and resolving power of current biochemical techniques and the extent to which they have been adapted to work with plant cells. No attempt will, however, be made here to assess the current status of analytical biochemistry! Attention will rather be directed to assessing how far plant cell culture can provide a good 'living system' for biochemical characterisation. The scope will be further restricted by dealing in a separate lecture with the problem of the genetic instability of such cell cultures.

By definition a cell culture is an unorganised system; in so far as there is variable aggregation of cells or qualitative differences between the cells the system departs from 'ideal'. This means that with cell cultures we are excluding those aspects of phenotypic expression which only emerge as a consequence of organised development (morphogenesis)

at the multicellular level. This also implies that it is a chosen
unnatural state in so far as the cells that are being studied only occur in
nature as constituent cells of the multicellular plant. The cells of such
cell cultures are very much alive, they are highly organised at the intracellular level but they do not correspond in their environment and hence
not in their metabolism with any cell in the living higher plant. However,
as will be discussed in my second lecture, such cells can be used to
initiate plants providing they have retained their genetic competence to do
so. Thus, in cell cultures we can study biochemical changes both compatible with and incompatible with their proper functioning within a viable
organism.

Since plant cell cultures can now be initiated from single cells –
are clones of recent origin from single cells – it will be assumed that we
are dealing with genetically homogeneous cell populations. This is justified despite the fact that the techniques to be discussed have been developed
with genetically heterogeneous cultures.

DEFINITIONS

Plant cell cultures are normally initiated from small surface-
sterilised explants (organ fragments) from plants. Some of the living
cells of the explant are induced to divide as a consequence of the injury
involved in excising the explant, combined with the provision of an appropriate mixture of essential nutrients and growth factors and an appropriate
physical environment (moisture, temperature, light). The result is the
development of an undifferentiated wound tissue (a callus). This is then
separated from the explant and grown into a callus culture (often referred
to as a tissue culture). This callus can be maintained indefinitely in
culture by fragmenting it at appropriate intervals (i.e. after an appropriate
period of incubation or culture passage) and transferring the fragments
(subculturing) singly to new vessels containing culture medium. Up to
this stage the culture medium used is normally solidified with agar so
that the callus sits in the medium and grows up into the air-space of the
culture vessel. As an alternative the callus may be supported on a filter-
paper bridge which 'wicks up' culture medium to the contact surface
between the callus and the filter paper.

Callus cultures can vary in texture and form from compact and
smooth to extremely irregular and friable (easily crumbled). The degree
of friability can often be increased by adjusting the levels of growth regulators (and particularly the auxin level) in the culture medium.

<u>Suspension cultures</u> (also referred to as cell cultures or cell suspension cultures) are obtained by transfer of callus fragments to agitated liquid medium and it is usually necessary to have very friable callus to obtain a finely dispersed suspension culture.

The period of incubation during which the suspension culture is developed from callus fragments is usually referred to as the initiation passage. During this passage not only do the callus fragments break up but the cells grow and divide until the depletion of some nutrient in the medium brings the increase in biomass to a stop (the culture enters a stationary phase). At some time before this the culture is used to initiate new cultures (Passage 1 suspensions) by pipetting off aliquots of the suspension into new flasks of culture medium. Where, as here, we transfer at each subculture a population of cells into a finite volume of nutrient medium the culture is termed a <u>batch culture</u>.

Even the most finely dispersed suspension cultures of higher plant cells contain a proportion of the cells associated together in aggregates (they are not truly free-cell cultures). The finer the suspension the smaller the average size of the cell aggregates (and the smaller the number of cells they contain) and in general the higher the proportion of the cell population present as individual free cells. Further the degree of cellular aggregation is not constant but changes significantly during the grand period of growth (growth cycle) of the batch culture; as the culture enters stationary phase cell aggregation is minimal, during the period of most active growth the aggregation is maximal.

BATCH CULTURE OF CELL SUSPENSIONS

Batch suspension cultures are most commonly maintained in conical flasks incubated on platform (orbital) shakers at speeds of 80 - 120 rpm. Closure of vessels by aluminium foil permits adequate gaseous exchange but reduces loss by evaporation compared with cotton plugs. Most commonly such stock suspensions are diluted on subculture by a factor of ca. x 10 and incubated until just before or just after entry into stationary phase (this usually means a passage duration of 21 - 28 days). This implies growth during each passage equivalent to 3 - 4 cell generations (e.g. increase from an initial density of 2×10^5 cells/ml^{-1} to 2×10^6). For experimental studies on growth, lower initial densities can be used thereby extending the period of growth (and number of cell generations). With sycamore cell suspensions for instance, cultures initiated at 2×10^3 cells/ml^{-1} can yield at stationary

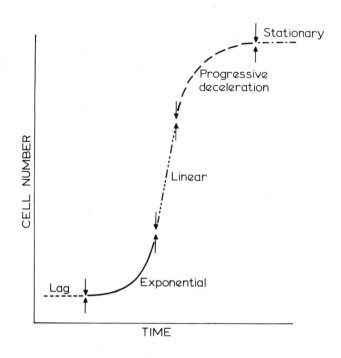

Fig. 1. Model curve relating cell number per unit volume of culture
to time in a batch grown cell suspension culture. Growth phases
labelled. (after Wilson, King and Street, 1971).

phase a density of 4×10^6 (ca. 11 cell generations). When growth in such
cultures is monitored by determination of cell number, cell dry weight
and packed cell volume per unit volume of culture, a growth curve of the
form shown in Fig. 1 is obtained.

Growth studies of this kind can be very valuable for the characterisation of cell lines. Criteria readily calculated include:

(i) <u>Specific growth rate</u> (μ) – the rate of increase of biomass per
unit of biomass during exponential growth

$$\mu = \log_e \frac{x}{t} + \log_e x_o$$

$$\log_e x = \mu t + \log_e x_o$$

where t = time interval, x_o = cell density at the beginning of the time interval, x = cell density after time t. By plotting t against $\log_e x$ a straight line is obtained of slope μ if the growth is exponential. (Plotting $\log_{10} x$ against time (t) gives slope = $\mu/2.303$).

From the value for μ the mean generation time g (usually synonymous with doubling time td) can be calculated.

(ii) <u>Biomass yield</u> per ml culture volume as the culture enters stationary phase. This can be expressed in terms of cell number, cell dry wieght, biomass volume (packed cell volume), protein, calorific value. By following utilisation of any particular nutrient, e.g. carbon source, N source and so on it is possible to calculate yield coefficients (cells formed per unit nutrient consumed).

(iii) <u>Mean cell volume</u> by dividing packed cell volume by cell number. Similarly calculated are values for mean dry weight and mean protein per cell.

(iv) <u>Duration of lag phase in relation to initial cell density</u>. As cell density is reduced lag phase is extended, and below a certain cell density (the <u>critical initial density</u>) the culture will fail to grow.

(v) <u>Viability in stationary phase</u> . Cell count data may remain steady for many days after the culture enters stationary phase or may quickly fall indicating the onset of cell lysis. Staining with 0.01% fluorescein diacetate (Widholm, 1972) can be used to monitor viability particularly where cell death is not associated with any cell lysis.

Studies of growth in such small scale flask cultures (volumes of culture medium in the range of 20 - 100 ml) are also most convenient for initial screening of cell lines for nutrient requirements, ability to utilise alternative carbon and nitrogen sources, responses to growth regulators (particularly phytohormones and vitamins) and to growth inhibitors (drugs and analogues of natural metabolites). Such studies are greatly facilitated by the development of fully-defined culture media supplying a utilisable sugar, a balanced solution of essential mineral salts and defined growth factors. Undefined supplements such as coconut milk, casein hydrolysates and yeast extracts are now little used; they can now nearly always be replaced by use of known phytohormones, vitamins, amino-acids, sugar alcohols, and nucleotides.

The number of samples which can be aseptically withdrawn for analysis from individual small cultures is strictly limited and often in

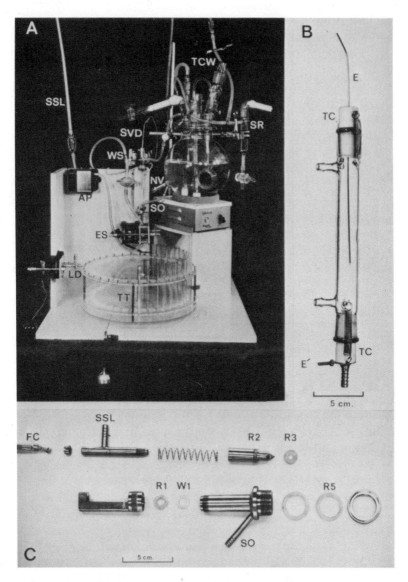

Fig. 2. Assembly for automatic sampling of a 4-litre batch culture.
A. View of complete assembly. Key: AP = air pump which clears the
sample volume detector (SVD) of liquid by a pulse of air; ES = solenoid
valve when open empties sample into collecting tube on turn-table; LD =
latching device, operated by a solenoid, which activates movement of
turn-table (powered by the brass weight shown hanging down below turn-
table); NV = needle valve (see C); SO = sample outlet line for needle valve;
SR = sample receiver permitting manual sampling of the culture; SSL =

studies designed to follow the progress of growth or nutrient utilisation
it is necessary to utilise a number of replicate cultures (and variation
between the replicates may prevent critical data being readily obtained).
Further, considerable biomass may be needed for comprehensive biochemical analysis or for assay of cell constituents present in very low
concentration. This has led to the development of larger scale batch
culture systems. A simple and effective scaling up to cultures of 5 1
capacity was achieved by spinning 10 1 culture bottles around an inclined
axis (Short, Brown and Street, 1969). With sycamore suspensions each
such culture yields 10^9 cells, 1.4 1 of packed cells and 40 g cell dry
weight.

Where platform shakers are used or where agitation is effected
by spinning the culture, sampling inevitably involves interruption of
agitation with consequent problems in obtaining small representative
samples. More important, it is not possible to vary at will in individual
cultures gaseous exchange and agitation nor to monitor continuously
culture pH, O_2 uptake and the evolution of CO_2 and other volatiles (measuring CO_2 evolution is essential to constructing carbon balance sheets of
the cultures). Again culture temperatures have to be regulated through
room temperature control or enclosure of platforms within incubators;
individual cultures cannot easily be controlled at different temperatures
or submitted to temperature regimes. To overcome these problems
batch culture vessels providing for controlled forced aeration and independent magnetic stirring have been developed (Miller et al., 1968; Veliky
and Martin, 1970; Wilson, King and Street, 1971). Such vessels have
proved particularly valuable in establishing and monitoring synchronously
dividing cell suspensions (King, Mansfield and Street, 1973; King et al.,
1974), when linked to electronically regulated sampling equipment (Fig. 2).

---

sterile saline line used to wash out sample volume detector and valve;
SVD = sample volume detector electrode; TCW = port carrying the temperature controlling glass coil; TT = turn-table; WS = solenoid controlling
the saline wash.   B. Sample volume detector showing details of construction: E and E' = electrodes; TC = teflon cones.   C. Units of
the needle valve separated out.

All after Wilson, King and Street (1971).

Hitherto a high and persistent level of division synchrony has only
been reported for sycamore cell suspensions using a starvation and re-
growth treatment. Current work on the location of the point of arrest
within the cell cycle induced by nitrogen starvation of sycamore cells looks
as if it will provide a criterion by which to recognise appropriate starvation conditions for other cell lines in which it is desired to induce division
synchrony by this approach. Further, the use of DNA synthesis inhibitors
(hydroxyurea, 5-fluorodeoxyuridine, 5-aminouracil) (Eriksson, 1967) or
appropriate with-holding of essential cytokinin (Jouanneau, 1971) may
prove valuable in inducing synchrony in other cell lines. The value of
synchronously dividing cultures is that they enable us to study control
events in the cell cycle, to analyse factors affecting growth rate in terms
of such control points and to study the kinetics of synthesis of particular
macromolecules. This will clearly be important to characterise mutants
affecting DNA and RNA synthesis, the synthesis of histones and of particular enzymes.

CONTINUOUS CULTURES - CHEMOSTATS AND TURBIDOSTATS

Studies of cellular composition, enzyme activities and activities of
basic metabolic processes in batch suspension cultures has shown that a
succession of metabolic patterns emerge and decline during the progress
of growth; the cells pass through a succession of short-lived physiological
states (Street, King and Mansfield, 1971). Even during the short phase of
exponential growth (constant doubling time) observed in standard batch
cultures the composition of the cells is continuously changing (Fig. 3 from
King, Mansfield and Street, 1973); biosynthesis is uncoupled from cell
division. This situation is a consequence forced upon the cells by the
continuous change in environmental conditions which is inevitable when
growth occurs in a closed system of finite dimensions. The use of open
continuous culture systems (in which an inflow of fresh medium is balanced by outflow of an equal volume of culture) offers by contrast the
possibility of achieving 'indefinite' periods of steady state growth (balanced growth where cell division rate is constant and linked to biosynthesis so that the cells also have constant composition and metabolic
activity) (King and Street, 1973). Wilson, King and Street (1971) demonstrated that functional continuous culture systems of both the chemostat and turbidostat type could be operated with a suspension culture of
sycamore and that steady states of long duration could be achieved by
this approach (Fig. 4 and 5). These steady states were characterised in
terms of growth rate (cell division rate, rate of increase of cell volume
and cell dry weight), cell morphology (cell size), cell composition

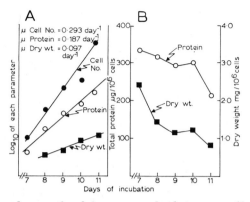

Fig. 3. Unbalanced growth of Acer pseudoplatanus cells during the exponential growth phase of a batch culture. A. Semi-logarithmic plot showing rates of change of cell number, total protein and cell dry weight per unit volume of culture. The slope of the line of best fit (calculated by linear regression analysis, $P < 0.01$) was used to determine the specific growth rate (μ) of each parameter. B. Changes in total protein content and dry weight of cells with time calculated from data in A. Data from King and Street (1973).

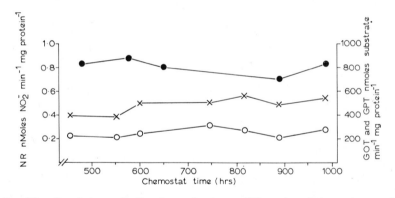

Fig. 5. Steady states of nitrate reductase (NR-●-), glutamate-oxaloacetate transaminase (GOT-x-) and glutamate-pyruvate transaminase (GPT-o-) activity in a chemostat culture of Acer pseudoplatanus cells. The culture was N-limited and was diluted at the rate of 0.094 day^{-1} (td = 178 hours). The steady-state biomass was characterized by a cell density of 2.32×10^6 cells ml^{-1} and a total-protein content of 705 μg ml^{-1}. GOT and GPT were measured by a coupled assay technique with α-oxoglutarate and aspartate (GOT) or alanine (GPT) as substrates. The oxaloglutarate (GOT) or pyruvate(GPT) generated was determined by monitoring the change in extinction at 340 nm in the presence of malic dehydrogenase (GOT) or lactic dehydrogenase (GPT). (Data from Young, 1973).

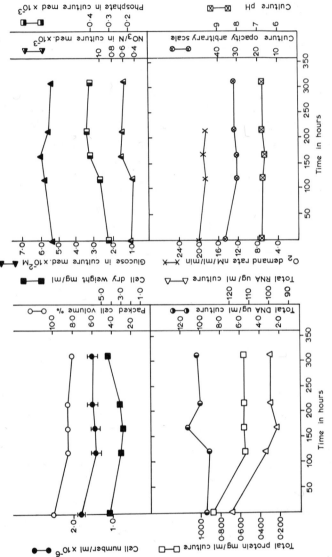

Fig. 4. A steady state established in a 4-litre chemostat culture of Acer
pseudoplatanus cells. The culture was diluted for c. 400 hours at a rate of
0.194 day^{-1}. Samples (50 ml) were withdrawn at intervals for biomass
measurements, nutrient analysis and respiration rate determinations.
Culture opacity and pH were monitored continuously in the culture vessel.
(Data from King and Street, 1973).

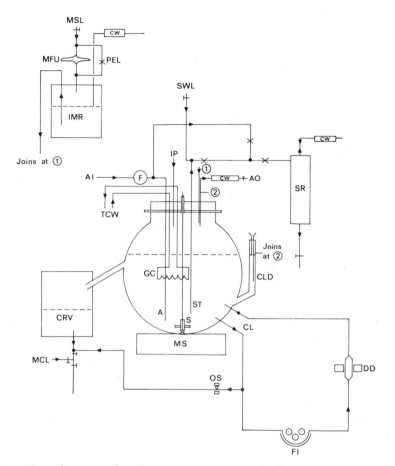

Fig. 6. Flow diagram for the open continuous culture system - chemo-stat of Wilson, King and Street (1971). Key: A = aerator; AI = air inlet; AO = air outlet; CL = circulation loop; CLD = constant level device; CRV = culture receiving vessel; CW = cotton wool filter; DD = density detector; F = minature airline filter; FI = flow inducer; GC = glass coil through which circulates water at controlled temperature (TCW); IMR = inter-mediate medium reservoir; IP = inoculation port; MS = magnetic stirrer motor; MSL = medium supply line; OS = outlet solenoid valve through which culture harvested in response to signal from the constant level device; S = PTFE-coated magnetic bar(s) carried on stainless steel rod; ST = sample tube connected to sample receiver (SR); SWL = sterile water line to wash-out SR.

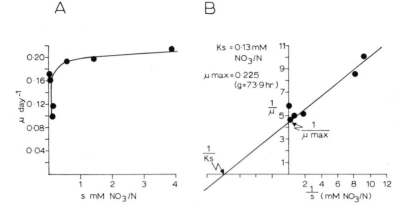

Fig. 7. Relationship between specific growth rate and steady state level of nitrate N/ in chemostat cultures of <u>Acer pseudoplatanus</u>. The double reciprocal plot (B) shows calculation of Ks and μmax for the data shown in A. The saturation type curve shown in A is that to be expected if NO_3/N is the limiting nutrient (from King and Street, 1973).

(protein, level of soluble nitrogen, soluble carbohydrate), cell metabolism (respiration rate and respiratory quotient), levels of a number of 'universal' enzymes) and yield coefficients (carbon and nitrogen conservation as cell material).

In the chemostat cultures (Fig. 6) the cultures were grown at a number of growth rates below the maximum growth rate by regulation of rate of medium input (and hence supply of a limiting nutrient) and it was shown that such cultures conformed to the Monod equation (Monod, 1950):

$$\mu = \mu max \frac{s}{Ks + s}$$

where s = equilibrium concentration of the limiting nutrient and Ks = a 'saturation constant' = the nutrient concentration at which specific growth rate (μ) is half its maximum value (μmax) (Fig. 7 and 8). These studies also showed that the cells had at each steady state a characteristic composition and metabolism (Fig. 4 and 5) and that the total output and effective yield (output per unit of energy source consumed) of any particular cell constituent (cellulose, protein, secondary metabolic product) depended upon the particular steady state achieved (Fig. 9). This implies that different cell lines can be compared in their biochemistry and physiology under conditions of equal rate of biomass production or their

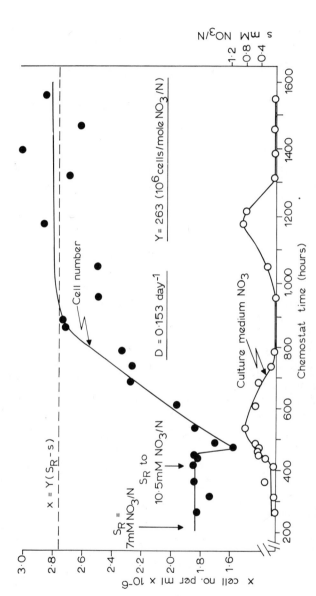

Fig. 8. Change in the biomass of a 4-litre chemostat culture of Acer pseudoplatanus cells following a change in the concentration of the limiting nutrient (NO_3/N) in the inflowing medium (S_R). The culture was diluted at a constant rate (D) 0.153 day^{-1} (td = 108 hours). The yield coefficient, Y, for the first steady state (ended after 420 hours) = 263 x 10^6 cells mole N^{-1}. s = steady state concentration of NO_3/N in the culture vessel, and hence in the outflow. The equation (Monod, 1950) relating equilibrium cell density (x) to the yield coefficient (Y) and the change in substrate concentration between input (S_R) and output (s) was used to calculate the expected change in x from increasing the level of S_R. Note the close agreement between the expected and recorded new equilibrium cell density. (From King and Street, 1973).

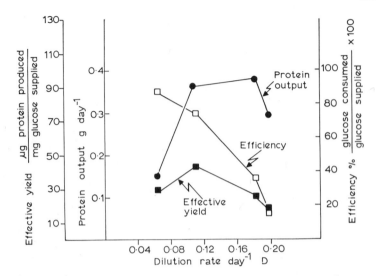

Fig. 9. The production of protein by a 4-litre chemostat culture of
Acer pseudoplatanus cells at different dilution rates. Protein output (Fx)
calculated from the flow rate (F in ml/day^{-1}) and the protein concentration
in the culture vessel (x in g ml^{-1}). (From King and Street, 1973).

growth rates and effective yields compared when the steady state for each
line is selected to maximise production, per unit of culture or per cell, of
some particular enzyme or metabolic product. Hitherto, such experiments
have been carried out over a wide range of growth rates but further study
is required to establish viable non-growing cultures by a transition from
an open to a closed continuous culture in presence of an appropriate limiting nutrient or inhibitor of cell division. The 'closed' continuous culture is one where supply of new medium is balanced by harvesting of an
equal volume of 'spent' medium (and not of culture). A system of this
type has been described (Wilson, King and Street, 1971) (Fig. 10) but has
not yet been operated to maintain viability over a prolonged period in a
non-growing culture. Such a system may be necessary to optimise production of particular secondary plant products.

    As explained above, chemostat cultures achieve steady states by
control of the rate of biomass production by the level of supply of a limiting nutrient; the cultures are grown at growth rates (μ) below the maximum growth rate (μmax). If the rate of medium inflow (dilution rate) is
raised to the point where μ approaches μmax, the culture approaches
the wash-out point (Fig. 11). For steady state growth where growth rate
is not limited by a particular nutrient, recourse is made to a turbidostat

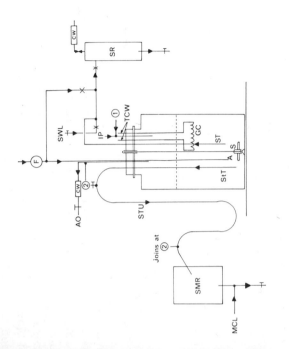

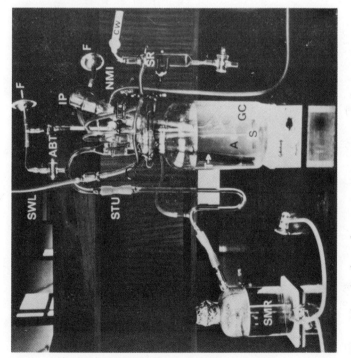

Fig. 10. A closed continuous system after Wilson, King and Street (1971). Key: A = aerator; ABT = air bleed for removal of air trapped in stilling tube; CW = cotton filter; F = filter; GC = glass coil; IP = inoculation port; NMI = new medium input; S = stirrer; SMR = spent medium reservoir; SR = sampling tube; StT = wide stilling tube; STU = syphon unit tube; SWL = sterile water line.

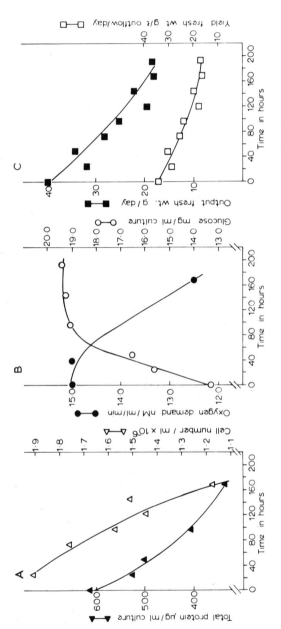

Fig. 11. 'Wash-out' of Acer pseudoplatanus cells from a chemostat culture diluted at a rate in excess of the critical dilution rate. The dilution rate was 'stepped-up' from 0.182 day^{-1} (steady state) to 0.274 day^{-1} at time = 0 hours and cells were washed-out at a rate of 0.038 day^{-1} indicating a critical dilution rate of 0.236 day^{-1}. A. Decay in cell number and protein per millilitre of culture. B. Decline in oxygen demand and increase in the concentration of glucose per ml of culture (input glucose concentration, S_R = 20 mg/ml). C. Decline in the total output of biomass per day and in the daily yield per litre of outflow (the latter is equal to the biomass concentration in the culture vessel). (From King and Street, 1973).

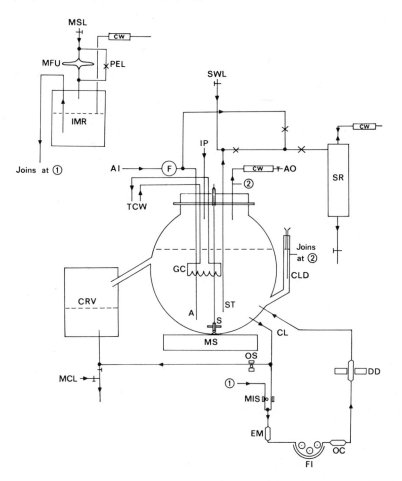

Fig. 12. Flow-diagram for the open continuous culture system - turbido-stat of Wilson, King and Street (1971). Key as Fig. 6. plus: EM = electrode module permitting insertion of pH electrode and/or oxygen electrode in circulation line; MIS = new medium input solenoid valve; OC = observation chamber the volume of which determines the volume of the pulse of new medium.

system (Fig. 12). Here a selected cell density (cells per unit volume of culture) (characterised by the light absorption or light scattering of the culture) is maintained by a pulse of new medium being called for when the density exceeds (by culture growth) the pre-set value. These steady state cultures therefore grow at μmax and at a predetermined density below a critical density (above this density the culture fails by depletion causing a fall in growth rate and a consequent demand not for more but for less new medium per unit time).

The μmax referred to here is not an absolute value corresponding to the highest potential growth rate characteristic of the genome but a μmax corresponding to the particular culture medium and other operating environmental factors (temperature, light, pH, gaseous exchange and so on). Such cultures therefore enable the growth and metabolic responses of cell lines to be studied where they are not controlled by a limiting supply (quantitative) of a major nutrient. This system is therefore particularly valuable if cell lines are to be characterised for their optimum growth temperature, optimum light regime, responses to growth hormones and other specific growth factors, relative growth with qualitatively different carbon and nitrogen sources and so on. By appropriate experimental techniques (Gould, Bayliss and Street, 1974) the effects of these variables can be assessed not only in terms of mean growth rate and cellular physiology of the culture but also in terms of the durations of the individual phases of the cell cycle.

CONCLUSION

Recent developments in technique enable the metabolism of cultured plant cells to be investigated under strictly defined environmental conditions. Of particular importance are those techniques which induce a high level of division synchrony in cell cultures and which enable steady states of growth to be maintained over extended periods and the transitions from one steady state to another to be closely monitored. Techniques of this degree of sophistication are essential for the proper characterisation of cell lines arising naturally in culture or achieved by the use of mutagens.

REFERENCES

Eriksson, T. Physiologia Pl. 19, 900-10. 1967.
Gould, A.R., Bayliss, M.W. and Street, H.E. J. exp. Bot. 1974 (in press).
Jouanneau, J.P. Expl Cell Res. 67, 329-37. 1971.
King, P.J., Cox, B.J., Fowler, M.W. and Street, H.E. Planta (Berl.) 117, 109-22. 1974.
King, P.J., Mansfield, K.J. and Street, H.E. Can. J. Bot. 51, 1807-23. 1973.
King, P.J. and Street, H.E. p. 269-337 in Plant Tissue and Cell Culture Ed. H.E. Street. Blackwell Scientific Publ., Oxford. 1973.

Miller, R.A., Shyluk, J.P., Gamborg, O.L. and Kilpatrick, J.W.
    Science, N.Y. 159, 540-2. 1968.
Short, K.C., Brown, E.G. and Street, H.E. J. exp. Bot. 20, 579-90.
    1969.
Street, H.E., King, P.J. and Mansfield, K.J. pp. 17-40 in Les cultures
    de tissus de plantes. Coll. Intern. CNRS 193. Strasbourg 1970.
    CNRS, Paris 1971.
Veliky, I.A. and Martin, S.M. Can. J. Microbiol. 16, 223-6. 1970.
Widholm, J.M. Stain Technol. 47, 189. 1972.
Wilson, S.B., King, P.J. and Street, H.E. J. exp. Bot. 21, 177-207.
    1971.
Young, M. J. exp. Bot. 24, 1172-85. 1973.

PLANT CELL CULTURES: PRESENT AND PROJECTED APPLICATIONS FOR STUDIES IN GENETICS

H.E. Street

Botanical Laboratories

University of Leicester, Leicester, LE1 7RH, U.K.

INTRODUCTION

This lecture falls into three main sections: (i) Plant tissue and cell cultures offer the possibility of regenerating plants from single cells (including cells regenerated from single or fused protoplasts - Cocking and Evans, 1973). The central problems associated with plant regeneration from callus and suspension cultures will therefore be outlined. (ii) The cytological stability of cells in culture is of critical importance whether our purpose is the use of tissue cultures for multiplication of a particular individual plant phenotype or to preserve a particular cell line or to reveal the phenotypic expression in the whole plant of such a cell line. It is also important if we wish to preserve the haploid states of cells unchanged during a programme of mutagenesis, mutant selection and multiplication. It is therefore necessary for us to be aware of the present state of knowledge regarding cytological instability and to assess how far it may be possible to stabilise the cytology of cells in culture or to circumvent this problem. (iii) The availability of haploid cells via anther and pollen culture (Sunderland, 1973a and Nitsch in this volume) requires attention to the potentiality of such cells and to the problems associated with their use as a source of naturally occurring and induced mutant cell lines. Here it is necessary to consider the use of mutagenic agents and the problems of selecting higher plant cell mutants.

TECHNIQUES OF PLANT REGENERATION FROM CULTURED CELL LINES

Shoot bud initiation

Skoog and his co-workers at Wisconsin, in studies directed to inducing and maintaining cell division in cylinders of tobacco stem pith, demonstrated the necessity of supplying the pith cells with both the plant growth hormone, auxin and a second cell-division factor or (as they termed it) cytokinin. They further showed that the initiation and the type or organ primordia formed from the resulting callus could be controlled by appropriate adjustment of the relative levels of the auxin and cytokinin. With high auxin - low cytokinin roots developed, with low auxin - high cytokinin shoot buds developed; at intermediate levels undifferentiated callus developed (Skoog and Miller, 1957). In these studies an unnatural cytokinin - kinetin (6-furfurylaminopurine) - was used but later work was to show that cytokinins occur naturally in all higher plants and are 6-substituted amino-purines. This dramatic demonstration of the control of organogenesis by the balance in concentration between two externally-applied hormones has continued to dominate our thinking regarding the nature of the control of organogenesis in vivo and in vitro.

Since the shoot buds initiated on the tobacco callus, when excised, readily formed adventitious roots it was possible to regenerate from the callus numerous tobacco plants. This therefore raised the possibility of a general technique of plant propagation: from explant to callus (which could be maintained and multiplied by subculture) to shoot buds to plants, through manipulation of the levels of known plant hormones incorporated in the culture media. However, as time has passed it has become clear, as Reinert (1973) has pointed out, that 'cultures from the medullary parenchyma of tobacco shoots are a somewhat special case so that the principle of regulation of organogenesis by quantitative changes in the ratio between specific compounds cannot be generalized to cover cultured tissues in general'. The situation can be summarised as follows: (i) when callus cultures are first initiated they often show spontaneous root initiation and rather less frequently (and often on separate cultures) shoot bud initiation; (ii)in most cases (though there are exceptions) the tendency for organogenesis declines as the callus or derived suspension cultures are serially propagated in culture. In such cases root initiation often still occurs when the culture has apparently lost its competence for shoot bud initiation; (iii) root initiation is often promoted by an appropriate level of externally applied auxin (particularly NAA or IAA); (iv) in some cases, as in tobacco, a cytokinin (or purine derivative possibly functioning as a cytokinin precursor) may promote but in other cases it suppresses bud initiation.

The unsatisfactory state of our knowledge of how to induce shoot bud initiation from cultured cells severely restricts current work on genetic manipulation via tissue and cell cultures. Future progress will depend upon extending our knowledge of the hormonal control of bud initiation (probably requiring the discovery of other naturally-occurring growth regulators additional to auxins, cytokinins, gibberellins and abscisins) and understanding more clearly the processes of dedifferentiation (achievement of totipotency) occurring during callus initiation.

Embryogenesis

Work dating from the pioneer studies of Steward, Mapes and Mears (1958) has led to the recognition of a quite different mechanism of plant regeneration in culture, a process of embryo formation from individual cultured cells. This process has recently been studied in detail in cultures of Ranunculus sceleratus (Thomas, Konar and Street, 1972), belladonna (Atropa belladonna - Konar, Thomas and Street, 1972) and carrot (Daucus carota - McWilliam, Smith and Street, 1974). There is however evidence, based upon less critical studies, that regeneration via embryogenesis occurs in a considerable number of callus and suspension cultures derived from diverse genera and families (Street, 1974). It could be that this pathway of plant regeneration will prove of wider application than that depending upon shoot bud initiation.

This somatic embryogenesis takes place from individual cells at the surface of callus cultures or at the surface of the cellular aggregates of suspension cultures. These embryogenic cells undergo a sequence of orderly segmentations to give rise to a globular bipolar embryo which during its later stages of development closely mimics the stages passed through during 'in ovule' embryology from the zygote. These somatic embryos become clearly distinct from the callus or aggregate, in which they arise, early in embryology and thus can be easily detached from the callus surface and normally float free from the aggregates in agitated suspension cultures. The released plantlets when transplanted to filter paper bridges and supplied with a culture medium of low sugar content yield young plants which can be readily grown on.

Provided a callus or cell culture has the competence to form embryos, the process of embryogenesis can usually be initiated by transfer

from a medium containing auxin (2,4-D) (a medium promoting undifferentiated proliferation) to a medium lacking auxin   Frequently very
large numbers of plantlets can be initiated (e.g. a 20 ml suspension culture of carrot may contain thousands of small plantlets after 21 days'
incubation in auxin-free medium). It was at one time thought that complex
media (containing undefined supplements like coconut milk) were necessary
for embryogenesis but by adopting the inorganic salt mixture of Murashige
and Skoog (1962) which supplies part of the nitrogen as ammonium, high
levels of embryogenesis are achieved now in defined media.

All plant cells which have retained the genome of the zygote unim-
paired during cellular differentiation are probably capable of embarking
upon embryogenesis (i.e. are totipotent). However, the realisation of this
potential (i.e. the acquiring of embryogenic competence) is clearly dependent upon appropriate cellular changes occurring during the initiation of
callus from the primary organ explant. Induction of cell division and
formation of callus is not synonymous with induction of embryogenic competence. In attempting to achieve plant propagation via embryogenesis
particular attention should therefore be directed to finding the appropriate
chemical and environmental stimuli which yield a callus, at least some of
the cells of which are embryogenically competent. It has frequently been
observed that calluses developed from immature zygotic embryos, from
embryos arising in culture and from haploid plantlets developed by anther
culture are particularly embryogenic. Perhaps a more profound 'dedifferentiation' is needed to produce embryogenically competent cells from
the mature tissue cells in root and shoot explants.

It is clearly important to establish the necessary conditions conducive to shoot bud initiation or embryogenesis in a wide range of species
if the potential of plant tissue and cell culture in plant breeding is to be
fully exploited.

THE CYTOLOGY OF CELLS IN CULTURE

"Plant tissues and cells,like their animal counterparts, display
more than the usual degree of nuclear irregularity when they are removed
from the stabilizing environment of the intact organism and plunged into
the alien environment of the culture vessel: variation and evolution in such
cell populations can therefore be a serious problem" (Sunderland, 1973b).
The above statement implies that changes in nuclear cytology actually
occur more frequently 'in vitro' than 'in vivo'. This is however still
uncertain, excepting of course instances where cultured cells have been

exposed to obviously unphysiological conditions (e.g. very high levels of
2,4-D). In a recent study of mitotic abnormalities in cultured carrot cells,
multipolar separations occurred frequently (and did not occur in root meristems of the species); lagging chromosomes and chromosome bridges
were observed both in the cultures and in root meristems but occurred at
higher frequency in the cultures (Bayliss, 1973). However it seems that
more important in accounting for the rapid appearance of chromosome
mutations and departure from the diploid (or haploid) chromosome number
is the selective action of the cultural environment. Abnormalities (which
'in vivo' would be associated with suppression of further division) are
either at no selective disadvantage and may be at a selective advantage in
culture. If this is so then such abnormal cells may be starting points for
a rapid and diverse breakdown of nuclear cytology (aneuploids quickly generating further and differing aneuploids).

It is common experience that old established callus and cell cultures have high modal chromosome numbers and are highly aneuploid
(Smith and Street, 1974; Bayliss and Gould, 1974). Sometimes the culture may contain almost exclusively a single modal chromosome number
but in many cases the cell population is heterogeneous. In the latter case
the proportions of cells with the different modal chromosome numbers may,
over many serial subcultures, remain almost constant. However, such a
culture may, when examined again after a further considerable period of
culture, contain a quite different spectrum of chromosome numbers. A
rise in specific growth rate is frequently observed during the early serial
passages following initiation and this can be correlated with changes in the
nuclear cytology of the cells suggesting a selection pressure for a high
growth rate genome. However the cytological changes which occur in established cultures are not necessarily associated with any significant change
in mean growth rate. This suggests that potential growth rate of a particular cytological 'deviant' may not be determinative in its survival or the
cause of the 'deviant' becoming dominant in the cell population of the culture. Smith and Street (1974) have described an experiment where a mixed
culture of carrot cells was experimentally established by mixing equal
numbers of cells from two recent single cell isolates (one with a diploid
and one with a tetraploid mode) and which had identical specific growth
rates in monoculture. During serial subculture the proportion of tetra=
ploid cells rose until ultimately the whole culture became tetraploid.
Such findings suggest that there are aspects of competition and interaction
between cells in mixed culture which are at present not understood.

Cultures which when first established show a high potential for
organogenesis or embryogenesis often show a decline in this potential

as they are serially propagated and many old established cultures have
a nil potential for such morphogenesis. Often as morphogenetic potential
declines the proportion of abnormal shoot buds or embryos rises. In the
case quoted above of the mixed carrot cell culture the diploid cell line had
a high embryogenic competence, the tetraploid line no such competence,
and the culture declined in embryogenic competence on serial subculture
and eventually had a nil competence. Selection pressure in culture is for
survival in the proliferating culture and this is often associated with a
loss of the capacity for organised development.

Although it may be possible to establish cultural conditions which
minimise cytological breakdown, it now seems clear that continuing
growth in culture will always be incompatible with the preservation of
mutant cell lines or the 'perfect' multiplication of plants of a selected
phenotype. Plant propagation via tissue and cell culture should therefore be achieved by procedures which minimize the period of unorganised
growth in culture. It now seems possible however that this need can be
met and cell lines stabilised by freeze-preservation. Carrot cell lines
have been successfully stored for extended periods at the temperature of
liquid nitrogen (-196°C). Cells which survive the initial controlled freezing (and this can be a very high percentage), fully retain their viability
for long periods at -196°C. Further, the surviving cells when restored
to ambient temperature by an appropriate thawing procedure are unaltered
in cytology, growth rate and potential for morphogenesis (Nag and Street,
1973).

The stability of the haploid condition in culture is of particular
importance where it is desired to use haploid cultures (of anther origin)
in mutagenesis work. Haploid lines of Atropa belladonna derived from
haploid plantlets of anther origin can under appropriate conditions remain
predominantly haploid over several successive culture passages although
eventually they become increasingly heterogeneous and ultimately come to
contain only cells of higher ploidy. (Rashid and Street, 1973). In other
cases (e.g. Nicotiana spp.) departure from haploidy may proceed more
rapidly. Here again we see the necessity to reduce to a minimum periods
in culture before applying techniques of mutagenesis, mutant selection and
regeneration. Recently Gupta and Carlson (1972) noted that p-fluorophenyl-
alanine (PFP) strongly inhibited growth of a diploid callus of Nicotiana
tabacum at concentrations without effect upon a haploid callus of the same
species. From this they suggested that PFP could be used to select preferentially the haploid cells from a mixed population of cells varying in
ploidy. We have recently examined this possibility in more detail using
diploid and haploid-derived cell lines of Nicotiana sylvestris (Dix and

Street, 1974) and shown that different cell lines differ significantly in their sensitivity to PFP inhibition but that it is the genotype of the cell line and not its ploidy level which determines resistance or sensitivity. Mixed cell populations whether resistant or sensitive to PFP inhibition did not change significantly in their ploidy composition in presence of PFP. This substance therefore does not offer us a convenient general technique for preferential selection of haploid cells.

Following up the isolation of haploid mutant cell lines it will be necessary to restore them to the homozygous diploid condition if plants regenerated are to be fertile. This may be achieved by exploiting the increase in ploidy which occurs spontaneously in culture. However, the cytology of diploid cells arising in this way has not been examined critically nor has the uniformity of diploid plants derived in this way from a culture of haploid single-cell origin. An alternative procedure is to use colchicine. To achieve diploidisation of pollen plantlets of <u>Nicotiana</u> <u>tabacum</u> 0.4% colchicine applied over 96 hours has been used. Studies of the meiotic behaviour of several diploid plants derived in this way has however shown a high frequency of nuclear aberrations (Nakata and Tanaka, 1970). When an <u>Atropa belladonna</u> suspension culture containing over 90% haploid cells was treated for 24 hours with medium containing 0.1% colchicine it yielded a reduced number of plantlets (compared to the untreated suspension) but 70% of these plantlets were diploid and showed no gross abnormality (Rashid and Street, 1973). Further work is now required to see how generally useful colchicine may be in producing a high yield of homozygous diploids from haploid cultures.

MUTAGENESIS AND THE SELECTION OF MUTANT CELL LINES

What is needed here would seem to be a programme built up of the following component steps: (1) preparation of actively growing cell suspension cultures (preferably haploid if mutagenesis is involved) consisting entirely or predominantly of free viable cells (or capable of giving a high yield of protoplasts which can be readily induced to regenerate single cells); (2)(a) application of an effective and appropriate mutagenic treatment to the cells or protoplasts or (b) fusion or genetic modification of the protoplasts followed by regeneration of viable cells; (3) a selection procedure leading to the development of callus colonies from just those single cells having the sought for genetic constitution; (4) diploidisation (if haploid cells have been used) and plant regeneration.

Other lectures in this School will be concerned with protoplast

technology and with techniques of genetic manipulation other than the use
of mutagens. Attention here will be directed to techniques of single-cell
cloning, mutagenesis and mutant selection in culture.

Single cell cloning techniques

Techniques of single cell cloning are based upon a technique of
plating out cells (or protoplasts) on agar in petri dishes (Bergmann, 1960).
The objective is to distribute evenly the cells or very fine cell aggregates
(suspension cultures) or protoplasts in a thin layer of agar-solidified medium at as low a plating density (cellular units per ml medium) as is compatible with high plating efficiency (PE). Plating efficiency (PE) is calculated from the equation:

$$PE = \frac{\text{No. of colonies developed per plate}}{\text{No. of cellular units incorporated per plate}} \times 100$$

Isolation of large numbers of representative single cell clones from a cell
suspension is only feasible if it contains only viable single cells and very
small aggregates (preferably of only 2 - 8 cells so that they are likely
themselves to be of single cell origin). With more aggregated suspensions
recourse must be made to: (1) aseptic filtration through an appropriate
mesh bolting cloth,or (2) the intermediate formation of protoplasts provided that the plating conditions yield a high proportion of viable cells
from the plated protoplasts (at present this is only the case in very few
instances with protoplasts derived from cultured cells - Cocking, 1973),
or (3) the incorporation aseptically into the culture medium of enzymes
used in protoplast preparation but now at very low concentrations sufficient
to only soften the cell walls and increase the degree of cell separation as
the suspension grows (see results of K.J. Mansfield quoted in Street, 1973).

The necessity of low density plating is to ensure that colonies do
not mingle or spread over other cells or cell aggregates before they are
large enough to be transferred from the plates to tubes of new medium for
further growth. For any cell line and culture medium combination there
is a critical inoculum density below which no growth of cells will take place
and a range of densities above this and before a density is reached which
gives the highest achievable PE. Two techniques have been developed to
lower the plating density at which this PE is achieved: (1) By 'feeding'
the plated cells by a 'nurse' callus from which growth-promoting substances diffuse into the layer of agar. To prevent overgrowing of plated

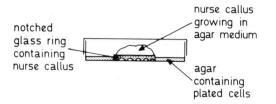

Fig. 1. Technique of using a 'nurse' callus to increase the plating efficiency of cells dispersed in agar at low cell density.

cells by the growing callus, the callus is confined within a notched glass ring centred in the petri dish (Fig. 1); (2) by using a medium 'conditioned' by having previously supported the growth of a high density culture as a constituent (up to 50% by volume) of the plating medium (Stuart and Street, 1969). Analysis of such 'conditioned' medium may enable a synthetic medium to be developed which is favourable to the growth of cells at low density. Such a medium has been developed for sycamore cell suspensions by enriching the standard minimal medium with amino-acids, kinetin and gibberellic acid, and alteration of the initial pH (Stuart and Street, 1971). Recent work on the growth of very dilute suspensions has also shown the importance of the CO_2 level in the gas atmosphere of the culture vessels, and very significant increases in PE have been obtained by raising this to 1% (unpublished data and results of K.J. Mansfield quoted in Street, 1973). Although this effect was first discovered in work with sycamore cell suspensions it has now been demonstrated for cultures of other species.

Cells may be spread out on the surface of the agar medium previously solidified in the dishes but under these circumstances cells (and particularly protoplasts) undergo harmful desiccation even when the dishes are sealed with parafilm or tape. Cells should therefore be distributed uniformly through the agar as rapidly as possible with the agar maintained liquid at a temperature not exceeding 35°C (0.6% Oxoid agar No. 3 or similar grade is satisfactory) and only a thin layer of agar plus cells plated (not more than 2 ml per 9 cm petri dish). Plates should be incubated in darkness (at least until colony growth has started) - if they need to be examined at intermediate times before harvesting colonies, this should be in low intensity diffuse light.

Mutagenesis

Experience here is at present very limited. Preliminary work has been undertaken with nitrosoguanidine (400 μg ml^{-1}) (Lescure, 1970) and ethylmethane sulphonate (EMS) (2.5 mg ml^{-1}/hr) (Carlson, 1973). Such mutagens should in short term treatments be used at dosages (concentration-duration) which are lethal to a high (and preferably predictable) proportion of the cells. Alternatively they should be allowed to act over longer periods at sufficiently low concentrations to permit continuing growth in culture. Basic studies on the toxicities of selected mutagens to a range of diploid and haploid cell lines from a range of species are now urgently needed to guide those attempting to induce mutation in cell cultures. The objective here is to obtain as high a proportion as possible of mutated cells in a drastically reduced but still numerous population. As will appear in the final section of this lecture, most variant cell lines have hitherto been selected from cultured cell populations whose heterogeneity has developed spontaneously in culture. Further, even when mutagens have been used it has not been satisfactorily demonstrated that the isolated variant cell lines arose by their action and could not have been isolated from the untreated culture. This is one of the reasons for current difficulty in deciding whether the variants described are properly to be regarded as mutants. Variants described have not even been submitted to critical cytological analysis.

Technique for selection of mutant cell lines

As indicated above the changed cell lines described have rarely been shown to be mutants and are perhaps better described, in most cases, as 'variant' cell lines. Widholm has put forward the following criteria as needing to be fulfilled if the change is to be regarded as due to mutation: (i) be stable in the absence of the selection agent; (ii) have occurred instantaneously; and (iii) have occurred in low frequency. A further, and critical criterion, would seem to be that the change is not lost during plant regeneration and is inherited through a sexual cycle and can be thus subjected to genetic analysis. This, of course, requires that fertile plants can be regenerated from the cell line.

Variant cell lines have so far been obtained showing: (i) less exacting growth requirements than the parent culture; (ii) enhanced resistance to drugs and anti-metabolites; (iii) lesions in biosynthesis. Consideration of these types will serve to illustrate the nature of the selections used in their isolation.

Sievert et al. (1961,1965) isolated by single cell cloning from a culture of the hybrid Nicotiana tabacum x N. glutinosa, 54 lines which could be differentiated by using media from which individual growth factors (auxins and coconut milk) were omitted or where glucose was replaced by other sugars. Only 8 of the 54 clones showed any growth on galactose and 2 of these showed good growth with this carbon source. Arya, Hildebrandt and Riker (1962) using normal and Phylloxera gall tissues of grape, also obtained single-cell clones differing in their ability to use different sugars and having different sugar concentration optima for growth. Fox (1963) isolated strains of tobacco callus differing from 'wild' type in relation to hormone requirement; one strain had no requirement for exogenous auxin, a second strain required neither auxin nor a cytokinin. Lescure (1970) isolated two strains of sycamore capable of growth in absence of 2,4-D and differing in their friability and degree of greening.

The above cases where cell lines autotrophic for auxin were isolated is of particular interest in view of the long known phenomenon of habituation (Limasset and Gautheret, 1950). A considerable number of tissue cultures when cultured in presence of IAA (particularly relatively high concentrations of IAA) have been shown to change in colony characteristics, to become auxin autotrophic and to acquire tumorous properties (capable of inducing tumours when grafted into the parent plant). With tissue cultures from some species habituation can be reproducibly induced, and sometimes by relatively short auxin (or kinetin) treatments (Bennici et al., 1972). There is also some evidence that this habituation can be reversed, though this evidence does not rigorously exclude that the reversal is not achieved by selection of normal (auxin-requiring) cells from a mixed population of normal and habituated cells (Syono and Furuya, 1974). Despite the fact that habituation has been known for about 25 years, the nature of the change induced is still obscure. The habituated tissue has a high level of endogenous auxin, but it is not known for certain whether this is due to enhanced auxin synthesis or a reduced rate of auxin destruction. More important, it is not certain whether the habituated cells are genetically modified (are mutant cells) or have simply a different, and very stable, enzyme activation pattern (a different pattern of gene expression). After all, the requirements of tissue cultures for any growth hormone (auxin, cytokinin, gibberellin), vitamin or other growth factor (sugar alcohol, purine, pyrimidine, amino-acid etc.) does not reflect lack of genetic information for their synthesis (since the whole plant has no need for their exogenous supply) but must simply reflect failure of the cells to meet their requirements for any such substance under the particular conditions of culture adopted. We must therefore always bear in mind that any variant cell line (and this applies to the 'drug resistant' lines to be mentioned below)

may arise by a change in expression of existing genes and that its mutant
nature is not established unless we are able to demonstrate its expression
in the phenotype of a derived plant and preferably also through a breeding
programme.

Heimer and Filner (1970) isolated a diploid tobacco cell line resistant to 100 μM threonine and reported that this variant occurred at a frequency of ca. 10^{-7} in the population. When cultured for long periods in
absence of the inhibitor it retained its resistance. Lines resistant to
streptomycin have been obtained from Petunia (Binding, Binding and Straub,
1970) and tobacco (Maliga, Breznovits and Martin, 1973) using haploid
cell cultures. Maliga et al. regenerated plants from their resistant lines
and showed that callus derived from leaf pieces of such plants was resistant.
Crossing experiments with the regenerated plants pointed to maternal inheritance of the resistance (implicating plastids or mitochondria as the site
of the resistance). This group of workers (Maliga, Breznovits and Martin,
1973) have also selected lines resistant to bromodeoxyuridine (BuDR) from
haploid tobacco callus. Resistance to streptomycin and to BuDR appeared
to occur at a frequency of ca. 10^{-6}. Lescure (1973) has selected from
diploid tobacco cultures, lines resistant to 8-azoguanine and Widholm
(1972) lines resistant to DL-5-methyltryptophane from diploid cultures of
carrot and tobacco. Carlson (1973) has isolated lines resistant to methionine sulphoxine (MSO) by treating haploid tobacco cells with ethylmethane
sulphonate (EMS) and shown that plants regenerated are less susceptible
to the wildfire pathogen (Pseudomonas tabaci). The nature of the apparent
relationship between resistance to MSO and the pathogen has not been worked out.

The final types of variant to be discussed are those which apparently have a lesion in a biochemical pathway. In 1970 Carlson reported
the selection of 6 leaky auxotrophic lines from a haploid tobacco culture
following treatment with the mutagen, EMS (2.5 mg ml^{-1} for 1 hr, killing
46-67% of the cells). Lines were recovered needing for normal growth
respectively hypoxanthine, biotin, p-aminobenzoic acid, arginine, lysine
or proline: the variants were leaky in so far as they grew slowly on unsupplemented medium. It was suggested that the leaky nature of the variants
may be due to Nicotiana tabacum being an allopolyploid and hence possibly
not being a functional diploid so that the anther-derived cells were not
functionally haploids. An interesting feature of this work was the use of
BuDR with the object of enriching the surviving population in auxotrophs.
This followed the evidence from work with mammalian cell cultures (Puck
and Kao, 1967) that BuDR in the dark followed by exposure to light was
only lethal to cells dividing in its presence. Following upon the mutagen
treatment, Carlson cultured the surviving cells on minimal medium for

96 hr (presumably a starvation treatment for the auxotrophs thereby bringing them into a non-dividing state) and then treated the culture with 10^{-5}M
BuDR for 36 hr in the dark and then exposed the culture to light (cool,
white fluorescence, 30 cm from 40 watt light) for 36 hr. The variants
were then selected from the surviving cells able to generate colonies on
supplemented media. This paper does not give any evidence as to whether
the mutagen was essential to obtain the variants or whether it increased
their yield. The 36 hr treatment with BuDR was stated to be lethal to the
growing original cell line but it was not tested against the cells of the original line brought to a non-dividing state by starvation of an essential nutrient (e.g. carbohydrate, phosphate, nitrogen). Evidence that it was acting preferentially on the 'wild-type' cells rests in the fact that a few cells
did survive the selection treatment; however, some of these surviving
cells were definitely not auxotrophs.

The above study by Carlson has been discussed at some length because it would clearly be of considerable importance if BuDR could be generally used as a selective lethal agent against cells which, following mutagenesis, are still capable of active growth on a minimal medium. Using
sycamore cell suspensions inhibited in growth by readily reversible starvation treatments (growth inhibition judged by a fall to a very low level in
the rate of S^{35} incorporation from sulphate into the TCA-insoluble fraction
of the cells) we have been able to demonstrate a general toxicity of BuDR
at the level used by Carlson but not a major contrast in the susceptibility
of growing versus non-growing cells. We are therefore of the opinion that
more work is needed to assess the value of BuDR in auxotroph selection
from plant cultures, just as more work is needed with haploid cells from
true diploids to see if non-leaky auxotrophs can be isolated.

REFERENCES

Arya, H.C., Hildebrandt, A.C. and Riker, A.J. Pl. Physiol., Lancaster
    37, 387-97. 1962.
Bayliss, M.W. Nature 246, 529-30. 1973.
Bayliss, M.W. and Gould, A.R. J. exp. Bot., 1974 (in press).
Bennici, A., Buiatti, A., Tognoni, F., Rosellini, D. and Giorgi, L.
    Plant and Cell Physiol. 13, 1-6. 1972.
Bergmann, L. J. gen. Physiol. 43, 841-51. 1960.
Binding, H., Binding, K. and Straub, J. Naturwissenschaften 57, 138-9,
    1970.
Carlson, P.S. Science, N.Y. 168, 487-9. 1970.
Carlson, P.S. Science, N.Y. 180, 1366-7. 1973.
Cocking, E.C. and Evans, P.K. The isolation of protoplasts, pp. 100-

120, in Plant Tissue and Cell Culture. Ed. H.E. Street,
    Blackwell Scientific Publ. Oxford, 1973.

Dix, P.J. and Street, H.E. Plant Sci. Letters , 1974 (in press).

Fox, J.E. Physiologia Pl. 16, 793-803. 1963.

Gupta, N. and Carlson, P.S. Nature (New Biol.) 239, 86. 1972.

Heimer, Y.M. and Filner, P. Biochim. biophys. Acta 215, 152-65. 1970.

Konar, R.N., Thomas, E. and Street, H.E. Ann. Bot. 36, 123-45. 1972.

Lescure, A.M. Soc. bot. Fr. memoires 353-65. 1970.

Lescure, A.M. Plant Sci. Letters 1, 375-83. 1973.

Limasset, P. and Gautheret, R. C.r. hebd. Séanc. Acad. Sci. Paris
    230, 2043-5. 1950.

McWilliam, A.A., Smith, S.M. and Street, H.E. Ann. Bot.38,243, 1974

Maliga, P., Sz-Breznovits, A. and Marton, L. Nature (New Biol.) 244,
    29-30. 1973.

Maliga, P., Marton, L. and Sz-Breznovits, A. Plant Sci. Letters 1,
    119-21. 1973.

Murashige, T. and Skoog, F. Physiologia Pl. 15, 473-97. 1962.

Nag, K.K. and Street, H.E. Nature 245, 270-2. 1973.

Nakata, K. and Tanaka, M. Jap. J. Breeding 20, Suppl. 1, 7-8. 1970.

Puck, T. and Kao, F. Proc. Natl. Acad. Sci. U.S.A. 58, 1227. 1967.

Rashid, A. and Street, H.E. Plant Sci. Letters 2, 89-94. 1974.

Reinert, J. Aspects of organisation - organogenesis and embryogenesis,
    pp. 338-355, in Plant Tissue and Cell Culture. Ed. H.E. Street,
    Blackwell Scientific Publ. Oxford, 1973.

Sievert, R.C. and Hildebrandt, A.C. Am. J. Bot. 52, 742-50. 1965.

Sievert, R.C., Hildebrandt, A.C., Burns, R.H. and Riberg, A.J.
    Pl. Physiol., Lancaster. 36, Suppl. XXIX. 1961.

Skoog, F. and Miller, C.O. Symp. Soc. exp. Biol. 11, 118-30. 1957.

Smith, S.M. and Street, H.E. Ann. Bot. 38, 223 - 241, 1974.

Steward, F.C., Mapes, M.O. and Mears, K. Am. J. Bot. 45, 705-8,
    1958.

Street, H.E. Single-cell clones, pp. 191-204, in Plant Tissue and Cell
    Culture, Ed. H.E. Street, Blackwell Scientific Publ. Oxford, 1973.

Street, H.E. in Textbook of Developmental Biology. Ed. C.F. Graham
    and P.F. Wareing. Blackwell Scientific Publ. Oxford, 1974.
    (in press)

Stuart, R. and Street, H.E. J. exp. Bot. 20, 556-71. 1969.

Stuart, R. and Street, H.E. J. exp. Bot. 22, 96-106. 1971.

Sunderland, N. (a) Pollen and anther culture, pp. 205-239; (b) Nuclear
    cytology, pp. 161-190, in Plant Tissue and Cell Culture. Ed.
    H.E. Street, Blackwell Scientific Publ. Oxford, 1973.

Syono, K. and Furuya, T. Plant and Cell Physiol. 15, 7-17. 1974.

Thomas, E., Konar, R.N. and Street, H.E. J. Cell Science 11, 95-109.
    1972.

HETEROGENEOUS ASSOCIATIONS OF CELLS FORMED IN VITRO

P. S. CARLSON[*] AND R. S. CHALEFF[†]

Biology Department, Brookhaven National Laboratory

Upton, New York 11973 U.S.A.

Abstract: Two experimental systems are described which explore
the applicability of in vitro culture to force associations
between cells of widely divergent origins. In one experiment, chimeral plants were induced to differentiate from
mixed calluses formed by coculturing cells of two tobacco
species. In another experiment, a symbiosis was forced
between cells of carrot and of the free-living nitrogen-
fixing bacterium, Azotobacter vinelandii.

1. INTRODUCTION

Tissue culture methodology permits associations between cells
of different genotypes to be constructed in vitro. In this
system the spectrum of such associations is limited only by the
growth requirements of the cultured cells and not by the complex
developmental and morphogenetic processes which are naturally
restrictive. We shall now discuss two examples of our attempts
to explore the potentialities of this technique. The first
describes a system in which cells of two different tobacco
species were brought together in culture to generate chimeral
calluses. In the second experimental system carrot and bacterial
cells were forced to grow together in a mutually dependent
symbiosis.

*Present address: Department of Crop and Soil Science, Michigan
State University, East Lansing, Michigan 48823, U.S.A.
†Present address: Department of Applied Genetics, John Innes
Institute, Colney Lane, Norwich NOR 70F, England.

A. Chimeral Plants:

Many varieties of plants are chimeral associations of
genetically dissimilar cells (Avery et al., 1959; Whitehead et
al., 1953). Although most of these varieties originated spontaneously, chimeras have been formed experimentally as the result
of grafting (Jorgensen and Crane, 1927; Neilson-Jones, 1969).
Cells from both scion and stock may contribute to callus tissue
which is formed at a graft union. Adventitious buds arising
from this callus occasionally produce chimeral shoots. This
experimental approach has limited chimeral production to combinations between species which are graft compatible and which
form callus at the graft union. It is hoped that these con-
straints will be lifted by the use of calluses grown in culture.
An experimental system may be designed in which genetically
distinct cells are able to proliferate contiguously and form a
chimeral association. Genetic markers and nutritional requirements may be exploited to identify the chimeral product of the
two constituent species. By transferring these chimeral calluses
to an appropriate growth medium, it should be possible to induce
the development of chimeral plants.

Although the cells of a chimeral association are in contact,
they remain genetically discrete and separable components of a
heterogeneous tissue. This form of association is distinguished
from a genetic hybrid which may result from fusion of the cytoplasm and nuclei of somatic cells. Much research has been
directed recently toward accomplishing fusion between protoplasts
derived from widely divergent and sexually incompatible species.
Heteroplasmic fusion events have been reported between protoplasts
of oat and maize (Power et al., 1970) and soybean and barley
(Kao and Michayluk, 1974). Indeed this approach is exciting and
offers a new tool for dissecting cellular and developmental
functions and for constructing new plant varieties. The experimental production of chimeral plants in vitro should provide a
complementary technique for developing new varieties of vegetatively propagated species.

The in vitro synthesis of chimeral plants requires three
sequential steps: 1) initiation, recognition, and maintenance
of chimeral callus; 2) regeneration of mature plants from chimeral
callus; 3) verification that the recovered plants are chimeral.
The experimental system to be described utilizes callus cultures
of Nicotiana tabacum and the amphiploid hybrid N. glauca x N.
langsdorfii. Throughout this study the very distinct morphologies
and hormonal requirements of N. tabacum and the amphiploid hybrid
were exploted as markers to identify the tissues of these two
forms.

Table 1

Hormone concentrations (μg/ml)

Species	Callus initiation and maintenance		Shoot induction		Root induction	
	IAA	2iP	IAA	2iP	IAA	2iP
Nicotiana tabacum	3.0	0.3	0.3	3.0	1.0	0
Amphiploid hybrid (GGLL)	0.1	0	0	0	N.A.[*]	

[*]Not accomplished.

2A. METHODS

Biological materials:

   Tissue was derived from Nicotiana tabacum cv. Wisconsin 38 and the amphiploid hybrid between Nicotiana glauca and Nicotiana langsdorfii (GGLL).

Media:

   Culture media contained the mineral salts and vitamin concentrations described by Linsmaier and Skoog (1965) with 4% sucrose as carbon source. The various media differed only in concentrations of auxins and cytokinins. Callus cultures were initiated by placing explants of pith tissue on the appropriate medium. All cultures were maintained at 22-24°C on a 16 hour light-8 hour dark cycle.

Hormone concentrations:

   Different levels of auxin and cytokinin are required for callus induction and maintenance, shoot regeneration, and root regeneration. These hormonal requirements are not the same for N. tabacum and the amphiploid hybrid (GGLL). The optimal concentrations of indoleacetic acid (IAA) as auxin and 6(γ,γ-dimethylallylamino)-purine (2iP) as cytokinin are listed in Table 1.

3A. RESULTS AND DISCUSSION

Chimeral callus:

   Chimeral callus is most easily obtained by placing pith slices of the two different genotypes adjacently and in contact

with each other on the medium containing 3 mg IAA/liter and 0.3
mg 2iP/liter. This medium promotes callus formation in both N.
tabacum and the GGLL hybrid. Once callus has proliferated, the
chimeral regions can be excised from the surrounding tissue and
subcultured. The distinct morphology and color of callus derived
from the two species allows the chimeral regions to be identified
visually. When cultured in the light N. tabacum forms a lighter
colored tissue than the amphiploid hybrid. With each successive
transfer, the two cell types which compose the callus become more
interdispersed.

In another approach to the construction of a chimeral callus,
suspensions of protoplasts of the two species were mixed and plated
together. This method was unsuccessful since the chimeral associations could not be identified positively from among the many
regenerated calluses. This result may reflect merely the difficulty in the recognition and not the formation of heterogeneous
associations. In fact, if very distinct genetic markers are
used, the plating of mixed cell suspensions may prove a more
efficient method of producing chimeral calluses.

Differentiation of mature plants:

Mature plants of Nicotiana tabacum may be recovered by
sequential transfer of callus tissue to media containing different
hormone concentrations. Higher relative levels of cytokinin are
used initially to promote shoot formation and subsequent exposure
to higher relative levels of auxin promotes root formation. In
contrast, shoots are organized on callus derived from the amphiploid hybrid in the absence of exogenous hormones. Root formation
has not been accomplished with this genotype (Table 1). The
difference in the exogenous hormone levels required to induce
organogenesis in the two genotypes was crucial to the efficient
recovery of chimeral plants.

Plants differentiated from a chimeral callus may be composed
of tissue from both or from only one of the two constituent
species. The number of chimeral individuals may be enriched by
a phenotypic rescue technique. The chimeral callus is placed on
a medium which favors organ development in tissue of only one of
the genotypes and shoots displaying a morphology characteristic
of the other genotype are selected. In this study approximately
300 separate chimeral calluses were cultured as visually identified chimeras for at least six months by transfer to fresh medium
every three weeks. When these chimeral calluses were forced to
differentiate, approximately 7000 shoots were recovered and
examined. Of these shoots 237 were selected as potential chimeras
and were regenerated into mature plants. Twenty eight of the 237
plants were confirmed to be truly chimeral by procedures described
in the following section.

Verification of the chimeral composition of the plants:

The most direct method of determining the chimeral nature of a plant is by demonstrating that cells of each tissue layer in the apex contain a chromosome number or morphology characteristic of a given genotype. However, chromosome numbers fluctuate greatly in cultured cells. Therefore, chromosome numbers are not reliable markers of the genotype of a tissue layer in chimeral plants obtained from in vitro cultures. The genotype of the tissue layers must be ascertained from other traits.

Previous research on several species of Solanaceae has demonstrated that the three germ layers in the apical meristem are independent and each contributes specific tissue to the developing organs. The T1 layer gives rise to the epidermis of the stem, the T2 layer gives rise to both the male and female gametes, and the corpus region gives rise to the central region of the pith (Avery et al., 1959). Thus, the genotype of each of the three germ layers may be deduced by examining distinguishing characteristics of the derivative mature tissue.

The morphology and density of epidermal hairs on the stem are species specific characters which are reliable indicators of the composition of the T1 layer (Neilson-Jones, 1969). Since the morphology and density of epidermal hairs of N. tabacum and the amphiploid hybrid (GGLL) differ (Goodspeed, 1954), the genotype of the T1 was determined from inspection of the epidermal hairs on the stem of the chimeral plant. This trait proved to be a distinct and autonomous characteristic of the epidermal tissue (i.e. T1 layer) in the chimeral plants.

The genotype of the T2 layer is the same as that of the progeny obtained from self-fertilization of the chimeral plant. In all cases, only one type of progeny, either N. tabacum or amphiploid hybrid, was recovered from the self-fertilization of a chimeral individual. Approximately 30 progeny obtained from selfing each presumptive chimeral plant were scored. This trait consistently reflected the genotype of the T2 layer.

The genotype of the corpus region was identified by explanting pieces of the central pith into in vitro culture. Pith tissues of the amphiploid hybrid will proliferate and form callus on medium containing 0.1 mg IAA/liter whereas pith from N. tabacum will not.

The compositions of 25 of the 28 chimeral plants recovered are described in Table 2. Not all possible chimeral associations of the two genotypes were recovered; although we know of no reason why these types should not be expected to appear if a

larger sample of chimeral plants were analyzed. Analysis of
three individuals was precluded by instability in the tissue
layers or failure to yield viable progeny following self-fertilization. The basis of this tissue instability is unknown, but was
not due to segregation in a mericlinal chimera. Many of the
chimeral plants displayed some instability in the composition of
their meristematic layers over long periods of growth and upon
vegetative propagation. The most frequently observed instability
was the replacement of amphiploid hybrid tissue by N. tabacum
tissue.

Table 2

Genotypic composition of the tissue layers in the
recovered chimeral plants produced between the
amphiploid hybrid (GGLL) and N. tabacum (Nt)

Number of individuals	Genotype of layer		
	First tunica layer	Second tunica layer	corpus
11	Nt	Nt	GGLL
0	Nt	GGLL	Nt
3	Nt	GGLL	GGLL
2	GGLL	GGLL	Nt
1	GGLL	Nt	GGLL
8	GGLL	Nt	Nt
3	Undetermined		
Total 28			

A range of morphologies intermediate between N. tabacum and
the amphiploid hybrid were observed among the chimeral plants.
In general, the T2 layer exerted the most distinct influence on
the gross morphology of the chimeral plants. The morphology of
leaves from the chimeral plants is illustrated in Fig. 1. Since
plants regenerated from in vitro cultures often show morphological
abnormalities, these photographs do not demonstrate definitively
the morphological deviations in leaves due to their chimeral
composition. It was impossible to distinguish reliably the
morphological differences attributable to chimeral associations
of cells from those attributable to the effects of in vitro
culture.

All recovered chimeral plants formed tumorous outgrowths on
the stem. Tumor formation is an autonomous genetic characteristic
of amphiploid hybrid tissue and the observation that all classes
of chimeral plants form tumors demonstrates that tumor production
is not confined to any single tissue layer in the mature plant.

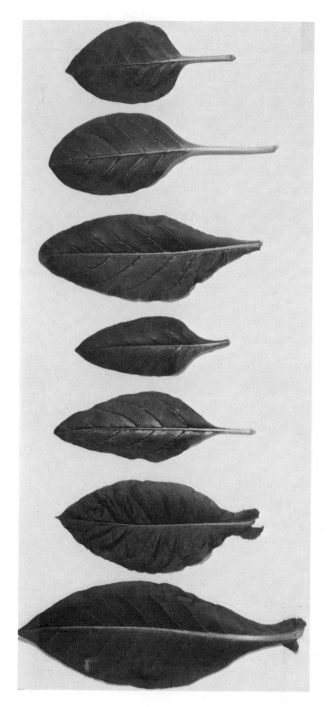

Fig. 1. The leaf morphology of N. tabacum, GGLL, and some of the chimeral plants containing tissue of both types. The composition of the T1, T2 and corpus regions are given for each individual. The N. tabacum leaf is on the left and the GGLL leaf is on the right. The composition of the leaves from left to right is: 1) T1, N. tabacum; T2, N. tabacum; corpus, N. tabacum; 2) T1, GGLL; T2, N. tabacum; corpus, N. tabacum; 3) T1, GGLL; T2, GGLL; corpus, N. tabacum; 4) T1, GGLL; T2, N. tabacum; corpus, GGLL; 5) T1, N. tabacum; T2, N. tabacum; corpus, GGLL; 6) T1, N. tabacum; T2, GGLL; corpus, GGLL; 7) T1, GGLL; T2, GGLL; corpus, GGLL.

We are now attempting to apply the _in vitro_ methods to the construction of a chimera composed of soybean and tobacco tissues. Several plants have been recovered which exhibit morphological characteristics of both of these evolutionarily remote species.

The procedures which have been outlined in this section represent an extension of earlier work in which callus formed at a graft union was used to facilitate chimera production. Although the technique of _in vitro_ chimeral callus construction releases the experimental synthesis of chimeral plants from the requirement of graft compatability, there are undoubtedly limits to the applicability of _in vitro_ methods. These methods may prove useful for constructing improved varieties of vegetatively propagated crops. Since these procedures permit the formation of chimeral plants from known parental types, it should be possible to combine the desirable characteristics of different genotypes into a single variety. Chimeras synthesized _in vitro_ may also provide a useful tool for the study of plant development. The contribution of each germ layer to mature organs may be followed in chimeras constructed from genetically dissimilar tissues containing appropriate identifying genetic markers.

B. Plant-bacterial associations:

In addition to constructing associations between plant cells of different genotypes, _in vitro_ culture methods may be used to bring together cells of more distant origins. A case in which this has been accomplished in nature is the agronomically important symbiotic relationship between many plant species and bacteria capable of reducing atmospheric nitrogen (Stewart, 1966; Bond, 1968). In several laboratories _in vitro_ systems are being developed for the study of these natural associations. The reduction of acetylene to ethylene, a sensitive assay of bacterial nitrogenase activity (Hardy et al., 1968), has been reported in Rhizobium-infected soybean cultures (Holsten et al., 1971; Phillips, 1974; Child and LaRue, 1974). In one instance, the bacteria were shown to be located within the cytoplasm of the infected plant cell (Holsten et al., 1971). The uptake of Rhizobium cells by isolated protoplasts of Pisum sativum has also been accomplished (Davey and Cocking, 1972).

We have attempted to define an experimental system for investigating the possibility of extending the nitrogen-fixing symbiosis to additional crop species. Tissue culture techniques have been used to force an association between the free-living nitrogen-fixing bacterium Azotobacter vinelandii and cells of carrot, Daucus carota. This system is based upon the establishment of a condition of mutual dependency between an auxotrophic strain of Azotobacter and carrot cells cultured on a medium lacking combined nitrogen. By selecting a free-living nitrogen-fixing bacterial species for these experiments, we hoped to bypass the complex interactions which have been evolved in natural symbioses.

2B. METHODS

Strains:

Daucus carota cultivar Danver's Half Long was obtained from the Fredonia Seed Company, Fredonia, New York.

The adenine-auxotrophic strain of Azotobacter vinelandii was acquired from the American Type Culture Collection (ATCC 25308).

A prototrophic strain of Azotobacter vinelandii, UW 59, was generously furnished by Dr. W. Brill.

Media:

Azotobacter cells were grown on a modified Burk's nitrogen-free medium which has been described elsewhere (Carlson and Chaleff, in preparation).

Carrot cells were grown on a Linsmaier and Skoog (1965) medium supplemented with 4% sucrose and containing 3 mg IAA and 3 mg 2iP per liter. NH_4NO_3 and KNO_3 were omitted from N-free medium. Medium which lacked NH_4NO_3 and contained 0.19 g KNO_3 per liter is referred to as low N medium.

T broth medium contained 10 g Bacto-tryptone, 5 g NaCl, 0.6 g $CaCl_2$, and 10 g glucose per liter (pH 7.0).

Penicillin:

A concentrated solution of K^+ penicillin G was filter sterilized and added to autoclaved medium to a final concentration of 50 mg per liter.

Callus formation:

Sections of carrot root tuber were excised aseptically and placed on solidified culture medium. The resulting calluses were subcultured on liquid medium of the same composition. All suspension cultures were incubated at 23° C under constant illumination.

Formation of Azotobacter - plant cell association:

Aliquots of a carrot cell suspension were transferred to
fresh liquid medium. Following a three day incubation these
cultures were inoculated with log phase cells of Azotobacter
vinelandii to a final concentration of 10^6 cells per ml. After
12 days the mixed cultures were washed and resuspended in N-free
carrot medium. The cultures were incubated for an additional
two weeks after which they were plated in N-free carrot medium
solidified with 1% Noble agar. The plates were incubated at 23° C
in a 16 hour light-8 hour dark cycle. The rare growing colonies
were selected as they appeared three to six months after plating
and were transferred to either N-free or low N medium. The
cultures were maintained on the same media and were transferred
approximately every six weeks.

Nitrogenase assay:

Approximately 50 mg fresh tissue were placed in 1 ml vials
which were then injected with 0.10 ml acetylene. The Azotobacter
controls contained approximately 8 (10^7) cells in 0.10 ml modified
Burk's medium. Reactions were stopped by the addition of 1.0 ml
0.1 N H_2SO_4. The ethylene content of samples was determined by
published gas chromatographic procedures (Burris, 1972) by
Richard Peterson in the laboratory of Dr. R. H. Burris.

Electron microscopy:

Tissue was fixed with glutaraldehyde and OsO_4. Samples were
embedded in epoxy resin and thin sections were stained with uranyl
and lead salts (Carlson and Chaleff, in preparation).

3B. RESULTS AND DISCUSSION

Growth studies:

Carrot cells are unable to survive in vitro in the absence
of combined nitrogen. When 1.9 mM KNO_3 is supplied as the sole
source of combined nitrogen, the carrot cell mass survives over a
four month period, but does not proliferate. Calluses derived
from Azotobacter-inoculated carrot cell suspensions increase in
fresh weight on these media. This increase is significantly
greater on the low nitrogen medium than on an N-free medium,
indicating that nitrogen is limiting to growth. On medium containing 20.6 mM NH_4NO_3 and 18.8 mM KNO_3 (standard concentrations),
no difference in growth rates is observed between uninoculated
calluses and inoculated calluses which are capable of growth on
N-free medium (Fig. 2). Although electron microscopy does not

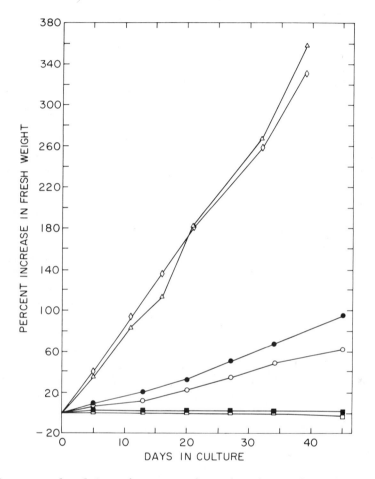

Fig. 2. Growth of <u>Azotobacter</u>-infected and uninfected control
carrot tissues on media containing different levels of combined
nitrogen. Calluses were grown on low N medium for 3 weeks before
being transferred to the medium indicated. Control carrot tissue
transferred to N-free (□), low N (■), or standard Linsmaier and
Skoog (Δ) medium. <u>Azotobacter</u>-containing carrot tissue transferred
to N-free (o), low N (●), or standard Linsmaier and Skoog (◊)medium.

reveal cell divisions in the <u>Azotobacter</u>-inoculated callus, thin cell walls are observed with sufficient frequency to suggest that the carrot tissue maintains a moderate rate of mitotic activity.

Reisolation of <u>Azotobacter</u> cells:

    <u>Azotobacter</u>-infected calluses capable of growth on N-free or low N medium were suspended in T broth and in Burk's minimal and adenine-supplemented media. After several days turbidity developed only in the adenine-supplemented Burk's medium. This suspension was plated and identified as the original <u>Azotobacter</u> adenine auxotroph with which the calluses had been inoculated. The absence of growth in T broth, which supports growth of a prototrophic <u>Azotobacter</u> strain, but not of the adenine-requiring strain, after a three week period indicates that the calluses contain no contaminating microorganisms. None of these three media became turbid when inoculated with control carrot callus.

Nitrogenase activity:

    <u>Azotobacter</u>-containing carrot tissue capable of growth on N-free medium evolves significantly more ethylene in the acetylene-reduction assay for nitrogenase than does the uninoculated control callus (Table 3). The increased ethylene production by the composite callus is observed only in the presence of acetylene and, therefore, cannot be due to endogenous ethylene synthesis by the plant tissue.

Table 3

Acetylene-reduction activity

Tissue	Medium	Incubation period (hr)	C_2H_2	nmol C_2H_4/ml gas
No tissue	--	24	+	0.17
<u>Azotobacter</u>	N free	1	+	1.91
Carrot	+N	24	-	0
Carrot	N free	24	-	0
Carrot	+N	24	+	0.31
Carrot	N free	24	+	0.30
Carrot-<u>Azotobacter</u>	N free	24	-	0
Carrot-<u>Azotobacter</u>	N free	24	+	1.84
Carrot-<u>Azotobacter</u>	N free	0	+	0.28

Penicillin treatment:

The ability of the inoculated callus to grow on N-free
medium is destroyed by the addition of penicillin G at a concentration which is known to kill Azotobacter cells (50 μg/ml).
Growth of either inoculated or uninoculated calluses on medium
containing normal levels of combined nitrogen is not inhibited by
the addition of penicillin. These observations indicate that the
ability of the inoculated callus to grow on N-free medium is
dependent upon the presence of functional bacterial cells in the
callus mass.

Electron microscopy:

Electron micrographs of inoculated carrot callus grown on
low N medium clearly establish the presence of bacterial cells in
the intercellular regions of the tissue (Fig. 3a-d). Azotobacter
cells are also found in the medium beneath the callus. No live
bacteria were observed within the carrot cells. Contaminating
microorganisms were not detected in either the callus or the
underlying medium.

The fine structure of the bacteria present in the cultured
tissue (Fig. 3a,b) is comparable in all essential details to that
of Azotobacter vinelandii (Vela et al., 1970). The bacterial
cells found within the callus contain a large number of internal
vesicles near the cell periphery. These vesicles are characteristic of Azotobacter vinelandii cells growing at the expense of
atmospheric nitrogen. Fewer vesicles are found in bacteria
utilizing NH_4 and none are visible in cells growing on NO_3
(Oppenheim and Marcus, 1970).

The independent lines of evidence which have been presented
suggest that a symbiosis has been forced in vitro between carrot
and Azotobacter cells. Only carrot cell cultures which have been
inoculated with Azotobacter are able to proliferate on medium
lacking combined nitrogen. These cultures have been maintained
for over one year on N-free medium without any reduction in growth
rate. Azotobacter-inoculated tissue regains its dependence on an
exogenous source of combined nitrogen in the presence of penicillin.
Penicillin does not affect the growth of control carrot or mixed
carrot-Azotobacter calluses on medium containing combined nitrogen.
Thus, it appears that a prokaryote is providing the carrot cells
with a source of reduced nitrogen. This conclusion is supported
by the significantly higher levels of acetylene-reduction activity
in the Azotobacter-inoculated calluses than in the uninfected
control calluses. Finally, the presence of Azotobacter cells in

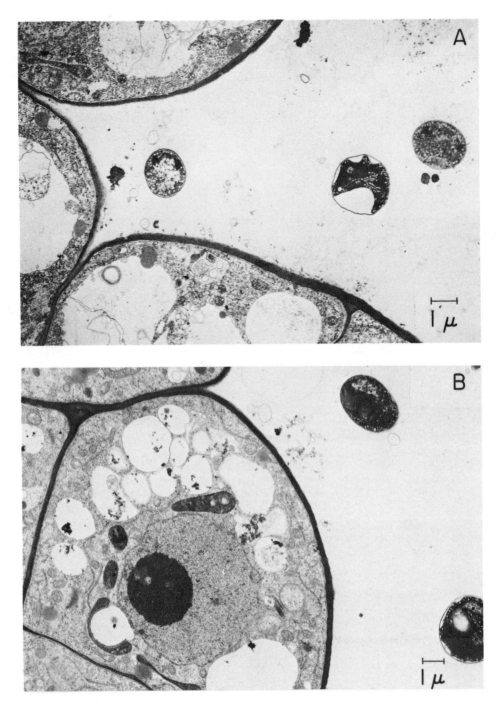

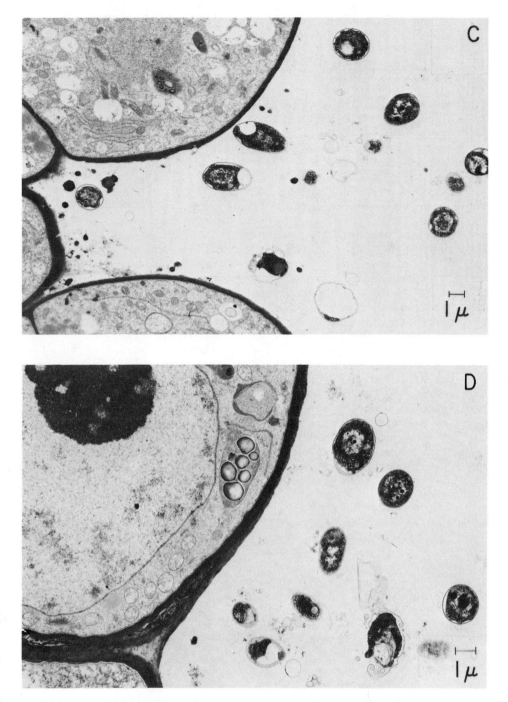

Fig. 3 a-d. Electron micrographs of carrot-<u>Azotobacter</u> composite callus.

the callus capable of growth on N-free medium was demonstrated by electron microscopy and by reisolation of the original _Azotobacter_ adenine auxotroph with which the calluses had been infected.

The association between cells of carrot and _Azotobacter_ was accomplished by designing a system in which the two components are able to survive only by entering into a relationship in which each complements a deficiency of the other. Presumably, carrot cells receive reduced nitrogen from _Azotobacter_ cells which, in turn, depend upon the carrot cells to satisfy their auxotrophic requirement for adenine.

The experiments reported here describe an incipient system which must be refined much further before any applications may be considered. The carrot-_Azotobacter_ association is not completely stable. Ocassionally, sectors of a callus will lose the ability to grow on N-free medium. Other calluses become overgrown by bacteria. Because these bacteria grow in the absence of both combined nitrogen and adenine, they are assumed to be prototrophic revertants of the original _Azotobacter_ strain. This latter form of instability may be controllable by using nonrevertible _Azotobacter_ strains in which essential genes have been deleted. The composite callus grows very slowly on either N-free or low N medium. We are attempting to increase the flow of reduced nitrogen to the plant cells by using _Azotobacter_ strains which are derepressed for nitrogenase synthesis.

An assessment of the agricultural usefulness of the carrot-_Azotobacter_ association must await the regeneration of mature plants from the composite calluses. Thus far, we have been unable to accomplish this. The use of genetic markers and nutritional requirements to force a symbiosis is a generalized procedure which should be applicable to all plant species which can be grown in culture.

REFERENCES

Avery, A. G., S. Satina, and J. Rietsema, (1959), _Blakeslee: The Genus Datura_ (Ronald Press Co., New York).

Bond, G., (1968), Some biological aspects of nitrogen fixation, in "Recent Aspects of Nitrogen Metabolism in Plants", eds. E. J. Hewitt and C. V. Cutting (Academic Press, New York), p.

Burris, R. H., (1972), Nitrogen fixation-assay methods and techniques, in "Methods in Enzymology", ed. A. San Pietro, (Academic Press, New York), Vol. 24, 415.

Child, J. J. and T. A. LaRue, (1974), A simple technique for the establishment of nitrogenase in soybean callus culture, Plant Physiol., _53_, 88.

Davey, M. R. and E. C. Cocking, (1972), Uptake of bacteria by
    isolated higher plant protoplasts, Nature, 239, 455.
Goodspeed, T. H., (1954), The Genus Nicotiana (Chronica Botanica
    Co., Waltham, Mass.).
Hardy, R. W. F., R. D. Holsten, E. K. Jackson and R. C. Burns,
    (1968), The acetylene-ethylene assay for N_2 fixation:
    laboratory and field evaluation, Plant Physiol., 43, 1185.
Holsten, R. D., R. C. Burns, R. W. F. Hardy and R. R. Hebert,
    (1971), Establishment of symbiosis between Rhizobium and
    plant cells, Nature, 232, 173.
Jorgensen, C. A. and M. B. Crane, (1927), Formation and morphology
    of Solanum chimaeras, J. Genetics, 18, 247.
Kao, K. N. and M. R. Michayluk, (1974), A method of high frequency
    intergeneric fusion of plant protoplasts, Planta, 115, 355.
Linsmaier, E. M. and F. Skoog, (1965), Organic growth factor
    requirements of tobacco tissue cultures, Physiol. Plant.,
    18, 100.
Neilson-Jones, W., (1969), Plant Chimeras (Methuen & Co., Ltd.,
    London).
Oppenheim, J. and L. Marcus, (1970), Correlation of ultrastructure
    in Azotobacter vinelandii with nitrogen source for growth,
    J. Bacteriol., 101, 286.
Phillips, D. A., (1974), Factors affecting the reduction of
    acetylene by Rhizobium-soybean cell associations in vitro,
    Plant Physiol., 53, 67.
Power, J. B., S. E. Cummins and E. C. Cocking, (1970), Fusion of
    isolated plant protoplasts, Nature, 225, 1016.
Stewart, W. D. P., (1966), Nitrogen Fixation in Plants (Athlone
    Press, London).
Vela, G. R., G. D. Cagle and P. R. Holmgren, (1970), Ultrastructure
    of Azotobacter vinelandii, J. Bacteriol., 104, 933.
Whitehead, T., T. P. McIntosh and W. M. Findlay, (1953), The
    Potato in Health and Disease (Oliver and Boyd, Edinburgh).

Research carried out at Brookhaven National Laboratory under
the auspices of the U. S. Atomic Energy Commission. The authors
thank Drs. R. H. Burris and M. C. Ledbetter for generously lending
their advice and laboratories to this project. The excellent
technical assistance of Ms. B. Floyd, Mr. J. Tilley, Mr. R.
Ruffing and Mr. W. Geisbusch also contributed to this research
as did the critical discussions with Drs. J. Polacco, D. Parke
and T. Rice.

PLANT REGENERATION AND CHROMOSOME STABILITY IN TISSUE CULTURES

WM, F, SHERIDAN

Division of Biological Sciences, University of Missouri

3 Tucker Hall, Columbia, Missouri 65201 USA

INTRODUCTION

Since the initial reports in 1939 independently by Gauthert, Nobecourt and White of the successful growth and subculturing of tissue cultures of carrot and tobacco, these two dicots and a multitude of others, including soybeans, bush beans, tomato, potato, belladonna, sycamore and Jerusalem artichoke have been extensively cultured and used for a variety of studies (see WHITE 1963). For almost 30 years following the initial successes with dicots, the tissue culture of monocots remained a rare event, such as the report on the aroid Amorphophallus (MOREL and WETMORE 1951).

By the late 1960's the situation began a rather sudden and rapid change which has resulted in the establishment of all of the major families of monocots in tissue culture. This sudden change probably results from three developments.

First was the development and widespread use of new media, with very high concentrations of mineral salts, particularly nitrate. This was mainly the medium of MURASHIGE and SKOOG (1962) or its slight modification (LINSMAIER and SKOOG 1965) and also the B-5 medium of GAMBORG and EVELEIGH (1968).

The second development was the general use of 2,4-D as an auxin in place of IAA or NAA for callus induction and subculture. With certain exceptions, the monocots not only respond better to 2,4-D but often require its presence in the culture medium for induction and maintenance of undifferentiated callus. This is especially

true of the cereals. At the present time all of the world's major
cereal crops are being grown in tissue culture.

The third reason for the sudden success in monocot tissue
culture was that many laboratories began to attempt such cultures.

Plant tissue cultures have been initiated and carried out
with many goals in mind. They have been used for physiological,
morphogenetic and cytological studies. Recent interests in the
culture of cereals and legumes have reflected the growing concern
for improvement of yield and seed protein quality in these crop
plants. If the techniques of culture, treatment and manipulation
currently employed for genetic and biochemical analysis of microbial systems could be applied to wheat, maize, rice, soybeans, and
other species, without losing the spectrum of techniques, particularly those associated with sexual reproduction, currently employed
in their study, then the utility of these plants in basic genetic
research and their improvement as agronomic crops is bound to increase.

Sooner or later in any discussion of the use of plant tissue
cultures for genetic studies, attention is bound to be focused upon
the possibility of regenerating normal plants from the cultured
cells. This question, in turn requires a consideration of chromosome behavior during culture and whether the chromosomes have remained stable. Chromosome stability is desirable since it is
likely to be a prerequisite for regeneration of plants. Although
this generalization is not absolute, it is nearly so and a stable
chromosome level is to be hoped for, particularly if normal fertile plants are to be obtained.

Our current state of knowledge of regeneration of plants
from callus or cell cultures will be reviewed. Studies on the regeneration of roots or other structures which fail to yield regenerated plants will not be considered. The formation of plants from
anther or pollen cultures will not be discussed since this topic is
considered elsewhere (see Nitsch, these Proceedings). A discussion
of chromosome behavior of plant cells in culture will then follow.
The third section of this paper will present my studies on long-
term lily callus cultures. The results of experiments on nutritional requirements, plant regeneration, and chromosome behavior
will be presented.

PLANT REGENERATION

Crucial to the extension of microbiological techniques for
the genetic manipulation of higher plants is the initial establish-

ment of tissues of these plants in sterile culture. The tissues
are induced to produce masses of undifferentiated cells, callus,
which is then subcultured on agar solidified media or grown as
suspension cultures in liquid media. These cells can be treated
with mutagens and mutant cells can be selected for in order to
establish mutant cell lines.

Success in regenerating plants from mutant cells in culture
should allow the achievement of a number of goals. These include
1) the study of mutant gene expression in differentiated plant
organs as well as in cells grown in culture; 2) the study of developmental mutants affecting embryonic events such as the "germ-
less" and "defective mutants" of maize as well as mutations affecting plastid development, photoperiod, phototrophic, geotrophic,
and other environmentally induced responses; 3) transmission of the
gene by sexual methods so that mutant alleles could be introduced
into other genetic lines; 4) the mapping and cytogentic analysis
of mutants by the techniques of classical plant genetics which are
dependent upon meiosis and recombination analyses. These could include the determination of dominance or recessiveness and gene interaction as well as linkage relationships; 5) improvement of food
and fiber quality, particularly seed protein quality.

Since 1957, hopes have been high that regeneration of plants
from cells in culture would be a rather simple and straightforward
matter of manipulating the relative amounts of phytohormones in
the culture medium and thereby produce shoots, or roots, or both
on command. These hopes resulted from the report by SKOOG and
MILLER (1957) that in cultures of Nicotiana tabacum, the adjustment
of auxin to cytokinin ratio resulted in shoot and root formation
reproducibly. Unfortunately, this principle does not hold true for
most other plant species, including some other Nicotiana species.

Even so, during the past two decades over 30 plant species
have been regenerated from callus or suspension cultures. These
include many ornamental plants that are now being propagated on a
commercial scale by tissue culture techniques. The propogation of
plants by tissue culture was recently reviewed (MURASHIGE 1974).

Plants may be regenerated from cells growing in culture by
either embryogenesis or organogenesis. In the former process,
embryos develop from the cultured cells in a fashion that is similar to that of zygotic embryos with the sequential appearance of
the different stages of development. When plants are regenerated
by organogenesis, a shoot is usually first regenerated followed by
the appearance of roots, or, the shoot is removed from the culture
and root formation occurs in soil. Totipotency and embryogenesis
in plant cell and tissue cultures were recently discussed by VASIL
and VASIL (1972).

REGENERATION IN DICOTS

The dicot tissue of carrot, one of the two original plant species established in culture, has been widely and intensively studied with regard to its capacity for regeneration. In the laboratory of F. C. Steward, he and his many co-workers have studied embryogenesis in suspended cell cultures. They stressed not only a stimulatory role in inducing growth and cell division on the part of such fluids as coconut milk, but proposed a requirement for coconut milk or similar materials in the induction of embryogenesis and furthermore, that this inductive effect had to be exerted on cells free from intimate contact with other cells, STEWARD, MAPES and MEARS (1958); STEWARD ET AL. (1963); STEWARD, KENT and HOLSTEN (1964).

It was shown, however, by HALPERIN and WETHERELL (1964) and HALPERIN (1966a and 1966b) that coconut milk "was a superfulous constituent of wild carrot cell cultures undergoing embryogenesis." That coconut milk is not required for embryogenesis in cultures of domestic carrot was shown by REINERT (1959) and KATO and TAKEUCHI (1963). HALPERIN (1966a) states that under certain circumstances coconut milk can, in fact, be inhibitory to carrot embryogenesis.

Considerable light was shed on this question by the report of SUSSEX and FREI (1968) who pointed out that the conflict may be the result of the change in response of carrot tissues to coconut milk as the tissue culture ages. They reported that a tissue culture of domestic carrot which had been continuously subcultured since 1956 did not produce embryoids on media containing coconut milk, but would produce embryoids in liquid media containint IAA when coconut milk was omitted. No embryoids were formed in the absence of IAA or on any agar solidified medium. They also observed that the addition of casein hydrolysate to the liquid medium reduced the time of embryoid appearance from about 7 to 8 weeks to 4 weeks. The embryoids could be grown into plants, some of which eventually flowered.

Sussex and Frei pointed out that the tissues used by Steward and his co-workers and by Halperin and Wetherell were newly explanted. Since the tissues had been grown through only a few subcultures, the tissues were still friable and probably contained initials of embryoids at the time they were used in experimental treatments, and the embryoids therefore had arisen spontaneously, and not in response to any particular treatment (SUSSEX and FREI 1968). They suggested, "it seems probable that the experimental treatment of these workers affected growth of preformed embryoids, rather than their initiation, and that coconut milk supported the subsequent growth of embryoids, although perhaps at a reduced rate." They then noted that the cultures used by REINERT (1959)

and themselves, were of relatively coherent texture and had been
in continuous culture for several years on media containing coconut milk with abundant subculturing, during which time, although
roots did appear there was no indication of a capability for embryoid production. They concluded, "it appears that in these tissues embryoids are initiated in response to particular experimental
conditions, notably, the omission of coconut milk from the medium."

The stimulatory effect of casein hydrolysate on carrot em-
byrogenesis in culture is in agreement with the observation of
REINERT, TAZAWA, and SEMENOFF (1967) who reported that the addition
of nitrogen compounds including potassium nitrate or ammonium nitrate had a stimulatory effect on embryoid production. They stated
"the fact that there was no qualitative difference between the
capacity of oxidized and reduced nitrogen to induce embryos demonstrates clearly that it is the concentration and not the form of
the nitrogen in the medium which is important."

The loss of totipotency of carrot cells growing in culture
was studied by REINERT AND BACKS (1968). They observed that callus
growing on the medium of Murashige and Skoog grew more rapidly and
lost the capacity for embryoid production sooner than callus growing on White's basal medium. They also observed that callus which
had lost its regenerative capacity could regain it when transferred to media lacking auxin (2,4-D in these experiments). This
capacity for regaining of regenerative capacity also disappeared
during subsequent subculturing. They concluded that the "gradual
loss in morphogenetic capacity of the cultures is probably caused
by the decrease of some stable information or substance which is
present in the freshly isolated explants and which slowly diminishes during growth in vitro", and that a certain balance between
nitrogen and auxin concentrations in the culture medium is essential for the formation of embryos.

A remarkable restoration of totipotency in long-term tissue
cultures of carrot was reported by WOCHOK and WETHERELL (1972).
They observed a three-fold increase in embryo number in long-term
cultures when kinetin was added to the medium at 0.1 micromolar
concentration. Higher concentrations had no effect or were inhibitory. When 2,4-d was added at 1 micromolar and kinetin at
0.1 micromolar concentrations, the frequency of embryo formation
was restored to the level observed in recently isolated cultures.

Tobacco callus has been a favorite material for tissue culture research since its inception. It was with this species that
SKOOG and MILLER (1957) analyzed the chemical regulation of organ
formation in tissue culture. They observed that the interactions
between IAA and kinetin and between these and other growth factors
determined the morphogenetic response. Higher ratios of auxin to

kinetin tended to result in root formation while higher kinetin to
auxin ratios resulted in bud production. Their results, which indicate a quantitative interaction rather than a qualitative interaction of growth factors in the regulation of growth, tend to argue
against the concept of organ specific hormones. Their results suggested that the achievement of regeneration of roots and shoots
from callus for any given species might be a rather straightforward
process of simply manipulating the proportions of auxin and kinetin
in the culture medium. Unfortunately, such has not been the case.
In the case of regeneration of geranium plants from callus (EL-NIL
and HILDEBRANDT 1971), the auxin to kinetin ratio was critical in
successful regenerating organoids which eventually developed into
shoots. Geranium callus was also shown to require an alternating
light-dark cycle in addition to having an appropriate auxin-
kinetin ratio in order to undergo differentiation and that "roots
were induced on differentiated shoots when the medium contained
more auxin and less kinetin, i.e. when proportions required for
shoot formation were reversed" (PELLAI and HILDEBRANDT 1969).

In many other instances, the situation is quite different,
with no organ or plantlet regeneration occurring despite the callus
being grown on media of a very wide auxin to kinetin range. Regeneration will also occur as in the case of carrot cells in certain circumstances where embryoids are formed upon subculturing into coconut milk free media or onto media low in auxin (SUSSEX and
FREI 1968), or in the case of endive (VASIL, HILDEBRANDT and RIKER
1964) where leafy green structures are formed when callus maintained on Hildebrandt's "D" medium containing 2,4-D and NAA is
transferred to "C" medium (same as "D" minus 2,4-D). However,
when these endive callus tissues were subsequently transferred to
the liquid medium of Murashige and Skoog (lacking any auxin) there
was much better differentiation and organ formation in the callus.
It is apparent that just as it usually requires the addition of an
auxin to a culture medium in order to achieve callus induction, so
it also requires a reduction or elimination of auxin from the medium in order to induce organ and plantlet regeneration.

Carrot petiole, when cultured on a 2,4-D containing solid
medium, produces many small spherical meristems. When 2,4-D is
omitted from the medium the globular and preglobular embryos are
permitted to develop into mature embryos (HALPERIN 1964). Not
only may the 2,4-D be critical as an auxin source, which is required
for callus induction, but clearly it is required to prevent embryo
development from the proembryonic meristems which are part of the
callus. A similar effect on organized growth in cultured wild
carrot tissue by CEPA (2-chlorethylphosphonic acid) was observed by
WOCHOK and WETHERELL (1971). They suggested that the disorganizing
effect of CEPA was the result of its degradation resulting in the
release of ethylene. They concluded "that polarity as expressed

by polarized cell growth is a prerequisite condition for the organization of organ primordia and that the establishment and maintenance of polarity is disrupted by ethylene."

Addition of the antiauxin 2,4,6-T (2,4,6-Trichlorophenoxyace-
tic acid) to the culture medium enhances the development of wild
carrot tissues into embryos following transfer from a 2,4-D containing medium, (NEWCOMB and WETHERELL 1970); however, embryo elongation was slowed down and root hair formation did not occur in
the presence of 2,4,6-T.

Callus of Brassica oleracea growing on Murashige and Skoog's
basal medium supplemented with 2,4-D and kinetin differentiated into entire plants when subcultured onto 2,4-D free medium. The
morphogenetic capacity decreased with time with shoot forming
capacity disappearing in six to eight and root forming capacity in
ten or eleven subcultures (LUSTINEC and HORAK 1970).

Differentiation of Tylophora indica callus into roots and
shoot buds on Murashige and Skoog's medium supplemented with coconut milk, casein hydrolysate,adenine, and 2,4-D was reported by
RAO, NARAYANASWAMI and BENJAMIN (1970). The callus also contained
globular and heart-shaped embryos which upon transfer to the same
medium (but auxin free), matured and grew into plants. They further observed that when the callus tissue containing embryos was
subcultured to a modified White's medium with a high 2,4-D content, it underwent complete dedifferentiation. This callus was
subcultured several times to avoid a residual effect of the previous
medium. When the callus was then subcultured onto a simple
Murashige and Skoog's medium without auxin or with low 2,4-D concentrations, embryogenesis was restored. The embryos, as in the
original callus, did not develop beyond the heart-shaped stage
however, unless transferred onto coconut milk medium. They noted
"This indicated that coconut milk, while being beneficial for enhanced growth of germinal and post-germinal phases of embryogeny,
was not essential for embryo initiation, and observation almost
similar to that recorded recently for carrot (SUSSEX and FREI
1968)." More recently (RAO and NARAYANASWAMI 1972) it was observed
that transfer of Tylophora callus to medium supplemented with
casein hydrolysate and lacking 2,4-D would allow the development
of proembryos to occur.

Callus development and embryogenesis has been reported for
Petunia inflata and Petunia hybrida (RAO, HANDRO and HARADA 1973).
The newly induced callus contained proembryos which grew into
mature embryos while remaining in the 2,4-D containing medium.
Upon transfer to auxin free medium the embryos grew into plantlets.
Embryogenesis was also observed to occur in suspension cultures
maintained in a 2,4-D containing medium. The downy thornapple

(Datura innoxia) is readily grown in callus culture on a slightly
modified Linsmaier and Skoog medium (ENGVILD 1973). The callus
cultures spontaneously formed shoots, a tendency that was increased
at high cytokinin to auxin ratios. Benzyl-aminopurine was the
cytokinin source. Callus cultures of Citrus sinensis, 'Shamouti'
Orange, were obtained by KOCHBA and SPIEGEL-ROY (1973). They used
unfertilized ovules as a source of tissue. The addition of malt
extract promoted embryoid formation.

Endosperm tissue cultures of Codiaeum variegatum, a member
of the Euphorbiaceae, were obtained by CHIKKANNAIAH and GAYATRI
(1974). They initiated the callus by placing seeds on a modified
White's medium containing coconut milk, casein hydrolysate, kinetin
and 2,4-D. In some instances, endosperm callus growing on this
same medium produced both roots and shoots. Another member of this
same family, Euphorbia pulcherrima, the Poinsettia, has been
studied in tissue culture by DE LANGHE, DEBERGH and VAN RIJK (1974).
They initiated callus from petioles or stem internodes on a modified Murashige and Skoog medium. They observed that the best callus formation was in the presence of NAA and dimethyl allyl amino
purine (2-i-p). Bud formation with the eventual formation of
shoots, which could be readily rooted, occurred when inositol was
added to the culture medium at 5 g/l and a high ratio of 2-i-p to
NAA was included in the culture medium. The higher the 2-i-p
level the faster buds appeared.

Tomato callus has been grown for many years and is of much
potential value for genetic studies because of the numerous mutants
available in the Lycopersicon genus. Plantlet formation from tomato leaf callus was reported by PADMANABHAN, PADDOCK and SHARP
(1974). They tested callus of three strains of Lycopersicon esculentum on a modified Murashige and Skoog medium. Shoot initiation
occurred within 30 days after subculturing onto a medium containing
4 mg/l each of IAA and kinetin. Other concentrations of these two
hormones failed to induce shoot regeneration. Most of the shoots
produced roots and became plantlets by 10 days after transfer to a
hormone-free medium. They observed that the shoot-forming potential was neither correlated with callus-forming potential nor
with vigor of strain.

Callus of several tomato varieties was cultured by DE LANGHE
and DE BRUIJNE (1974). They used stem explants for callus induction. Shoots were obtained when high amounts of zeatin or coconut milk were included in the culture medium. Callus tissues
that had been subcultured more than 30 times and that were more
than one year old retained the capacity to regenerate plants.
Observation of more than 200 plants suggested that no genetic
aberrations occurred prior to or during the regenerative process.

Another group of plants which until recently have resisted all attempts at regeneration of plantlets in culture are the legumes. These plants are of extreme importance because of their high protein content and because their amino acid composition complements that of the cereal grains. Shoot formation from the callus tissue of hormone-treated cowpea leaves was noted by INDIRA and RAMADASAN (1967). They induced callus at the base of the petiole of the trifoliate leaves of 10 day old cowpea seedlings by submerging them in water containing IAA. Upon transfer to a mineral solution containing IAA, shoot primordia developed from the callus. Roots also were formed and plants were obtained. Although this callus was not subcultured and grown independent of the leaf petiole, and therefore is not a case of plant regeneration from independent callus cultures, the regeneration of plants in this study is nevertheless significant, since it clearly demonstrates the capacity of the callus to produce shoot primordia.

The production of alfalfa plants from callus tissue cultured on Miller's medium was reported by SAUNDERS and BINGHAM (1972). They observed that callus initiation from immature anthers or immature ovaries was readily obtained when the culture medium contained 2.0 mg/l each of 2,4-D, NAA, and kinetin. Callus growing on this medium would produce buds when transferred to a basal medium but addition of inositol and yeast extract stimulated formation of buds and plantlets. They observed a difference in response among different genotypes and suggested that "many genotypes, if capable at all of in vitro morphogenesis, have specific medium requirements" (SAUNDERS and BINGHAM 1972).

Another legume, and one of considerable dietary importance, is Pisum sativum. Recently, shoot formation was obtained in pea callus cultures by GAMBORG, CONSTABEL and SHYLUK (1974). They compared the B-5 medium of GAMBORG and EVELEIGH (1968) with that of MURASHIGE and SKOOG (1962). The B-5 medium was superior for shoot production and benzyladenine, when added to the medium over the range of 0.2 to 5 micromolar concentration, had a stimulatory effect. Root formation did not occur regularly but some whole plants were obtained.

b. REGENERATION IN MONOCOTS OTHER THAN GRASSES

Although the development of successful tissue culture of monocots lagged considerably behind that of dicots, once monocots were established in culture, considerable progress was made in regenerative studies. Asparagus callus was induced under continuous il-

lumination on Linsmaier and Skoog's medium supplemented with 2,4-D
and kinetin. When the callus was transferred to liquid medium
containing low 2,4-D and kinetin concentrations, the callus developed many small globular embryoids which grew into normal banana
shaped embryos. When transferred to a solid medium of the same
composition as the liquid medium, the small embryoids grew and attained geotropic orientation. The embryos often dedifferentiated
again unless they were subsequently transferred onto a simpler
medium (Difco orchid agar) upon which plantlets were produced. The
plantlets eventually were transferred to soil. As embryogenesis
proceeded and embryo growth followed, a need for progressively
lower and lower concentrations of auxin and kinetin in the culture
medium was observed (WILMAR and HELLENDORN 1968).

In his study of regeneration of Asparagus plants from protoplast derived callus, BUI-DANG-HA (1974) obtained shoot formation
only when the culture media contained 6-benzylaminopurine in combination with either IAA or NAA. Embryoids, some of which grew
into plants, were observed to form when tissues grown on a medium
containing a high ratio of cytokinin to auxin were transferred to
a growth substance-free medium.

Callus of Lilium longiflorum grows readily on agar solidified
Linsmaier and Skoog's medium with or without IAA added to the medium, but rarely regenerates plants (SHERIDAN 1968). However,
upon being subcultured into liquid medium of the same composition
and growing to a high density, hundreds of lily plantlets can be
produced in each culture flask. Callus growing in liquid media containing only mineral salts and sucrose as well as callus growing in
liquid media with organic supplements and a low IAA content both
have a great propensity for plantlet production. Lily callus is
exceptional among monocots in two respects. It does not require
2,4-D or even high IAA concentrations in order to induce callus
formation or growth. Also, plantlets readily form as outgrowths
on large callus clumps, and there is clearly no requirement for the
dispersal of cells into small clumps or single cell suspensions
(SHERIDAN 1968). These callus lines, which were established in
1967 have continued to grow at essentially the same growth rate and
to regenerate plants throughout the past seven years of subculture
(SHERIDAN 1974).

Growth and organogenesis in tissue cultures of Allium cepa
was studied by FRIDBORG (1971). He grew callus on the agar solidified B-5 media of GAMBORG AND EVELEIGH (1968). Shortly after isolation of the tissue, organ regeneration was vigorous, but the
ability of the callus to regenerate buds decreased so that by the
end of a year of subculture they were exceptional. Low 2,4-D or
its absence was optimum for organ regeneration with cytokinin slightly
stimulating the formation of leafy buds. In contrast to lilies and
several other species, liquid cultures developed only roots and no
bud or leaf formation was observed in liquid cultures.

In their recent studies, FRIDBORG AND ERIKSSON (1974) observed that the medium of NORSTOG (1973) was much more effective for shoot regeneration from Allium callus than the medium of MURASHIGE AND SKOOG (1962) or the B-5 medium of GAMBORG AND EVELEIGH (1968). They suggested that this was probably due to its high content of organic nitrogen. They also reported that shoot regeneration was observed only in newly isolated cultures. A similar report on Allium was that of MACKENZIE, DAVEY AND FREEMAN (1974), who observed that shoot development was restricted to recently initiated (10 months in culture) onion callus and was absent from well established (4 years in culture) callus. SELBY AND COLLIN (1974) established 20 clones of callus from each of the three onion varieties, Red Italian, Rijnsburger and White Lisbon. They evaluated the clones at the sixth and eighth subculture and concluded that some clonal differences, such as degree of friability and pigmentation were established in this preliminary period of subculturing. HAVRANEK AND NOVAK (1973) studied bud formation in callus cultures of garlic, Allium sativum. They observed that 2,4-D prevented regeneration, which would occur in its absence. NAA had a similar but weaker effect.

The induction of callus and subsequent formation of buds and roots on the callus of Haworthia was reported by KAUL AND SABHARWAL (1970). The most prolific response was obtained on a modified White's medium supplemented with coconut milk. Addition of low concentrations of IAA or kinetin did not have any significant effect on the callusing or differentiation processes. They subsequently cultured Haworthia callus on Murashige and Skoog's medium and reported that on this medium root and shoot formation were controlled by the auxin to cytokinin ratio (KAUL AND SABHARWAL, 1972).

Among the Iridaceae, Gladiolus has been studied with regard to its regenerative capacity. ZIV, HALEVY AND SHILO (1970), using a modified Murashige and Skoog medium, induced callus formation on thin discs of young inflorescence stems of Gladiolus. They succeeded in obtaining root primordia on a high NAA and low kinetin medium, followed by bud or cormlet formation upon transfer to a media containing kinetin and lacking or low in NAA. SIMONSEN AND HILDEBRANDT (1971) also studied morphogenesis of Gladiolus callus on a modified Murashige and Skoog medium. Poor or no callus growth occurred when this medium was supplemented with coconut milk or when callus was placed on Hildebrandt's T, C, or D media. Callus differentiated into plants more frequently on agar solidified media than in liquid media. Differentiation of plants was most common on the basal medium lacking any auxin and with a low kinetin level. Mixed cultures of callus and differentiating plants were produced on the basal medium supplemented with kinetin and NAA.

Regeneration of plantlets from callus transferred to media containing lower auxin was successful with several genera in the laboratory of HUSSEY (1974). These included Ornithogalum, Muscari,

Scilla, Hyacinthus, Ipheion, Freesia and Narcissus.

BARRETT AND JONES (1974) were able to regenerate plantlets from
callus cultures of the oil palm, Elaesis guineesis. The callus
was cultured on Murashige and Skoog's medium supplemented with NAA
and casein hydrolysate. The reduction of NAA level in the medium
stepwise resulted in the appearance of embryoids which in some instances developed in plantlets.

Plantlet formation from callus of the aroid Anthurium andreanum
was obtained by PIERIK (1974). By omitting 2,4-D from the culture
medium regeneration was obtained. Organ formation and development
was strongly enhanced by light. Optimum callus growth was obtained
in liquid media in continuous dark.

c. REGENERATION IN GRASSES

Organ differentiation in tissue cultures of sugarcane was
studied by BARBA AND NICKELL (1969). When freshly isolated callus
tissue was subcultured onto Murashige and Skoog's medium containing
either low levels or lacking 2,4-D there was formation of roots
and shoots. Although Murashige and Skoog's medium was inferior to
White's medium in supporting callus growth, it was as reported by
VASIL, HILDEBRANDT AND RIKER (1964) for endive "infinitely superior" to White's medium in "fostering differentiation of shoots or
roots, or both in freshly isolated sugarcane tissues. When a tissue culture was isolated on W (White's) medium and the callus that
was formed subcultured more than once on this medium, it apparently irreversibly lost its ability to differentiate shoots. Sugarcane cultures on MS (Murashige and Skoog's medium) but subsequently grown for more than one subculture (3-4 weeks each) on W medium
also apparently irreversibly lost their ability to differentiate
shoots." They also observed that the addition of kinetin or coconut milk did not aid growth or differentiation while high auxin
levels inhibited both phenomena.

Subsequent to the above work, HEINZ AND MEE (1970) induced
plant regeneration from sugarcane callus cells following colchicine
treatment of suspension cultures. They induced callus on Murashige
and Skoog's medium containing 2,4-D (HEINZ AND MEE 1969) and coconut milk. After treatment with colchicine in liquid medium of the
same composition but lacking 2,4-D they placed the cells on solid
medium lacking 2,4-D. Within 30 days plants began to differentiate
from the cell cultures. These were later transferred to soil and
grown in pots.

By simply transferring brome grass callus from the B-5 liquid
medium containing 2,4-D to the same medium lacking 2,4-D, GAMBORG
CONSTABEL, AND MILLER (1970) obtained embryos. This process occur-

red equally well in the dark and in the light, but in all cases the
embryos were albino. They were unable to induce green tissue despite
varying the nitrate and sucrose concentrations, adding gibberellic
acid or kinetin, and exposing to natural light.

TAMURA (1968) used nineteen varieties of rice including Japanese, Indian and European types in his study on regeneration from
callus. Seeds were placed on White's medium supplemented with
yeast extract and 2,4-D. Callus formed in the dark and was subcultured twice on the same medium before being placed on organ forming
media. Several different media were tested. The most effective
medium was that of Linsmaier and Skoog's supplemented with 2mg/l of
IAA, 4mg/l of kinetin, 20g/l of sucrose and 8g/l of agar. After
two weeks of incubation in the light, many green buds were visible
on the surface of the callus. After the buds had grown and the
second leaves extruded, they were subcultured onto the same medium
in which kinetin was omitted and IAA was reduced to 0.2mg/l. Roots
formed and the plants were successfully transferred to pots and
grown to maturity. Many of the plants were albino and ceased to
grow in culture after four of five leaves expanded.

KAWATA AND ISHIHARA (1968) studied regeneration of rice plants
from callus isolated from root tips and subcultured for nine months
to a year on a modified Murashige and Skoog medium supplemented with
1 mg/l of 2,4-D, 20 g/l of sucrose and 10g/l of agar. When the
callus was subcultured onto the same medium lacking auxin, roots
readily formed. Callus subcultured onto the same medium containing
0.1, 1.0 or 10.0 mg/l of IAA also formed buds at 1.0 mg/l. At this
concentration of IAA, 5% sucrose or 1% casein hydrolysate in the
media aided in bud formation. Their media differed from that of
TAMURA (1968) primarily in that Tamura included kinetin and inositol
in his medium, but omitted casein hydrolysate.

The barley and wheat suspension cultures of GAMBORG AND
EVELEIGH (1968) frequently differentiated and produced roots. This
tendency could be increased by replacing the 2 mg/l of 2,4-D in the
medium with IAA or NAA at the same concentration. Lines were
selected which gave suspension cultures and after continued subculturing the cells could no longer be induced to produce roots.

In their studies on the culture of wheat callus, SHIMADE,
SASAKUMA AND TSUNEWAKI (1969) observed that root formation occurred
in all of their kinds of media except those containing no growth
factors or supplemented with 2,4-D at 1 to 5 mg/l or higher. Their
basal medium was White's which they supplemented with a variety of
factors including coconut milk, yeast extract, casein hydrolysate,
2,4-D, IAA and kinetin in their studies on callus growth and organ
formation in wheat. Shoots were formed in six calluses but none
of the growth factors were found to be specifically effective in
shoot differentiation.

The application of 2,4-D as well as several other materials used as herbicides, to wheat plants in spray form, induced multiple shoots in developing embryos of wheat (FERGUSON AND MC EWAN 1970). Treatment during the first week of embryo development was necessary, with later treatment giving rise to callused seedlings. A similar observation was made by NORSTOG (1970) on cultured barley embryos. When excised immature embryos were cultured on a medium containing 0.1 mg/l of kinetin, they frequently developed embryolike structures as outgrowths from the embryo. Embryos cultured on the same medium lacking kinetin did not develop such outgrowths.

Sorghum callus, after initiation and two subcultures on Murashige and Skoog's medium supplemented with 2,4-D and coconut milk, when transferred to the same medium containing 5 mg/l of NAA, initiated green buds which eventually formed roots and plantlets (MASTELLER AND HOLDEN 1970). The plantlets were eventually grown to maturity.

The effects of various auxins on callus induction and organogenesis from the callus were studied by using various tissues of rice, Oryza sativa L. cv. Kyota Asahi (NISHI, YAMADA AND TAKAHASHI 1973). Callus was successfully induced by 2,4-D, NAA and IAA with tissues from seed, root, shoot, anthers and ovary. Shoots and roots were regenerated from all types of callus by transfer to auxin-free media. Cytokinins were not required for organogenesis. It was suggested that auxin is the only exogenous factor that determines dedifferentiation and redifferentiation in rice plant tissue cultured in vitro.

Two recent developments hold promise for regeneration of plants in two of the cereals, barley and maize, which heretofore have been completely resistant to all efforts. CHENG AND SMITH (1974) cultured "Himalaya" and "Mari" barley on a modified Murashige and Skoog medium containing both an auxin source and a cytokinin. When they transferred cultures to hormone-free media, organogenesis occurred and normal diploid plants were obtained.

Green at the Allerton Maize Genetics Conference in March 1974 described his success in regenerating maize plants from callus cultures. He used a modified Linsmaier and Skoog medium containing asparagine and 2,4-D to induce callus from scutellum of immature maize embryos. Such callus, when subcultured onto the same medium remained undifferentiated and proliferated. Upon transfer to low 2,4-D media, the callus produced numerous green shoots and roots. Complete plants have been obtained and transferred to pots. This success was obtained with A 188, a Minnesota inbred line. Whether this approach will be generally applicable awaits further study.

SUMMARY AND CONCLUSIONS

Many plants can now be regenerated from callus or suspension cultures. However, many other species have resisted all attempts at regeneration. The most important areas where success has remained quite limited are studies with legumes and cereals. Recent developments with both groups of plants are promising.

The induction of callus cultures nearly always requires the addition of auxin to the culture medium. In cases of plant regeneration by embryogenesis, although embryos may sometimes form in the presence of exogenous auxin, their subsequent development usually requires its omission from the culture medium. This is especially true when the exogenous auxin is 2,4-D.

The regeneration of plants by organogenesis probably results from altering the composition of the culture medium or environmental factors in such a way as to remove a repressive condition rather than provide an inductive one. Consequently, the plant tissue proceeds to express a potential previously held in check but now released. This is indicated by the frequent success resulting from the omission of all phytohormones from the culture medium. It seems likely that many, if not most tissue cultures are totipotent, at least during the early stages of subculture. Most plant species progressively lose their regenerative capacity during repeated subculture.

That phytohormones are involved in both embryogenesis and organogenesis is evident from the reports on rejuvenation of long term cultures by the addition of cytokinins or by other alterations in the culture medium, as well as the observations on tobacco, tomato, and geranium demonstrating critical concentration requirements of auxin and cytokinin for regeneration of plants by organogenesis. Other components of the culture medium besides the phytohormones are important as well. The concentration of mineral nutrients, particularly nitrogen compounds, the concentration and kinds of amino acids, the amount of inositol, and other constituents all have been implicated in the regeneration of plants.

Success at regeneration through either embryogenesis or organogenesis may depend on two conditions. First, the removal of repressive conditions that were imposed during initiation of the tissue culture, and second, the provision of a suitable culture medium and environment for the functioning of the basic cellular metabolism so that the liberated genetic potential can express itself. Effort should focus on the development of culture media which allow the initiation and maintenance of plant regeneration in long term cultures.

CHROMOSOME STABILITY OF TISSUE CULTURES

In his study of long-term callus cultures of Pisum sativum, TORREY (1967) observed a progressive loss in organ forming capacity that was paralleled by increasing abnormalities in chromosome constitution with a greater frequency of aneuploidy. He suggested that "the loss in organ forming capacity is correlated with the increase in abnormality of chromosomal constitution."

There are two general types of departure from the normal diploid chromosome number which may occur in cultured cells. One is the formation of polyploid cells containing multiples of the basic chromosome number. The second type is the occurrence of aneuploid cells which would contain some number of chromosomes different from a simple multiple of the basic chromosome number.

In the first case, tetraploid callus might be expected to regenerate tetraploid roots and in fact was observed to do so by TORREY (1967). That tetraploid and octaploid cells of callus cultures may in fact originate by induction of division in polyploid cells preexisting in the original explant which was used for callus induction was reported by BENNICI et al. (1971) in their study of Haplopappus gracilis. They also observed that after 18 subcultures, those cultures grown on lowest NAA containing media (1mg/l) had 100% polyploid mitoses, while cultures grown on the highest NAA concentration (4 mg/l) for the same number of subcultures had the lowest number of polyploid mitoses (19%). Aneuploids were rarely seen at any time during the subculturing sequence.

In cases where the polyploid level becomes very high, the tissues may lose their regenerative capacity because of a loss in ability for normal cell division. However, a more frequent cause for loss of regenerative capacity is the second type of chromosomal abnormality, aneuploidy. It is clear from the work of MURASHIGE AND NAKANO (1965, 1967) with tobacco callus that, although aneuploid cells do not completely lose all regenerative capacity, the capacity is severely reduced with root formation practically disappearing and shoot formation substantially reduced. That aneuploid cells are not necessarily impaired in their ability to undergo division in culture, and in fact may have some selective advantage in the cultural milieu, is evident from their accumulation during subculturing in several plant tissue culture systems (TORREY, 1967; MURASHIGE AND NAKANO 1965, 1967; KAO, et al. 1970; SACRISTAN and MELCHERS 1969; SMITH AND STREET 1974).

The lack of aneuploidy in cultures of Haplopappus gracilis (2n=4) (KAO et al. 1970; BENNICI et al. 1971) contrasts with the condition of many other species in culture which have been examined in that most other plants have a higher number of chromosomes and

often exhibit aneuploidy. This is true of peas (2n=14), TORREY,
(1967); Triticum monococcum (2n=14), T. aestivum (2n=42), sweet clover
(2n=16) and soybean (2n=40) (KAO et al. 1970); tobacco (2n=48)
(MURASHIGE AND NAKANO 1965, 1967); and sugarcane (2n=106) (HEINZ AND
MEE 1971). It is noteworthy that in the case of sugarcane (HEINZ AND
MEE 1971) found that one clone of callus produced plants which were
aneuploids and ranged in chromosome number from 108 to 128 but observed that another callus line which was diploid produced only diploid plants, indicating a high degree of chromosome stability. A
fairly stable species in culture is Crepis capillaris, which was
studied by SACRISTAN (1971). Although she noted a marked tendency
for haploids to become diploid and for diploid cultures to become
tetraploid Crepis callus nevertheless showed little tendency to become aneuploid.

Because of the earlier observations of frequent aneuploidy,
particularly in tobacco, there has been a tendency to generalize that
plant cells in culture usually become aneuploid. Although this is
certainly true of some species, and possibly even a majority of them,
there are enough known exceptions that this general conclusion is
certainly no longer valid.

Two kinds of data are available which demonstrate a greater
complexity of chromosome behavior in plant cell cultures than that
previously described. First, it is evident that some species, both
dicots and monocots, remain quite stable in culture. Although there
are no absolutely stable chromosomal systems known (either in plants
or tissue cultures) the degree of chromosomal stability of several
plant tissue culture systems is more than adequate for most genetic
and developmental experiments.

The Haplopappus and Crepis cultures described above have very
little aneuploidy and the degree of polyploidization is low enough
to allow for recovery of haploid or diploid clones and plants. Although Haplopappus has not yet been regenerated, conditions for regeneration of Crepis are known (SACRISTAN 1971). Helianthus annuus according to unpublished work of Tommerup and Butcher (cited
by SUNDERLAND 1973) remained diploid for at least nine months in
culture.

Two species of Vicia have been studied with regard to chromosome behavior in culture. O'HARA AND BAYLISS (1974) reported that
Vicia hajostara is quite unstable, and rather quickly develops into
aneuploid mixtures. But with Vicia faba, SHAMINA and FROLOVA (1974)
have shown that lines which are stable and have a 50:50 ratio of
diploid and tetraploid cells can be maintained for at least 4 years.

Among the monocots, Allium cepa appears to remain diploid in
culture for periods up to a year (Selby and Collin, personal communication). This stability is also indicated by the ability of Al-

lium cepa to regenerate plants for about the same period of time
MACKENZIE, DAVEY AND FREEMAN 1974).

The most stable monocot reported to date is Lilium longiflorum
(SHERIDAN 1968, 1974). After seven years in callus culture most of
the callus lines have remained diploid and continued to regenerate
diploid plants.

The second type of data now available, which prompts a re-
evaluation of any generalization on chromosome behavior in tissue
culture, are the recent studies on chromosome behavior of different
cells growing under different culture conditions. It appears that
chromosome behavior in plant cell culture is a complex phenomenon
and is little understood. BAYLISS (1973) studied two suspension
culture lines of Daucus carota (2n=18) and compared their frequencies
of mitotic abnormalities with those observed in root tips of the
same species. The undifferentiated suspension cultures showed a
significantly higher frequency of lagging chromosomes, multipolar
separations and bridges than the root meristems. Furthermore, when
samples of the cultures were transferred to a 2,4-D free medium to induce embryogenesis, there was a reduced incidence of mitotic abnormalities. It was not possible, however, to distinguish the effect of
removing 2,4-D with regard to abnormality. The reduced frequency of
abnormality could conceivably result from either effect. In Lilium,
however, which can be grown in continuous culture as undifferentiated
callus in the absence of any exogenous auxin source, it is clear that
the induction of differentiation is not necessary for the presence of
a low frequency of mitotic abnormalities (SHERIDAN 1974).
low frequency of mitotic abnormalities (SHERIDAN 1974).

Carrot cells usually become aneuploid during repeated subculture and progressively lose their embryogenic potential (SMITH
AND STREET 1974). Nevertheless, diploid and tetraploid lines can be
selected for which retain a constant chromosome number and retain
also a high embryogenic potential, a phenomenon not associated with
aneuploid carrot cell lines (BAYLISS 1973; SMITH AND STREET 1974).
BAYLISS (1973) and Street (personal communication) have suggested
that the selective features of the culture system are what determine
the ultimate chromosome constitution of a plant cell culture. If
this is true, and it certainly is reasonable, then by proper manipulation of the culture milieu, the establishment and maintenance of
desired ploidy levels, particularly haploid and diploid lines, in
long-term cultures may become feasible. That such results are possible is evident from the success in selection of diploid tobacco
(FOX 1963) and carrot (BAYLISS 1973) lines which have remained stable
after many subcultures as well as the report of several lily lines
which have remained diploid for over seven years (SHERIDAN 1974).
Chromosome behavior in plant tissue cultures has been recently reviewed by SUNDERLAND (1973).

SUMMARY AND CONCLUSIONS

Cells of many plant species become aneuploid or polyploid upon repeated subculture. The degree of aneuploidy and polyploidy is dependent on the species being cultured but also appears to be strongly influenced by the culture conditions. Although some species may rapidly become aneuploid under all culture conditions, others, such as tobacco and carrot, have yielded both stable diploid lines and aneuploid lines. Other species, such as Haplopappus, Crepis and others are rather stable while Lilium is highly stable.

Those conditions that favor rapid growth and suppress differentiation, particularly the inclusion of 2,4-D in the culture medium, may tend to increase aneuploidy. A search for conditions that stabilize the chromosome number and tend to preserve euploidy should focus upon those cultural and environmental conditions that preserve regenerative capacity and avoid high auxin levels and rapid growth rates.

Not very much is really known about the behavior of chromosomes of plant cells in culture. Much work needs to be done, particularly in evaluating the effects of different culture conditions, auxin levels, and environmental factors on chromosome behavior. These studies are needed both for short term and long term cultures.

LONG-TERM LILY CALLUS CULTURES

In 1967 several lines of Lilium longiflorum var. Ace were established in sterile culture (SHERIDAN 1968). Callus was initiated from stem apices which after removal of all primordia and surface tissue, were placed on the medium of LINSMAIER AND SKOOG (1965) containing 1 mg/l of IAA. The resulting callus was subcultured two or three times on the same medium and then used to initiate the seven lines (I-VII) described below in Table 1.

Table 1. Modifications of Linsmaier and Skoog Medium

Callus Line	I	II	III	IV	V	VI	VII
Mineral salts and sucrose	+	+	+	+	+	+	+
Inositol 100mg/l			+	+	+	+	+
Thiamine 0.4mg/l				+	+	+	+
Agar 8g/l		+	+		+		+
IAA 1mg/l						+	+

Early in the subculture sequence the subculture period was about one to two months in duration. Subsequently this was extended in some instances to six months in the case of liquid cultures and to widely varying periods including slightly over a year in the case of agar-grown cultures. The growth rates of the callus lines cultured in liquid media have been essentially the same throughout the first six years of culture. (Fig. 1A). The average fresh-weight yield in grams at the end of each subculture period was respectively I, 12.9; IV, 9.6 and VI, 12.7. In spite of the variability in length of culture period, and to some extent, the varying explant size during early subcultures, these results are similar.

The growth rates of the callus lines cultured on agar-solid-ified media were even more striking in their similarity, regardless of medium composition (Fig. 1B). The average fresh weight yield in grams of these lines at the end of each subculture period was, respectively, II, 9.4; III, 9.7; V, 10.0 and VII, 9.6. (The cal-culations excluded the results of the initial subculture period.)

An examination of Figures 1A and 1B reveals similar growth rates among liquid-grown and agar-grown cultures, both with regard to their increase in fresh weight during each culture period and when average growth rates were observed during short culture periods (when maximum growth clearly was not realized) as well as during prolonged culture periods when the callus grew to nearly 20 grams or more per flask. Therefore, the similarity is not the result of allowing the cultures to reach a growth plateau before collecting and weighing.

Two conclusions seem clear. First, the lily callus can continue to grow on a culture medium consisting of water, mineral salts, and sucrose (with or without agar) at a similar rate of growth for over six years. Second, the addition of inositol and thiamine alone or in combination with auxin is not required for lily callus growth and at the concentrations used in this study does not significantly affect the growth rate of these callus lines.

The lily callus lines have retained, with only infrequent ex-ceptions the dilpoid number of 24 chromosomes throughout the several years of subculture. During the last six months between five and ten dividing cells were examined from two callus sublines grown on Medium I, four sublines grown on Medium II, two sublines grown on Medium III, and three sublines grown on Medium VII. Five additional sublines grown on these media were examined using samples of one to three cells. In every case, except for some of the Medium II sublines all dividing cells were observed to contain 24 chromosomes.

The callus lines have not been absolutely stable, however, since what seems to be an isochromosome has appeared in several sub-

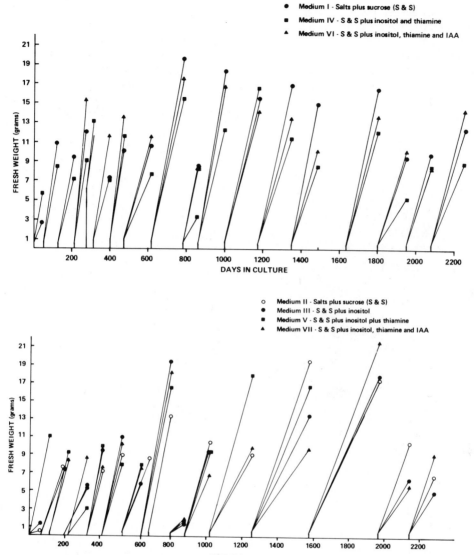

Fig. 1. Fresh weight increase of lily callus during continuous sub-culture. The starting fresh weight is indicated by the height of the vertical line at the beginning of each subculture period. 125 ml Erlenmeyer flasks containing 50 ml of medium were used for all cultures. Each point represents the average of 2 to 20 replicas. The average number of replicas was: I, 9; IV, 8; VI, 9; II, 6; III, 7; V, 6; and VII, 8. Fig. 1A (upper) Growth in liquid media. Fig. 1B (lower) Growth on agar-solidified media. Note that no weight was obtained for callus on Medium III for the subculture period ending at 1250 days. All of the callus on Medium V grew into plants during the subculture period ending at 1960 days in culture.

lines grown on Medium II. This small chromosome, which appears to
have been derived from the short arm of one of the acrocentric
chromosomes, is one of the 24 chromosomes present in two of the
sublines grown on Medium II and is present in addition to the 24
chromosome complement in four sublines grown on this medium. Complete counts have been obtained in only one or two cells in these
four sublines, but the presence of the isochromosome was readily
apparent in many additional cells which were insufficiently spread
for complete counts.

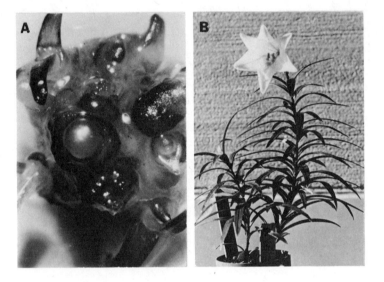

Fig. 2. Regenerated lily plants. A. Plantlet formation on liquid-
grown lily callus. B. Lily plant grown to maturity from plantlet
regenerated on agar-grown lily callus.

        Since the beginning of their culture, the liquid-grown callus
lines have displayed the capacity to regenerate plantlets. Plantlets were rarely produced during the usual culture period in liquid
media, but large numbers of plantlets were produced after a prolonged culture period when the callus masses had grown to a high
density in the culture medium (Fig. 2A). The regenerative response
has fluctuated rather widely. From 10 to over 100 plantlets have
been commonly observed in flasks containing callus grown for three
or four months or longer. There has been no marked change in
frequency of plantlet production over the years, but no constant
record of plantlet formation has been kept. Similarly, there has
been no pronounced difference in frequency of plantlet formation
between the three liquid-grown callus lines. However, line I has
appeared to be somewhat more prolific in this respect.

The lily callus lines grown on agar-solidified media have occasionally regenerated plantlets. The frequency of regeneration
is much lower than that of liquid-grown callus, with the average
production being one plantlet or less per flask per culture period.
The frequency of plantlet production does seem to increase as the
culture ages during a subculture period, but rarely are there more
than four or five plantlets produced per flask. Some of these
plantlets have been transplanted to soil in pots and grown for two
years in the greenhouse to the mature flowering stage (Fig. 2B).
When plantlets form in these cultures, they continue to grow, while
callus growth slows or ceases. If such cultures are left without
subculturing, the plantlets develop extensive roots and numerous
leaves, form bulbs, and callus death usually occurs. This sequence
resulted in the termination of callus line V during a 13-month
subculture period.

Root tips of seven regenerated plants were examined with at
least ten dividing cells being counted for each plant. Five plants
were diploid. One plant which was regenerated from callus growing
on Medium II and which contained the isochromosome in addition to
the normal complement, was identical to the callus in chromosome
makeup. The seventh plant was tetraploid. The latter plant may
have arisen from a rare tetraploid cell in a callus or it may have
undergone a spontaneous doubling early in its regeneration.

The growth of most plants in tissue culture has required the
presence of auxin in the culture media (see GAUTHERET 1955). A
number of exceptions to this generalization have been reported and
those tissues which are capable of growing in culture without an
external source of auxin may be conveniently considered under the
following headings: (1) numerous tumor tissues such as crown-gall
tumor (WOOD AND BRAUN 1961) which are produced in response to a
bacterium or some other external agent, (2) the genetic tumor tissue of the Nicotiana langsdorffii X N. glauca hybrid and the N.
suaveolens X N. langsdorffii hybrid (WHITE 1939 and SCHAEFFER AND
SMITH 1963), (3) maize endosperm tissue which can be grown on auxin-
free media (STRAUS 1960 and GRAEBE AND NOVELLI 1966), (4) the
"habituated" tissue strains which are derived from auxin requiring
tissues that have undergone numerous transfers and have acquired the
capacity to grow on auxin-free media (GAUTHERET 1955); the habituated tissues change in their appearance by becoming transparent and
friable and decreasing in their capacity for differentiation. A
similar type of autonomy is the O-1 tissue strain derived from a
callus tissue of Nicotiana tabacum after several years of culture
and which differs from the parent strain both in its chromosome
number and in the fact that it no longer requires auxin. (FOX
1963), (5) normal tissue of carrot which was reported by GAUTHERET
(1955) to grow in the absence of auxin, but he noted that other
workers found it necessary to provide auxin in the culture medium
for the growth of carrot tissue.

Except for tumor tissues, such as crown gall tumor (WOOD AND BRAUN 1961), plant tissues have not been previously reported to grow on a culture medium containing only mineral salts and sucrose. The successful growth and repeated subculturing of lily callus on a medium containing only sucrose and mineral salts is clearly established in this investigation.

The lily callus lines described in this report appear to be exceptional in their response to growth in sterile culture. The simplicity of nutrient requirements and lack of response to the addition of organic or hormonal supplements is unusual. The fact that these lines were established shortly after callus initiation, their chromosomal normalcy and their regenerative capacity all argue against their being "habituated" lines. Rather, the stability of these characteristics indicate that they have remained normal throughout the seven years the callus has been growing in culture. To my knowledge, there is no previous report of such a long-term stable culture of normal plant tissues possessing these properties.

In considering a possible explanation for the stability of the lily callus, three points may be noted. The lily callus in comparison to many other plant callus lines, grows rather slowly. The callus has remained green-pigmented throughout the culture period. And all of the media tested were rather simple in composition inasmuch as they lacked complex organic supplements such as casein hydrolysate, yeast extract, or coconut milk.

The growth on the vitamin- and hormone-free media indicates that the callus must be able to synthesize these substances. The greenness of the tissue suggests that the cells are similar in their metabolic capacity to those of leaves. The capacity of the lily plant to make its own growth factors is patent. The lily callus cells, which were derived from green stem tissue of a vegetative plant appear to also have these capacities. The slow growth of the callus probably results from the endogenous levels of growth factors in the callus. Although it has not been attempted, faster growth rates might be obtained by supplementing the culture media. It has been observed that kinetin at low concentrations is not stimulatory and at higher concentrations is inhibitory in this regard (SHERIDAN 1968). Nonetheless, the slow rate of growth together with the selective pressure exerted by the simplicity of the culture media may be supposed to have resulted in a selection for normal diploid cells during the series of subcultures described in this report. Whatever the reason for the comparative autonomy and stability of these callus lines, that they do in fact have these characteristics seems established. These lines may be useful for regeneration, chromosomal, nutritional and other studies. Callus explants are available to interested investigators.

SUMMARY AND CONCLUSIONS

Several callus lines of <u>Lilium</u> have been maintained in continuous subculture on agar solidified and in liquid media since 1967. Growth on media containing only sucrose and mineral salts was the same as when inositol, thiamine or IAA were included. Most callus lines have remained diploid and have retained the capacity to regenerate normal diploid plants.

These callus lines are exceptional in their simplicity of culture requirements, chromosomal stability and regenerative capacity. There is no previous report of such a long-term stable culture of normal plant tissues possessing these properties. These lines may be useful for regeneration, chromosomal, nutritional and other studies.

REFERENCES*

BARBA, R. and L. G. NICKELL 1969 Nutrition and organ
    differentiation in tissue cultures of sugarcane,
    a monocotyledon. Planta 89: 299-302.

BARRETT, J. N., and L. H. JONES 1974 Development of
    plantlets from cultured tissues of oil palms (Elaeis
    guineensis) Abst. #218. I.C.P.C.A.T.C.

BAYLISS, M. W. 1973 Origin of chromosome number varia-
    tion in cultured plant cells. Nature 246: 529-530.

BENNICI, A., M. BURATTI, F. D'AMATO and M. PAGLIAI 1971
    Nuclear behavior in Haplopappus gracilis grown in
    vitro on different culture media. Proceedings of
    3rd Int. Tissue Culture Conf. Centre Nat. Rech.
    Sci. 193: 245-250.

BUI-DANG-HA, D. 1974 Regeneration of complete plants
    of Asparagus from protoplasts cultures. Abst. #261.
    I.C.P.C.A.T.C.

CHENG, T. Y. and H. H. SMITH 1974 Contributions toward
    an in vitro genetic system for Hordeum vulgare.
    Abst. #68. I.C.P.C.A.T.C.

CHIKKANNAIAH, P.S. and M. C. GAYATRI 1974 Organogenesis
    in endosperm tissue cultures of Codiaeum variegatum
    Blume. Curr. Sci. 43: 23-24.

de LANGHE, E. and E. de BRUIJNE 1974 Massive propagation
    in vitro of tomato plants with maintenance of genetic
    stability. Abst. #42. I.C.P.C.A.T.C.

de LANGHE, E., P. DeBERGH AND R. van RIJK 1974 In vitro
    culture as a method for vegetative propagation of
    Euphorbia pulcherrima. Z. Pflanzenphysiol. 71:
    271-274.

*I.C.P.C.A.T.C. when used in a reference refers to the
Abstracts of the 3rd International Congress of Plant Cell
and Tissue Culture held at Leicester, England, July, 1974.

EL NIL, M. M. A., A. C. HILDERBRANT 1971 Differentiation of virus symptomless geranium plants from anther culture. Plant Disease Reporter 55: 1017-1020.

ENGVILD, K. C. 1973 Shoot differentiation in callus cultures of Datura innoxia. Physiol. Plant. 28: 155-159.

FERGUSON, J. D. and J. M. McEWAN 1970 The chemical induction of supernumerary shoots in the developing embryos of wheat. Physiol. Plant. 23: 18-28.

FOX, J. E. 1963 Growth factor requirements and chromosome number in tobacco tissue cultures. Physiol. Plant. 16: 793-803.

FRIDBORG, G. 1971 Growth and organogenesis in tissue cultures of Allium cepa var. proliferum. Physiol. Plant. 25: 436-440.

FRIDBORG, G. and T. ERIKSSON 1974 Morphogenesis in callus cultures of Allium cepa. Abst. #245. I.C.P.C.A.T.C.

GAMBORG, O. L. and D. E. EVELEIGH 1968 Culture methods and detection of glucanases in suspension cultures of wheat and barley. Can. J. Biochem. 46: 417-421.

GAMBORG, O. L., F. CONSTABEL, and R. A. MILLER 1970 Embryogenesis and production of albino plants from cell cultures of Bromus inermis. Planta 95: 355-358.

GAMBORG, O. L., F. CONSTABEL and J. P. SHYLUK 1974 Organogenesis in callus from shoot apices of Pisum sativum. Physiol. Plant. 30: 125-128.

GAUTHERET, R. J. 1955 The nutrition of plant tissue cultures. Ann. Rev. Plant Physiol. 6: 433-484.

GRAEBE, J. E., and G. D. NOVELLI 1966 A practical method for large-scale plant tissue culture. Ex. Cell Res. 41: 509-520.

HALPERIN, W. 1964 Morphogenetic studies with partially synchronized cultures of carrot embryos. Science 146: 408-410.

HALPERIN, W. 1966a Alternative morphogenetic events in cell cell suspensions. Amer. J. Bot. 53: 443-453.

HALPERIN, W. 1966b Single cells, coconut milk and embryogenesis in vitro. Science 153: 1287-1288.

HALPERIN, W., and D. F. WETHERELL 1964 Adventive embryony in tissue cultures of the wild carrot Daucus carota. Amer. J. Bot. 51: 274-283.

HAVRANEK, P. and F. J. NOVAK 1973 The bud formation in the callus cultures of Allium sativum L. Z. Planzenphysiol. 68: 308-318.

HEINZ, D. J. and G. W. P. MEE 1969 Plant differentiation from callus tissue of Saccharum species. Crop Sci. 9: 346-348.

HEINZ, D. J. and G. W. P. MEE 1970 Colchicine induced polyploids from cell suspension cultures of sugarcane. Crop Sci. 10: 696-699.

HEINZ, D. J. and G. W. P. MEE. 1971 Morphologic, cytogenetic and enzymatic variation in Saccharum species hybrid clones derived from callus tissue. Amer. J. Bot. 58: 257-262.

HUSSEY, G. 1974 Tissue culture responses of bulbs and corms. Abst. #260. I.C.P.C.A.T.C.

INDIRA, P. and A. RAMADASAN 1967 Shoot formation from the callus tissue of hormone treated cowpea leaves. Curr. Sci. 22: 616-617.

KAO, K. N., R. A. MILLER, O. L. GAMBORG and B. L. HARVEY 1970 Variations in chromosome number and structure in plant cells grown in suspension cultures. Can. J. Gen. and Cytogen. 12: 297-301.

KATO, H., and M. TAKEUCHI 1963 Morphogenesis in vitro starting from single cells of carrot root. Plant and Cell Physiol. 4: 243-245.

KAUL, K. and P. S. SABHARWAL 1970 In vitro induction of vegetative buds on inflorescence segments of Haworthia. Experientia 26: 433-434.

KAUL, K. and P. S. SABHARWAL 1972 Morphogenetic studies on Haworthia: establishment of tissue culture and control of differentiation. Am. J. Bot. 59: 377-385.

KAWATA, S., and A. ISHIHARA 1968 The regeneration of rice plant Oryza sat. var. in the callus derived from the seminal root. Proc. Japan Acad. 44: 549-553.

KOCHBA, J. and P. SPIEGEL-ROY 1973   Effect of culture media on embryoid formation from ovular callus of 'Shamouti' Orange (Citrus sinensis), Z. Pflanzenzuchtg. 69: 156-162.

LINSMAIER, E. M., and F. SKOOG 1965   Organic growth factor requirements of tobacco tissue cultures. Physiol. Plant. 18: 100-127.

LUSTINEC, J. and J. HORAK 1970   Induced regeneration of plants in tissue cultures of Brassica oleracea. Experientia 26: 919-920.

MacKENZIE, I. A., M. R. DAVEY, and G. G. FREEMAN 1974   Structure, differentiation and flavour production of onion callus isolates. Abst. #255. I.C.P.C.A.T.C.

MASTELLER, V. J., and D. J. HOLDEN 1970   The growth of and organ formation from callus tissue of Sorghum. Plant Physiol. 45: 362-364.

MOREL, G., and R. H. WETMORE 1951   Tissue cultures of monocotyledons. Am. J. Bot. 38: 138-140.

MURASHIGE, T. 1974   Plant propagation through tissue cultures. Ann. Rev. Plant. Physiol. 25: 135-166.

MURASHIGE, T., and R. NAKANO 1965   Morphogenetic behavior of tobacco tissue cultures and implications of plant senescence. Am. J. Bot. 52: 819-827.

MURASHIGE, T. and R. NAKANO 1967   Chromosome complement as a determinant of the morphogenetic potential of tobacco cells. Am. J. Bot. 54: 963-970.

MURASHIGE, T., and F. SKOOG 1962   A revised medium for rapid growth and bioassays with tobacco tissue cultures. Physiol. Plant. 15: 473-497.

NEWCOMB, W., and D. F. WETHERELL 1970   The effects of 2,4,6-Trichlorophenoxyacetic acid on embryogenesis in wild carrot tissue cultures. Bot. Gaz. 131: 242-245.

NISHI, T. Y. YAMADA, and E. TAKAHASHI 1973   The role of auxins in differentiation of rice tissue cultures in vitro. Bot Mag. (Tokyo) 86: 183-188.

NORSTOG, K. 1970   Induction of embryolike structures by kinetin in cultured barley embryos. Develop. Biol. 23: 665-670.

NORSTOG, K. 1973 New synthetic medium for the culture of
    premature barley embryos. In Vitro 8: 307-308.

O'HARA, J. and M. W. BAYLISS 1974 Chromosomal variation
    in cultured plant cells. Abst. #279. I.C.P.C.A.T.C.

PELLAI, S. K., and A. C. HILDEBRANDT 1969 Induced differ-
    entiation of geranium plants from undifferentiated
    callus in vitro. Amer. J. Bot. 56: 52-58.

PIERIK, R. L. M. 1974 Physiological and genetical factors
    controlling plantlet formation in callus tissues of
    Anthurium andreanum Lind. Abst. #141. I.C.P.C.A.T.C.

PADMANABHAN, V., E. F. PADDOCK and W. R. SHARP 1974
    Plantlet formation from Lycopersicon esculentum leaf
    callus. Can. J. Bot. 52: 1429-1432.

RAO, P. S., S. NARAYANASWAMI, and B. D. BENJAMIN 1970
    Differentiation ex ovulo of embryos and plantlets
    in stem tissue cultures of Tylophora indica.
    Physiol. Plant. 23: 140-144.

RAO, P. S. and S. NARAYANASWAMI 1972 Morphogenetic
    investigations in callus cultures of Tylophora
    indica. Physiol. Plant. 27: 271-276.

RAO, P. S., W. HANDRO and H. HARADA 1973 Hormonal con-
    trol of differentiation of shoots, roots and embryos
    in leaf and stem cultures of Petunia inflata and
    Petunia hybrida. Physiol. Plant. 28: 458-463.

REINERT, J. 1959 Uber die Kontrolle der Morphogenese und
    die Induktion von Adventivembryonen an Gewebekul-
    turen aus Karotten. Planta 53: 318-333.

REINERT, J., and D. BACKS 1968 Control of totipotency
    in plant cells growing in vitro. Nature 220: 1340-
    1341.

REINERT, J., M. TAZAWA and S. SEMENOFF 1967 Nitrogen
    compounds as factors of embryogenesis in vitro.
    Nature 216: 1215-1216.

SACRISTAN, M. D. 1971 Karyotypic changes in callus cul-
    tures from haploid and diploid plants of Crepis
    capillaris. Chromosoma 33: 273-283.

SACRISTAN, M. D. and G. MELCHERS 1969 The caryological analysis of plants regenerated from tumorous and other callus cultures of tobacco. Molec. Gen. Genetics 105: 317-333.

SAUNDERS, J. W. and E. T. BINGHAM 1972 Production of alfalfa plants from callus tissue. Crop Sci. 12: 804-808.

SCHAEFFER, G. W., and H. H. SMITH 1963 Auxin-kinetin interaction in tissue cultures of Nicotiana species and tumor-conditioned hybrids. Plant Physiol. 38: 291-297.

SELBY, C., and H. A. COLLIN 1974 Clonal variation in growth patterns and biosynthesis of flavor compounds in tissue cultures of onion. Abst. #283. I.C.P.C.A.T.C.

SHAMINA, Z. B., and L. V. FROLOVA 1974 Chromosomal instability in the long term cultivation of plant tissues in vitro. Abst. #281. I.C.P.C.A.T.C.

SHERIDAN, W. F. 1968 Tissue culture of the monocot Lilium. Planta 82: 189-192.

SHERIDAN, W. F. 1974 Plant regeneration from and chromosome stability in seven year old callus cultures of lily. Abst. #43. I.C.P.C.A.T.C.

SHIMADA, T., T. SASAKUMA, and K. TSUNEWAKI 1969 In vitro culture of wheat tissues. I. Callus formation, organ redifferentiation and single cell culture. Can. J. Gen. and Cytogen. 11: 294-304.

SIMONSEN, J. and A.C. HILDEBRANDT 1971 In vitro growth and differentiation of Gladiolus plants from callus cultures. Can. J. Botany 49: 1817-1819.

SKOOG, F., and C. O. MILLER 1957 Chemical regulation of growth and bud formation in plant tissues cultured in vitro. Symp. Soc. Exp. Biol. 11:118-131.

SMITH, S. M. and H. E. STREET 1974 The decline of embryogenic potential as callus and suspension cultures of carrot (Daucus carota L.) are serially subcultured. Ann. Bot. 38: 223-241.

STEWARD, F. C., M. MAPES, and K. MEARS 1958 Growth and
    organized development of cultured cells. II. Organi-
    zation in cultures grown from freely suspended cells.
    Amer. J. Bot. 45: 705-708.

STEWARD, F. C., L. M. BLAKELY, A. E. KENT, and M. O. MAPES
    1963 Growth and organization in free cell cultures.
    Brookhaven Symposia in Biology 16: 73-88.

STEWARD, F. C., A. KENT, and R. HOLSTEN 1964 Growth and
    development of cultured plant cells. Science 143:
    20-27.

STRAUS, J. 1960 Maize endosperm tissue grown in vitro.
    III. Development of a synthetic medium. Am. J.
    Bot. 47: 641-647.

SUNDERLAND, N. 1973 Nuclear Cytology, Chapter 7. In
    Plant Tissue and Cell Culture. ed. by H. E. Street.
    Univ. of Calif. Press. Berkeley. pp. 161-190.

SUSSEX, I. M. and K. A. FREI 1968 Embryoid development
    in long-term tissue cultures of carrot. Phytomorpho-
    logy 18: 339-349.

TAMURA, S. 1968 Shoot formation in calli originated from
    rice embryo. Proc. Japan Acad. 44: 544-548.

TORREY, J. G. 1967 Morphogenesis in relation to chromo-
    somal constitution in long-term plant tissue cultures.
    Physiol. Plant. 20: 265-275.

VASIL, I. K., A. C. HILDEBRANDT and A. J. RIKER 1964
    Endive plantlets from freely suspended cells and cell
    groups grown in vitro. Science 146: 76-77.

VASIL, I. K. and V. VASIL 1972 Totipotency and embryo-
    negesis in plant cell and tissue cultures. In Vitro
    8: 117-127.

WHITE, P. R. 1939 Potentially unlimited growth of excised
    plant callus in an artificial nutrient. Am. J. Bot.
    26: 59-64.

WHITE, P. R. 1963 The cultivation of animal and plant cells.
    The Ronald Press Co., New York. 2nd edition.

WILMAR, C. and M. HELLENDORN 1968   Growth and morphogenesis
     of Asparagus cells cultured in vitro.   Nature
     217: 369-370.

WOCHOK, Z. S., and D. F. WETHERELL 1971   Suppression of
     organized growth in cultured wild carrot tissue by
     2-chloroethylphosphonic acid.   Plant and Cell
     Physiol.   12: 771-774.

WOCHOK, Z. S. and D. F. WETHERELL 1972   Restoration of
     declining morphogenetic capacity in long-term
     tissue cultures of Daucus carota by kinetin.
     Experientia 28: 104-105.

WOOD, H. N., and A. C. BRAUN 1961   Studies on the regula-
     tion of certain essential biosynthetic systems in
     normal and crown-gall tumor cells.   Proc. Nat. Acad.
     Sci. (U. S.) 47: 1907-1913.

ZIV, M., A. H. HALEVY, and R. SHILO 1970   Organ and plant-
     lets regeneration of Gladiolus through tissue culture.
     Ann. Bot. 34: 671-676.

SINGLE CELL CULTURE OF AN HAPLOID CELL : THE MICROSPORE

Colette NITSCH

Physiologie Pluricellulaire C. N. R. S.

GIF (91190) FRANCE

Important advance in genetic has been achieved as a result of the work with bacteria, unicellular haploid cells because of their short life cycle and low nutrient requirement. These advantageous in bacteria may now be expected in higher plants if one works with microspores : unicellular haploid cells .

The very interesting report of Guha and Maheshwari (1966), showing that anther culture of Datura innoxia produced embryo like structures ; opened a new field of research. These embryos are derived from pollen therefore from an haploid cell. Progress toward the obtention of haploid plants using this finding, moved forward quickly . In 1967 J. P. Bourgin and J. P. Nitsch succeeded in raising haploid plants of Nicotiana tabacum and N. sylvestris to the flowering stage. It is indeed possible today to obtain a fully differentiated plant with shoots and roots in two weeks time starting from a single microspore .

The aim of our report is to present the conditions which have been found necessary for success. Namely how can one grow a plant from an haploid cell. The first part deals with anther culture, to understand the mechanism , the second with the culture of isolated pollen grains, the real goal which will be useful in genetic studies .

I. HAPLOIDS PRODUCED FROM ANTHER CULTURE

1. Several years of studies enable us to determine the conditions by which it is possible to obtain haploid plants from anther culture

297

a. State of the mother plants. The plant from which the anthers are excised should be grown in the most suitable environment for good flowering. Therefore it is important to adapt temperature and light regime for each species. As an example, we found that Datura innoxia anthers yield more haploid plantlets if the mother plants is grown in a high light intensity at 24 °C (67 % of anthers yield embryos) than if it is grown at 17 °C (31 % of the anthers yield embryos). Provided the plant receives optimal nutrient, changes in day length were not found to appreciably affect the number of embryos. The age of the plant has only a relative effect if it is kept actively flowering in preventing seed formation. This is achieved by cutting off old flower buds (Fig. 1) .

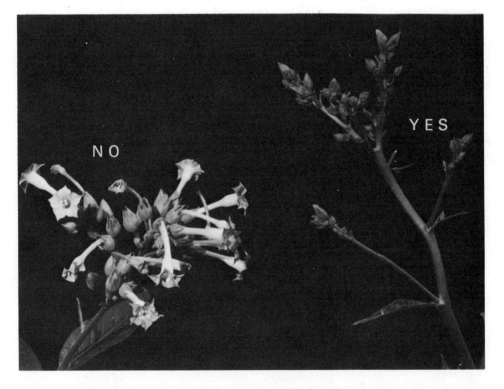

Fig. 1 - Nicotiana Tabacum : seeds developing on the plant at the left of the picture are inhibitory for good pollen production .

b. Stage of pollen development . Extensive trials on several
species by different workers have shown that the most important
point in the technique is to excise the stamens at the proper stage
of development. Stamens planted at the tetrad stage or when
starch is being produced in the pollen grains fail to produce
embryos. The crucial stage occurs at the moment when microspores are nearing the first mitosis. It is therefore rather crucial
to follow, for each species, the evolution of the microspore and,
if possible, to find a relationship between bud and pollen development. As an example Fig. 2 shows the case of Nicotiana sylvestris
Feulgen technique for staining the nucleus in order to follow its
evolution is best for most species. A fixation in acetic acid : ethanol (1 : 3) followed by 10 minutes hydrolysis in IN HCl at 60° (the
time may vary between species) and 2 hours in the Schiff's reagent.
By using aceto-carmin staining, one can easily overlook the exact
stage, owing to the reduced staining property of the vegetative nucleus at an early state of differentiation .

c. Cultures conditions. The minimal medium for culture is
quite simple : 2 % sucrose solidified by 0.8 % agar. On this medium a relatively low percentage of Nicotiana or Datura anthers
form embryos, but these embryos do not develop beyond the globular stage. One key element for the complete development of the
embryos is iron; zinc, manganese or other minor elements can
not substitute for iron- Iron deficiency in higher plants is known
to bring about an abnormally high level of arginine. In fact, when
arginine is added to the optimal medium, production of embryos
is nearly suppressed. This effect occurs at the globular stage, the
second week of culture. If arginine is given to the cultures during
the first or the third or fourth week only, embryo development
occurs normally. This should be related to the observations in
several reports where the authors mention the first stage of embryo development but that no differentiation from the globular to
the heart shape embryo could be obtained. The passage from globular to heart shape is a critical step where the culture medium
is decisive. Practically in order to study the culture conditions,
it is important to prepare a large number of anthers extracted
from flower buds of about the same age and randomise them before putting the anthers onto the medium. Even in the same bud, the
stage of pollen development is not synchronized, consequently by
planting the anthers of one bud per dish may bring false conclusions.
An aliquot number of anthers, from the mixed population planted,
should also be stained to control the actual state of the pollen.
Most anthers will grow as well on liquid medium as on medium solidified by agar however, the amount of liquid medium has to be
adjusted to the size of the dish as well as the number of anthers
to allow good aeration. Shaken culture does not seem suitable .An
other advantage of liquid medium is the facility to sterilize by
filtration which is advisable when working out a new medium .
Anthers grown in the dark will initiate embryos as well as in the

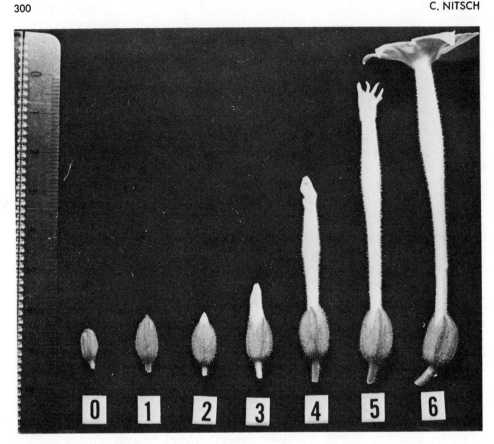

maximum number of anther yielding embryos (35 %) with flowers
taken between bud 2 and 3 .

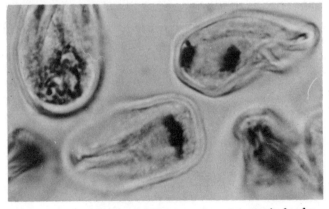

Feulgen staining of the grains in such buds .

Fig. 2

light but after 2 weeks in culture the light is necessary for normal development of the plantlets.

2. Improvement of the induction of microspores toward embryogenesis

The pollen grain which is the origin of the male gameto-phyte in higher plants follows a very well known developmental sequence from the mother cell to mature pollen grain. The mother cell : a diploid cell, by the process of meiosis divides into a tetrad consisting of four haploid cells included in a callose matrix. After disruption of the callose, uninucleate haploid cells called microspore are liberated. The microspores undergo what is u-sually referred to as the first pollen mitosis. At cytokinesis, two unequal cells are formed. A large cell with diffuse and low staining capacity nucleus, the vegetative cell, and a small cell with condensed nucleus easily stained, the generative cell which will divide once more to give the two gametes (Fig. 3) .

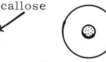
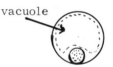

mother cell   tetrad   microspore

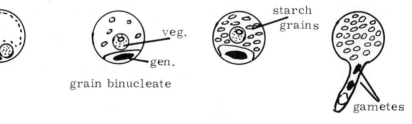

grain binucleate

pollen tube

Fig. 3 : Normal evolution of a pollen grain of Nicotiana .

The first observations made, following the development of microspores into embryoids, showed a low percentage of grains having an equal division at the first mitosis instead of the usual asymetric division. From Sax's work on Tradescantia it is known that a shock given to the plant at the time of mitosis modifies it. The action by which one cuts the flower bud off the plant may be considered as a shock given to the pollen. This may be the reason why the microspores which are at that moment in mitosis, instead of developing normally toward gametogenesis have a different evolution. The normal mitosis has been disrupted and gives, two equal cells . Sax showed that a sudden change in temperature modifies the mitosis. Treating the flower bud at low temperature for 2 to 3 days after it as been cut off the plant and before one dissect out the anthers, increases the number of microspores with 2 equal cells (Nitsch & Norreel, 1973) . In the same maner the number of embryos produced is greater as it is shown in the table below

Pretreatment of buds		Percentage of anthers yielding embryos	Percentage of microspores with 2 identical nuclei
Datura	0	63	3
	48hrs at 3°	95	22
Nicotiana	0	28	2.4
	72hrs at 7°	75	6.5

The cold treatment is given to the bud kept in a humid atmosphere, thus it prevents its driing out (Debergh& Nitsch, 1973), the best result is obtained when the cold shock is given in the dark .

The low temperature has also an effect when it is given to the grain just after the mitosis. When the grains have one vegetative cell and one generative cell not fully differentiated. In such a case the cold treatment enhances the division of the vegetative cells whereas the generative cell degenerates. In other word the cold shock increases the yield of embryo originated from pollen in two ways, first by its action on the mitosis, second by extending the time during which the grain is able to have a vegetative development instead of a reproductive cycle .

The technique of anther culture has been successful for the production of haploid plants with a rather limited number of plants (Sunderland, 1973). So far, the Solanacae seem to respond the best to produce embryos directly from the unicellular microspores. Other genera which produce haploids plants in anther culture start by producing an undifferentiated callus which has then to be induced toward shoots and roots formation. The regeneration of buds from callus as not yet been possible with many species. Moreover the undifferentiated cells of the callus are know to undergo numerous modifications at the chromosome level (Sacristan & Melchers, 1969). This makes impossible any genetic study on such material. We are therefore, naturally guided to consider the limitation of anther culture for the production of haploid plants

3. The limits of anther culture

a. Many species have been experimented out to produce haploids plants by the anther culture technique with no success. Theoritically we see no reason why it should not be possible to succeed in modifiing the evolution of the microspore in all species. The lack of response may come either from an unsufficient induction of the microspore toward embryogenesis or from the presence in the anther tissue of inhibitory substances which prevent any growth inside that tissue. In such case taking the pollen out of the anther should give positive results. This cell could freely express its totipotentiality.

b. Anther culture of graminae (Niizeki & Oono 1968, Nitzsche 1970, Chapham 1971 and 73, Tsun-Wen & Han 1973, Picard 1973) Cruciferae (Kameya & Hinata 1970, Wenzel & Thomas 1974) or Liliacae (Pelletier, 1972 ; Doré, 1974) have been partly successful, a low percentage of haploid plants have been obtained. In all cases the induction was achieved with high hormone concentration in the medium. High auxin and cytokinin is known to induce callus formation from the somatic cells originating mostly from the connective tissue. This induces also haploid callus originating from the pollen. The difficulty then arises from the presence side by side of diploid and haploid tissue. The competition between the two types of growth is generally in favor of the diploid tissue (Fig. 4). It is also known (Nishi & Yamada 1973) that a medium containing growth substances causes deadifferentiation. So that we came to the following conclusion ; anther culture may be beneficial for the induction of the microspore toward the vegetative cycle but, and specially if the induction has to be done by hormones, the microspore will have a better chance to pursue its vegetative development if it is taken out of the somatic tissue at a very early state. The most obvious question was then : how to grow isolated microspores ?

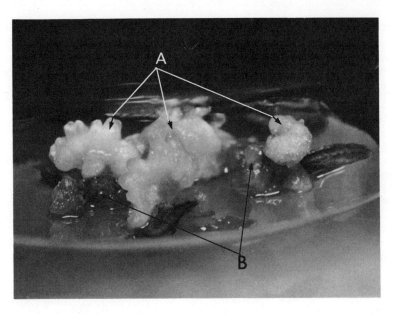

Fig. 4 : Anther culture of Hyacinth . Competition between the development of the callus originating from the somatic tissue (A) and
the haploid tissue originating from the pollen (B) .

II. SINGLE CELL CULTURE OF POLLEN GRAINS

From what has been written above, we come to the conclusion that
the first step toward the production of haploid plants is the induction of the microspore toward the vegetative cycle. The inductive
period can last from 2 to 8 days and is given on the flower bud or
on the intact anther . The microspores are isolated from the anthers when   the occurrence of equal division as been verified by
staining with Feulgen .

1. From anther to pollen culture (in Nicotiana for example)

     a. Technique for microspores isolation . 50 anthers floating
in the inductive medium in an erlenmeyer are emptied into a 30ml
beaker, the pollen is squeezed out of the anthers by applying pressure on them with the piston of a syringe. To separate the pollen
from the anther tissue, the medium is poured out of the beaker
onto a nylon sieve (fig. 5)

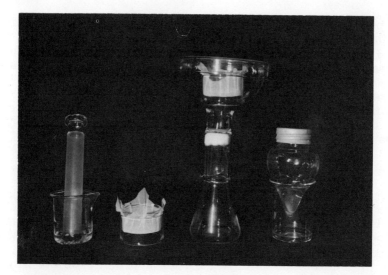

Fig. 5 :   Filtration by nylon sieve (Scrynell : Zurich benteltuch fabrick CH 8803 Eüschlikon Zurich Switzerland) ; holes 48 microns in diameter for Nicotiana or Datura, 25 microns for tomato, 150 microns for cupressus etc.

        The solution thus obtained contains the pollen grains together with fine debris. To separate a clean preparation of single pollen grains, the solution is centrifuged down at 800 to 1,000 r. p. m. for 3 to 5 minutes. The supernatant containing the fine particules is discarded while the pollen is resuspended into fresh medium and centrifuged again twice in order to take out any inhibitory substances coming from the anther tissue. The pollen is then taken back into the culture medium, (at a concentration of 10^4 cells per ml), which is placed into 5 cm in diameter pyrex petri dishes, 2.5 ml per dish. Some of the plastic dishes are not suitable specially if this volume is not enough to completely cover the bottom of the dish. It is indeed necessary for the pollen not to be immersed to deeply into the medium .

        b. Culture medium. As we mentioned earlier, the microspore has to be induced before it is taken out of the anther. The culture medium used for isolated pollen is therefore a medium which should allow the growth of the pollen towards embryos .

        The first study made concerning this medium was to mimic the nutrient contained in the anther tissue of Nicotiana or Datura since the pollen was able to develop to a complete plant inside these anthers. Moreover it has been shown by Sharp in 1972 and Pelletier in 1973 that it was somewhat possible to grow tomato and petunia isolated pollen using the nurse culture technique. The nurse tissue being anther or similar tissue. In 1973 we have shown that a water extract of anthers containing pollen grains at a young stage of embryogenesis, added in the culture medium was sufficient to pursue the complete development of the microspore into a plant. In 1974 the analysis of the extract showed that some amino acids (serine and glutamine) as well as a carbohydrate : myo-inositol are capable of substitute for the anther tissue. The induced microspores of Datura or Nicotiana are therefore grown isolated from the anther on the following medium . For 1 liter of media : NH_4NO_3: 2,900 mg + KNO_3 : 3,800 mg + $MgSO_4,7H_2O$: 740 mg, $CaCl_2$: 664 mg + KH_2PO_4 : 272 mg + FeEDTA 5 ml of a solution of (EDTA Na_2 : 7.45 gm + $FeSO_4,7H_2O$: 5.57 gm/l) + 20 gm saccharose + 5 gm myo-inositol + 100 mg L-serine + 800 mg glutamine, pH adjusted to 5.8, growth substances added to this medium will not be beneficial for embryo development. On the contrary we found that by the addition of auxin or cytokinin in the medium, we decrease the number of embryo growing and increase the time necessary for its development .

To adapt this technique, described for the solanacae, to other genera it seems necessary to study in details the mechanism and to find the real origin of the embryos .

2. Origin of embryogenesis in the pollen

It is indeed rather difficult to know which type of pollen become embryo since we have not yet been able to follow the development of one microspore continuously to its corresponding embryo . The approach we therefore used, was to follow statistically, during the course of its development, the number of each different type of grain and the number of embryos obtained at the end .

To do this, we have prepared an experiment of 20 dishes each containing 25 x 10^3 microspores. 2 dishes were used every day for staining by Feulgen and 500 to 800 grains were observed and classified as having, one nucleus, two nuclei one vegetative + one generative, two identical nuclei or being dead (Fig. 6) . It was striking to see that the percentage of grains in early mitosis at the beginning of the experiment, the percentage of grains having two identical nuclei and the percentage of 4 cell pro-embryos as well as 20 cell embryos range of about the same value namely 6 to 8 % .

Before drawing any conclusion, we have analysed 300 pro-embryos staining them with Feulgen to observed from which type of cells they were made. The results were the following .

Pro-embryos with 4 cells	4 identical	3 vegetative + 1 generative	2 vegetative 2 generative	1 vegetative 2 generative
100	67	21	8	4

It is clear that the highest percentage of embryos come from grains which started with a symetrical division. Therefore we can suggest that the first step toward androgenesis is really to trigger the microspore toward a symetrical division at the time of the first haploid mitosis. The second possibility can be to inactivate the generative nucleus to make it degenerate and save the vegetative cell which will therefore pursue a vegetative growth. In the Solanum family the highest percentage of embryos come from the microspore and is induced at the time of the first mitosis . The other way may for another family be more valuable this is the reason which make us follow step by step, in staining it, the evolution of the nucleus during the inductive phase. We have mostly been decribing induction done by physical means . It should nevertheless be possible to induce vegetative development of the microspore by chemical treatment, possibly in killing selectively the generative cell .

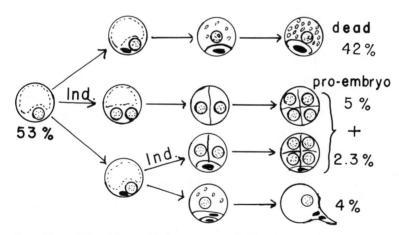

Fig. 6 : For Nicotiana Tabacum : 53 % of the grains are at the microspore state, 8 % of which in early mitosis at the time of the cold shock . A = 42 % of these microspores die in culture ; B = 5% become pro-embryos with 4 equal cells ; C_1 = 2.3 % have an induction post-mitosis; C_2 = 4% follow the normal reproductive pathway.

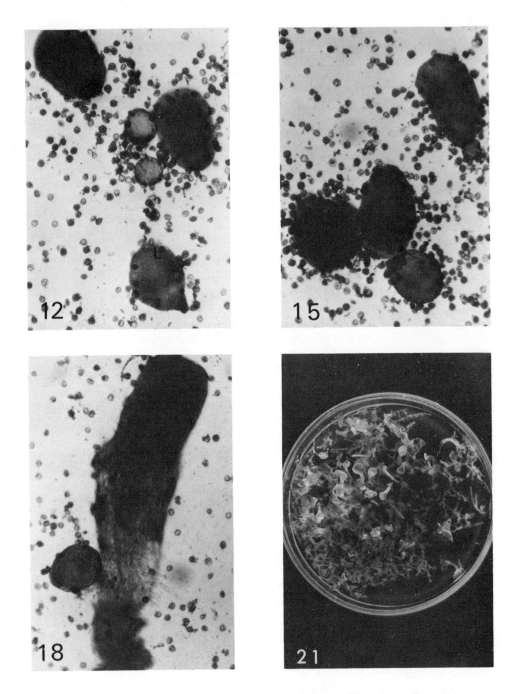

Fig. 7 : Number of days of Nicotiana pollen in culture .

III. CONCLUSION

The results of this new technique provide a method for obtaining haploid plants in a very large number, starting from a single cell . The whole process taken place within a relatively short time (Fig.7) Geneticists will no doubt benefit from it for their work on mutation as well as on transformation. The single cell culture allows an easy plating for screening mutants or drug resistant plants in the same way as it is done with bacteria. The availability of monoploid individuals would also lead to the production of homozygous strains which could be crossed to hybrids having the increased vigor brought about by heterosis .

The biochemistry of the differentiation of plant will also benefit from this results. It is indeed now possible, starting from one cell : the microspore, to follow day by day the succession of events which will lead to the whole plant. The absence of iron in the medium which blocks the embryo at the globular stage, namely with all cells of the same type, is a possible line of biochemical investigation towards the understanding of the mechanism which makes one cell become a shoot and the other one a root .

The achievement in this study for the production of haploids is only dealing with the solanacae. The understanding of the mechanism with this family of plant should be remembered in working with other species . Two steps are critical : first is a good induction of androgenesis ; second is the importance of the amino acids in the culture medium for the growth of the young embryos . A complete biochemical study of the part played by the amino acids in this system will open a new line of research for understanding differentiation at the cellular level .

IV. LITERATURE

J. P. Bourgin and J. P. Nitsch. 1967 - Obtention de Nicotiana haploides à partir d'étamines cultivées in vitro . Ann. Physiol. Vég. 9 : 377-382 .
D. Clapham. 1971 - In vitro development of callus from the pollen of Lollium and Hordeum. Z. Pflanzenzuch. 65 : 285-292 .
D. Clapham. 1973 - Haploid Hordeum plants from anthers in vitro. Z. Pflanzenzuch, 69 : 142-155 .
P. Debergh and C. Nitsch. 1973 - Premiers résultats sur la culture in vitro de grains de pollen isolés chez la Tomate . C.R. Ac. Sci. Paris 276 D : 1281-1284 .
C. Doré. 1974 - Production de plantes homozygotes mâles et femelles à partir d'anthères d'asperge cultivées "in vitro" . C.R. Acad. Sci. Paris 278 D : 2135-2138 .

S. Guha and S.C. Maheshwari. 1966. Cell division and differentiation of embryos in the pollen grains of Datura in vitro. Nature 212 : 97-98.

T. Kameya and K. Hinata. 1970 - Induction of haploid plants from pollen grains of Brassica. Jap. J. Breed 20 : 82-87.

H. Niizeki and K. Oono. 1968 - Induction of haploid rice plant from anther culture. Proc. Japan Acad. 44 : 454-457.

T. Nishi, Y. Yamada and E. Takahashi. 1973 - The role of auxins in differentiation of Rice tissues cultured in vitro. Bot. Mag. Tokyo 86 : 183-188.

C. Nitsch. 1974 - La culture de pollen isolé sur milieu synthétique. C.R. Ac. Sci. Paris 278 D : 1031-1034.

C. Nitsch and B. Norreel. 1972 - Factors favoring the formation of androgenetic embryos in anther culture. Genes, enzymes and populations. A. Srb ed. Plenum press 2 : 128-144.

C. Nitsch and B. Norreel. 1973 - Effet d'un choc thermique sur le pouvoir embryogène du pollen de Datura cultivé dans l'anthère ou isolé de l'anthère. C.R. Ac. Sci. Paris 276 D : 303-306.

W. Nitzsche. 1970 - Herstellung haploider Pflanzen aus Festuea-Lolium-Bartenden. Naturwissenschaften 57 : 199-200.

G. Pelletier, C. Raquin and G. Simon. 1972 - La culture in vitro d'anthères d'Asperge. C.R. Ac. Sci. Paris 274 D : 848-851.

G. Pelletier. 1973 - Les conditions et les premiers stades de l'androgenèse in vitro chez Nicotiana tabacum. Mem. Soc. Bot. Fr. Coll. Morphol. : 261-268.

E. Picard. 1973 - Influence de modifications dans les corrélations internes sur le devenir du gametophyte mâle de Triticum aestivum L. C.R. Ac. Sci. Paris 277 D : 777-780.

M.D. Sacristan. 1967 - Auxin-Autotrophie und Chromosomenzahl. Molec. and Gen. Genetics 99 : 311-321.

K. Sax. 1937 - Effect of variations in temperature on nuclear and cell division in Tradescantia. Am. J. of Botany 34 : 218-225.

W.R. Sharp, R.S. Raskin and H.E. Sommer. 1972 - The use of Nurse-culture in the development of haploid clones of Tomato. Planta 104 : 357-361.

N. Sunderland. 1973 - Pollen and anther culture. "Plant tissue and cell culture" H.E. Street ed. Blackwell Scientific Publications p. 205-240.

O. Tsun-Wen, H. Han, C. Chia-Chung and T. Chun Chik. 1973 - Induction of pollen plants from anthers of Triticum aestivum L. cultured in vitro. Scientia Sinica 16 : 79-95.

G. Wenzel and E. Thomas. 1974 - Observations on the growth in culture of anthers of Secale cereale. Z. Pflanzenzuch in Press.

PLANT PROTOPLASTS AS GENETIC SYSTEMS

E. C. Cocking

Department of Botany, University of Nottingham

University Park, Nottingham NG7 2RD, England

Work on isolated plant protoplasts has progressed very rapidly since the first international meeting held on higher plant protoplasts in Versailles in 1972[1]. Indeed, whereas earlier symposia on protoplasts in general included short sections on those from higher plants[2] there are probably now more workers studying higher plant protoplasts than those from micro organisms. As we shall see there has been a major resurgance of interest during the past few years in higher plant protoplasts as genetic systems. At the Versailles Meeting it was evident that some of the foundations for this had been established. Much effort since then has gone into the fuller development of protoplasts as genetic systems, and I will try in this chapter to assess the extent to which this work has been successful and also try to indicate where difficulties still exist.

An attempt will be made to provide some perspective rather than just a summary of additional progress since the Versailles Meeting.

ISOLATION

It is particularly noteworthy that an ever increasing number of isolations of protoplasts directly from plant leaves has been reported[3,4], and there is no doubt that leaves are often ideal for the isolation of large quantities of uniform populations of protoplasts. Protoplasts can of course be isolated from callus and suspension cultures but there is no doubt that the ability to isolate protoplasts directly from the plant is a great advantage. The range of enzymes now available commercially is very extensive

(see [4]) but initially it is best to utilise a cellulase mixture
such as Onozuka or Meicelase, and a cell separating enzyme
mixture such as Macerozyme. These can either be used
sequentially or as a mixture and are available commercially (see [5]).
Initially when attempts are being made to isolate protoplasts for
the first time from the leaves of a particular species, mixtures
of cellulases and Macerozyme should be employed. Usually it is
better to remove the lower epidermis by peeling to facilitate the
entry of the enzymes. High yields of viable protoplasts can often
be obtained from leaf material and, depending on the species,
between 1×10^5 to 1×10^7 protoplasts can be obtained per gram
fresh weight of leaf material [5]; and this ability to obtain large
single cell populations of eukaryotic cells has commended
protoplasts to the geneticist as an attractive system for genetical
studies. However, there are still many problems not fully resolved.
Some leaf systems yield protoplasts with a marked tendency to
contamination by bacteria even though steps are taken to surface
sterilise the leaves. With certain varieties of petunia this can
be a major difficulty. The addition of antibiotics such as
ampicillin to the enzyme mixture can often help greatly [6] but many
antibiotics are toxic to protoplasts. Routinely we add ampicillin
to the enzyme mixture used for the isolation of petunia and
tobacco [6]. The isolation of protoplasts directly from plant organs
such as leaves is sometimes very sensitive to the growth conditions [7]
of the plant. For tobacco for instance it has been noted that
the most important factors, apart from the actual stage of the
plant, appear to be:
1. Illumination: intensities in excess of 25,000 lux cause
problems due in part to starch accumulation which makes the
protoplasts easily damaged during preparation.
2. Temperature: high temperatures encountered very occasionally
during summer (in excess of 38°C) and low temperatures (below
19°C) caused unspecified damage, and again the protoplasts burst
during or shortly after preparation.
3. Insecticides: the use of sprays was usually disasterous.
·Even the nicotine vapour treatment that was used occasionally
to control aphids etc., made the leaves unsuitable for protoplast
work for the next 1 or 2 days.

In our experience it would seem likely that the same principle
holds for other species although the exact environmental
influences will vary. Thus there is no doubt that each particular
species and even the particular variety being utilised for
genetical studies needs an extensive study of the conditions for
the reproducible isolation of large quantities of protoplasts.
Subsequent culture of the isolated protoplasts is often critically
dependent on the growth conditions of the plants from which
protoplasts have been isolated and for each new species
investigated the optimum conditions have to be decided largely
by trial and error. Guidelines exist for a few species such as

petunia and tobacco[6] but these need to be established more
comprehensively for Arabidopsis, the Brassicas, the legumes and
the cereals. It does not of course follow that all isolated leaf
protoplasts are capable of division and there is no doubt that
further studies are needed on the isolation and culture of
protoplasts from callus and suspension culture cells. In
particular the ready isolation of protoplasts from crown gall
cell suspension cultures may be very useful in more fully
elucidating basic causes of tumourigenesis; since although the
growth of the crown gall cell suspensions is independent of an
exogenous supply of growth regulators, their isolated protoplasts
are dependent at least initially on a supply of growth regulators
for the initiation of division[8]. As I shall discuss later the
ready isolation of epidermal protoplasts[9], and the combined use of
callus and mesophyll protoplasts, has provided a good visual marker
for fusion product identification in somatic hybridisation studies.
Although most culture of protoplasts is now carried out in
nutrient agar using the basic methodology of Bergmann, it is
necessary for mutagen work to have protoplasts in liquid suspension.
Protoplasts, however, differ in the readiness with which they can
be cultured in liquid media and as will be discussed later
difficulties may arise in this respect.

At Nottingham we have worked extensively with *Nicotiana
tabacum* and *Petunia hybrida* and these two genera are currently
being employed in fusion, selection and somatic hybridisation
studies. The detailed procedures for the isolation of protoplasts
from the mesophyll of these two species are illustrated
diagrammatically in Fig.1. A typical practical protocol for the
isolation of tobacco mesophyll and petunia mesophyll protoplasts
is as follows (abstracted from Power, Frearson and Hayward)[6]:
1. Surface sterilise leaves in 5% v/v 'Domestos' solution for
   30 min.
2. Wash thoroughly in sterile tap water.
3. Remove the lower epidermis (N.B. This material can be used as
   a source of epidermal protoplasts).
4. Using a scalpel, cut out regions of the leaf where the epidermis
   has been removed and place these pieces, exposed surface
   downwards, on the surface of C.P.W. medium maintained in 14 cm
   petri dishes. Leave for 1-2 h.
5. Remove C.P.W. from below the leaf pieces and replace with the
   appropriate filter-sterilised enzyme solution (20 ml/dish).
   Tobacco:
   4% w/v Meicelase   )
     0.4% w/v Macerozyme dissolved) pH adjusted to 5.8
            in C.P.W. medium   ) with 5N HCl

   Petunia:
   2% w/v Meicelase   )
     0.2% w/v Macerozyme dissolved) pH adjusted to 5.8
            in C.P.W. medium   ) with 5N HCl

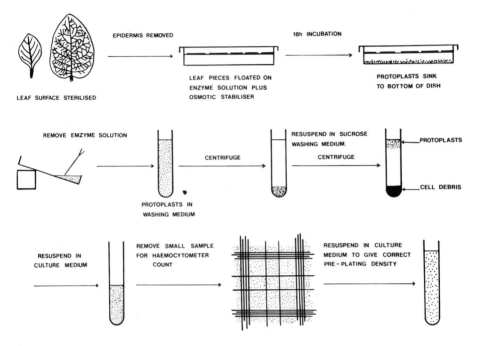

Fig. 1.   Isolation of Protoplasts (e.g. Petunia and Tobacco Mesophyll)

6. Incubate overnight at 27°C (18 h).
7. Using forceps, agitate leaf pieces to release the protoplasts.
   Tilt the dish and allow protoplasts to settle out for 30 min.
8. Remove enzyme solution and transfer the protoplasts to a medium
   size centrifuge tube, suspend in C.P.W. and spin at 35 x g
   (5 min).
9. Remove supernatant and resuspend protoplasts in 20% w/v sucrose
   (containing C.P.W. Salts). Spin 50 x g (10 min).
10. Resuspend protoplasts in F_5 medium and determine yield by
    haemocytometer count.

   Although still at an early stage in its refinement the
isolation of pollen tetrad protoplasts provides potentially very
useful haploid protoplasts for mutagen treatment, fusion and
cultural studies[18]. The method depends on the degradation of the
callose (β1-3 glucan) of the tetrad by the β1-3 glucanase present in the
Helicase enzyme complex. It is also possible to isolate protoplasts
from more mature pollen grains[11]. A typical protocol for the
isolation of pollen tetrad protoplasts from tobacco is as follows

(abstracted from Davey and Bush)[6]:
1. Prepare 5 ml of cell wall degrading enzyme mixture consisting
   of 1% w/v Helicase, 10% w/v sucrose and C.P.W. salts, pH 5.4.
2. Excise developing buds from tobacco flower heads, selecting
   buds about 5 x 10 mm in size. Peel back the sepals with fine
   forceps and split the corolla longitudinally to expose the 5
   developing anthers in the bud.
3. Remove 2 anthers from each bud. Place each anther separately
   on a glass slide, add 1 drop of water, cut off the basal end
   of the anther with a sharp scalpel and gently crush the anther
   with a glass spatula or scalpel blade. The anther contents are
   expelled as a milky coloured fluid. Examine under the light
   microscope to see the stage of pollen grain development. If
   both anthers contain tetrads, then use the remaining 3 anthers
   from the bud for protoplast isolation. If pollen grains are
   present select a younger bud; if only pollen mother cells are
   found then excise a slightly larger bud.
4. Place a drop of enzyme solution (about 0.1 ml) on a cavity slide
   and crush the pollen tetrads from one of the 3 remaining anthers
   into the enzyme mixture using the procedure described in 3
   above. Remove the remains of the anthers. Gently swirl the
   cavity slide to aggregate the tetrads in the centre of the
   depression and follow protoplast release under the light
   microscope. The isolation may be scaled up by incubating
   anthers in enzyme solution contained in small embryo dishes.
   (Use about 5 anthers/1 ml enzyme). Protoplasts can be washed
   by replacing the enzyme mixture with 10% w/v sucrose containing
   C.P.W. salts. Finally the washing medium is replaced by a
   suitable culture solution.

CULTURE

     Our knowledge of the culture of isolated protoplasts is still
somewhat limited and it will first be useful to try to assess the
extent that these limitations are restricting the use of protoplasts
as genetic systems. Often protoplasts can be readily freed from
contamination by cells and general debris by simple washing and
flotation procedures but sometimes this is difficult, particularly
when dealing with protoplasts isolated from cultured cells.
However, the recent very elegant fractionation procedures of
Kanai and Edwards[12], which have enabled the separation of mesophyll
protoplasts from C_3, C_4 and Crassulacean acid metabolism plants
using an aqueous dextran-polyethylene glycol two phase system,
should now greatly improve the facility with which purer preparations
of protoplasts can be obtained.

     A prerequisite for the use of protoplasts in fusion and
somatic hybridisation, and in uptake studies, is that they should
be able not only to be isolated reproducibly and aseptically, but

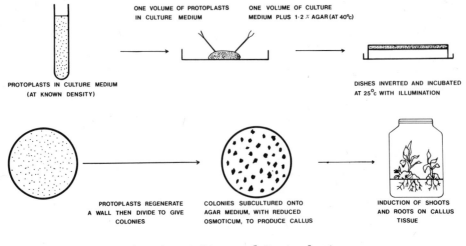

Fig. 2.   Culture of Protoplasts

that they should also be able to be cultured reproducibly at a
high plating efficiency.   Fortunately very marked progress has
been made and reproducible high plating efficiency is now possible
both for tobacco and for petunia.   Many other species are actively
being investigated in numerous laboratories throughout the world.
Evans and Cocking[4] have pointed out the help that studies on the
culture of walled cells (particularly those isolated directly from
leaves) have provided.   The pattern of development to be expected
is now clear.   The isolated protoplasts first synthesise *de novo*
at their surfaces a cell wall primarily made up of cellulose and
pectin[13,14], and either concomitantly, or subsequently, in suitable
culture media they will divide to form cell aggregates and finally
callus.   Whole plant regeneration can result (see Fig.2).
Although this complete pattern has been obtained for several
species including tobacco, carrot and petunia, as stressed by
Halperin[15] further advances in our understanding of embryogenesis
and organogenesis *in vitro* will be necessary if we are to recover
viable plants from isolated protoplasts and any modified cells
produced from them.   Intensive effort is being applied to the
culture of protoplasts from those species which are of interest
in uptake or fusion studies.   Indeed, this is now the major
bottleneck in the very major momentum of work in this field.   Cell
wall regeneration is no longer a major problem and usually this
will proceed readily although sometimes, particularly with

protoplasts isolated from cultured cells, special additions are
necessary[16]. The choice of suitable media for the division of
these regenerated protoplasts is, however, still largely empirical
and there is an urgent need for a rationalisation of the approach
at this level.

In general, except for special microscopic observations, small
scale microdrop and special culture chamber methods are best avoided.
Genetic studies require large populations (several million) of
protoplasts which can be plated at known densities. The elegant
procedure originally introduced by Bergmann is the basic procedure
employed. This is illustrated diagrammatically in Fig.2. At
Nottingham we have found 5 cm tight-lidded Falcon dishes ideal for
plating. Microscopic examination is readily carried out without
removing the lid from the dishes. Problems still exist if large
scale liquid cultures are required. Such liquid cultures are
necessary if mutagen treatment is being carried out as a
preliminary to the transfer of the treated regenerated cells to
nutrient agar. Protoplasts differ greatly in the ease with which
they can be cultured in liquid media. For instance, tobacco is
very tolerant and will grow well. Indeed if left undisturbed the
protoplasts will form colonies which adhere strongly to the
bottom of the Falcon dishes. Petunia does not, however, grow well
in liquid media.

UPTAKE

The extent to which nucleic acids, virus particles, organelles
or micro organisms can be taken up into protoplasts is clearly of
basic importance in any assessment of the use of isolated
protoplasts as genetic systems. Extensive efforts are currently
being made to obtain definitive evidence for transformation in
higher plants and no attempts will be made to discuss this
particular aspect. It is very evident, however, that more
detailed knowledge of the entry of macromolecules, virus particles,
organelles and micro organisms is required. Much attention has
centred[17] on the introduction of purified macromolecules into living
cells, and on the uptake of nucleic acids into plant cells and
more recently into isolated protoplasts. While there is some
evidence that greater uptake may be possible into protoplasts than
into walled cells it should be noted that nucleic acids are known
to be taken up intact into the protoplasts of various intact plant
tissues[18]. The basic attraction of isolated protoplasts is
therefore not so much in relation to uptake of nucleic acids *per se*
but in relation to the readiness with which large numbers of
individual cells can be subjected to treatment. The interaction
between viruses (and their nucleic acids) and isolated
protoplasts has attracted a major research effort. Isolated
protoplasts have played a key role in this work since normally

the cell wall acts as a very efficient barrier to the penetration
through it of virus particles. Virus particles can therefore be
readily presented directly to the plasmalemma. Isolated higher
plant protoplasts offer an excellent system in which to study virus
infection and replication since there is the potential of
obtaining efficient and synchronous infection. Indeed many
laboratories now have major virus research programmes based on
protoplast infections with particular viruses[19]. Because
infection is dependent on the controlled interaction between virus
and plasmalemma considerable attention has recently been given
to the actual mechanism of the infection process. Parallel to this
more specialised problem of the interaction between an increasingly
wide range of different viruses and protoplast systems there has been
considerable work on endocytosis in isolated protoplasts.

The observations of Mahlberg[20] on the phenomenon of secondary
vacuolation in living cells, which involves the invagination of
the plasma membrane in walled plant cells leading to the formation
of peripheral or endocytotic structures are noteworthy. These
observations provided a major stimulus for a more detailed
ultrastructural investigation using isolated protoplasts. With
isolated tomato fruit protoplasts, it was possible to show
unequivocally using polystyrene latex particles and the freeze
etch technique that endocytosis was taking place[21]. Uptake
involved an adsorption phase followed by invagination of the plasma
membrane. In 1969 it was suggested from studies on the infection
of isolated tomato fruit protoplasts[22] that the pinocytic vesicles
in which removal of the protein capsid of the virus is probably
occurring are likely to be cellular infective centres, but the
possibility cannot be excluded of undetected infecting particle(s)
entering isolated protoplasts by a route other than the pinocytic
vesicle. The entry of particles by a route other than that of
endocytosis is further complicated if adequate evidence of
cellular integrity is not provided in ultrastructural studies[23].
There is no doubt that viruses can be taken up into endocytotic
vesicles in a wide range of different protoplast systems[24,25].
Whether, when particles are detected entering isolated protoplasts
by other routes[26], this means that infection via endocytosis is
excluded, is unresolved, and probably unresolvable, until the
actual infective particle or particles can be identified
ultrastructurally. Much more knowledge is required of
endocytosis and its extent in different protoplast systems and
also its dependence on temperature and the influence of polycations
such as poly-L-ornithine, which is essential for the infection of
tobacco leaf protoplasts by negatively charged viruses[27], but not
for the infection of tomato fruit protoplasts[22]. Recent studies
using microelectrophoretic methods[28,29] which have demonstrated
the extent to which the charge on the surface of isolated
protoplasts (which is usually negative) can be altered by the
external milieu, are particularly pertinent. The similar

difficulty of interpretation of the observations of every event
in cell-animal virus interactions should be noted[30].

These studies on virus infection have all utilised RNA plant
viruses. They have demonstrated the facility with which protoplasts
can be utilised in synchronous infection studies to elucidate the
various stages in protein virus coat and nucleic acid replication.
Comparable studies with the few DNA plant viruses could also help
to provide basic information relevant for transformation and
transduction attempts with higher plant protoplasts.

There have as yet been only very few investigations of the
uptake of organelles such as chloroplasts or nuclei or micro
organisms into selected protoplasts. Studies here at Nottingham
have indicated that it is very difficult to get uptake of particles
much greater than 0.5μ into protoplasts by endocytosis. Optical
observations of uptake can be misleading and fine structural
observations are required for confirmation of visual observations.
Unfortunately all reports of transplantation of chloroplasts and
nuclei into isolated protoplasts have been based on visual
observations using light microscopy[31,32]. Transplantation of cell
organelles would be a very helpful method for genetic manipulation
and for experiments on problems of developmental biology and of
extra chromosomal inheritance. As we shall see later the selection
of such 'modified protoplasts' will be a prior requisite before
such genetic manipulations can become a reality. Another
fundamental problem to be resolved is whether or not such large
organelles as chloroplasts and nuclei can be transplanted better
by fusion than by uptake. This work[31] has suggested that
chloroplasts and nuclei isolated directly from protoplasts are
better than more conventionally isolated chloroplasts for uptake
into protoplasts. It seems very likely to the writer that what may
be involved is fusion between the chloroplast membrane and the
plasma membrane. This is indicated by the fact that lysozyme, a
known slight inducer of fusion, is required for transplantation.
Work on transplantation using known fusion inducer (see later)
might give greatly enhanced transplantation, if transplantation is
primarily by fusion.

The uptake of micro organisms by isolated protoplasts has been
more rigorously investigated. It has been shown that bacteria such
as *Rhizobia* can be taken up into vesicles in the cytoplasm of
protoplasts as a result of engulfment of the bacteria into
invagination of the plasma membrane during plasmolysis[33]. This
plasmolytic uptake could also be a method for uptake of other
micro organisms such as the free nitrogen fixing bacteria such as
Azotobacter and the blue green algae. Electron microscopic studies
show clearly that uptake is involved and not fusion. Since as we have
seen protoplasts can regenerate a wall and divide the potential of
studies such as these for the establishment of endosymbiotic
relationships is great.

FUSION AND SOMATIC HYBRIDISATION

As has been recently discussed by Nickell and Heinz current
interest in the fusion of isolated protoplasts is high because of
the potential of this technique for fusion of somatic cells from
distantly related plants to produce new plants. These workers have
pointed out, however, that such approaches are of limited practical
use at present and that much has to be done to develop techniques
for application to specific problems.

The actual technique of protoplast fusion is now well
established. Several fusion inducers can be used such as sodium
nitrate[34], polyethylene glycol[35] and high pH calcium[36]. For inter-
species fusion careful adjustment of the actual fusion conditions
is necessary to ensure the subsequent viability of the fused
protoplasts; and although frequently extensive fusion can be
obtained with polyethylene glycol and high pH and calcium treatments
considerable loss of viability may result. Although the actual
mechanism of fusion induction is not as yet clear, it would seem
likely that the readiness with which protoplasts adhere as a
result of the treatment with the fusion inducing agent results
from a reduction in the negative charge on the surface of the
isolated protoplasts.

Fusion of protoplasts from different genera is readily
achievable and fusion results in the formation of heterokaryons
which contain the nuclei of the two genera. Heterokaryons can be
readily identified if the nuclei are different in their staining
properties. The following method for the preparation of
heterokaryons of *Nicotiana otophora* and *Nicotiana tabacum* outlines
the general practical procedures involved (abstracted from Evans,
Berry, Banks and Safwat)[6]:
1. Surface sterilise leaves by 30 min wash in 5% Domestos. Remove
   Domestos with five washings in sterile water.
2. Remove areas of lower epidermis with fine forceps. Cut out
   these peeled areas with a scalpel and place them, peeled side
   down, on the surface of a thin layer of 13% w/v mannitol in
   C.P.W. salts in a petri dish. After at least 30 min exposure
   to the mannitol solution, the mannitol is replaced with enzyme
   solution. The leaf pieces are incubated in the dark for 18 h.
   The petri dish is then agitated and the leaf pieces shaken to
   liberate the protoplasts.
3. The protoplasts are sedimented at 100 x g for 5 min and
   resuspended in mannitol in C.P.W. salts and sedimented again.
   The mannitol is replaced with 21% w/v sucrose and the protoplasts
   resuspended. Centrifugation at 200 x g for 5 min brings
   protoplasts to the surface and sediments cells and debris. The
   floating protoplasts are removed with a pasteur pipette and
   resuspended in an excess volume of mannitol in C.P.W. salts.
   After further sedimentation the protoplasts are suspended in a

known volume of mannitol in C.P.W. salts and a small sample
taken for counting.

4. The two types of protoplasts are mixed in the ratio 1:1, and
   sedimented at 100 x g for 5 min. The mannitol solution is
   replaced with 40% polyethylene glycol in F_5 medium previously
   warmed to 37°C. After incubation for 40 min a sample is
   examined for cell fusion. If the level of fusion is low at this
   time the incubation is continued. When frequent cell fusions
   have occurred, the criterium for fusion being the same as that
   used for the cereal leaf protoplasts described in Section A (see [6]),
   the polyethylene glycol is removed by successive washings in
   F_5 culture medium. A sample is fixed overnight in formaldehyde
   solution and the remainder cultured in liquid F_5 medium. Samples
   are fixed at 24 h intervals.
5. The fixed protoplasts are sedimented and the supernatant
   removed. A drop of sediment is transferred to a slide and a
   drop of carbol fuchsin stain is added. The sample is covered
   with a coverslip which is gently tapped to spread the
   protoplasts. The slide is then squashed and made permanent.
6. The slide is examined for heterokaryons. *Nicotiana otophora*
   nuclei are clearly distinguishable by the presence of
   heterochromatin blocks absent from nuclei of *Nicotiana tabacum*.

The general procedure employed for the fusion of protoplasts
when they are being subsequently cultured in somatic hybridisation
studies is outlined in Fig.3.

The demonstration[37] that the fusion of protoplasts from
Nicotiana glauca and *Nicotiana langsdorfii* with sodium nitrate,
followed by a special solution procedure dependent on a knowledge
of the growth characteristics of the sexual hybrid, resulted in the
formation of a few in a million somatic hybrids highlighted the key
importance of adequate selection in somatic hybridisation studies
(for a comprehensive discussion see[38]).

Many attempts are currently being made in several laboratories
to devise really adequate selection procedures. Moreover such
selection procedures should not be dependent on a knowledge of
the properties of the sexual hybrid since the practical application
of somatic hybridisation lies in crossing species which it is not
possible to cross sexually. Such selection procedures should also
be readily applicable to a wide range of different genera. Recently
Cocking *et al*. have devised a possibly generally applicable
procedure which makes use of naturally occurring differential drug
sensitivities of protoplasts to drugs such as amino acid analogues
and growth substances which is now enabling an assessment to be
made of their complementation capabilities. The approach makes
use of complementation selection as used in microbiology in which
only the heterokaryon or hybrid is able to grow in the presence of

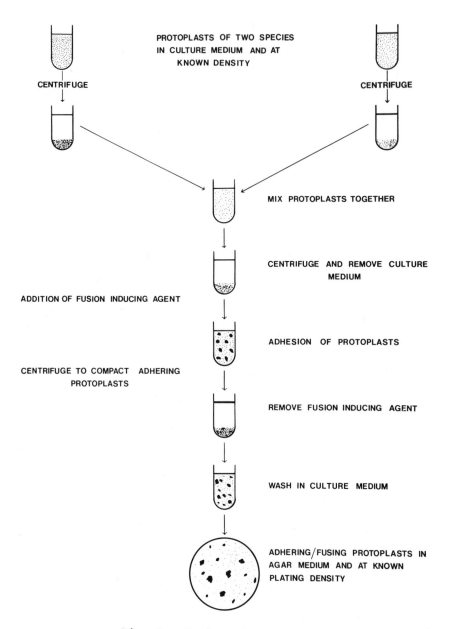

Fig. 3.   Fusion of Protoplasts

Category	TOBACCO	PETUNIA
1	P.E. ⩾ 30%	P.E. ⩾ 20%
2	P.E. ⩾ 15% → P.E. < 30%	P.E. ⩾ 10% → P.E. < 20%
3	P.E. < 15% → occasional colony formation	P.E.< 10% → occasional colony formation
4	High viability with no division	
5	Majority of protoplasts dead. No viable colonies	

L-HOMOARGININE HCL (μg/ml)

0	10·0	25·0	50·0	100·0
TOB 1	2	2	2	2
PET 1	2	3	4	5

DL-7-AZATRYPTOPHAN (μg/ml)

0	0·5	1·0	2·5	5·0	7·5	10·0	50·0	100·0
TOB 2	2	2	2	2	2	2	2	3
PET 2	1	2	2	2	3	3	5	5

4-CL-PHENOXYISOBUTYRIC ACID (μg/ml)

0	0·1	0·5	1·0	2·5	5·0	10·0	25·0	50·0
TOB 2	2	2	2	2	2	2	2	5
PET 2	2	3	5	5	5	5	5	5

CIS-TRANS ABSCISIC ACID (μg/ml)

0	0·005	0·025	0·05	0·1	0·5
TOB 2	2	3	5	5	5
PET 2	2	2	2	2	2

ETHANOL (×)

0	0·5	1·0	1·5	2·0	2·5
TOB 2	4	4	4	4	5
PET 1	1	2	2	2	3

Drugs producing substantial differential sensitivities between petunia and tobacco. In the case of the first group of drugs (homoarginine, 7-azatryptophan and 4-Cl-phenoxyisobutyric acid) petunia is more sensitive than tobacco.
The second group of drugs (abscisic acid and ethanol) show the converse situation with petunia being substantially less sensitive than tobacco.

Fig. 4.   Categories for the Assessment of Protoplast Growth Response

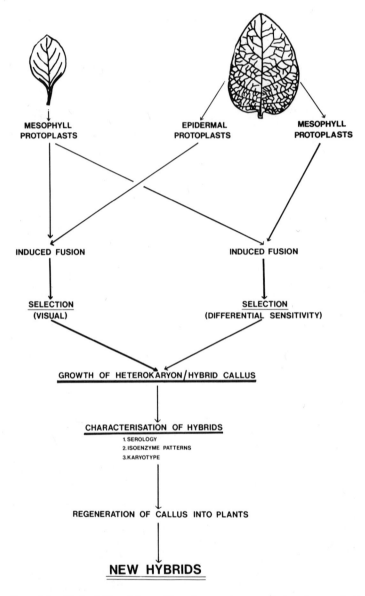

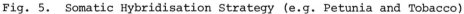

Fig. 5.   Somatic Hybridisation Strategy (e.g. Petunia and Tobacco)

both of the drugs. Neither parental line can grow under these
conditions. The attraction of this complementation approach is
that it is not dependent on any knowledge of a sexual hybrid, and
that several drugs can be readily selected for complementation
assessments. For petunia and tobacco, which cannot be crossed
sexually, we were readily able to select abscisic acid and ethanol
for favourable differential petunia growth and homoarginine,
azatryptophan and 4-Cl-phenoxyisobutyric acid for favourable
differential tobacco growth[39]. (Fig.4). The use of such
naturally occurring differential sensitivity methods is also
attractive because it eliminates the need to produce mutant cell
lines and also because such selection procedures are likely not to
be dependent on the ploidy level of the species being employed.

The general somatic hybridisation strategy which is emerging
is outlined in Fig.5. Visual selection, based for instance on the
fusion of chloroplast containing leaf protoplasts with those from
the colourless epidermal protoplasts, or cultured cell protoplasts,
can be used initially for light microscopic characterisations and
any initial observations on nuclear behaviour. Sometimes this may
also enable observations on heterokaryons resulting from the fusion
of protoplasts of two species which are not culturally compatible
(i.e. will not grow in the same culture medium), and may enable
any tendency for nuclear fusion to be detected by chromosomal
analysis of any mitotic figures. Nevertheless, an effective somatic
hybridisation strategy requires the growth of each of the parental
lines, a stringent selection procedure (based for instance on
complementation of naturally occurring differential sensitivities
of the two species) and a rigorous characterisation of any
presumptive hybrids by isoenzyme pattern methods and detailed
karyotyping. Even when this has been achieved such 'raw hybrids',
which will often be amphidiploids, will be needed to be subjected
to an extensive breeding programme (see Cocking[38]).

ACKNOWLEDGEMENT

The original experimental work presented in this review was
supported by a grant from the Agricultural Research Council.

BIBLIOGRAPHY

[1] Morel, G., *Colloques internationaux C.N.R.S. No.212, Protoplastes et Fusion de Cellules Somatiques Végétales* (Paris 1973).

[2] Cocking, E.C., and Pojnar, E., *Acta Facultatis Medicae Universitatis Brunensis (Proc. 2nd Int. Symp. Yeast Protoplasts, Brno 1968)*, 37, 159 (1970).

[3] Nickell, L.G., and Heinz, D.J., in *Genes, Enzymes and Populations* (edit. by Srb, A.M.) 2 (Plenum Press, New York, London, 1973), Chapter 9.

[4] Evans, P.K., and Cocking, E.C., in *New Techniques in Biophysics and Cell Biology* (edit. by Pain, R., and Smith, B.) 2 (John Wiley, Chichester, 1974) In the press.

[5] Wakasa, K., *The Japanese Journal of Genetics*, 48, 279 (1973).

[6] Cocking, E.C., and Peberdy, J.F., *The Use of Protoplasts from Fungi and Higher Plants as Genetic Systems - A Practical Handbook* (Department of Botany, University of Nottingham, 1974).

[7] Watts, J.W., and King, J.M., in *64th Annual Report John Innes Institute*, p. 78 (Norwich, 1973).

[8] Scowcroft, W.R., Davey, M.R., and Power, J.B., *Plant Science Letters*, 1, 451 (1973).

[9] Davey, M.R., Frearson, E.M., Withers, L.A., and Power, J.B., *Plant Science Letters*, 2, 23 (1974).

[10] Bhojwani, S.S., and Cocking, E.C., *Nature New Biology*, 239, 29 (1972).

[11] Cocking, E.C., and Evans, P.K., in *Plant Tissue and Cell Culture* (edit. Street, H.E.) Chapter 5, Botanical Monographs 11 (Blackwell, Oxford, 1973).

[12] Kanai, R., and Edwards, G.E., *Plant Physiology*, 52, 484 (1973).

[13] Cocking, E.C., in *Dynamic Aspects of Plant Ultrastructure* (edit. Robards, A.W.) Chapter 8 (McGraw-Hill, Maidenhead, 1974)

[14] Willison, J.H.M., and Cocking, E.C., *Protoplasma*, in the press.

[15] Halperin, W., *Canadian Journal of Botany*, 51, 1801 (1973).

[16] Wallin, A., and Eriksson, T., *Physiologia Plantarum*, 28, 33 (1973).

[17] Gurdon, J.B., *Nature*, 248, 772 (1974).

[18] Ledoux, L., *Uptake of Informative Molecules by Living Cells* (North-Holland Publishing Company, Amsterdam, 1972)

[19] Zaitlin, M., *Advances in Virus Research*, in the press.

[20] Mahlberg, P., *American Journal of Botany*, <u>59</u>, 172 (1972).

[21] Willison, J.H.M., Grout, B.W.W., and Cocking, E.C., *Bioenergetics*, <u>2</u>, 371 (1971).

[22] Cocking, E.C., and Pojnar, E., *Journal of General Virology*, <u>4</u>, 305 (1969).

[23] Burgess, J., Motoyoshi, F., and Fleming, E.N., *Planta (Berl.)*, <u>111</u>, 199 (1973).

[24] Honda, Y., Matsui, C., Otsuki, Y., and Takebe, I., *Phytopathology*, <u>64</u>, 30 (1973).

[25] Hibi, T., and Yora, K., *Annals of the Phytopathological Society of Japan*, <u>38</u>, 350 (1972).

[26] Burgess, J., Motoyoshi, F., and Fleming, E.N., *Planta (Berl.)*, <u>112</u>, 323 (1973).

[27] Takebe, I., and Otsuki, Y., *Proceedings of the National Academy of Sciences, USA*, <u>64</u>, 843 (1969).

[28] Grout, B.W.W., and Coutts, R.H.A., *Plant Science Letters*, <u>2</u>, 397 (1974).

[29] Pilet, P.E., and Senn, A., *C.R. Acad. Sc. Paris, Série D*, <u>278</u>, 269 (1974).

[30] Dales, S., *Bacteriological Reviews*, <u>37</u>, 103 (1973).

[31] Potrykus, I., *Zeitschrift für Pflanzenphysiologie*, <u>70</u>, 364 (1973).

[32] Potrykus, I., and Hoffmann, F., *Zeitschrift für Pflanzenphysiologie*, <u>69</u>, 287 (1973).

[33] Davey, M.R., Cocking, E.C., and Bush, E., *Nature*, <u>244</u>, 460 (1973).

[34] Power, J.B., Cummins, S.E., and Cocking, E.C., *Nature*, <u>225</u>, 1016 (1970).

[35] Kao, K.M., and Michayluk, M.R., *Planta (Berl.)*, <u>115</u>, 355 (1974).

[36] Keller, W.A., and Melchers, G., *Zeitschrift für Naturforschung*, <u>28</u>, 737 (1973).

[37] Carlson, P.S., Smith, H.H., and Dearing, R.D., *Proceedings of the National Academy of Sciences, USA*, <u>69</u>, 2292 (1972).

[38] Cocking, E.C., in *Scienza & Tecnica 74*, p.199 (Arnoldo Mondadori, Milano, 1974).

[39] Cocking, E.C., Power, J.B., Evans, P.K., Safwat, F., Frearson,E.M., Hayward, C., Berry, S.F., and George, D., *Plant Science Letters*, in the press.

INDUCTION OF AUXOTROPHIC MUTATIONS IN PLANTS

G. P. RÉDEI

Department of Agronomy, University of Missouri

117 Curtis Hall, Columbia, Mo. 65201 USA

INTRODUCTION

Auxotrophic mutants in microorganisms have contributed most importantly to the rapid development of genetics and biochemistry in the last three decades. Their usefulness is not limited to elucidation of the genetic control of biochemical pathways but they are indispensable for the study of protein synthesis, regulation, various mechanisms of information transfer, the nature of mutation etc.

Nutritional mutants are expected to be equally useful in higher organisms yet the lead of microbial genetics was followed in this area with a considerable lag period.

With a few exceptions, the nutritional mutations of mammalian cells have limited value because the exact nature of the genetic lesions involved is incompletely known. Mammalian cell genetics is still struggling with severe technical problems inasmuch as the isolation of auxotrophs can be practiced only with hypoploid special cell lines requiring complex media (containing serum). Several of the mutations exhibit a complex nutritional requirement (CHU, SUN and CHANG 1972), indicating that probably simultaneous alterations are responsible for their appearance. Though ingenious methods have been developed for their mapping by the use of somatic hybridization (RUDDLE 1973), the mammalian cells cannot be differentiated into complete organisms and subjected to traditional analysis. The problems of auxotrophy in mammalian cells have been reviewed recently in detail (THOMPSON and BAKER 1973).

Induction of auxotrophic mutations in higher plants is under
study for about 20 years (LANGRIDGE 1955) yet verified obligate requirement has been found only in the thiamine pathway (RÉDEI 1960,
1962, 1965; FEENSTRA 1964; LI and RÉDEI 1969a) where to date about
200 independent mutations have been isolated at several loci, controlling different steps in the biosynthesis (RÉDEI, unpublished).

Leaky nutritional mutations in higher plants have been reported in barley (WALLES 1963) where some of the biochemical mechanisms
involved seem to be more complicated than anticipated (LAND and
NORTON 1970). Several leaky auxotrophs were obtained in tobacco
cell cultures (CARLSON 1970) and in tomato (BOYNTON 1966). In the
latter species an obligate pyrimidine mutant was also discovered
(LANGRIDGE and BROCK 1961).

A number of other auxotrophs of higher plants (reviewed by
NELSON 1967) require confirmation.

This sketchy survey indicates that much needs to be done in
the field of isolation nutritional mutations in angiosperms if
higher plant genetics wishes to catch up with the developments in
microbial genetics. There is an obvious need for biochemical mutants suitable for thorough analysis of molecular mechanisms in
gene function at a level comparable to what is being done in bac-
(e.g. BRONSON, SQUIRES and YANOFSKY 1973, LI and YANOFSKY 1973) or
yeast (SHERMAN and STEWART 1971). There is an obvious need for
clear, selective markers for backmutation, recombination, DNA-mediated information transfer and for other novel approaches in genetics.

THE BIOLOGICAL MATERIAL

Mutations in higher plants can be induced in haploid or diploid cells. Both pollen and egg cells have been successfully
treated with a variety of mutagens. Recently haploid cell cultures
(CARLSON 1970, CHALEFF, this publication) or protoplasts (COCKING
1972) offered promises for mutational use. Since these areas will
be separately dealt with during these series of lectures, my discussions will be limited to the classical approaches of mutagenesis
in higher plants.

ORGANIZATION OF THE GERMLINE

The total lifecycle of angiosperms includes both sporophytic
and gametophytic phases. The former is di- or polyploid and multicellular. Mutagens applied to the sporophytic generation have somewhat different consequences. Since the vaste majority of the muta-

tions are recessive, in contrast to haploids, the generation treated does not reveal the mutations induced. The earliest possible
stage of detection follows the gametophyte generation. Unfortunately
there are very few mutations which can be identified at this stage
and even fewer could possibly be isolated even if detected.

The effectiveness of a mutagenetic treatment can be assesed by
examination of the immature fruits, about 11-13 days after pollination, (MÜLLER 1963) collected from the plants, emerging from treated seeds or even when the sporophyte was treated at later developmental stages. Lethal embryos or color-deficient cotyledons can
be readily seen when the siliques are opened up with the aid of
sharp forceps. By this procedure we can save the cost involved in
planting the second generation. This method has, however, limited
usefulness for isolation of mutations for future genetic manipulations.

For the identification and isolation of auxotrophic mutants,
we plant the seeds harvested from the plants developed from the mu-
tagen-treated material. In this second (M_2) generation the recessive mutants can be easily detected and identified with a limited
degree of accuracy. Since usually the seed is exposed to the muta-

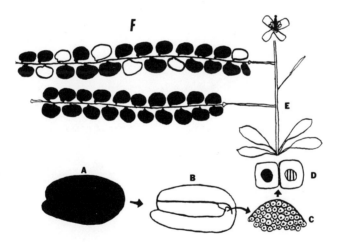

Figure 1.   Semidiagrammatic illustration of the consequences of ex-
            posing the seed to an effective mutagenic treatment. A:
            mature seed covered with the seedcoat. B: removal of the
            seedcoat reveals the folded two cotyledons (top) and the
            radicle (below); at the base of the arrow the small apex
            is visible. C: the apex enlarged. D: the two cells of the
            germline. E: the plant body. F: two fruits (carpels re-
            moved) corresponding to the two cells of the germline;
            note the segregation in only one of the fruits.

gen the segregation is not 3:1 in this population. On seed-treat-
ment some of the fruits will produce only wild type progenies and
others will segregate in an approximately mendelian ratio in the
M_2 generation, derived from a single seed. In other words, one may
say that an effectively treated seed becomes a genetic chimera
(Figure 1).

In an experiment with X-rays and ethyl methanesulfonate the
following segregation ratios were actually observed for wild type
and mutant: 4878:707 and 9346:1636, respectively, in several hundred
families. Combined, this corresponds to an approximately 6.1:1
ratio, obviously different from 3:1. It is not too far off, however, from 7:1. The 7:1 ratio can be readily understood as being
the result of lumping together 3:1 and 4:0 as illustrated on the
diagram (Fig.1).

Thus, by this very simple genetic technique we can determine
the number of cells in the apical meristem at the time of the treatment, capable of contributing to the seed, produced by the chimeric
plant. If the seed is exposed to a mutagen several days after imbibition or the growing plant is treated with the mutagen, the
ratios observed in the M_2 may vary considerably because by the time
of the treatment the number of cells in the germline has increased.
The figures, given above, were obtained with Arabidopsis and other
plants may have differently constructed apices, containing higher
number of cells in their germline even in the dormant seed. This
number of cells which produce the seeds of the plant was called
genetically effective cell number, GECN (LI and RÉDEI 1969).

GECN has to be determined on the basis of mutations with normal transmission. Wide genetic ratios may result also from poor
transmission of mutations associated with chromosomal defects or
gametophyte factors, functioning as segregation distorters. Thus,
it may be necessary to see that in the families, used for the determination of GECN, in M_3 or in more advanced generations the seg-
gregation is 3:1 in the progenies of the heterozygotes. Alternatively one may use the M_3 to see that for each recessive mutant
two heterozygotes occur.

The GECN may vary from 1 to 10 even in the seed. The theoretical M_2 segregation ratios corresponding to various GECNs can be calculated by formula $(4n-1):1$; n=GECN. Thus a 7:1 ratio indicates
that in the apical meristem there were two cells and a 39:1 proportion reveals ten cells capable to produce seed progeny. GECN is
constant for a particular ontogenetic stage but it may appear different if the mutagen has a delayed effect.

CALCULATION OF MUTATION RATES

If we know the ploidy of the germline cells and the GECN has
been determined, the mutation rate can be calculated in a manner

comparable through phylogenetic boundaries. The general formula is as follows:

$$R = \frac{M}{S \times GECN \times P \times D}$$

where R= mutation rate, M= number of M_2 families segregating for recessive mutations, S= surviving families, GECN= genetically effective cell number of the treated tissues, P= correction factor for ploidy, D= dose of the mutagen applied under standard conditions.

This method estimates mutation frequency on the basis of the survivors and ignores the controversial class of lethals which may be due to genetic as well as to physiological causes. Auxotrophic mutations are not expected to be lethal in a cell surrounded by tissues of normal metabolism.

This method makes possible to avoid or asses some of the biases of mutation rate estimation in higher plants. The greatest advantage of it is, however, that it expresses mutation rate on genome basis, and thus the results are comparable under a variety of conditions, irrespective of the genetic system or developmental stage of the of the organisms to be compared.

In an experiment of mutation induction without selective screening, in Penicillium (a fungus) 2×10^{-4} mutations were found for thiamine auxotrophy in a large scale experiment (BONNER 1946). In Arabidopsis a similar experiment revealed a mutation frequency for the same requirement as 3×10^{-4} (LI and RÉDEI 1969a). These are remarkably close figures for organisms so distant on the evolutionary scale. Besides, the conditions of treatments were different in time and location though apparently both laboratories used optimal mutagenic exposures for the organisms concerned.

This similarity in mutability of 'homeologous' loci in different organisms is expected if their respective enzymes are similar proteins. There is good evidence that amino acid composition and sequence is largely preserved during evolution of proteins (MARGOLIASH 1963) and the genetic code is universal (YČAS 1969).

GENERAL PRINCIPLES OF ISOLATION OF MUTATIONS

THE M_1 POPULATION

Mutations are rare events thus large populations have to be screened to find the desired types. The search for spontaneous mutations is impractical when a large number of powerful mutagens are available (RÉDEI 1970).

Before decisions concerning M_1 size could be made, we have to know or anticipate the rate of mutation at particular loci of interest. If mutation frequency information in a particular species is

not available, we have to turn to other organisms and use the principles outlined above for estimation of mutation rates. This procedure may not be practical, however, in all cases because in green
plants the mutation spectrum for nutritional requirement is very
narrow for some not entirely understandable reasons (LI, RÉDEI and
GOWANS 1967). In fungi and bacteria the frequency of induced mutations for requirement of vitamins and amino acids is in the 10^{-3} to
10^{-4} range.

If the mutation rate per genome is known, the size of the population (M_1) can be calculated with the formula: $(f)^n = P$ (MATHER
1957), where f is the reciprocal of the mutation rate, n= the population size required to recover at least one mutant with the probability specified by P. If we wish to obtain a thiamine mutant
which is expected at a frequency of 3/10,000 genomes of the germline, the necessary genome population to be screened for finding at
least one with 0.01 probability is:

$$n = \frac{\log 1 - \log 100}{\log 9997 - \log 10000} = \frac{-2}{-0.00013} = 15384$$

Since we arrived at the conclusion earlier that the germline in the
seed of Arabidopsis consists of two diploid cells, actually we have
to treat with the mutagen only 15384/4 = 3846 seeds to recover at
least on thiamine mutant with a 99% chance provided we screen in
M_2 large enough populations not to miss any mutation induced.

THE M_2 POPULATION

The size of the M_1 population determines the number of mutations induced while the recovery of the mutants depends on the number of individuals tested in each M2 progeny. The required size of
individual M_2 populations to detect at least one mutant among the
descendents of heterozygous or chimeric M_1 plants at selected levels
of probability can be determined with the same formula that was used
to estimate the size of the M_1 generation. If we wish to know how
many plants should be screened among the descendents of a heterozygous M_1 plant in M_2, to detect at least one recessive mutation at
0.999 probability, the calculation is as follows:

$$(3/4)^n = 1/1000 \text{ or using logarithms } n \log (3/4) = \log (1/1000)$$
$$\text{that is } n(-0.125) = 3.000 \text{ or } n = \frac{-3.000}{-0.125} = 24$$

If the genetically effective cell number is 2, we start with $(7/8)^n$;
for some other GECNs the appropriate values for both recessive and
dominant mutants are listed in Table 1. With the same procedure
the required M2 sizes for other probabilities can also be determined.
Table 2 lists the minimal M_2 sizes at various probabilities and for

Table 1.   Absolute number of individuals required in M_2 to recover
           at least one mutant with .999 probability at various
           GECNs.   R: recessive, D: dominant mutations.

	Genetically effective cell numbers						
	1	2	3	4	6	8	10
	Number of individuals required in M_2						
R	24.0	51.7	79.4	107.1	162.2	219.0	272.7
D	5.0	9.9	24.0	33.3	51.7	70.3	88.5

cases of different GECNs, in percentage of that required for 0.999
P.   The expression of M_2 sizes in percents involves the some biases,
especially at larger GECN values.   Thus, if exact figures are want-
ed, it is advisable to calculate the figures as shown for each case.
In most practical experiments, the figures shown in Table 2 are
sufficiently close to the real values.   The use of the tables is as
follows: if we wish to screen M_2 populations permitting the recovery
of at least one recessive mutant with only 0.500 P and the GECN is
2, we take from Table 1 the value given as 51.7 and multiply it with
0.10, as read from Table 2, and we see that an average of 5.2 individuals should be classified.

These tables may be useful in planning some practical experiments.   A closer scrutiny of the data reveals furthermore that if
we use a population size in M_2 what we called 100% (Table 2) because it gives us a very high (.999) probability of recovery of at
least one mutant, we will have to plant and classify at GECN=1 an
M_2 of 24 individuals (Table 1).   If we are satisfied with only
0.250 probability of recovery, the required number of individuals
in M_2 falls between 5.2 to 3.2% of 24 which is approximately 1

Table 2. M_2 sizes at various levels of probabilities, expressed at
           percent of that required at .999 P to recover at least one
           mutant, recessive or dominant.

P	.999	.990	.950	.900	.800	.500	.300	.200	.100
M_2 sizes	100	66.7	43.4	33.3	23.3	10.0	5.2	3.2	1.5

single plant. By reduction the size of individual M_2 progenies from 24 to 1, we can save space for 24 times larger number of families and the total population to be classified still remains the same as before. The 24 fold increase in number of families provides us now a 24 x 0.250 chance of recovery of mutations, i.e. a 6 fold higher efficiency compared to the procedure aiming at 0.999 P recovery of mutants in individual families. Thus the effectiveness of mutation recovery can be plotted against the probability of recovery of at least one mutant in family, and we can graphically compare this with the relation of probability of recovery of at least one mutant in M_2 to the relative size of an M_2 family (Figure 2).

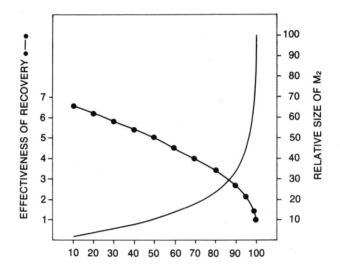

Figure 2.   Comparison of the probabilities of recovery of at least one mutant in a mutation carrier progeny (M_2) with the effectiveness of mutation recovery (left ordinate) and with the relative size of individual M_2 populations. Note that the effectiveness of isolation independent mutations decreases with increased probability of recovery of the mutations induced. The probability of detecting all mutational events in single families is, however, rapidly increasing as the number of individuals per M_2 increased. The conclusion is, that in order to get the maximal number of independent mutations, one should screen large number of families of minimal size.

It should be noted that in a large size individual M_2 one generally recovers the mutations in multiple copies whereas if only a single plant is used in M_2, maximally one mutant can be recovered from a mutational event. This may turn out to be of substantial advantage since we need initially only one fertile mutant plant. When we find many in the progeny of a single M_1 plant of multicellular germline, we have to make special tests to ascertain that all these mutants are identical. This cannot be determined by phenotypic criteria alone in many instances.

THE COST OF A MUTATION

On theoretical ground, the conclusion was reached that maximal effectiveness in mutation induction can be accomplished if maximal number of M_1 plants are tested with minimal size M_2 offspring. What is 'maximal' or 'minimal' under the conditions of a laboratory requires some qualifications. The practical proportion of M_1 number and M_2 size can be easily determined if the cost of a mutation in space, labor and funds is assessed.

A simple example illustrates how the cost of a mutation can be determined. According to Tables 1 and 2, if GECN=1, 24 M_2 offspring of a single M_1 carrier (altogether 25 plants) can yield at least 1 mutant (1 mutation) with 0.999 P. Assuming that the cost of production of plants is the same in both generations, and the total expenditure involved in the 25 plants is 100 units, the cost of the single mutation recovered is 100/1. If we plant only 2.4 plants in an average M_2 yet use 10 M_1 families the total number of plants to be handled increases to 34 and the total cost grows proportionally to 136 units. According to expectations (Figure 2) of mutant recovery, now we isolate 5 mutants. Thus the cost per mutation becomes 136/5 = 27.2. In Table 3 the cost of mutations is tabulated for various sizes of M_2 (compare probability and size information given in Table 2) and three different M_1 : M_2 cost ratios. The optimal experimental conditions (population sizes) for a certain laboratory can be determined either by direct calculation according to the principles indicated or by interpolation, using the information of Table 3.

The obvious conclusion is that it is very expensive to try to recover all mutations induced, and it is far more economical to reach a good compromise between M_1 and M_2 sizes. It is also important to estimate with a reasonable accuracy the cost of the two generations. We have to devise means to reduce the cost of production of the M_1 plants and make it possible to grow them in maximal number. The yield of seed can be reduced to a minimum. In the M_2, screening should be selective if possible and identification of the mutations should be carried out at the earliest possible stage of the experiments.

Table 3. Cost of a mutation at various probabilities of recovering
of at least one mutation per M_2, and 3 M_1 : M_2 cost ratios.

Cost of M_1 : M_2	Probabilities of recovery								
	.999	.99	.95	.90	.80	.50	.30	.20.	.10
	Cost of a mutation								
5:5	100	68.7	47.9	40.0	33.0	27.3*	29.9	35.6	54.8
9:1	100	76.5	61.8	57.2	55.3*	69.2	103.4	148.2	283.9
1:9	100	67.5	45.8	37.4	29.6	20.9	18.7	18.5*	20.0

*indicates the most efficient conditions of isolation

Table 4. M_1 plant representation at random seed withdrawal from
bulk harvest according to the cumulative terms of Poisson
series.

Cumulative representation	Average number of seeds withdrawn									
	1	2	3	4	5	6	7	8	9	10
0	36.8	13.5	5.0	1.8	0.7	0.2	0.1	.	.	.
1	63.2	86.5	95.0	98.2	99.3	99.8	99.9	.	.	.
2	26.4	59.4	80.1	90.8	96.0	98.3	99.3	99.7	99.9	.
3	8.0	32.3	57.7	76.2	87.5	93.8	97.0	98.6	99.4	99.7
4	1.9	14.3	35.3	56.7	73.5	84.9	91.8	95.8	97.9	99.0
5	0.4	5.3	18.5	37.1	56.0	71.5	82.7	90.1	94.5	97.1
6	0.1	1.7	8.4	21.5	38.4	55.4	69.9	80.9	88.4	93.3
7	.	0.5	3.3	11.1	23.8	39.4	55.0	68.7	79.3	87.0
8	.	0.1	1.2	5.1	13.3	25.6	40.1	54.7	67.6	78.0
9	.	.	0.4	2.1	6.8	15.3	27.1	40.7	54.4	66.7
10	.	.	0.1	0.8	3.2	8.4	17.0	23.8	41.3	54.2

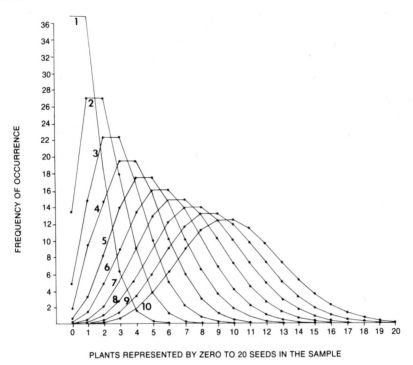

Figure 3.   The representation of individual M_1 plants by various
numbers of seed in M_2 after random withdrawal on an average from 1 to 10 seeds from a bulk harvest of large
number of plants. The chart was constructed on the
basis of Poisson distribution. The actual distribution
would fit better to multinomial series which is extremely difficult to handle in case of large numbers. For
all practical purposes, this is an acceptable and useful
approximation of the actual distribution.

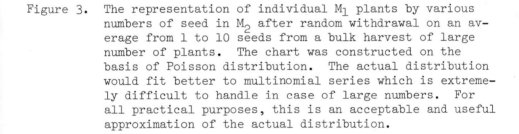

        Considerable amount of labor can be spared if we do not treat
the material by the pedigree method. The M_1 can be harvested in
bulk and the desired average number of seed may be withdrawn for
M_2 test. The representation of M_1 individuals in the sample will
approximate the Poisson distribution as shown on Figure 3. or Table
4.

        As it can be seen after withdrawing an average of single seed
per M_1 plants over 1/3 of the treated population will be entirely
missed in M_2 and approximately 8% of the M_1 will be represented by
3 or more seeds. Yet the success of mutation isolation will not

be much affected. A recent calculation of the results of some hypothetical experiments indicated that in a combined M_1 and M_2 population of identical total number of plants the efficiency of mutation isolation by the classical pedigree method was 0.198 while the pedigree selection according to the suggested improvements was expected to give a coefficient of 0.966 and the bulking procedure appeared very close with a factor of 0.913 (RÉDEI 1974).

AN ACTUAL EXPERIMENTAL TEST OF THE PROCEDURES OUTLINED

Approximately 1200 seeds were exposed to 0.2% ethyl methanesulfonate for 15 hrs, then washed and planted. Each plant was harvested separately. Subsequently 1000 seeds were planted in each of the five series in such a way that 1, 2, 4, 8 and 24 seeds represented in M_2 the 1000, 500, 125 and 42 M_1 plants, respectively. In each series the mutations were scored several times up to the time of flower initiation. Though the experiment was limited in size, the results were in good agreement with the expectations, i.e. the large families, represented by 24 plants in M_2 permitted the recovery of more mutations per family than the small ones (Table 5). The predicted values were arrived at by multiplying the frequency of mutations per family in the 24 seed population with the appropriate recovery factors for GECN=2.

Though the frequency of mutation per family was the highest in the large families, in absolute numbers more independent mutations were recovered in the small individual populations combined (Table 6). We may note again that the total number of M_2 offspring

Table 5. Mutation recovery as a function of the size of individual M_2 populations. Experimental test of the suggested procedures of isolation of mutations. GECN=2.

Number of seeds planted per M_2 families	Number of families planted	Number of survivors	Mutations per families	
			Observed %	Predicted %
24	42	713	26.2	26.5
8	125	771	18.4	17.4
4	250	784	12.0	11.0
2	500	832	8.0	6.2
1	1000	763	3.6	3.3

was nearly the same in all series (Table 5, Column 3). The number
of M_1 individuals varied greatly among the series (Table 5, Column
2), being largest when the size of an M_2 population was reduced to
the minimum. Based on the principles discussed above in detail,
the cost of a mutation was determined in each series at three M_1:
M_2 cost ratios. Actually, I believe, in an experiment where the
purpose is not to test the technique rather to induce useful mutations the 1:1 ratio appears to be the most realistic with the procedures generally used. Yet at all cost ratios, mutation induction
was more economical when small M_2 and large number of M_1 is used
(Table 6). Even the largest M_2 (24) in the test contained only
about half as many individuals as would have been required for a
recovery at the 0.999 P level (see Table 1). Even at the worst
cost ratio shown (4:1) the 24-size M_2 procedure cost almost twice
as much as the ones with 8 or 4 seeds. At the more realistic 1:1
cost ratio, in the 2-seed M_2 families the expense involved in the
production of a mutation is almost a third of that what is required
with 24-seed M_2 procedure.

Table 6. The number of mutations recovered in a series of experi-
          ments where the total M_2 offspring planted was 1000 per
          series but the size of individual M_2 families varied from
          24 to 1. The cost of a mutation was estimated at three
          M_1: M_2 cost ratios.

Number of plants in individuals M_2 progenies	Number of mutations recovered	Cost of a mutation at M_1: M_2 cost ratios		
		1:1	2:1	4:1
24	11	95.1	99.3	106.9
8	23	49.3	54.8	65.7*
4	30	42.0	50.4*	67.2
2	40	37.8*	50.4*	75.6
1	36	56.0	84.0	140.0

*indicates the lowest cost of a mutation in the series.

INDUCTION OF THIAMINE AUXOTROPHS IN ARABIDOPSIS

After discussing the general principles of isolation of induced mutations, the specific methods of isolation of auxotrophs
may be expected. Unfortunately, I am unable to tell how to produce
the variety of nutritional mutants in angiosperms, common to bacteria
and fungi. In Arabidopsis - and as far as I know, in other diploid

photoautotrophic green plants – mutants with obligate requirements
for single defined metabolites supplied exogenously, exist only in
the thiamine pathway. To date approximately 200 thiamine auxotrophs
have been isolated in our laboratory at at least four loci. Yet no
other nutritional mutants, requiring normal metabolites have been
found. Thus the spectrum of auxotrophs in Arabidopsis is significantly different from that in bacteria or fungi (Figure 4). In an
experiment where no selective screening was employed, BONNER (1946)
isolated in Penicillium 18 thiamine mutants and 17 times as many
other identified auxotrophs. If this experiment can be used as a
valid sample of induced mutability in a fungus, and we are willing
to accept the data as 'expected' in the higher plant Arabidopsis,
we should have now over 3000 other than thiamine auxotrophs but
none are available.

The method of induction and isolation of auxotrophs applies
thus only to thiamine mutants of Arabidopsis.

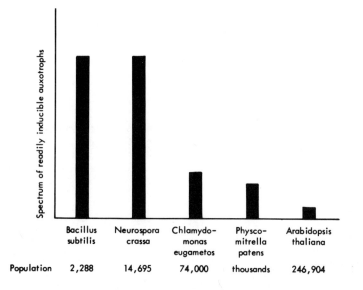

Figure 4.   Spectrum of vitamin, amino acid and nucleic acid precur-
            sor auxotrophs in a few representative organisms where
            data are available from experiments, conducted without
            selective screening techniques (on the basis of data by
            LI, RÉDEI and GOWANS 1967). Since the compilation was
            made, almost 5 times more thiamine mutants have been iso-
            lated in Arabidopsis yet the proportions shown have not
            changed.

All the mutations induced in my laboratory were obtained from seed treatment. In the past, we used 12 kR x-rays to 24 hrs imbibed seed. Recently we are inducing mutations with ethyl methanesulfonate (0.2% in water, 15 hrs, followed by 4 hrs washing in running water).

For mutagenic treatment the seed is tied into cloth bags, containing also a few glass beads to prevent floating. The seed should be loosely packed, making allowance for swelling during the treatment. This way we can avoid clumping of the wet seed. For planting the seed is taken out from the bags after washing and it is suspended in a cold viscose agar solution. The quantity of agar may vary, depending on the batch (approximately 0.15% may be satisfactory). The agar should be cooled after solubilization with continuous stirring to prevent the formation of lumps. We generally use 5 ml solution per pot and distribute this volume with the aid of a separatory funnel. This way we can layer in uniform distribution approximately 100 seeds on the surface of each pot, well watered earlier. Commonly we treat 100,000 seeds, estimated on weight basis (1000 seeds weighs 18-22 mgs, depending on the genotype and origin). Such an M_1 population can be planted in less than an hour time by a single person.

The M_1 should be raised under continuous illumination; under such conditions even larger number of plants can be grown per pot. If we want to sample all plants we should allow about 6-7 weeks for maturation.

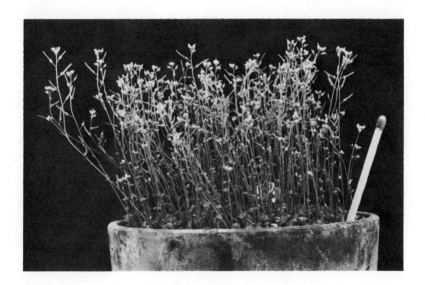

Figure 5. Over 100 M_1 plants grown to maturity in a 5 inch pot.

The harvesting can be done by bulk; pots or groups of pots can
be treated separately. Dividing the material into smaller groups
is advisable in order to recognize mutants which were produced by the
same mutational event. Thus if two pyrimidine mutants occur in a
population of 100, the greatest chance is that they are identical
in origin. The subdivision of the seed helps in recognizing contaminations of all kind and some sort of 'fluctuation test' (LURIA
and DELBRÜCK 1943) can be applied. To facilitate the recognition
of contaminants from previous experiments, we used to treat material
carrying appropriate markers.

For M_2 screening we may plant again 100 or more seeds per 5
inch pots. Thiamine mutants can be recognized early (Figure 6B).
Even thousand seedlings per pot is not too many for the recognition
and isolation of thiamine mutants (Figure 6A). The thiamine mutants
germinate with normal green cotyledons, and unless they are leaky,
and only a very small percent of the total is, they fail to develop
normal green additional leaves (Figure 6A). Often they die within
10 days after germination because the thiamine supply in the cotyledons is used up. The leaky ones or the temperature-sensitive
mutants under non-restrictive conditions may grow to various extent
but they display chlorophyll deficiency symptoms in most of the
cases (Figures 7, 8).

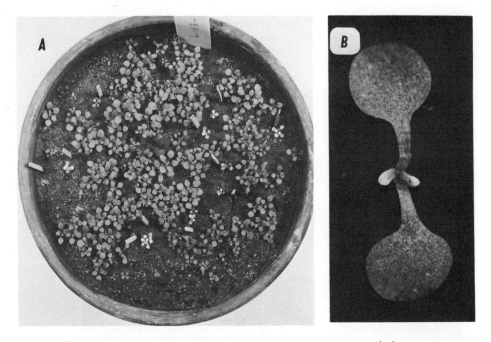

Figure 6. Segregation for thiamine auxotrophy in M_2 (A). Typical
          thiamine mutant at the cotyledonous stage (B); note the
          white rosette leaf initials.

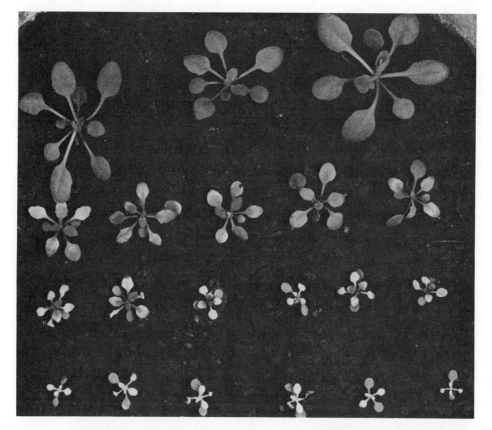

Figure 7. Different degrees of thiamine deficiency; top wild type.

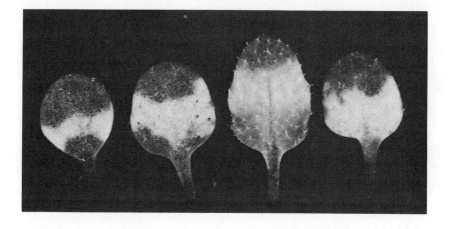

Figure 8. Banded leaves, frequently observable on thiamine mutants.

The thiamine mutants - as soon as they can be classified - are marked by toothpicks, and after their neighbors are discarded a dilute thiamine solution is dropped on each plant. Usually we feed all suspected auxotrophs with a mixture of thiamine, nicotinic acid amide, yeast extract, yeast hydrolysate and casein hydrolysate. The feeding continues twice weekly until maturity. As soon as there is enough seed, the nutritional requirement is verified in aseptic agar cultures on basic and "complete" media.

The basic solution contains salts (mgs/l double distilled water: NH_4NO_3 40, $MgSO_4.7H_2O$ 20, $CaH(PO_4)_2.H_2O$ 20, KH_2PO_4 20, K_2HPO_4 10, $FeC_6H_5O_7.3H_2O$ 0.5), 2% glucose or sucrose and enough agar to just solidify the medium. The complete medium includes in mgs/l thiamine 20, nicotinic acid amide 20, yeast extract 10, yeast hydrolysate 10, casein hydrolysate 50 and 2% coconut milk. Note that the concentration of this organic mixture is about 1/100 of that what is fed to the soil-grown plants. If the plants respond favorably to the organic supplements then thiamine and later its precursors are tested. At the moment only thiamine is available commercially; 2-methyl-4-amino-5-aminomethyl pyrimidine or better the 2-methyl-4-amino-5-hydroxymethyl pyrimidine and 4-methyl-5-beta hydroxyethyl thiazole can be obtained as a gift upon request from some of the major chemical companies (e.g. Merck, LaRoche). The commercially sold oxythiamine serves as a good thiazole source after autoclaving.

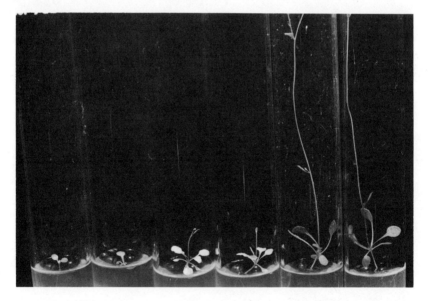

Figure 9. Thiamine mutants on minimal (four test tubes on the left), and on complete media (two tubes on the right). Note the two leaky mutants in the center, they grow to some extent but produce only minimal amounts of leaf pigments.

Some of the thiazole and intact thiamine requiring mutants
are subject to catabolite repression when fed by glucose or maltose
(LI and RÉDEI 1969d).

The nutritional requirement test is followed by allelism test.
This genetic test provides some information on the position of the
genetic block even if the required chemical compounds are unavailable. F_1 hybrids of non-alleic mutants grow like wild type in the
absence of thiamine or its precursors (Figure 10A). If in the F_1
the growth is only slightly improved we are dealing with allelic
complementation (Figure 10B). Allelic complementation is common
among the temperature sensitive mutants (LI and RÉDEI 1969c).

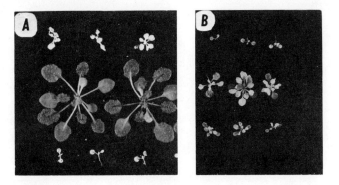

Figure 10.   Non-allelic (A) and allelic (B) complementation among
             thiamine mutants. The parental types are in the top
             and bottom, the F_1 hybrid plants in the central hori-
             zonal row.

SUMMARY

Obligate auxotrophic mutations in angiosperms have been limited
to the thiamine pathway. In Arabidopsis thiamine mutations occur
at about the same frequency as in microorganisms yet so far no other
verified nutritional mutants are available. The most effective
method of mutation production involves the mutagenic treatment of
maximal number of M_1 plants and their offspring is screened in minimal size M_2. The efficiency of isolation can be further improved
by bulking and mass testing procedures. Convenient formulas and
table are provided to plan efficient mutation experiments. Thiamine mutants are described in sufficient detail to facilitate their
recognition.

ACKNOWLEDGEMENT

Contribution from the Missouri Agricultural Experiment Station.
Journal Series Number 7062 . Approved by the Director.

LITERATURE CITED

BONNER, D. 1946 Production of biochemical mutations in Penicillium.
    Amer. J. Bot. 33: 788–91.

BOYNTON, T. E. 1966 Chlorophyll-deficient mutants in tomato re-
    quiring vitamin B_1. I. Genetics and physiology. Hereditas 56:
    171–99.

BRONSON, M. J., C. SQUIRES and C. YANOFSKY 1973 Nucleotide se-
    quences from tryptophane messenger RNA of Escherichia coli:
    the sequence corresponding to the amino-terminal region of the
    first polypeptide specified by the operon. Proc. Nat. Acad.
    Sci. U.S. 70: 2335–9.

CARLSON, P. S. 1970 Induction and isolation of auxotrophic mutants
    in somatic cell cultures of Nicotiana tabacum. Science 168:
    487–9.

CHU, E. H. Y., N. C. SUN and C. C. CHANG 1972 Induction of auxo-
    trophic mutations by treatment of Chinese hamster cells with
    5-bromodeoxyuridine and black light. Proc. Nat. Acad. Sci.
    U. S. 69: 3459–63.

COCKING, E. C. 1972 Plant cell protoplasts – isolation and develop-
    ment. Ann. Rev. Plant. Physiol. 23: 29–50.

FEENSTRA, W. J. 1964 Isolation of nutritional mutants in Arabidop-
    sis thaliana. Genetica 35: 259/69.

LANGRIDGE, F. 1955 Biochemical mutations in the crucifer Arabidop-
    sis thaliana (L.) Heynh. Nature 176: 260–1.

LANGRIDGE, J. and R. D. BROCK 1961 A thiamine-requiring mutant of
    the tomato. Aust. J. Biol. Sci. 14: 66–9.

LAND, J. B. and G. NORTON 1970 The nature of the leucine require-
    ment of the barley mutant Xan-b[61]. Genet. Res. Camb. 15: 135–
    7.

LI, S. L. and RÉDEI, G. P. 1969a Thiamine mutants of the crucifer,
    Arabidopsis. Biochem. Genet. 3: 163–170.

LI, S. L. and G. P. RÉDEI 1969b Estimation of mutation rate in
    autogamous diploids. Radiation Bot. 9: 125–31.

LI, S. L. and G. P. RÉDEI 1969c Allelic complementation at the
    pyrimidine (py) locus of the crucifer, Arabidopsis. Genetics
    62: 281–8.

LI, S. L. and G. P. RÉDEI 1969d Gene locus specificity of the glu-
    cose effect in the thiamine pathway of the angiosperm, Ara-
    bidopsis. Plant Physiology 44: 225-9.

LI, S. L., and G. P. RÉDEI and C. S. GOWANS 1967 A phylogenetic
    comparison of mutation spectra. Molec. Gen. Genet. 100: 77-
    83.

LI, S. L. and C. YANOFSKY 1973 Amino acid sequence studies with
    the tryptophan synthetase chain of Salmonella typhimurium.
    Proc. Nat. Acad. Sci. U.S. 248: 1830-6.

LURIA, S. E. and M. DELBRÜCK 1943 Mutation in bacteria from virus
    sensitivity to virus resistance. Genetics 28: 491-511.

MARGOLIASH, E. 1963 Primary structure and evolution of cytochrome
    c. Proc. Nat. Acad. Sci. U. S. 38: 672-9.

MATHER, K. 1957 The Measurement of Linkage in Heredity. Methuen &
    Co. London.

MÜLLER, A. J. 1963 Embryonentest zum Nachweis recessiver Letalfak-
    toren bei Arabidopsis thaliana Biol. Zbl. 83: 133-63.

NELSON, O. E., Jr. 1967 Biochemical genetics of higher plants.
    Ann. Rev. Genet. 1: 245-68.

RÉDEI, G. P. 1960 Genetic control of 2,5-dimethyl-4-aminopyrimidine
    requirement in Arabidopsis thaliana. Genetics 45: 1007.

RÉDEI, G. P. 1962 Genetic block of "vitamin thiazole" synthesis
    in Arabidopsis. Genetics 47: 979.

RÉDEI, G. P. 1965 Genetic blocks in the thiamine synthesis of the
    angiosperm Arabidopsis. Amer. J. Bot. 52: 834-41.

RÉDEI, G. P. 1970 Arabidopsis thaliana (L.) Heynh. A review of the
    genetics and biology. Bibliographia Genet. 21: 1-151.

RÉDEI, G. P. 1974 Economy in mutation experiments. Zeitschr.
    Pflanzenzücht. in press.

RUDDLE, F. H. 1973 Linkage analysis in man by somatic cell gene-
    tics. Nature 242: 165-7.

SHERMAN, F. and J. W. STEWART 1971 Genetics and biosynthesis of
    cytochrome c. Ann. Rev. Genet. 5: 257-96.

THOMPSON. L. H. and R. M. BAKER 1973 Isolation of mutants of cultured mammalian cells. Pp. 209-81. Methods in Cell Biology, Prescott, D. M., Ed., Vol. 6. Acad Press, New York.

WALLES, B. 1963 Macromolecular physiology of plastids, IV. On amino acid requirements of lethal chloroplast mutants in barley. Hereditas 50: 317-44.

YČAS, M. 1969 The Biological Code. North-Holland Publ. Co. Amsterdam.

IN VITRO SELECTION FOR MUTANTS OF HIGHER PLANTS

R. S. CHALEFF* AND P. S. CARLSON[†]

Biology Department, Brookhaven National Laboratory

Upton, New York 11973 U.S.A.

Abstract: Tobacco plants resistant to wildfire disease have
been regenerated from methionine sulfoximine-resistant
calluses selected in vitro. The intracellular concentration
of free methionine is elevated in two of the three mutant
plants. Three rice cell lines which are resistant to the
lysine analogue, S-(β-aminoethyl)-cysteine have also been
isolated in vitro. Analyses of free and protein-incorpor-
ated amino acid composition reveal increased levels of
several amino acids in the variant cell lines.

1. INTRODUCTION

Genetic studies of microorganisms have achieved a highly
sophisticated and refined level. The relative ease with which
defined mutants are isolated in these unicellular forms has permitted the elucidation of biochemical and developmental pathways.
Investigations of microorganisms also have contributed largely
to our present understanding of the molecular mechanisms which
mediate the expression of genetic information. In contrast,
defined biochemical mutants of higher plants are not isolated
readily. This experimental distinction is due primarily to the
differences in biological organization between microbes and
higher plants. Bacteria and fungi have extended haploid phases

*Present address: Department of Applied Genetics, John Innes
Institute, Colney Lane, Norwich NOR 70F, England.
  †Present address: Department of Crop and Soil Science,
Michigan State University, East Lansing, Michigan 48823 U.S.A.

and small nutrient reserves which permit the immediate phenotypic
expression of genetic variation. The ability to grow large, homogeneous populations with short generation times on defined media
makes possible the application of selective screens to enormous
numbers of genomes. The organizational features, which have
nearly restricted the molecular genetical approach to microbes,
are now becoming available to higher plants. Cells of many plant
species may be cultured under defined conditions (Street, 1973);
techniques exist for obtaining haploid cell lines (Chase, 1969;
Nitsch, 1972; Sunderland, 1973); and whole plants may be differentiated from cultured cells (Vasil and Vasil, 1972; Reinert,
1973). With the ability to manipulate experimentally higher plant
cells as microorganisms, it should be possible to dissect the
functioning of these more complex forms. This understanding could
then be applied to effect agronomically beneficial changes in
important crop species.

A. Mutants which overproduce amino acids:

Several experiments have illustrated the feasibility of
applying microbial selective systems to cultured cells of higher
plants to achieve directed modification of plant genomes. In one
experiment, mutants of Nicotiana tabacum resistant to the wildfire
disease were recovered (Carlson, 1973). This disease of tobacco
is caused by a bacterial pathogen, Pseudomonas tabaci, which
produces a toxin structurally similar to methionine (Braun, 1955).
Resistant plants were obtained by screening populations of
haploid tobacco cells and protoplasts for the ability to grow in
a medium containing an inhibitory concentration of the methionine
analogue, methionine sulfoximine (MSO). MSO is an analogue of
the wildfire toxin which elicits the formation of the same characteristic halos on tobacco leaves as does the natural bacterial
toxin (Braun, 1955).

Haploid plants of Nicotiana tabacum cv. Wisconsin 38 were
obtained from anther culture. Populations of haploid cells and
protoplasts were isolated from these haploid plants (Carlson,
1970) and were treated with 0.25% ethyl methanesulfonate for
1 hour and plated. After 2 weeks the cultures were overlaid
with a medium containing 10 mM MSO. Surviving calluses were
recovered, grown in the absence of the analogues, and then
retested for resistance to 10 mM MSO. One callus (mutant 1)
which was stable in expression of MSO resistance was recovered
from among $1.9 (10^7)$ viable cells. Two additional stably resistant clones (mutants 2 and 3) were isolated from a population of
approximately $2.7 (10^7)$ viable protoplasts. Diploid plants were
regenerated from each of the three calluses and their chromosomal
composition was confirmed cytologically. Each mutant plant was
crossed to a wild type to give heterozygous F_1 progeny. The F_1

progeny were self-fertilized to produce an F_2 generation. One hundred F_2 seedlings from each of the three crosses were germinated sterilely and tested for resistance to MSO. The results are presented in Table 1. The pattern of transmission of mutant 1 is complex and approximates a 9:3:3:1 ratio which is expected from

Table 1

Growth of 100 F_2 seedlings on
medium containing 10 mM
methionine sulfoximine

Mutant no.	No growth	Slight growth	Normal growth
1	59	37	4
2	31	51	18
3	36	42	22

two independently segregating recessive loci with additive effects. The patterns of transmission of mutants 2 and 3 appear simpler and are best explained by single semidominant loci yielding a 1:2:1 ratio. As the mutants were derived from mutagenized cells and there is the possibility of extensive genetic damage, these ratios must be considered preliminary. Crosses between mutants 2 and 3 indicate that they may be allelic. However, since these two mutants were isolated in separate experiments, they must result from two distinct mutational events. All three mutants are less susceptible than the parent plant to the pathogenic effects of bacterial infection (Carlson, 1973).

The levels of free amino acids in fully expanded leaves of wild type tobacco and of the three homozygous mutants are presented in Table 2A. The level of free methionine is specifically increased in mutants 2 and 3, but not in mutant 1. The concentrations of free amino acids in leaves of heterozygous plants derived from crossing the homozygous mutants to wild type are shown in Table 2B. That the amount of free methionine in the heterozygous strains of mutants 2 and 3 is half of that observed in the homozygous mutant plants is consistent with the semidominant resistance phenotype of these two mutants and suggests that resistance may be related to endogenous levels of free methionine.

The recovery of tobacco plants resistant to wildfire disease reveals the potentiality of selection for toxin resistance in vitro as a generalized procedure for obtaining disease resistant

Table 2

Concentrations of certain free amino acids in tobacco leaves
(nmol per gram fresh weight)

Strains	Methionine	Glycine	Alanine	Proline
A) Homozygous				
Havana Wisconsin 38	0.4 ± 0.2	1.3 ± 0.3	1.8 ± 0.3	0.3 ± 0.1
Mutant 1	0.3 ± 0.2	1.4 ± 0.3	1.7 ± 0.5	0.4 ± 0.2
Mutant 2	1.9 ± 0.5	1.7 ± 0.5	2.0 ± 0.4	0.5 ± 0.2
Mutant 3	2.4 ± 0.6	1.2 ± 0.2	1.5 ± 0.3	0.4 ± 0.2
B) Heterozygous				
Mutant 1/+	0.5 ± 0.2	1.6 ± 0.4	2.1 ± 0.5	0.3 ± 0.2
Mutant 2/+	0.9 ± 0.4	1.5 ± 0.3	1.7 ± 0.4	0.5 ± 0.2
Mutant 3/+	1.5 ± 0.7	1.1 ± 0.3	1.9 ± 0.5	0.3 ± 0.2

Fully expanded young leaves were deveined and homogenized at room
temperature. An equal volume of 10% trichloroacetic acid was added to
the homogenate. The acid soluble supernatant was applied to an automated
amino acid analyzer.

varieties. These results also demonstrate that mutants of higher
plants in which the regulation of amino acid biosynthesis is
altered may be recovered in vitro. This latter conclusion has
been extended by additional research. Widholm (1972a,b) has
isolated cell lines of tobacco and carrot which are capable of
growth in the presence of a normally inhibitory concentration of
5-methyl tryptophan. Crude extracts of the resistant cell lines
contain a species of anthranilate synthetase which is less sensitive to feedback inhibition by tryptophan and 5-methyl tryptophan
than is the wild type enzyme. Endogenous levels of free tryptophan
in resistant cell lines of tobacco and carrot are 15 times and
27 times higher, respectively, than the wild type levels. Thus,
it is evident that in higher plants the endogenous concentration
of a specific metabolite may be increased by selecting for resistance to a structural analogue of that metabolite. It follows,
therefore, that by using analogues of amino acids essential to
human nutrition, variants of crop species which produce elevated
levels of these compounds may be induced and selected in culture.

B. Experiments with cultured rice tissue:

        The seed endosperm protein of rice is of inferior nutritional
quality because of relative insufficiencies of lysine, threonine,
and isoleucine. In higher plants these amino acids and methionine,
which is also nutritionally essential, are derived from aspartate
via the biosynthetic pathway outlined in Fig. 1 (Miflin, 1973).
The activity of the first enzyme, aspartokinase, appears to be
regulated through feedback inhibition primarily by lysine and
to a lesser degree by threonine (Bryan et al., 1970; Furuhashi
and Yatazawa, 1970; Henke et al., 1974). Aspartokinase activity
in cell free extracts of rice shoots is also sensitive to feedback
inhibition by the lysine analogue S-(β-aminoethyl)-cysteine (SAEC)
(Halsall et al., 1972). These observations suggested that resistance to SAEC could be utilized to select for rice mutants in which
lysine biosynthesis is released from regulatory control. Furthermore, it was anticipated that a mutation conferring analogue
resistance would be semidominant. Thus, the experiment could be
carried out with cultured diploid cells by a procedure similar to
that used by Widholm (1972a,b).

2. MATERIALS AND METHODS

Strains:

        Seeds of Oryza sativa (C.I. 8960-S) were obtained from the
U.S. Department of Agriculture/Agricultural Research Service,
Stuttgart, Arkansas, U.S.A.

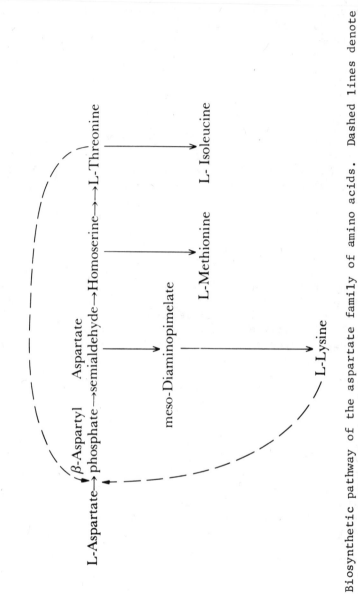

Fig. 1. Biosynthetic pathway of the aspartate family of amino acids. Dashed lines denote hypothetical patterns of feedback inhibition.

Culture conditions:

Callus cultures were maintained either in liquid or on solid medium containing the mineral salts and vitamin concentrations described by Linsmaier andSkoog (1965) supplemented with 3% sucrose and 0.5 mg 2,4-D, 5.0 mg indoleacetic acid, and 0.3 mg kinetin per liter. Callus cultures were obtained from seed by the procedure of Yamada et al. (1967). All cultures were incubated in the dark at $27 \pm 1^{\circ}$ C.

Mutant induction and selection:

Small cell aggregates from suspension cultures were incubated in liquid medium containing 1% ethyl methanesulfonate for 1 hour. The cultures were then washed twice and resuspended in fresh medium. Cultures were incubated for 10 days following mutagenesis to ensure genetic segregation and phenotypic expression of any mutational event. The tissue was then plated on medium supplemented with 2 mM SAEC, a concentration of the analogue which kills wild type cells. Resistant clones were selected as they appeared over a two month period.

Amino acid analysis:

Callus tissue was harvested on a Buchner funnel, washed thoroughly with distilled water, and lyophilized for several days. The dried tissue was ground with a Wylie mill and lyophilized for an additional day. Free amino acids were extracted in water at 85° C using a glass homogenizer. Samples were concentrated to dryness and redissolved in 0.2 N sodium citrate buffer (pH 2.2). Total amino acid composition was determined by hydrolyzing a sample of lyophilized callus tissue in 6 N HCl for 22 hours according to the procedure of Moore and Stein (1963). All samples were analyzed on an automated amino acid analyzer.

3. RESULTS

Three variant rice cell lines were selected which survive and grow very slowly in the presence of 2 mM SAEC. The intracellular concentration of free amino acids in these three variant cell lines and in the wild type are presented in Table 3. The three variant lines contain elevated levels of three of the amino acids derived from aspartate as well as of leucine, valine, tyrosine, and alanine. Threonine was not resolved by the chromatographic system which used sodium citrate buffer. The largest increases, which were observed in the levels of free isoleucine and leucine, are not as great as the tryptophan increases reported by Widholm (1972a,b) in 5-methyl tryptophan-resistant lines of tobacco and carrot. However, these increases

Table 3

Free amino acid pools of rice tissue cultures
(expressed as nmols/mg dry weight)

Amino acid	Wild type	EMS-5	EMS-6	EMS-8
Lysine	7.67	14.07	14.84	19.47
Histidine	10.76	6.21	5.97	6.96
Arginine	5.90	5.97	8.74	10.99
Glycine	6.89	11.17	17.27	17.89
Alanine	1.82	22.35	8.40	23.75
Valine	2.84	8.18	12.02	14.25
Methionine	0.71	1.86	1.80	2.06
Isoleucine	0.79	3.10	6.44	7.04
Leucine	0.80	3.88	6.26	6.67
Tyrosine	0.97	2.87	2.74	3.64
Phenylalanine	10.22	6.91	5.41	7.51
Total nmol per mg dry wt	104.10	182.32	149.31	193.06

are comparable with the specific increase in free methionine
observed in methionine sulfoximine-resistant tobacco leaves (Table
2). If the variant rice cell lines are presumed to be heterozygous, since they were isolated from diploid tissue, any changes
in the free amino acid concentrations should be comparable with
those in the heterozygous mutant strains of tobacco (Table 2B).
It is seen that free lysine, methionine, and valine are increased
by the same factor as is methionine in the heterozygous tobacco
mutants.

The increase in free lysine is not sufficient to explain
the increase in total lysine content of approximately 30 nmoles
per mg dry weight which is realized in the variant cell lines. The
total amino acid composition of the wild type and variant rice
cell lines are presented in Table 4. These data were obtained
from acid hydrolysis of callus tissue and represent the sum of
free and protein-bound amino acids. The data in Table 4 are
expressed as mole per cent of total amino acid content and,
therefore, reflect protein quality. The per cent differences
from the wild type values are given in brackets. The increases
in the relative levels of lysine, isoleucine, leucine, and valine
evidence the improved quality of total cell protein in the three
variant lines. That analogue resistance has selected for strains
altered not only in endogenous concentrations of free amino acids,

Table 4

Total amino acid composition of rice tissue cultures
(expressed as per cent moles of total)

Amino acid	Wild type	EMS-5	EMS-6	EMS-8
Lysine	5.19	6.54(+26.0)	5.86(+12.9)	6.26(+20.6)
Histidine	2.49	2.13(-14.5)	2.05(-17.7)	2.12(-14.9)
Arginine	4.19	4.69(+11.9)	4.72(+12.6)	4.78(+14.1)
Aspartate	11.37	10.55(- 7.2)	9.85(-13.4)	9.91(-12.8)
Threonine	5.26	5.02(- 4.6)	5.13(- 2.5)	5.04(- 4.6)
Serine	6.91	6.79(- 1.7)	6.65(- 3.8)	6.73(- 2.6)
Glutamate	8.86	11.15(+25.8)	9.91(+11.9)	10.12(+14.2)
Proline	5.49	5.40(- 1.6)	5.93(+ 8.0)	5.58(+ 1.6)
Glycine	17.50	12.05(-31.1)	13.69(-21.8)	13.12(-25.0)
Alanine	9.33	10.15(+ 8.8)	9.70(+ 4.0)	10.20(+ 9.3)
Valine	6.37	6.94(+ 8.9)	7.42(+16.5)	7.23(+13.5)
Isoleucine	3.97	4.41(+11.1)	4.44(+11.8)	4.45(+12.1)
Leucine	6.79	7.87(+15.9)	7.88(+16.1)	7.81(+15.0)
Tyrosine	2.21	2.56(+15.8)	2.89(+30.8)	2.80(+26.7)
Phenylalanine	4.08	3.75(- 8.1)	3.91(- 4.2)	3.85(- 5.6)
		Per cent protein		
	22.9	25.8 (+12.9)	23.2 (+1.6)	28.3 (+23.7)

but also in the relative amount of each amino acid incorporated
into protein, is an interesting and unexpected result.

There is also some indication that the total amount of protein is higher in EMS-5 and EMS-8 than in the cell line from which
these variants were isolated (Table 4). However, these differences in protein content should be interpreted with caution,
since they were somewhat variable and the extent of dehydration
may not have been constant for the lyophilized samples upon which
the dry weight determination was based. Differences also were
noted in the amino acid compositions between several wild type
rice cell lines, but not within a given cell line. This variability may be due to physiological differences, making valid
only a comparison between analyses of variant cell lines and
the original untreated cell line from which they were derived.
Analogue resistance selects merely for expression of a specific
phenotype. The mechanisms which effect this phenotype will
remain unknown until mature plants are differentiated and
subjected to genetic analysis.

The growth responses of the wild type and variant cell lines
to several mixtures of exogenous amino acids should provide
further information concerning the nature of the phenotypic differences and also enable selective conditions for the isolation of
additional variants to be optimized. The results in Table 5
represent the growth of the wild type and three variant cell
lines following a 22 day incubation period on a culture medium
supplemented with combinations of lysine, threonine, methionine,
and isoleucine. A mixture of lysine and threonine inhibits
growth of rice callus tissue presumably by feedback inhibition
of aspartokinase and resultant starvation for methionine (Furuhashi
and Yatazawa, 1970; Fig. 1). EMS-6 is insensitive to this effect.
EMS-8 is less sensitive than wild type to inhibition by lysine
alone and growth of EMS-6 is unaffected by the addition of 4 mM
lysine to the medium. Whereas 2 mM lysine partially diminishes
the inhibitory effect of 2 mM SAEC on the wild type cell line,
the growth response of EMS-5 to the analogue is unaltered by
lysine. In general, growth of EMS-5 is affected more adversely
by exogenous amino acids than is that of the wild type tissue.
This is particularly evident in the response of these cell lines
to 2 mM isoleucine. The differences in growth responses of the
three variants to the mixtures of amino acids make it probable
that independent events are responsible for the observed phenotypes. Although there is no apparent difference between the
variant and wild type cell lines after 22 days in the presence
of 2 mM SAEC, a differential growth response is evident after
6-8 weeks which permits variants to be selected in culture. The
analogue-resistant phenotype of the three variant cell lines has
been expressed stably in vitro for more than one year, even
following extensive periods of subculture in the absence of the
analogue. The results in Table 5 indicate that variants similar
to EMS-6 could be recovered efficiently on a medium supplemented
with lysine and threonine. These experiments are now in
progress.

4. DISCUSSION

Previous studies have shown that cultured cell lines of
higher plants containing elevated levels of specific amino acids
may be selected in vitro (Widholm, 1972a,b; Carlson, 1973).
Genetic analysis of plants differentiated from MSO-resistant
tobacco calluses suggests that the changes in free amino acid
content are due to a stable Mendelian-inherited mutational event
(Carlson, 1973). This paper reports the selection in culture of
variant cell lines of rice in which the quality and perhaps the
quantity of cell protein are altered favorably. Unfortunately,
these variants were isolated from rice tissue which had been
maintained in culture for too long a period and no longer retained

Table 5

Growth responses of wild type and variant cell lines
to exogenous amino acids

Amino acids	Wild type	EMS-5	EMS-6	EMS-8
2 mM Lys	17.5	10.4	147.1	91.3
2 mM SAEC	1.1	0.5	1.7	0
2 mM SAEC 2 mM Lys	15.5	0.1	50.5	17.1
4 mM Lys	11.5	0.1	105.3	57.5
2 mM Ile	61.8	0	50.5	6.7
2 mM Thr	18.6	9.9	96.6	0
2 mM Met	8.2	0.4	20.5	12.8
2 mM Thr 2 mM Met	17.7	0	29.0	5.9
2 mM Lys 2 mM Thr	0	0.4	112.5	0
2 mM Lys 2 mM Thr 2 mM Met	43.5	0	95.2	26.8
2 mM Met 2 mM Thr 2 mM Ile	13.6	0	39.2	0
2 mM Lys 2 mM Thr 2 mM Ile	2.2	0	49.6	9.0
2 mM Lys 2 mM Thr 2 mM Met 2 mM Ile	20.8	0.2	54.3	4.4
No supplements	100(15.85 mg)	18.71 mg	8.87 mg	10.93 mg

Initial inoculum = 0.85 mg dry weight; numbers represent per
cent of growth (increase in dry weight) on unsupplemented
medium.

its morphogenetic apacity (Nishi et al., 1968). However, it is
hoped that these experiments have served to define conditions
which will permit the selection of similar variants in totipotent
tissue of rice and other food crops. It is not known whether
these changes in protein quality and quantity will be reflected
in the seed endosperm. This question is crucial and can be
answered only by studying plants obtained from variant cell
lines selected in vitro.

REFERENCES

Braun, A. C., (1955), A study on the mode of action of the wild-
    fire toxin, Phytopathology, 45, 659.
Bryan, P. A., R. D. Cawley, C. E. Brunner and J. K. Bryan, (1970),
    Isolation and characterization of a lysine-sensitive asparto-
    kinase from a multicellular plant, Biochem. Biophys. Res.
    Commun., 41, 1211.
Carlson, P. S., (1970), Induction and isolation of auxotrophic
    mutants in somatic cell cultures of Nicotiana tabacum,
    Science, 168, 487.
Carlson, P. S., (1973), Methionine sulfoximine-resistant mutants
    of tobacco, Science, 180, 1366.
Chase, S. S., (1969), Monoploids and monoploid-derivatives of
    maize, Bot. Rev., 35, 117.
Furuhashi, K. and M. Yatazawa, (1970), Methionine-lysine-threonine-
    isoleucine interrelationships in the amino acid nutrition of
    rice callus tissue, Plant Cell Physiol., 11, 569.
Halsall, D., R. D. Brock, and J. B. Langridge, (1972), Selection
    for high lysine mutants, CSIRO Div. of Plant Industry
    Genetics Report, p. 31.
Henke, R. R., K. G. Wilson, and J. W. McClure, (1974), Lysine-
    methionine-threonine interactions in growth and development
    of Mimulus cardinalis seedlings, Planta, 116, 333.
Linsmaier, E. M. and F. Skoog, (1965), Organic growth factor
    requirements of tobacco tissue cultures, Physiol. Plant.,
    18, 100.
Miflin, B. J., (1973), Amino acid biosynthesis and its control
    in plants, in "Biosynthesis and its Control in Plants", ed.
    B. V. Milborrow, (Academic Press, London), 49.
Moore, S. and W. H. Stein, (1963), Chromatographic determination
    of amino acids by the use of automatic recording equipment,
    in "Methods in Enzymology", eds. S.P. Colowick and N. O.
    Kaplan, (Academic Press, New York), Vol. 6, 819.
Nishi, T., Y. Yamada, and E. Takahashi, (1968), Organ rediffer-
    entiation and plant restoration in rice callus, Nature,
    219, 508.
Nitsch, J. P., (1972), Haploid plants from pollen, Z. Pflanzen-
    zucht., 67, 3.

Reinert, J., (1973), Aspects of organization-organogenesis and embryogenesis, in "Plant Tissue and Cell Culture", ed. H. E. Street, (University of California Press, Berkeley), 338.

Street, H. E., (1973), Plant Tissue and Cell Culture, (University of California Press, Berkeley).

Sunderland, N., (1973), Pollen and anther culture, in "Plant Tissue and Cell Culture", ed. H. E. Street, (University of California Press, Berkeley), 205.

Vasil, I. K.,and V. Vasil, (1972), Totipotency and embryogenesis in plant cell and tissue cultures, In Vitro, 8, 117.

Widholm, J. M., (1972a), Cultured Nicotiana tabacum cells with an altered anthranilate synthetase which is less sensitive to feedback inhibition, Biochim. Biophys. Acta, 261, 52.

Widholm, J. M., (1972b), Anthranilate synthetase from 5-methyl tryptophan susceptible and resistant cultured Daucus carota cells, Biochim. Biophys. Acta, 279, 48.

Yamada, Y., K. Tanaka, and E. Takahashi, (1967), Callus induction in rice, Oryza sativa L., Proc. Japan Acad., 43, 156.

Research carried out at Brookhaven National Laboratory under the auspices of the U. S. Atomic Energy Commission. The authors are extremely grateful to Dr. L. J. Greene for generously lending his advice and laboratory facilities to this project. The excellent technical assistance of Ms. R. Shapanka, Ms. B. Floyd, Mr. J. Tilley, and Mr. N. Alonzo also contributed to this research as did critical and helpful discussions with Drs. J. Polacco, D. Parke, and T. Rice.

ISOZYMES AND A STRATEGY FOR THEIR UTILIZATION IN PLANT GENETICS

I. ISOZYMES : GENETIC AND EPIGENETIC CONTROL

MICHEL JACOBS

Laboratorium voor Plantengenetica
Vrije Universiteit Brussel
B - 1640 St. Genesius-Rode

1. INTRODUCTION

One of the most crucial problem facing the plant geneticist is the elucidation of the mechanisms which enables information coded in DNA to determine the morphology of an organism. Early studies in this field, made on flower color mutants and their associated pigments (1,2) were limited by the fact that conclusions about genotypes were almost entirely based on phenotypic observations, and concerned morphological or complex physiological characteristics. However, in the last fifteen years, the impact of the "one gene-one enzyme" hypothesis of Beadle, Tatum and Horowitz has led to a new development of the biochemical genetics of higher plants by giving rise to studies that correlate differences in genotypes with enzyme variations and consider the earliest stages in the transcription and translation of the genetic code. Ten years ago most of our examples would be drawn from microorganisms, but now what emerges from higher plants forms an impressive bulk of data.

Two main types of approach have been used to study the link between genotype and phenotype. First, we can mention the establishment of correlations between a mutation with known developmental effects and biochemical modifications. Although mutant types have not been grasped so easily by plant physiologists than by microbiologists as experimental tools, a good body of literature on biochemical investigations with plant mutants is now available. Nelson (3) is his excellent review, has compiled the most significant contributions about :
- mutations affecting the photosynthetic apparatus.
- mutations affecting the synthesis of storage proteins in maize.

- mutations affecting the carotenoïd synthesis
- mutations affecting some growth factors.
- mutations affecting the characteristics of the plant nutrition.
- mutations affecting developmental processes.

The second approach consists in means of distinguishing between active enzymes which differ only in net charge or/and size and was the consequence of the emergence of new techniques :

1) the development of zone electrophoresis (Kunkel and Tizelius, 4) which has allowed a significant improvement in the resolution of proteins, specially with the use of starchgel as migration support (Smithies, 5) and later of polyacrylamide gel in which separation occurs on charge and size basis (Ornstein and Davies, 6).

2) The use of histochemical staining methods for proteins and enzymes associated with zone electrophoresis (Hunter and Markert 7) which has led to the obtention of a zymogram in which protein bands are located on the basis of their enzyme activity.

As results of the application of these techniques, enzymes with more than one electrophoretically distinct form have been detected in numerous plants (Shannon, 8, Scandalios, 9) It is now well established mainly by the work of Allard and his collaborators (10) that among plant populations a large proportion of the genome is subject to variation.

The mechanisms of gene mutation can account for the generation of numerous alleles at a single locus. However, we have to be aware that the electrophoretic method, depending on detecting differences in charges between the various forms of a protein, can pick up only a limited proportion of all the existing allelic versions of a protein. Not all amino acid substitutions result in changes in electrophoretic migration, nor do all point mutations results in amino acid substitution. About 25 % of all point mutations would be expected to have no effects in relation to the degeneracy of the code. A smaller proportion (2-6 %) should cause a loss or alteration of enzyme activity in the case of the non-sense mutation. In most cases (70 - 75%) mutations will lead to the insertion of a different amino acid in the polypeptide chain. Shaw (11) had estimated that 28 percent of the nucleotide possible substitutions will cause the replacement of one amino acid by another acid having a different electrical charge. Indirect alterations of the charge may also be the consequence of a modified configuration of the molecule due to amino acid substitution in the protein chain. Thus electrophoretic variants are the reflect of only a part of the existing polymorphism and a electrophoretic allele may include several genic variants with the same net charge. We have thus to keep in mind that the amount of heterozygocity defined by these techniques is in fact underestimated.

Several other techniques than electrophoresis are also used to characterize variants proteins such as :
- immunological techniques
- biochemical properties (activity, kinetic properties effects of inhibitors, thermal stability, substrate affinities,

coenzyme preferences, etc...)
- gelfiltration ion exchange chromatography
- finger printing analysis.

The most satisfactory way to define the amount of genetic variability at a defined locus should be the knowledge of the amino acid
sequence of the proteins controlled by its different alleles. For
plant enzymes however, sequencing techniques are time consuming and
costly and purification of the enzymes a quite tedious process.
In an attempt to discover other forms of the genetic variability,
it is worthwhile to mention the report of heat-sensitive allozymes
of xanthine dehydrogenase in the virilis group of Drosophila.
Bernstein et al (12) have revealed many more additional alleles at
the locus controlling this enzyme than previously obtained by electrophoretical studies (1,74 times as many alleles in the case of
xantine dehydrogenase).

Anyway, potentially every enzyme can exist in isozyme forms and
this assumption has been already verified for several hundred enzymes
in various organisms, and it is our purpose to describe in this lecture a number of different systems which can account for the occuren-

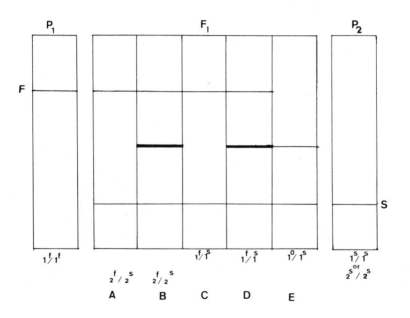

Fig. 1.
    Diagram showing isozyme patterns of the parents and their F₁
hybrids. (a) non-allelic isozyme genes without interaction.(b)
non-allelic isozyme genes with interaction.(e) allelic isozyme
genes without interaction (d) allelic isozymes genes with interaction (e) allelic isozyme genes with one gene silent.
1^F-1^S : allelic genes 1^F-2^S non-allelic genes.

ce of multiple molecular forms of an enzyme, making a clearcut distinction between genetically controlled enzyme variants, the isozymes,
and multiple molecular forms which are the result of secondary modifications of a single molecular species, thus due to epigenetic
changes. (table 1)

Examples of different systems shall be discussed and they can
be classified into five categories as shown in figure 1.

2. GENETICALLY CONTROLLED ISOZYMES

1. Multiple forms due to separate genes acting without interaction (non-allelic isozymes).

The simplest case to explain the occurence of different
isozymes on a zymogram is represented by separate genes coding
for separate enzymes. This was observed for esterases in maize.
The series of E_1, E_2, E_3, E_4 genes was described by Schwartz (13)
ans extended from E_5 to E_{10} by Mac Donald and Brewbaker (14). In
Avena fatua, Clegg and Allard (15) have reported five esterase loci,
each including two alleles.

2. A most interesting type of genetic relationship resulting
in the formation of multiple enzyme forms involves interaction between products of different genes (hybrids between non-allelic
isozymes).

In this category is represented the most famous and widely studied isozyme system in animals, lactate dehydrogenase. In most verte-
brates, lactate dehydrogenase occurs with a pattern of from one to
five bands in function of the tissue. It has been proposed (Appella
and Markert (16) that the five possible isozymes are produced as a
result of the random association into tetramers of subunits specified
by two different genes.

According to the hypothesis, LDH-1 contains four B subunits and
LDH-5 contains four A subunits; the other three bands contain different combinations of A and B subunits. This was demonstrated by dissociation and reassociation into tetramers of the two different subunits A and B of LDH. Markert (17) found that when equal proportions of
purified LDH-1 and LDH-5 are mixed, dissociated by freezing in NaCl,
then reassociated and subjected to electrophoresis, all five isozymes
are generated in the expected proportions (1:4 : 6:4 : 1).

In maize an alcoholdehydrogenase system have been reported in
which the observed pattern should be result of interaction between the
products of two different, unlinked genes Adh_1 and Adh_2 where products
dimerize to give three sets of ADH enzymes: the two homodimers (set I
and III) and the heterodimer (set II)(fig.2) (Schwartz, 18, Freeling
and Schwartz, 19). Adh_2 gene produces a protein which in normal conditions shows no activity, but the heterodimers (set II) are sufficiently
active to give a visible band after overstaining. Anaerobic conditions
as immersion of the entire seedling in water mediate a rapid accumulation of ADH specified by Adh_1 and Adh_2 genes. The arguments presented to
sustain the hypothesis - Set II is a heterodimer composed of products
specified by each of the two Adh genes - are the following :

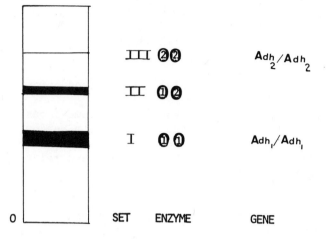

Fig. 2
     Diagram of the electrophoretic pattern of alcohol dehydrogenase
isozymes specified by two homozygous genes. 0 denotes the origin (after Freeling and Schwartz, 19)

     - all ADH enzymes behave as dimers and have a similar molecular
size.
     - all variants with an altered electrophoretic migration of the
set I enzymes give a correlated change in set II enzymes.
     - induced mutations in set I simultaneously alter the migration
of set II enzymes.
     - a mutation of Adh_2, induced by ethyl methane sulfonate, alters
set III and set II enzymes only. The mutant was first recognized by
the presence on the zymogram of three set II bands instead of the two
expected in an Adh_1^F/Adh_1^S, Adh_2^N/Adh_2^N heterozygote.
This mutant, designated Adh_2^F, was confirmed by its action on set III
enzymes after induction of enzymes by an anaerobic treatment. Adh_2^P
confers a slower migration rate to set III bands and also to set II
bands. A segregation test gives all expected dimers after self-polli-
nation of the double heterozygote. Adh_1 and Adh_2 appear to segregate
independently.
     Another very striking example of "collaboration" between the pro-
ducts of non-allelic isozyme genes was reported by Hart (20) with regard to alcohol dehydrogenase in hexaploid wheat. He has determined
the Adh phenotypes in the 40 nulli-tetrasomic lines available in the
variety "Chinese Spring". Three Adh phenotypes, I, II, III, differing
with respect to the presence or absence of Adh bands and their relative staining intensities, were observed among the 40 strains. The results
indicate that genes coding for ADH subunits are located in the chromosomes 4A, 4B and 4D - the homeologous chromosomes from each of the
three diploid progenitors. Genetic studies had provided evidence which
suggests that each of these isozymes is a dimer. An analysis of the

relationship between the chromosomal constitution and the zymogram
phenotype of each of the lines points out that :
- chromosome 4A contributes to the production of bands 1 and 2
- chromosome 4B and 4 D are both involved in the production of band
  3
- chromosome 4D, 4B and 4A all involved in the production of band
  2.
Results agreed with the idea that the 4A chromosome locus codes
for monomer α, the 4B locus for β and 4D for δ with random association of the monomers to produce six combinations of active dimers.
It is supposed that the isozyme ADH-1 which migrate relatively fast
is composed of $\alpha\alpha$ dimers, the intermediate isozyme ADH-2 of $\alpha\beta$ and $\alpha\delta$
and the slow migrating ADH-3 isozyme represented by $\beta\beta$, $\delta\delta$ and
$\beta\delta$ dimers.
Thus, in that case, a dimerization process between three subunits
code by triplicate genes give rise to the active ADH isozymes

3. There are many examples of enzyme systems by plants in which
different alleles produce enzyme forms that differ in electrophoretic migration (allelic isozyme) , with, in the simplest case, no interactions between the products of the different alleles. We have
met this type in Arabidopsis leucine amino peptidase (Jacobs, 21).
There are two forms of the peptidase 1 enzyme which have been found
to be specified by different alleles. The peptidase 1^F allele produces an enzyme which migrates faster toward the anode in electrophoresis than the enzyme produced by the peptidase 1^S allele. In heterozygotes, only the parental bands are represented. The absence of hybrid band does not automatically imply that the isozymes are monomers.
This type is observed in many enzyme species of several plants.

4. Now, in many systems, the products of different alleles may
combine to form hybrid enzymes when the alleles are present in heterozygous condition. The E_1 esterase of maize were the first hybrid-
forming enzymes to be described by Schwartz (22). The E_1 gene displays seven alleles. In heterozygotes between any two of the seven alleles, in addition to the parental bands, a third band with an intermediate migration rate is observed. The interpretation of this banding
pattern is that the E_1 esterase are dimers, each containing two homologous subunits . In heterozygotes, the random dimerization of f.i. S
and F subunits produces SS and FF autodimers but also SF allodimers
which migrate to a position intermediate between the two autodimers.
If the dimerization is random, the two autodimers must be found in
equal amounts, with twice as much of the allodimer. The observed
pattern in heterozygote approaches the expected binomial distribution
of 1:2:1

An analogous relationship has been described for maize catalase by Scandalios (23). There are six alleles of the catalase Ct_1

gene, with distinct electrophoretic mobilities. In heterozygotes, between any two of the six alleles, five isozymes are found,three of which are hybrid enzymes and the interpretation of this pattern is that the enzyme is a tetramer. A biochemical confirmation of the hypothesis involved dissociation and reassociation of catalase subunits. In vitro hybridization of catalase isozymes was accomplished by mixing any two of the variant catalase in 1,0 M NaCl, freezing to -20° C and thawing. The subunits of catalase dissociate and reassociate randomly with each other to form five isozymes in approximately the expected binomial distribution : 1 : 4 : 6 :4: 1, suggesting random combination of the presumed dissociated monomeric subunits.

It is worthwhile to mention that another catalase gene, Ct_2, generate products which interact with catalase 1 isozymes to form hybrid molecules (24). Thus catalase isozymes isozymes in maize can be generated by both intragenic and intergenic association of the products.

However, the absence of hybrid bands characterized by an intermediate migration rate between the ones of the parental isozymes does not necessary imply that the allelic isozymes are monomeric. Such a case is illustrated by the mode of inheritance of acid phosphatase isozymes in Arabidopsis. Three electrophoretically distinct groups of acid phosphatase AP_1 , AP_2 and AP_3 have been found in Arabidopsis. These groups differ in their relative migration rates towards the anode and in their levels of activity (Jacobs and Schwind, 25,26).

The AP_1 pattern shows four bands (numbered from 1 to 4 starting with the least anodal) and contains about 70 % of the activity of acid phosphatases present in the leaves. The intensity of the AP_1 bands is graded so that band 3 has the highest activity, bands 1 and 2 a lower comparable activity and band 4 is only slightly active.

Three types of electrophoretic variants of acid phosphatase were discovered among 155 geographical races. We have designated theses types as S (slow), I (intermediate) and F (fast) in order of electrophoretical mobility with respect to the anode. Each electrophoretic variant contains a set of four bands which in comparison to each other are displaced in a parallel fashion from S to I and from I fo F towards the anode. The value of this displacement is twice the distance between two successive bands so that the patterns overlap between S and I types and I and F types.
The three possible heterozygous hybrids (S/F, I/F, S/F) show both group of isozymes each of which comes from the homozygous parents. On a zymogram of a cross between a S and a I type (fig. 3) 6 bands are present instead the expected eight parental bands which can be explained by overlapping between bands 3^S and 1^I and between bands 4^S and 2^I. An hybrid between F type and S type displays 8 bands on the gel as there is no overlapping between the two parental sets.

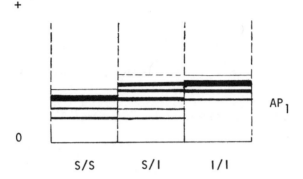

Fig. 3 Diagram of a zymogram showing the hybrid pattern obtained
from the cross between a S and a I variant.

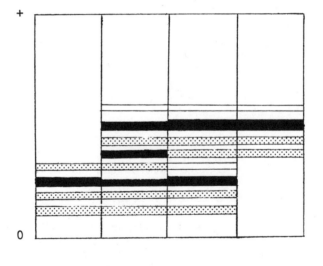

Fig. 4. Schematic picture of the acid phosphatase patterns in S/S
and F/F homozygotes, in a S/F heterozygote and in a 1:1
mixture of F and S extracts. (S & F)

Hybrid enzymes with a electrophoretic mobility differing from those of the parental bands do not appear in heterozygotes. It seems unlikely that the isozymes are composed of subunits which could randomly associate to generate the active enzymes. However, the distribution of activity between the bands of the heterozygote does not correspond to that expected from the addition of the parental bands (fig. 4). This pattern can be obtained with mixtures in a 1 : 1 ratio of extracts from the F and S types.

The particular distribution of activity in the heterozygote can be considered as indication of a dimeric constitution for the enzyme, with a restriction in the dimerization process to subunits belonging to the same corresponding bands in the three migration types S, I and F. Table 1 gives an example of a possible subunit composition of the isozymes in the case of the heterozygotes S/F and the intensity distribution of the bands in heterozygotes suggests that each subunit retains its characteristic activity in the heterodimer. Thus here the combinations 3^S3^I or 3^S3^F give the densest bands, the bands 1^S1^I, 1^S1^I, 2^S2^F and 2^S2^I are less dense and the bands 4^I4^S, 4^S4^F are the least intense.

In the F_2 generation all three possible types (the two parental and their corresponding heterozygote) were found in progenies in proportions showing a close agreement with the expected 1 : 2 : 1 ratio. The data presented in table 2 are consistent with the hypothesis that the AP_1 variants are controlled by three alleles at one locus (AP_1^S, AP_1^I, AP_1^F) acting without dominance.

Table 1.

Proposed subunit composition in AP_1 homozygotes and heterozygotes.

Genotypes.

Bands	I/I	S/I	S/S	S/F	F/F
4^F				4^F4^F	4^F4^F
3^F				3^F3^F	3^F3^F
$4^1 - 2^F$	4^I4^I	4^I4^I		$2^F2^F + 4^F4^S$	2^F2^F
$3^I - 1^F$	3^I3^I	$3^I3^I + 4^I4^I$		$1^F1^F + 3^F3^S$	1^F1^F
$2^I - 4^S$	2^I2^I	$2^I2^I + 4^S4^S + 3^S3^I$	4^S4^S	$4^S4^S + 2^F2^S$	
$1^I - 3^S$	1^I1^I	$1^I1^I + 3^S3^S$	3^S3^S	$3^S3^S + 1^F1^S$	
2^S		$2^S1^S + 1^I1^S$	2^S2^S	2^S2^S	
1^S		1^S1^S	1^S1^S	1^S1^S	

Table 2.

Segregation observed in the progeny of crosses made to determine
the inheritance of AP_1 variation.

Parent			AP_1 patterns of offspring				Total	Probability of χ^2 value
Female		Male	F	I	S	Heterozygote		
F	X	F	14	0	0	0	14	-
F	X	I	39	32	0	74	145	0.70>P>0.60
I	X	F	27	30	0	53	110	0.60>P>0.50
I	X	I	0	22	0	0	22	-
I	X	S	0	16	15	36	67	0.90>P>0.80
S	X	F	125	0	130	233	488	0.70>P>0.60
S	X	I	0	24	25	59	108	0.90>P>0.80

2.5. Another example related to allelic isozyme system is that in
which different alleles of a gene are responsible for the presence
or absence of enzyme activity. Examples of either spontaneous or
induced null mutants have been gathered by O'Brien (27). In Drosophila over 30 genes have a known gene product. Fourteen of them
present "silent" alleles which either produce no enzyme or produces an enzyme form which is more or less completely inactive. The
selection of such mutants has been elegantly carried out in Drosophila by Sofer and Hatkoff for alcoholdehydrogenase mutants (28).
They have exposed mutagenized flies to a secondary alcohol, penti-
tol. The flies with a wild-type level of ADH should oxidize the
alcohol into a poisonous ketone. Types with no ADH activity should
survive. They have obtained a mutation frequency of 0.012% for null
alleles at that locus.

In Arabidopsis we have discovered among previously isolated
morphological mutants a type characterized by the lack of AP_1 activity. This mutation did not affect the isozymes controlled by the
AP_2 and AP_3 loci and at the AP_1 locus eliminates all the bands simul-
teneously. Numerous mutants for one locus Acph-1 have been gathered by Bell and Mac Intyre in Drosophila using a spot test assay to
determine the activity of large numbers of mutagenized flies (29).
The frequency of induced mutations was about 0.3 %. The use of such
null mutants should allow to determine the effects of the loss of
one enzyme's activity on the development or the physiology of the
plant.

Schwartz (30) has studied the nature of alcohol dehydrogenase null
mutants of maize that produce no or only a such reduced amount of
hybrid enzyme in heterozygotes. Deletion or mutated gene with a reduced activity cannot explained this behaviour because an immunological test shows that the Adh_1^0 homozygotes produce substances
which react immunologically with antibodies of purified maize ADH.
The possibility of negative complementation which should render the
heterodimer inactive was ruled out by the comparison of activity
in S/O and S/F kernels. If negative complementation were involved,
the mutant heterozygote should contain much less than one-half of
the activity of the non-mutant type. However, the Adh_1^S/Adh_1^0 kernels
contained approximately half of the ADH activity of the Adh_1^S/Adh_1^F
sibling kernels (1942 versus 3907 units al of extracts).

The proposal is that the mutant subunits are structurally altered such that the Adh_1^0 subunits do not dimerize with the wild type
subunits or preferentially self-polymerise. This behaviour can be
interpreted as a consequence of changes in protein configuration possibly due to base substitutions in DNA after the mutagenic treatment.

3. NON-GENETIC MULTIPLE FORMS OF ENZYMES

In this discussion we have considered until now genetically controlled isozymes. The reason for multiple band pattern can also be
produced by secondary alterations of a single protein. Such situations can appear after the completion of a genetical analysis which
reveal that a series of bands on the zymogram is under the control
of one locus as f.i. after the obtention of mutants that change si -
multaneously the electrophoretic pattern or the activity of the multiple bands. Such an example of the formation of multiple enzyme forms
by a single allele is provided by alkaline phosphatase in Escherichia
coli (Schlessinger et al, 31) Four distinct bands have been observed
in electrophoresis and single mutations lead to electrophoretic mobilities which differ from those of the wild type, without altering the
spacing between the isozymes.

Different systems have been proposed to explain the origin of
these molecular varieties starting from one enzyme. We can mention:
- formation of aggregates by polymerisation of a single polypeptide chain.
- conjugation of a protein with different amount of small charged compounds (ligands) playing the role of coenzyme molecules.
- partial degradation of an enzyme (cleavage of peptide bond
by protease leading to terminal deletion of amino acid residues)
- formation of subclasses as evidence of conformational isozymes
of high stability.

I wish only to develop the problem of conformational differences
between isozymes which is particularly fascinating in relation to the
control of the configuration of a protein.
By conformers, I mean the ability of protein molecules with a similar
amino acid composition and sequence to assume a mixture of more than
one thermodynamically stable forms. Same enzymes may differ in con-

figuration by folding in various way of the polypeptide which may
conduct to differences in exposed charges and this allow the separation by electrophoresis (Epstein and Schechter, 32).

Conformational differences has been proposed to explain the
isozyme variation of chicken mitochondrial malate dehydrogenase
(Kitto et al, 33,). Schwartz (34) has proposed that the electrophoretic differences between the allelic isozymes of the E_1 esterase
in maize are a consequence of differences in conformation.
Evidence for conformational changes in grape eatechol oxydase was
reported by Lerner et al (35) This enzyme from Vitis vinefera was
resolved into several forms on acrylamide gel electrophoresis.
Short exposure to acid pH or urea induces a rapid 4-10 fold activation of the enzyme. Such treatments also induce marked changes
in the electric behaviour of the enzyme. There is a conversion of
the fast moving bands F to the slow ones S. The conclusion was
that the apparent dissociation of F into S bands might be the result of considerable changes in the distribution of charges on the
enzyme surface. Unfolding and possibly refolding of polypeptide
chain into a new conformation, resulting from exposure to urea or
acid pH, might caused here the reduced mobilities of the bands.
Analysis of the behaviour of the different bands upon migration in
different concentrations of acrylamide gels suggested that the F
bands have indeed similar molecular weights but differ in charge
distribution. (Harel et al, 36).

REFERENCES
(1) Haldane, J.B.S. 1942 . New paths in genetics pp 47-82, Harper,
    New York
(2) Lawrence W.J.F. and J.R. Price, 1940. The genetics and bioche-
    mistry of flower color variation. Biol. Rev. Cambridge Phil.
    Soc. 15 : 35-38.
(3) Nelson O.E. and B. Burr, 1973. Biochemical genetics of higher
    plants. Ann. Rev. Plant Physiol., 24: 493-518.
(3) Kunkel, H.G. and Tiselius, A. 1951
    J. Gen. Physiol. 35-89.
(5) Smithies, O. 1955. Zone electrophoresis of serum in starch gels.
    Biochem. Journ. 61 : 629
(6) Ornstein and Davies, B.J. 1962.Disc electrophoresis, Distilla-
    tion Products. Industries, Rochester.
(7) Hunter, R.L. and Markert, E.L. 1957. Histochemical demonstration
    of enzymes separated by zone electrophoresis. Science 125 :1294.
(8) Shannon L.M., 1968. Plant Isoenzymes. Ann. Rev. Pl. Physiol.19:
    187-210.
(9) Scandalios, I.G. 1969. Genetic control of multiple molecular
    forms of enzymes in plants : a review. Biochem. Genet. 3: 37-
    79.
(10)Allard R.W. and A.L. Kahler. 1971. Allozyme polymorphisms in plant
    populations. Stadler Symposia, 3 : 9-24.

(11) Shaw, C.R. 1969. Isozymes : Classification, frequency and sig-
     nificance. Int. Rev. of Cyt. 25 : 297.
(12) Bernstein S.C., L.H. Throckmorton and J.L. Hubby. 1973. Still
     more genetic variability in natural populations. Proc. Nat.
     Acad. Sci. U.S.A., 70 : 3928-3931
(13) Schwartz D., L. Fuchsman and K.H.M.Grath, 1965. Allelic iso-
     zymes of the pH 7.5 esterase in maize. Genetics, 52 : 1265-
     1268.
(14) Mac Donald T. and J.L. Brewbakker, 1974. Isoenzyme Polymorphism
     in Flowering Plants ix The E_5-E_{10} esterase loci of maize. The
     Journal of Heredity, 65: 37-42.
(15) Clegg M.T. and R.W. Allard, 1973. The genetics of Electrophore-
     tic variants in Avena. The Journal of Heredity, 64: 3-6.
(16) Appella, E. and C.L. Markert, 1961. Dissociation of lactate
     dehydrogenase into subunits with guanidine hydrochloride.
     Biochem. Biophys. Res. Communic. 6: 171-6.
(17) Markert, C.L.1963. Lactate dehydrogenase isozymes : dessocia-
     tion and recombination of subunits. Science 140 : 1329-30.
(18) Schwartz D., 1966. The genetic control of alcohol dehydrogenase
     in maize : gene duplication and respression. Proc. Nat. Acad.
     Sci. U.S.A., 56 : 1431-1436.
(19) Freeling M. and D. Schwartz, 1973. Genetic relationships between
     the multiple alcohol dehydrogenases of maize. Biochemical Genet.
     8 : 27-36.
(20) Hart G.E., 1970. Evidence for triplicate genes for alcohol de-
     hydrogenase in hexaploïd wheat. Proc. Nat. Acad. Sci. U.S.A.,
     66: 1136-1141.
(21) Jacobs, M. 1974. Contrôle génétique des isozymes de la leucine
     aminopeptidase chez Arabidopsis thaliana. Bull. Soc. Roy. Bot.
     Belg. in the press.
(22) Schwartz D., 1960. Genetic Studies on Mutant Enzymes in Maize:
     Synthesis of Hybrid Enzymes by Heterozygotes. Genetics, 46:
     1210-1215.
(23) Scandalios J.G., 1969. Genetic control of multiple molecular
     forms of catalase in maize. Annals of the New York Academy of
     Science, 151: 274-293.
(24) Scandalios J.G., E.H. Liu and M.A. Campeau, 1972. The effects
     of intragenic and intergence complementation on catalase struc-
     ture and function in maize : a molecular approach to heterosis.
     Archives of biochemistry and biophysics, 153: 695-705.
(25) Jacobs, M. and Schwind, F. 1973. Genetic control of isozymes
     of acid phosphatase in Arabidopsis thaliana. Plant Sci. Letters
     1 : 95-104.
(26) Jacobs, M. and Schwind, F. 1974. Biochemical genetics of Ara-
     bidopsis acid phosphatases polymorphism, tissue expression and
     genetics of AP_1, AP_2 and AP_3 loci. 3rd Int. Conf. on Isozymes,
     C.L. Markert, ed. Academic Press, N.Y. (in press).

(27) O'Brien, S.J., 1973. On Estimating functional gene number in Eukaryotes. Nature New Biology, 242 : 52-54.

(28) Sofer W.H. and M.A. Hatkoff, 1972. Chemical selection of alcohol dehydrogenase negative mutants in Drosophila. Genetics, 12 : 545-549.

(29) Bell J.B., R.J. Mac Intyre and A.P. Olivieri, 1972. Induction of null-activity mutants for the acid phosphatase-1 gene in Drosophila melanogaster. Biochemical Genetics, 6 : 206-216.

(30) Schwartz D., 1971. Dimerization Mutants of Alcohol Dehydrogenase of Maize. proc. Nat. Acad. of Sciences 68(1): 145-146.

(31) Schlesinger M.J. and L. Andersen, 1968. Multiple molecular forms of the alkaline phosphatase of Escherichia Coli. Annals of the New York Academy of Science, 151 : 159-170.

(32) Epstein, C.J. and A.N. Schechter. 1968. An approach to the problem of conformational isozymes. Ann. N.Y. Acad. Sci. 151: 85-101.

(33) Kitto, G.B., P.M. Wasserman, and N.O. Kaplan. 1966. Enzymatically active conformers of mitochondrial malate dehydrogenase. Proc. Nat. Acad. Sci. U.S.A. 56: 578.

(34) Schwartz, D. 1965. Genetic studies on mutant enzymes in maize. VI. Elimination of allelic isozyme variation by glyceraldehyde treatment. Genetics 52: 1295-1302.

(35) Lerner H.R., A.M. Mayer and E. Harel. 1972. Evidence for conformational changes in grape catechol oxidase. Phytochemistry, 11 : 2415-2421.

(36) Harel E., A.M. Mayer and E. Lehman. 1973. Multiple Forms of Vitis Vinifera Catechol oxidase. Phytochemistry, 12: 2649-2654.

ISOZYMES AND A STRATEGY FOR THEIR UTILISATION IN PLANT GENETICS

II. ISOZYMES AS A TOOL IN PLANT GENETICS

Michel JACOBS

Laboratorium voor Plantengenetica
Vrije Universiteit Brussel
B-1640   Sint-Genesius-Rode

Since 1961, the year where the National Academy of Sciences of the United States of America has sponsored a first symposium on the multiple molecular forms of enzymes, numerous reports have appeared which relate isozymes to various topics and this establishment of electrophoretic variants of enzymes in various organisms has led to a number of research applications in genetics, biochemistry and physiology. A review of recent advances in plant genetics mainly based on the use of isozymes in the goal of this paper. We shall first describe research areas where isozymes have played and still play a major role.

I. Isozymes and developmental genetics

They have been used as tracers to determine gene activity in a changing cell or tissue environment, as :

- different tissues of organs of a plant, different stadia of the life cycle of plants, or during the differentiation of a tissue (1,2).
- under the influence of physiological treatments : hormones, irradiation, wounding, or after infection by a pathogen(3)
- according to the intracellular localization (4)

II. Isozymes as a means to study gene expression and its regulation in eukaryotes.

III. Isozymes and the study of the interactions between the products of genes (intra- and intergenic complementation, molecular basis of heterosis)

IV. Physiological significance of isozymes

V. Isozymes as a tool in somatic cell genetics

VI. Isozymes and population genetics.

Electrophoretic separation of proteins and enzymes provides means for revealing genetically controlled variations at a biochemical level in plant populations. Isozymes have been used as gene markers in the study of natural variation in plant populations, especially to study the selection pressure in relation to environmental conditions (Allard, 5)

VII. Isozymes and the study of evolution.

Three topics among others could be sited :
- the study of evolutionary relationships of non-allelic isozyme genes in various species (6)
- the study of evolutionary relationships of related species by comparing their pattern of variation. The best examples in plants concern the phylogenetic origin of polyploid species as tobacco, coton or wheat (7,8)
- the identification of cultivars by means of isozyme patterns (9)

We shall now illustrate the usefulness of isozymes whose genetics is well understood in some of the research areas previously mentioned.

1. Gene regulation and gene dosage effects in higher plants.

Among various models which try to take into account the characteristics of the regulation system in higher organisms, one of them named the "competition model" is mainly based on the study of intensity ratios of allelic isozymes of alcoholdehydrogenase in maize. Allelic isozymes with different electrophoretic mobilities (a slow form S and a fast form F) have been used to make a distinction in heterozygotes between the activity levels specified by each of the two parental genomes. The starting point was the observation that the two alleles F and S of the alcoholdehydrogenase (Adh$_1$) gene showed different activities according to the developmental stages. With equal activity, the three isozymes should occur in a 1 : 2 : 1 ratio, with the allodimer FS twice as active as the FF and SS autodimers. It is the case in mature scutella, but in young scutella and seedlings, a more intense FF band than expected is obtained. A similar situation is observed in the developping endosperm.

Schwartz (70) has proposed a model to account for differential gene activity in diverse tissues of an organism. It is a competition model of gene regulation whereby the level of activity of a gene is dependent upon interaction and competition with other genes. It has the following features :
1) the amount of enzyme synthetized in a cell is limited by the concentration of some specific factor.
2) the limited factor acts at the gene level to control the activity; the more factor, the higher the gene activity.
3) A group of genes can be activated by the same limited factor, but the cell contains a number of different factors with high specificity.

4) The unrepressed genes within each group compete with each other
for the limited factor; the activity of each gene within the
group is determined by its capacity to compete (<u>competitive
ability</u>) with other genes in the same group for the limited
factor.

5) The relative competitive abilities of the genes in a group are
not fixed but can vary depending on the cellular environment.

The start point for experimental evidence was thus that in Adh_1^F /
Adh_1^S heterozygotes, in the scutella of the seed at late stages in
development the isozymes are formed in a 1: 2 : 1 ratio which translated in model terms means that the Adh_1^F and the Adh_1^S alleles compete equally well for the limited factor. In the endosperm, young
scutella and seedlings one observes that the Adh_1^F allele specifies
65-70 % of the total activity. That the competition for the limited
factor had to occur at the gene level was infered from the alcool
dehydrogenase pattern in mature pollen grains. The amount of enzyme
in pollen from F_2 plants obtained by selfing a Adh_1^F/Adh_1^S plant
was estimated to be the same for the three possible genotypes. No
hybrid enzyme is formed in pollen of the Adh_1^F/Adh_1^S heterozygote plants.
This indicates that the enzyme must have been produced <u>after</u> haploï-
dization. However, a sample of pollen grains from heterozygotes contain
much more FF isozymes than SS. If the enzyme in the pollen was formed
before that haploidization took place, all three enzymes FF, FS, and
SS would be present in each haploid grain. Thus the competition must
have occured at the diploid stage when both alleles were present in the
same cells and since enzyme was not synthetized until after haploïdi-
zation, the competition must be between the genes for a factor which
controls m-RNA synthesis and thus at the transcription level.

Schwartz has also presented evidence that the competition can also
occur between non-allelic genes, namely between the Adh_1 and Adh_2 genes.
If Adh_1 is the only competitor, then the level of enzyme in F/F and S/S
plants should be the same. However, if another gene (Adh_2 after derepressing anaerobic treatment) is competing with Adh_1 for the same limiting
factor, then F/F and S/S plants should not show the same amount of activity. The comparison between conditions where Adh_2 is repressed or derepressed shows indeed that the ADH level in the S/S plants is lower than
in F/F plants. Adh_1^F would thus compete better than Adh_1^S.

Another argument concerns the variation of the competitive ability
of genes according to the cell environment. A combination of spectropho-
tometric and electrophoretic analysis was used to establish that the
Adh_1^F and the Adh_1^S alleles compete unequally in the seedling but equally in the mature embryo. The study was performed with a Adh_1^0 allele,
which produce an inactive enzyme, and was derived from Adh_1^S by mutagenic treatment. If there is no competition between Adh_1^F and Adh_1^0 for
the limited factor or that the competitive abilities are similar, the
enzyme level in Adh_1^F/Adh_1^0 heterozygotes should be the half of that in
plants which contain two alleles which specify active enzymes. In the
case of competition, with a better competitive ability for Adh_1^F than

for Adh_1^O, the relative enzyme level in the Adh_1^F/Adh_1^O heterozygote should be higher, with more than half of the limited factor used in the synthesis of the active F subunit. The results are in agreement with the idea that competitive abilities of the Adh_1^F and Adh_1^O alleles vary according the stage of development. Moreover the relative competitive abilities can be changes by treatment with plant hormones.

Cultures of Adh_1^S/Adh_1^F root sections on nutrient agar show the typical intense FF band associated with a low activity of the SS band. If abcissic acid is added in the medium, the intensity ratio approximates 1 : 2 : 1, ratio found in the mature embryo. It is interesting to note that abcissic acid is a dormancy hormone which accumulates in fruits and other organs during late stages of development.

The competition model offers thus an explanation for the change in activity of different Adh_1 alleles. The molecular basis for the modification in competititive ability is however difficult to approach.

Efron (11,12) has identified a supplementary locus Adh_r, with two allelic forms Adh_r^N and Adh_r^L which controls the intensity of ADH isozymes. The Adh_r and Adh_r loci are linked on the first chromosome. The Adh_r^{rS} allele specifies equal activity levels of both the Adh_1^F and Adh_1^{rS} enzymes. By studying the relative activity of the isozymes during the development of heterozygous Adh_1^F/Adh_1^S scutella and endosperm in the absence or the presence of the allele Adh_r^L, it has been shown that the Adh_r^L allele reduced the gene activity of the allele Adh_1^S but did not affect the activity of the allele Adh_1^F. The interpretation of the data is based on Schwartz's limiting factor hypothesis; the Adh_r^L allele should present the increase in the amount of limited factor and the resulting competitition between the alleles Adh_1^F and Adh_1^S should lead to the synthesis of more subunits F than S. Adh_r^L was dominant over Adh_r^N regarding its effect on the activity of Adh_1^S. The locus Adh_r which repress the production of an enzyme may be considered as a regulatory gene.

Varied intensity ratios of allelic dimer isozymes in heterozygotes were found in rice peroxydase specified by the Px_1 locus (Endo, 13). In heterozygotes between the three known alleles, an hybrid band occurs normally in a ratio 1: 2: 1. However some F_2 segregants show deviation from the normal intensity ratio, due to some differential activation of the alleles in the heterozygote. Endo has inferred that at least two regulatory gene loci for Px_1 alleles are involved in these hybrids.

Another facet of gene function which can be approached by using isozymes as markers is gene dosage effects. Examples of such dosage effects are quite clear in some of the cases already presented, specially for alcohol dehydrogenase and catalase isozymes in maize triploid endosperm. Carlson (14) has used <u>Datura</u> trisomics to localize to chromosomes genes coding for enzymes. This method was based upon the finding that the activity of a given enzyme in a particular trisomic was more or less 150 % of that in the diploid plant, which indicates that the structural locus coding for that enzyme was located on the

triplicate chromosome in this line. Smith (15) has applied the same
method to six anodal isozymes of peroxydase in <u>Datura stramonium</u>. The
relative intensity of the bands in the trisomics was determinated
by densitometry. Significant differences of intensity were found according to the trisomic and the reactions to the presence of a triplicate chromosome fall in one of the following categories.

     1) An enzymatic activity which reachs 133 % of that of
the diploïd.

     2) A reduction of activity to two/third of the diploïd
type.

     3) An enzymatic activity equivalent to that present in
the diploid.

These results were interpreted as indication of a balance between
the amount of structural genes and the amount of regulatory genes,
controlling the synthesis of a particular peroxydase.

    2. Physiological significance of isozymes.

    Another aspect in some way related to the topics regulation
concerns the physiological role of isozymes. In other words, what is
the basis for the existence of isozymes. Two main hypotheses have
been presented. Enzyme polymorphism should represent a type of adaptation to the variation of substrates in the environment (Gillepsie
and Kojima, 16). In fact, enzymes of broad specificity are far more
variable than those enzymes which utilize specific metabolically
produced substrates. A second hypothesis, proposed by Johnson (17),
suggests that regulatory enzymes defined as enzymes of regulatory
importance in a metabolic pathway are more polymorphic than the
non-regulatory enzymes. The polymorphism should achieve a fine control of the reaction catalysed by the enzyme. Thus isozymes may
reflect distinct metabolic activities inside the plant and are associated with regulatory mechanisms in metabolism. A possible example
concerns the fact that different molecular forms of a protein should
function in different metabolic pathways which have common enzymatic steps. In various species, four forms of phosphoenolpyruvate
carboxylase have been identified. Each of the four forms is associated with a different metabolic pathway and can be distinguished
on the basis of kinetic characteristics and chromatography on DEAE-
cellulose (18)

    3. Interactions between gene products.

    Another important problem which can be examined by using isozy-
mes concerns the molecular basis of heterosis considered as the result of interaction between two alleles of a given gene locus.
Schwartz and Laughner (19) have used the fact that some Adh alleles
found in the nature produced active but relatively unstable enzyme
forms as the alleles S, F and C^t while the allele c^m produced isozymes
which were highly stable but showed very little activity. A F subunit is more stable to treatment with high temperature or pH above

10 as a dimer with a C^m subunit than in the form of a FF homodimer (20). The products of the two alleles interact in the heterodimer to give an active and stable alcohol dehydrogenase.

The effects of intragenic and intergenic complementation on catalase structure in maize have been also associated with heterosis by Scandalios et al (21) Hybrid catalases between allelic genes of the Ct_1 locus have been subjected to biochemical analysis (specific activity, temperature sensitivity, photosensitivity). In most instances, the heterotetramers generated by either intragenic or intergenic complementation exhibit improved physico-chemical properties over the less efficient parental molecules. Hybrid proteins may thus confer an advantage to the organism carrying them.

Efron (22) has also presented evidence for a better balance in the products of a single gene, controlling alcohol dehydrogenase activity in two different tissues of maize. A cross between a Adh_1^S/Adh_1^S line with low activity in the scutellum and high level of activity in pollen was crossed with an Adh_1^F/Adh_1^F line with a relatively low activity in the pollen and a relatively high activity in the scutellum. Thus, each of the homozygous parental lines shows low ADH activity in one of the tissues. The heterozygous S/F hybrids present intermediate levels of ADH activity in both tissues. Low activity of an enzyme in a certain tissue may be a limiting factor for the development and the development of this tissue may thus become less rate limiting in F_1 hybrids. The cumulative effects of many such heterozygous loci could be expressed as heterosis.

A second aspect related to this topic concerns case of interallelic complementation in higher plants. Schwartz (23) has shown that in maize the shrunken 1 locus on chromosome 9 controls the synthesis of a major protein in the developing endosperm. On the basis of electrophoretical and immunological analysis, it was possible to demonstrate that this protein is lacking in sh_1/sh_1 mutant, which cause the shrunken kernel instead of the plump phenotype. Sixteen sh_1 mutants induced by ethyl methane sulfonate treatment were characterized immunologically and electrophoretically by Chourey (24). Ten mutants do not show the presence of cross reacting material and the Sh_1 protein bands is absent on the gel. The six other mutants are CRM$^+$; four of them specify a protein with the same electrophoretical mobility as Sh_1 protein controlled by the normal allele; the remaining CRM$^+$ mutants exhibit a Sh_1 band with a modified migration rate; the sh_1^F allele controls the faster migrating band and the sh_1^S allele the slower migrating band. F_1 hybrids were made between all the mutants. Complementation based on the occurrence of plump seeds was observed only where the sh_1^S allele is combined with sh_1^F or with one of the four others CRM$^+$ mutant types. Starch-gel electrophoretic analysis of the sh_1^S/sh_1^F hybrid showed only the two parental bands, F and S, without hybrid band. The function of Sh_1 protein in the endosperm is not known. Various possibilities may account for the absence of an hybrid band : monomeric protein, very small amount of hybrid protein sufficient to give a normal phenotype, dissociation of the hybrid protein in subunits during the extraction or electrophoresis. This remains until now the first report of an interallelic complementation at the protein level in higher plants.

Bell and Mac Intyre (25) have used fifteen null mutants of the gene Acph-1 in Drosophila melanogaster induced after EMS treatment to try to identify non-sense mutations in this species, mainly on the basis that to identify such mutants by microorganisms no complementation occured with most other mutations at the locus and that antigenically CRM⁺ with antibodies against the wild-type gene product was absent. The complementation analysis based on the recovery of acid phosphatase activity in heteroallelic heterozygotes was performed on polyacrylamide gel electrophoresis on which it was possible to eliminate phosphatase activities contributed by other loci by observing the concerned zone (Acph-1). Only three of the Acph-1 null alleles showed neither leakiness nor any evidence of complementation with the other alleles. The CRM levels of these three mutants were virtually zero.

4. Somatic cell genetics

Recent progress in plant cell and tissue cultures associated with the techniques of isolation and fusion of protoplasts have opened new ways in studies of the genetic structure of eukaryotic cells.

Since a lot of enzymes are polymorphic and that so many enzymes exist, the isozymes represent a potentially large class of markers which might play a major role in the study of the following areas although the literature on isozymes of plant cell cultures is still very limited.

1° as markers for characterizing cell lines,isozyme patterns can be very stable in vitro and remain similar after numerous subculturing.

2° as a mean in somatic cell hybridization of distinguishing hybrid cells from the parental ones. This possibility was pointed out in the case of two species of Datura (D. innoxia and D. metel) characterized by a clear differential mobility exhibited by two of the mitochondrial isozymes (26)

3° In the study of gene interaction in somatic hybrids as beautifully demonstrated with the use of mammalian cells. We are interested to know if one paternal genome will express itself in a mixed cytoplasm in the presence of a foreign genome. In hybrids between relatively non-related species, shall the characteristics proteins of both parental types be synthetized or not. In the case of somatic hybridization between two species of Nicotiana reported by Carlson et al (27), the peroxidase pattern of the somatic hybrid represented the sum of the parental patterns but, in this case a sexual hybrid could be also obtained. The eventual absence of one or the other parental type of variant would indicate a misfunctioning in the chain of events between the transcription of the parental genes and the formation of a specific protein. Gene dosage effects could be also studied by the use of isozymes as they can be traced in

androgenic haploids, diploid cells and polyploïd lines.
4° In the study of the differential expression of the genome in cell
or/and tissue culture compared to normal morphogenesis.
     Changes of acid phosphatase$_1$ isozyme patterns have been descri-
bed in calli or cells in suspension of Arabidopsis thaliana.
     Jacobs (28) has observed a decrease of the activity of the two
first anodal bands which are well represented in whole plants.
5° The incorporation in protoplasts of allien organelles as mitochondria and chloroplasts might allow the study of the interaction
between nuclear and cytoplasmic genomes. What should be the expression at the isozyme level of a cell containing organelles coding for
an electrophoretic variant of a particular enzyme (Chaleff, 29).
6° The study of the influence of environmental factors on the evolution of a defined isozyme system.
The synthesis of different types of soluble acid phosphatases in rice
plant cell cultures in response to changes in the concentration of
phosphate in the culture medium has been reported (30). Three major
zones of activity 1, 2 and 3 have been identified on polyacrylamide
gels in extracts of cells which were cultivated on a control medium.
When the cells were incubated in a phosphate-deficient medium, the
electrophoretic pattern showed a noticeable change, namely the ratio
of isozyme 1 to the others decreased. When the cells are transfered
on a phosphate-rich medium, isozyme 3 decreased followed by isozyme 2.
Such a phosphate-phosphatase isozymes regulatory system may play an
important role in the regulation of phosphorus metabolism in the rice
plants callus cells. Thus isozymes are useful to examine the genetic
and epigenetic mechanisms of enzyme induction and synthesis, of enzyme
repression or depression and to determine the adaptative or constitutive nature of enzymes.
7° As abundantly exemplified in this symposium, the suspension cell
cultures offer a valuable tool to induce and detect mutant types.How-
ever, most of the systems presented are depending on the finding of
a tricky selection technique as resistance mutants or of the availability of haploid cell lines.
The use of isozymes might lead to look for mutants non-selectively
provided that many enzymes are investigated at the same time (which
is quite possible f.i. for dehydrogenases). Isozymes variants can be
induced in a high frequency by appropriate chemical mutagens; their
genetic control is generally relatively simple and in many instances
genes controlling isozymes are codominantly expressed. The results
of such mutagenic treatment shall be thus visualized on the zymogram as a change in the electrophoretic mobility of bands or as the
energence of hybrid bands. Here, it is worthwhile to mention the advantage to use diploid eukaryotic cells instead of haploid bacterial
cells. 2 sets of genes are represented and if a correlation between
an electrophoretical change and the activity of an enzyme does exist,
these is still a real chance in diploid plant cells to get the variant
under the form of an heterozygote. Until now, they are no report of

a systematic induction of electrophoretic variants in plants. Using
the alcohol dehydrogenase system and its three natural alleles S, F
and C^t , Schwartz (personal communication) has obtained three chemically induced variants, O, U and W : a null mutant and two variants in the
electrophoretic mobility.
8° The selective loss of plant chromosomes in somatic cell hybrids
have not yet been reported although fusion between correlated species
as barley and soja have been reported (31). The existence of such an
experimental system should allow to investigate gene regulation and
gene mapping problems. The loss of a particular chromosome of a species A may be correlated with the loss of a particular isozyme from
the hybrid and demonstrated by gel electrophoresis which permits the
localization of the corresponding gene.

REFERENCES

(1) Scandalios J.G. and L.G. Espiritu, 1969. Mutant aminopeptidase of
Pisum sativum. Molecular and General Genetics, 105: 101-112.

(2) Jacobs, M. and Schwind, F. 1974. Biochemical genetics of Arabidopsis acid phosphatase polymorphism, tissue expression and genetics of
$\overline{AP}_1$, AP_2 and AP_3 loci. 3rd Int. Conf. on Isozymes, C.L. Markert, ed.
Academic Press, N.Y. (in press).

(3) Chourey P.S. H.H. Smith and N.C. Combatti. 1973. Effects of X
irradiations and indoleacetic acid on specific peroxidase isozymes
in pith tissue of a Nicotiana amphiploid. Am. J. Bot. 60 : 853-857.

(4) Longo G.P. and J.G. Scandalios, 1969. Nuclear gene control of mitochondrial malic dehydrogenase in maize. Proc. Nat. Acad. Sci. U.S.A.,
62 : 104-111.

(5) Allard R.W. and A.L. Kahler, 1971. Allozyme polymorphisms in plant
populations. Stadler Symposia, 3 : 9-24.

(6) Gottbier, L.D. 1974. Gene duplication and fixed heterozygosity for
alcohol dehydrogenase in Clarkia franciscana. Proc. Nat. Acad. Sci.
U.S.A. 71 : 1816-18.

(7) Sing C.F. and C.J. Brewer, 1969. Isozymes of a polyploid series of
wheat. Genetics, 61 : 391-398.

(8) Johnson B.L., 1972. Seed protein profiles and the origin of the
hexaploid wheats. Ann. J. Bot. 59 : 952-960.

(9) Te Niedenhuis, B. 1971. Estimation of the proportion of inbred
seed in Brussels sprouts hybrid seed by acid phosphatase isoenzyme
analysis. Euphytica 20 : 498-507.

(10) Schwartz D., 1971. Genetic control of alcohol dehydrogenase : a
competition model for regulation of gene action. Genetics, 67 : 411-
425.

(11) Efron, Y. 1970. Alcohol dehydrogenase in maize : genetic control of enzyme activity. Science 170 : 791-3.
(12) Efron Y. 1971. Regulation of the activity of alcohol dehydrogenase isozymes during the development of the maize kernel. Molecular and General Genetics, 111 : 97-102.
(13) Endo T. 1973. Isozyme loci and a Strategy of Differentiation in Plants. Seiken Zihô, 24 : 89-104.
(14) Carlson, P.F. 1972. Locating genetic loci with aneuploids. Mol. Gen. Genetics 114 : 273-280.
(15) Smith H.H. and M.E. Conklin, 1974. Effects of Gene Dosage on Peroxidase Isozymes in Datura stramonium Trisomics 3rd Int. Conf. on Isozymes, C.H. Markert, e.a. Academic Press. N.Y. (in press).
(16) Gillispie, I. and K. Kojima. 1968. The degree of polymorphisms in enzymes involved in energy production compared to that in non specific enzymes in two Drosophila anassanae populations. Proc.Nat. Acad. Sci. U.S.A. 61 : 582.
(17) Johnson, G.B. 1974. Enzyme polymorphism and metabolism. Science 184: 28-37.
(18) Ting I.P. and C.B. Osmond, 1973. Multiple forms of plant phosphoenolpyruvate carboxylase associated with different metabolic pathways. Plant Physiol. 51 : 448-453.
(19) Schwartz D. and W.J. Laughner, 1969. A molecular bases for heterosis. Science, 166 : 626-627.
(20) Schwartz D., 1973. Single gene heterosis for alcohol dehydrogenase in maize : the nature of the subunit interaction. Theoretical Applied Genetics, 43 : 117-120.
(21) Scandalios J.G. E.H. Liu and M.A. Campeau, 1972. The effects of intragenic and intergenic complementation on catalase structure and function in maize : a molecular approach to heterosis. Archives of biochemistry and biophysics, 153 : 695-705.
(22) Efron Y. 1973. Specific Differences in Maize Alcohol Dehydrogenase : Possible Explanation of Heterosis at the Molecular Level. Nature New Biology, 241 : 41-42.
(23) Schwartz, D. 1960. Electrophoretic and immunochemical studies with endosperm proteins of maize mutants. Genetics 45 : 1419-27.
(24) Chourey P.S. 1971. Interallelic complementation at the Sh_1 locus in maize. Genetics, 68 : 435-442.
(25) Bell J. and R. MacIntyre, 1973. Characterization of Acid Phosphatase- 1 Null Activity Mutants of Drosophila melanogaster, Biochemical Genetics, Vol. 10 n° 1 : 39-55.
(26) Ganapathy P.S. and J.G. Scandalios, 1973. Malate dehydrogenase isozymes in haploid and diploid Datura species : their use as markers in somatic cell genetics. The Journal of Heredity, 64: 186-188.
(27) Carlson, P.S. H. Smith and R.D. Dearing. 1972. Parasexual interspecific plant hybridization. Proc. Nat. Acad. Sci. U.S.A. 69:2292-4.
(28) Jacobs M. 1975. In preparation.

(29) Chaleff, R. 1974. Heterogenous association of cells formed in vitro (this symposium).

(30) Igave I., M. Nishio and F. Kurasawa, 1973. Occurrence of Acid Phosphatase isozymes Repressible by inorganic Phosphate in Rice Plant Cell Cultures, Agr. Biol. Chem. 37(4): 941-943.

(31) Kao, K.N. F. Constabel, H.R. Michayluk and O.L. Gamborg, 1974. Protoplast fusion and growth of intergeneric hybrid cells. Abstract 148, 3rd Int. Cong. Plant Tissue and Cell Culture, Leicester.

PHYSICO-CHEMICAL ASPECTS OF CHROMATIN AND CHROMOSOME STRUCTURE

E. Fredericq

Institut de Chimie Physique

Université de Liège, SART-TILMAN
B-4000   LIEGE - BELGIUM

The genetic material of all higher organisms is constituted by a complex of DNA and proteins called chromatin. The purified chromatin isolated in vitro is also called nucleohistone or deoxy-ribonucleoprotein. In a few cases, i.e. in sperm nuclei, the basic constituents or histones are replaced by a class of still more basic proteins, the protamines which will not be considered here. In lower organisms such as protozoans, yeasts etc DNA is also associated with basic proteins which differ from the histones of higher organisms. Even in bacterial lysates proteins are found associated with DNA but it has not been proved that they were part of a native complex and even so they are quite distinct from histones.

In view of its fundamental importance chromatin has been the subject of numerous physicochemical studies especially in the past 15 years, since simple procedures have been described for obtaining it in solution. The present lecture intends to give a survey of our present ideas on the structure of chromatin in vitro (1,2) and of the hypotheses concerning its arrangement in chromosomes (3-6). Although most of the results we shall refer to were obtained using animal tissues, all our present knowledge demonstrates that very great similarities exist in the chromatin structure and properties of all eukaryotic organisms and studies performed in the case of some vegetal cells gave results quite similar to those obtained on organisms situated very far apart on the phyllogenic scale.

THE CHROMATIN COMPONENTS

It is difficult to estimate the exact content of a substance which is not a well-defined molecular entity and this explains the discrepancies between results of analysis of chromatin of the same

Table 1

Composition of chromatins from various origins. (Results are given as weight ratios referred to DNA).

Material	Histones	Non-Histones	RNA	Ref.
Calf thymus	1.14	0.33	0.007	(7)
	1.15	0.25		(8)
	0.95	0.33	<0.005	(9)
	1.15	0.50		(10)
	1.0	0.2		(11)
Chicken erythrocytes	0.82	0.45	<0.01	(12)
	1.18	0.32		(13)
Rat liver	1.0	0.67	0.043	(14)
	1.05	0.63		(15)
	1.0	1.0		(11)
Pea bud	1.30	0.10	0.11	(7)
Pea embryonic axis	1.03	0.29	0.26	(7)
Sea urchin gastrula	1.04	1.15	0.08	(16)

species (Table 1). Chromatin is composed of well-characterized DNA, basic proteins or histones and acidic proteins whose nature and number are unknown. Some RNA is found in metabolically active cells such as those from liver but it is not proved that it is an essential part of chromatin. It may be temporarily associated with it during its synthesis.

The weight ratio of histone to DNA is fairly constant and close to 1.2. The amount of non-histone proteins is much more controversial and depends not only on the cell origin but on the method used for its estimation. It varies from 0.1 to 2 weight-parts protein to one part DNA. In general the methods used for these analyses are likely to overestimate the acidic fraction since they are based on a preliminary extraction of histones which is very difficult to achieve completely. Moreover the histones because of their strongly basic nature easily bind acidic compounds and it is not clear whether all non-histones found in chromatin after its isolation are true components or contaminants (8,17) : cytoplasmic proteins which may be present if the nuclei have not been carefully purified before the extraction, enzymes taking part in the genetic function and more or less temporarily associated to DNA etc... In calf thymus which has a very reduced metabolic activity, the proportions of non-histone proteins are relatively low and vary from a few to 25 percents (17, 18)(see table 1) according to the author. In chromatin from other tissues much higher proportions have been reported.

DNA

　　DNA structure and characteristics are too well-known for being
described in detail here. We shall only point out a few features
particularly important in the present instance.

　　The DNA double-helix in aqueous media mainly exists in the "B
conformation" with its base pairs perpendicular to the long axis of
the molecule, a diameter of 20 Å and a pitch of 34 Å . In a few
cases it takes a somewhat more compact "C conformation" with a
slight tilting of the plane of the base pairs. These structures
present two external grooves of different size which can both accomodate proteins bound to DNA.

　　The negative charges of the phosphate groups are regularly
spaced on the outside of the double helix. This point is important
since these groups are candidates as fixation sites for the positively charged histones. These base pairs regularly stacked inside
the molecule have little possibilities for interactions with external ligands.

Histones

　　These basic proteins form essentially five distinct classes
which are found in approximately equal amounts in the chromatin
of most eukaryotes. They are all constituted by a single polypeptide chain of relatively small size, the molecular weight ranging from
11 000 to 21 000 (table 2). They are characterized by the typical
value of their ratio of lysine to arginine residues and by a large
excess of total basic over acidic groups ; around 25 % of their residues are basic. This confers a very high isoelectric point near
11 which is rather exceptional among all proteins. It is also
worthwhile mentioning that some fractions display a high content
in some particular amino acid capable of playing a role in the structure such as proline (in F1), threonine and serine in F2B, glycine
in F2A1, cystine in F3. The sequence of amino acids in histones has
been established almost completely in the five fractions of different
living species. It is remarkable that some fractions in particular
F2A1 display an almost identical sequence in organisms as far apart
as calf thymus and pea bud for instance (20). Fraction F1 is the
most differentiated in this respect. This fraction is fairly different from the others in many properties : exceptional content in lysine, higher molecular weight, more disordered conformation and weaker binding to DNA.

　　In all histones the amino acid sequence reveals an "asymmetric
or polar character" i.e. a concentration of basic residues in about
one half of the polypeptide chain, sometimes even in a smaller part.
This region bearing a large number of positively charged groups is

Table 2

Characteristics of histone fractions (3,19).

	F1	F2B	F2A2	F2A1	F3	Ref
M.W.	21 000	13 800	15 000	11 300	15 000	(3)
$\frac{Lys}{Arg}$	20	2.5	1.1	0.8	0.7	(3)
COO^-(%)	6.2	13.7	16.4	12.1	15.7	(19)
NH_3^+(%)	28.6	23.2	22.7	25.2	23.7	(19)

the most disordered because of the electrostatic repulsions between the groups. It is that part which presents the maximum of interaction with DNA and is called for this reason "the sticking part" of histones. The less basic part has a much more balanced composition recalling that of well-structured proteins. It is there that helical conformations are concentrated. Actually it has been shown that isolated histones at low ionic strength adopt a random coil conformation but except F1 acquire a fairly large helical content when the ionic strength is raised or when they are combined to DNA : 35-40 % (21) or 50 % (22) α-helix. The helical parts are supposed to play a role in histone-histone interactions and bring about the formation of aggregates in vitro(23,24).

Non-histone proteins.

An important role has been attributed to acidic proteins in the control of genetic functions since histone which have a very restricted diversity seem to lack the specificity required for playing such a role. Important experimental evidence has been obtained in the past few years in favour of this hypothesis (25). Unfortunately there are at the present time no precise data about the amount and nature of these proteins and practically nothing is known about their structure. No safe method has been described for their isolation or even for their detection. Different procedures used for their extraction from chromatin yield heterogeneous preparations where a very large number of acidic components can be generally detected. Most of these procedures require the use of denaturing agents such as urea, guanidine, detergents, strong bases etc. Moreover the non-histones are unstable, being rapidly degraded or aggregated in the usual buffer systems.

It seems very likely that the numerous components detected are due partly at least to the presence of possible contaminants : (i)

the enzymes taking part in DNA and RNA syntheses and metabolism may
be normally or artificially associated to chromatin during the isolation procedure ; (ii) cytoplasmic or nuclear acidic proteins may
be present ; (iii) variable aggregates of histones and non-histones
may be formed and still increase the apparent number of components,
either on the basis of electrophoretic or molecular weight analysis.
In a recent work from this laboratory, we isolated by a mild procedure a few fractions with a low number of components which had a
very strong acidic character and some contaminants appearing as aggregates of histones and non-histones (17). The main components
had molecular weights near 13000 and 25000 and ratios of acidic
over basic residues equal to 4.

    In view of our great ignorance regarding the nature of non-his-
tones and their significance as chromatin components, it is evident
that we cannot put forward any hypothesis about their role in chromatin structure and we shall not examine them in the next paragraph
which will treat the question. The only point that we can mention
is that according to our experience acidic proteins favor the formation of chromatin gels in vitro (17,26).

CHROMATIN STRUCTURE

    When considering physico-chemical studies on chromatin, it is
necessary to define the exact nature of the material investigated
which may considerably differ according to the way of isolation(26).
In the order of increasing complexity (1), there is first the solubilized chromatin (often called nucleohistone) which has been mostly
used for physico-chemical measurements requiring true solutions : it
consists of chromatin mechanically disrupted, soluble at low ionic
strength (0.01) ; a less degraded material is obtained in vitro in
the form of a diluted gel which is dispersed at very low ionic strength
only (0.001) and then we have chromatin threads or fibers mostly
useful for X-ray studies. In this series of increasing complexity,
there is an increasing number of components (or contaminants ?) like
acidic proteins and RNA and an increase in cross-links. Finally,
there is the native material in situ which will be described in the
last part of this lecture.

    It is impossible here to discuss in detail the numerous works
recently published on the subject and we shall just give a brief outline of the main features which appear from this complex sum of data.

    1. The DNA backbone preserves its main double-helix conformation
in chromatin but in a more compact form. In particular it has been
shown that the plane of the base-pairs is no more perpendicular to the
long axis in nucleohistone gels or solutions. This has been generally
interpreted as arising from the formation of a superhelix. Although
it seems reasonable to assume a supercoiling of the chain in chromatin

threads and still more in chromosomes, the exact parameters of the superhelix are still subject to controversy (27,28). The model proposed by Pardon and Wilkins (28) has a pitch of 120 Å and a diameter of 100 Å which is at least in agreement with the size of subunits found in chromosomes (see below). From circular dichroism measurements, other authors interpret the tilting of the base pairs as due to the passage of DNA to a "C conformation" in chromatin (29).

2. Histones are irregularly fixed on the DNA backbone since their positive groups cannot be in spatial coincidence with the regularly sequenced phosphate groups. It is assumed that the polar parts of the histones dispose their basic groups with maximum contacts with the phosphates whereas apolar parts mostly in α-helix conformation protrude towards the outside providing possibilities of hydrophobic interactions between neighbouring chains or parts of chains (22,23) (Fig. 1).

3. The very lysine-rich F1 fraction has a particular disposition. This fraction is the first to be selectively removed by an increase in ionic strength, leaving chromatin relatively unaltered. It remains in disordered conformation. It has been shown that it forms interlinks between DNA fibrils in condensed chromatin.

4. Divalent cations such as Mg and Ca bring about a compaction of chromatin structure but their possible role as inducers of supercoiling has been recently challenged (30). Although no precise scheme has been firmly established the following picture can be drawn taking into account the major experimental findings :

The fundamental chromatin thread is constituted by the DNA double helix around which are wrapped the four lysine-poor histones. An interesting recent suggestion (31) is that the very arginine-rich fractions F2A1 and FIII are wrapped in the narrow groove, in analogy with what happens in nucleoprotamines, with their basic groups neutralizing about one third of the total phosphate groups and their central helical parts having strong hydrophobic interactions with inner parts of the DNA. The high disproportion of positive charges and helical fragments would produce a periodical perturbation on the DNA backbone which is the driving force for super coiling. The moderately arginine-rich histones would be situated in the large groove providing additional neutralization of the remaining phosphates (one third of the total). They would have a weaker binding and a lesser effect on the general conformation.

It is also interesting to point out that the helix conformation can be changed by slight modifications of the ionic environment or by enzymatic modifications of groups such as acetylation. This would provide a possibility of control of the genetic function by the for-

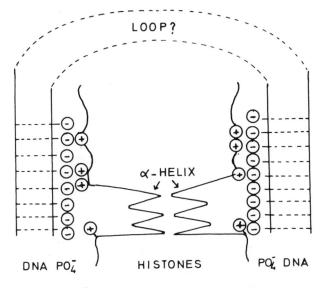

Fig.1.Model of chromatin structure. Two parallel DNA strands (or
      two parts of the same chain)are shown. Two histone molecules
      have electrostatic bonds with the DNA phosphates in the di-
      sordered part of their polypeptide chains. The helical parts
      provide hydrophobic interactions between the neighbouring his-
      tones.

mation or deformation of supercoiling (31) bringing about repression
and derepression effects respectively, in conformity with the role
attributed to histones according to recent theories.

Unicity and homogeneity of the chromatin backbone.

   Is the chromatin of one chromosome constituted by one unique thread
and is this thread perfectly homogeneous or constituted by alternating patches of free DNA and of nucleoprotein ? These two important
problems are still open to discussion.

   As regards the continuity of the DNA backbone, it is interesting
to notice that in the case of one short chromosome (that of yeast)
single DNA molecules have been isolated which contain the entire
DNA amount of the chromosome (32).

This is not necessarily true for larger entities and moreover does not prove that the double helix has a perfect continuity. In fact, since this conformation has a very limited flexibility, it is very likely that the double helix has some interruptions in its regular structure allowing for loops or local folding of the DNA backbone. All that we can say at the present time is that no extranucleotide link has never been identified in a chromatin or DNA strand.

The problem of the compositional homogeneity of chromatin is still more controversial particularly with regard to the presence and the amount of free DNA zones in the thread. An approach which has extensively been used in this field is to compare the action of different compounds and of enzymes on DNA in the free state or in chromatin. Different conclusions were drawn according to the method used and the amount of accessible DNA was found to vary between 10 and 50 %. In studying the binding of numerous dyes to DNA and to chromatin (33), we found that there is generally about one third of the total DNA which is reactive toward dyes but the characteristics of the reaction are not similar to those of free DNA and vary from one type of dye to another. We conclude that there are in chromatin parts of the DNA more reactive than the others, probably because of a non-homogeneous repartition of the proteins but that there is no truly "free" DNA in the sense of a double helix identical to the isolated compound.

The presence of DNA parts possessing different accessibility to various agents strongly suggests a heterogeneous structure of the chromatin thread as regards the repartition of histones and their binding to DNA. This is supported by other recent experimental findings according to which it is possible to obtain by sonication or by limited nuclease digestion fragments of chromatin having different protein and RNA content (34,35) and different degree of compactness (11,36). This suggests in chromatin the alternance of extended and compact DNA parts differing in their genetic activities and would be of great interest in relation with proposed models of chromosomes.

NATURE OF DNA-PROTEIN INTERACTIONS.

That histones are bound to DNA by important electrostatic bonds has always been a postulate of chromatin structure. Experimentally it has been demonstrated that 80 % of histone basic groups are not titratable (37) and dye binding indicates that the major part of DNA phosphates are bound in chromatin (1). However the existence of other bonds is also suggested by the very high ionic strength required for operating the dissociation of histone fractions except F1 from DNA. No evidence has been presented for the presence of hydrogen bonds but we have some good reasons to believe that hydrophobic interactions may be present. In particular there is an interesting correlation between the action of concentrated salts as dissociating

agents for nucleohistone and as breakers of hydrophobic bonds, resulting from their action on water structure (1). Such bonds
would also provide more possibilities for specificity of interactions between DNA and histones. In this respect we have investigated the reversibility of DNA-histone combination, by studying
under controlled conditions the dissociation and reassociation of
nucleohistone in salt media. We concluded that there is a limited
specificity of combination i.e. histone fractions are recombined in
a non-random order but do not display the exact structural features of the original material and this indicates that there is
not a strict reversibility in the combination, i.e. not a complete
specificity of interaction.

THE CHROMOSOME.

    Many models of chromosome structure have been proposed on the
basis of genetic and cytological considerations (4-6). In this
section we shall only discuss the results of direct observations
and of physico-chemical measurements.

    As we have seen above we can figure out that chromatin is main-
ly constituted by a very long thread of nucleoprotein in which the
DNA backbone is twisted in a superhelix with a width near 100 Å.
The problem is to determine how this huge thread is disposed in order to form the compact and condensed organites which are the fundamental genetic units i.e. the chromosomes. We shall restrict ourselves to the case of the metaphase chromosomes typical of most eukaryotic cells, although many interesting deductions have been made
from studies on other types of chromosome such as for instance the
giant species which were for a long time the only possible source
of information.

    Electron microscopic studies have detected the existence of
two main types of fibers according to the method used for the treatment of the material under observation, one 250 Å wide and one 100 Å
wide. It is generally accepted that the 250 Å fiber is the main
constituent of the chromosomes being probably formed either by one
100 Å thread in a second superhelical folding bringing about an increased width (38-40) or by the union of two unitary threads parallel
or torsed together (4). In the latter case we can also imagine that
the two threads are separated or are parts of a single unit looped
at one end (Fig. 2).

    It is interesting to point out that one can calculate the degree
of packing that such a thread must present in order to accomodate
the whole content of the nucleus DNA. In one human chromosome for
instance 73000 μ of pure DNA must be accomodated in 723 μ of the
250 Å fiber which necessitates a packing ratio of 100 (41). It is
actually difficult to obtain a fiber of such a width by a regular

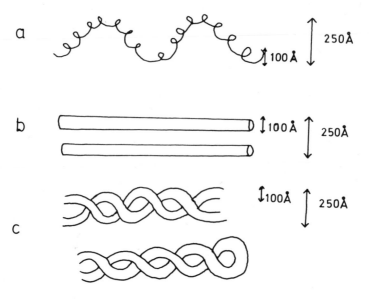

Different models for the formation of the 250 Å fiber
by one or two 100 Å threads.

superhelical torsion of the DNA double helix (42) and this points
towards the existence of more compact structures that we shall de-
pict below.

The metaphase chromosome consists of two chromatides united
by the centromere (Fig. 3) and the problem is mainly to see how the
250 Å thread is packed in each chromatide. We shall take the problem now starting from the other end, i.e. from the direct observation of the chromatide. The refinements of optical microscopy have
permitted very interesting observations which avoid the drawbacks
of the electron microscopic technique in the treatment of samples.

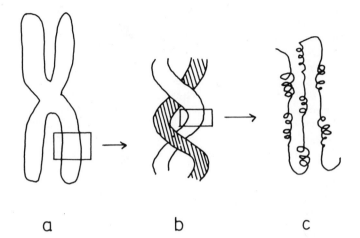

a   b   c

Figure 3.   Structure of the metaphase chromosome.
            a. Overall picture.
            b. Enlargement of a chromatide branch showing the two chro-
               monemes.
            c. Enlargement of one stretched chromoneme.

     Two main theories have been presented :
1. The chromatide is constituted by a unique 250 Å thread, a "chromoneme" folded in a tertiary superhelical order ; the folding could
   be transverse or longitudinal (38).
2. The chromatide is constituted by the union of several chromonemes
   either parallel (43) or torsed together.

     Two important progresses have been recently realised in refined
optical techniques which afford important new elements. First the
"scanning video" (Frederic 1969) based on an electronic treatment of
optical micrographs gives an analysis of photographic contrast by a
television device which allows a resolution of 100 Å. By this method Frederic observes very distinctly the presence of two chromonemes torsed together in a chromatide. In each chromoneme is seen

an alternance of relatively despiralized regions and more packed
ones containing lumps of loops ; these loops themselves appear
after stretching as constituted by 200-300 Åthreads. Consequently,
each chromoneme would consist of a parallel packing of alternatively extended and looped chromatin threads.

Secondly the "Q banding" technique introduced by Caspersson
and his school (1968) is based on the binding of fluorochromes
(mostly acridine derivatives) by the chromosomes on regions which
show a regular alternance of bands with a typical emission of fluorescence. This was observed in a great number of animal and vegetal chromosomes. The sequence and the brilliance of the fluorescent bands are remarkably reproducible for each chromosomal pair of
a species and constitute a unique pattern allowing its identification. The exact origin of the fluorescent bands is not yet very
clear : various causes have been proposed such as the nature of
base sequences and repetitiveness in DNA, the nature and amounts
of protein present, the secondary structure of DNA etc...(for a recent discussion see (46)). At any rate this indicates that some
regular structural features alternate along the chromatide, and
combined with the data of the "scanning video" demonstrates the
existence of zones of different compactness. This would also re-
join the theoretical model of Crick (47) according to whom there
would be along the chromosome an alternance of fibrous DNA which
has the coding properties and of globular DNA which has the control
and recognition function ; the latter would have a branched and
looped structure stabilised by strong interactions with proteins.

Crick theory also postulates the unicity and the continuity of
the chromoneme. However the presence of only one chromoneme per
chromosome is difficult to reconcile with its genetic behaviour.
This problem like this of the DNA continuity awaits for further experimental evidence.

REFERENCES

Note : In view of the extremely abundant literature on the subject,
       we mention here only references of particular significance
       for our purpose or very recent work. The reader will find
       exhaustive account of the literature in recent reviews
       on chromatin (1-3) or chromosomes (3-6).
(1) Fredericq, in Histones and Nucleohistones, edited by D.M.P. Phil-
    lips, Plenum Press, London and New York 1971, pp.135-186.
(2) R.T. Simpson, Advan. Enzymol., 38, 41-108 (1973).
(3) J.A. Huberman, Ann. Rev. Biochem., 42, 356-378 (1973).
(4) H. Ris in Handbook of Molecular Cytology, edited by A. Lima-de-
    Faria, North Holland, Amsterdam (1969), pp. 361-380.
(5) D.E. Comings, Advan. Hum. Genet. 3, 237-431 (1972).
(6) J. Frederic and C. Distèche, Arch. Biol., 84, 115-145 (1973).

(7) J. Bonner, M.E. Dahmus, D. Fambrough, R.C. Huang, K. Marushige and D.Y.H. Tuan, Science, 159, 47-56 (1968).

(8) E.W. Johns and S. Forrester, Eur. J. Biochem., 8, 547-551 (1969).

(9) R. Chalkley and R.H. Jensen, Biochemistry, 7, 4380-4388 (1968).

(10) H.H. Ohlenbusch, B.M. Olivera, D. Tuan and N. Davidson, J. Mol. Biol., 25, 299-315 (1967).

(11) R.T. Simpson and G.R. Reeck, Biochemistry, 3853-3858 (1973).

(12) C.W. Dingman and M.B. Sporn, J. Biol. Chem., 239, 3483-3492 (1964).

(13) R.F. Itzhaki and H.K. Cooper, J. Mol. Biol. 75, 119-128 (1973).

(14) K. Marushige and J. Bonner, J. Mol. Biol., 15, 160-174 (1966).

(15) H.V. Samis, Jr., D.L. Poccia and V.J. Wulff, Biochim. Biophys. Acta, 166, 410-418 (1968).

(16) R.J. Hill, D.L. Poccia and P. Doty, J. Mol. Biol., 61, 445-462 (1971).

(17) R. Hacha and E. Fredericq, Eur. J. Biochem., in the press.

(18) G.M. Goodwin and E.W. Johns, FEBS Letters, 21, 103-104 (1072).

(19) E.W. Johns in Ciba Foundation Symposium on Homeostatic Regulators, edited by G.E.W. Wolstenholme and J. Knight, Churchill Ltd, London, 1969, pp. 128-140.

(20) R.J. Delange, D.M. Fambrough, E.L. Smith and J. Bonner, J. Biol. Chem., 244, 319-334 (1969).

(21) R.T. Simpson and H. Sober, Biochemistry, 9, 3103-3109 (1970).

(22) M. Boublik, E.M. Bradbury, C. Crane-Robinson and E.W. Johns, Eur. J. Biochem., 17, 151-159 (1970).

(23) E.M. Bradbury, P.D. Cary, C. Crane-Robinson, P.L. Riches and E.W. Johns, Nature New Biol., 233, 265-267 (1971).

(24) E.M. Bradbury and H.W.E. Rattle, Eur. J. Biochem., 27, 270-281 (1972).

(25) S.C.R. Elgin, S.C. Froehner, J.E. Smart and J. Bonner, Advan. Cell Mol. Biol., 1, 1-57 (1971).

(26) E. Fredericq and C. Houssier, Eur. J. Biochem., 1,51-60 (1967).

(27) S. Bram and H. Ris, J. Mol. Biol., 55, 325-336 (1971).

(28) J.F. Pardon and M.H. Wilkins, J. Mol. Biol., 68, 115-124 (1972).

(29) T.Y. Shih and G.D. Fasman, J. Mol. Biol., 52, 125-129 (1970).

(30) A.S. Pooley, J.F. Pardon and B.M. Richards, J. Mol. Biol., 85, 533-549 (1974).

(31) P. DeSantis, E. Forni and R. Rizzo, Biopolymers, 13, 313-326 (1974).

(32) J. Blamire, D.R. Cryer, D.B. Finkelstein and J. Marmur, J. Mol. Biol., 67, 11-24 (1972).

(33) J. Bontemps and E. Fredericq, Biophys. Chem., in the press.

(34) A.A. Sharygin, A.A. Myulberg and I.P. Ashmarin, Biochemistry (SSSR), 38, 873-879 (1974).

(35) T.N. Priyatkin and A.I. Komkova, Biochemistry (SSSR), 38, 919-921 (1974).

(36) R. Rill and K.E. Van Holde, J. Biol. Chem., 248, 1080-1083 (1973).

(37) I.O. Walker, J. Mol. Biol., 14,381 (1965).

(38) E.J. Dupraw, Nature, 209, 577-580 (1966).

(39) J.G. Gall, Chromosoma, 20, 221-233 (1966).

(40) S.L. Wolfe, J. Cell. Biol., 37, 610-620 (1968).

(41) E.J. Dupraw, P.D. Bahr and G.F. Bahr, Act. Cytol., 188-205 (1969).

(42) G.F. Bahr, Exp. Cell. Res., 62, 39-49 (1970).

(43) J.G. Abuelo and D.E. Moore, J. Cell Biol., 41, 73-90 (1969).

(44) J. Frederic, Chromosoma, 28, 199-210 (1969).

(45) T. Caspersson, S. Farber, G.E. Foley, J. Kudynowski, E.J. Modest, E. Simonsson, U. Wagh and L. Zech, Exp. Cell. Res., 49, 219-222 (1968).

(46) J. Bontemps and C. Distèche, Chromosoma, in the press.

(47) F. Crick, Nature, 234, 25-27, (1971).

ISOLATION AND GRADIENT ANALYSIS OF DNA

Pol CHARLES

Cell Biochemistry-Radiobiology Department
Centre d'Etude de l'Energie Nucléaire
C.E.N./S.C.K., B-2400, MOL - Belgium

Many methods have been proposed for the isolation and purification of DNA from different materials.
Unfortunately, there does not seem to exist an universally applicable procedure whereby DNA can be isolated and purified from
any organism or tissue none being ideally suited to all situations.
The methods must be checked and adapted to each material. The one
discussed hereunder has been developed for the following reasons :
- Large quantities of DNA are needed for our experiments and preference is given to methods allowing a treatment of large
  amounts of material.
- Rapidity and minimal manipulation of the DNA are important.
- Yields must be high and the final preparation has to be representative of the DNA present in the starting material.
- The DNA must be as pure as possible and high molecular.

Preparation of the material for DNA extraction.

Viruses and phages are sensitive to detergent. Sodium dode-
cyl-sulfate (SDS) or Sarkosyl (NL-97 from GEIGY) at a concentration of 0.1% produces the lysis of the particules in suspension with an immediate release of nucleic acids and proteins into
the medium.

Different bacteria are sensitive to detergent but for most
of them, enzyme digestion is needed before treatment with a detergent.

Lysozyme digests the wall of gram-positive bacteria (such as
B.subtilis). With gram-negative bacteria (such as *E.coli*) lysozyme does not digest the wall and wall fragments usually remains
attached to the cell membrane. In all cases, the cell membrane
becomes available for detergent action.

Other classes of microorganisms such as **streptomyces** are very
resistant to lysis. Grinding in a mortar is required before enzyme digestion and detergent lysis.

With mammalian tissues,homogeneisation can be easily achieved
by using mechanical homogenizers such as Virtis or Ultra-Turrax
while free mammalian cells are readily sensitive to detergent.

With plants, more drastic treatments are generally needed :
such as the use of the French press or the grinding in the presence of solid CO_2 or liquid nitrogen. Of course, during these manipulations, precautions must be taken to limit the action of the
nucleases released in the medium.

Ordinarily, homogeneisation can be made in a saline-EDTA solution (0.15 M NaCl + 0.1 M EDTA, pH 8.0) EDTA inhibits the more
important DNase activity by chelating the activating ions (Mg,..).
Sodium lauryl sulfate also inhibits enzymes and denatures proteins.
We generally add pronase, a proteolytic enzyme with a broad action
spectrum (final concentration : 2 mg/ml) and allow the digestion
to proceed for 1 - 2 hours. (When large DNase activities are expected, this first digestion should be short - 30 min.).

Nucleic acids are then precipitated by adding 2 volumes ethanol.

The fibrous precipitate is recovered with a glass rod and
redissolved in diluted SSC (0.015 M NaCl + 0.0015 M trisodium
citrate).

When the precipitate is granular and difficult to wind on
the glass rod, centrifugation is needed. Concentrated polymerized
DNA require several hours to dissolve into an homogeneous solution. RNase is then added to a final concentration of 50 µg/ml
and the mixture is incubated at 37° for 1 hr; then treated with
pronase (2 mg/ml) for 2 hrs at 37°.

DNA purification can be continued with either :
  a) ultracentrifugation in CsCl gradient (Marmur 1961; Flamm,
     Birnstiel and Walker, 1969).
or b) molecular filtration on agarose gel (Loeb and Chauveau,1969)

In the first case, CsCl is added to the medium and the solution is centrifuged at 33.000 rpm during 63 hrs at 25°C. We use fixed angle rotors such as rotor 40 (Spinco) or 65 Ti (Martin-Christ). In each tube, 4.5 ml of CsCl solution containing 1 to 2 mg of DNA are used. When larger amount of DNA must be prepared the rotor 30 (SPINCO) or the rotor 40 (Martin-Christ) can be used. In this case, 10 ml of CsCl solution containing 5 to 6 mg DNA per tube can be centrifuged.
Before filtration on agarose, the NaCl concentration has to be adjusted to 2 M by the addition of dry NaCl to dissociate nucleoproteins.

Typical preparations obtained with the two methods are presented in fig.1 to 6. By selecting the convenient CsCl concentration and centrifugation conditions, RNA sediments at the bottom of the tube, proteins floats at the top of the gradient and DNA bands near the center of the gradient. DNA and proteins are well separated by filtration on agarose 4B. Highly polymerized DNA is excluded from the gel, while proteins and acidosoluble components are eluted later.

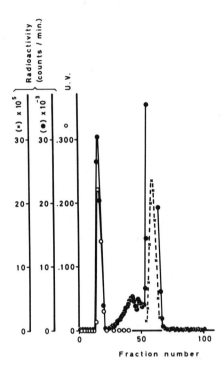

Fig.1

Agarose filtration of thymidine ^{3}H labelled phage lambda DNA.
Phage particules are suspended in saline-EDTA pH 8.0.
Sarkosyl is added (0.1% final) and after addition of proteinase
K (MERCK) (50 µg/ml) the solution is incubated at 37° for 1 hr.
Ionic strength is adjusted to 2 M by addition of crystals of
NaCl. After centrifugation at 5.000 rpm for 10 min., the clear
supernatant (10 ml) is layered on the agarose column.
Column Pharmacia K 26/40.
Bed dimensions : 2.5 x 40 cm
Bed volume : 200 ml
Eluant : NaCl 2 M ; Flow rate : 0.7 ml/min = 8 ml/cm^{2}h.
Sample volume:80 drops=3.5 ml.O—O—O : U.V.absorption
                              ●—●—● : radioactivity; X—X—X

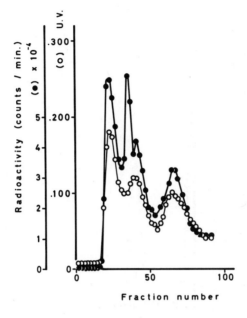

Fig.2

Preparation of tritiated bacterial DNA by agarose filtration.
E. coli strain P4 x JE x 8 ur⁻ was cultured in a mineral medium
containing uracil -6-^{3}H.
The bacteria are collected at the beginning of the stationary
phase by centrifugation. They are suspended in saline-EDTA,pH 8.0;
lysozyme is added (0.4 mg/ml) and the mixture is incubated at 37°C
for 1 hr. Complete lysis is obtained with sodium lauryl sulfate
(1%). Pronase (2mg/ml) is added and the visquous solution is incubated at 37° for 2 hrs.
NaCl is added (2 M final) and the solution is centrifuged for
10 min. at 5.000 rpm. The clear supernatant (10 ml) is added to
the agarose column. The elution conditions are as in fig.1
O—O—O : U.V. absorption
●—●—● : radioactivity.

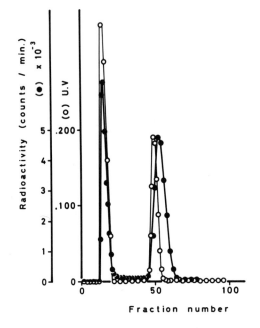

Fig.3

Preparation of tritiated plant DNA by filtration on sepharose 4B.
Plants grown aseptically in the presence of tritiated thymidine
were cut in small pieces. Pigments were extracted with alcohol at
-30° and ether. Liquid nitrogen was added and the material was
ground to dust in a mortar.
DNA was prepared as indicated in the text.
Elution conditions were as in fig.1.
O—O—O : U.V. absorption
●—●—● : radioactivity.

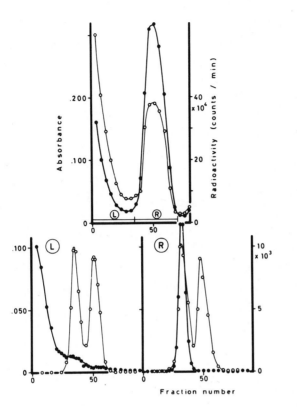

Fig.4

Preparation and analysis of tritiated bacterial DNA by isopycnic
ultracentrifugation.
Streptomyces coelicolor (strain ura A : 1) was cultured in a mineral medium containing uracil 6³H.
Pigments were removed with ether denatured ethanol and acetone.
DNA was prepared as indicated in the text.
Solid CsCl was added to the solution to obtain an initial density
of 1.730 g/cm³ (1.33 g CsCl per ml of solution - n_D = 1.7022).
The solution was centrifuged in 10 ml nitrocellulose tubes. Each
tube containing 4.5 ml of solution is overlayed with liquid paraffin to stabilise the gradient and to prevent tube collapse Isopycnic equilibrium was obtained after 63 hr at 33.000 rpm in a fixed
angle rotor. After centrifugation, each tube was punctured with
a needle n° 15 G and about 100 fractions of 2 drops each were

Fig.4 (cont.)
collected in scintillation vials. Tubes are eluted under a constant pressure of paraffin oil at a rate controlled with a micro-
metric screw. To every second fraction, 1 ml of distilled water
was added and the U.V. spectrum was recorded in a recording spec-
trophotometer (Cary model 14). The difference 260 - 310 mµ being
taken as a measure of the nucleic acid content.

The radioactivity of the fractions were then estimated by
adding 7.5 ml Instagel Packard and measuring the radioactivity in
a Packard 3380.

When the DNA is highly polymerized, its elution is accompanied by a sharp increase of the viscosity.

Result is represented on the upper part of the figure.(absorbance O—O—O or radioactivity ∎—∎—∎ being plotted versus
fraction number).

The fractions (L) of the left hand part of the gradient were pooled and recentrifuged in a swing-out rotor (SW 39) with
two density reference DNA's (Micrococcus lysodeikticus - 1.731
g/cm^3 and B.subtilis - 1.703 g/cm^3).
The fractions (R) of the right hand part of the gradient were
pooled and diluted 5 times with 0.01 M NaCl. DNA was precipitated by adding 2 vol. ethanol. After redissolution in dilute
SSC, an aliquot of the DNA solution was centrifuged in a swing-
out rotor in the presence of one density reference DNA (B.subti-
lis 1.703 g/cm^3).
The R fractions produce a sharp peak of radioactivity of clean
streptomyces DNA. No significant radioactivity is observed outside this peak.

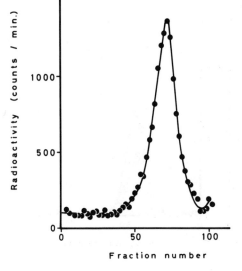

Fig.5

Preparation of tritiated plant DNA by isopycnic ultracentrifugation.
DNA was prepared as indicated in fig.3
1.27 g CsCl was added per ml of solution - n_D = 1.3998
The conditions of centrifugation and fractionation were the same
as in fig.4
The fractions containing DNA were pooled and after dilution (5
times) with 0.01 M NaCl, DNA was precipitated by adding 2 vol.
ethanol and redissolved in sterile 0.01 M NaCl.

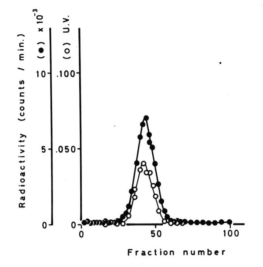

Fig.6

Analysis by ultracentrifugation in CsCl of tritiated plant DNA
prepared by filtration on agarose 4B.
50 µg of plant [³H] DNA (cf. fig.3) were centrifuged in a spinco-
rotor 40 at 33.000 rpm for 63 hrs at 25°C.
The solution was fractionated as indicated in fig.4.
It can be seen that the radioactivity exactly covers the U.V.
peak and that no significant radioactivity can be found outside the peak.
O—O—O : U.V. absorption
●—●—● : radioactivity

ANALYSIS OF THE MATERIAL OBTAINED WITH THE TWO METHODS.

I. Purity.

DNA preparations considered as pure, always contain traces
of RNA and proteins or amino-acids. To estimate the amount of
RNA and proteins contaminating the DNA solution we prepared DNA
from two different strains of *B. subtilis* :
1. *B. subtilis* wild type 168 cultured in a medium containing
   ^{3}H-5-uridine (a good precursor of RNA).
2. *B. subtilis* strain GSY 276 try$^-$ ilva$^-$ cultured in presence
   of ^{3}H-DL-valine.

Results :

1. *B. subtilis* 168 ^{3}H-5-uridine treated cells (Fig.7)

   A. CsCl preparation (7A)

      The DNA prepared by this method has a specific radio-
      activity of 1 x 10^{6}dpm/microgram. This radioactivity
      represents about 3.0% of the acidoprecipitable radio-
      active material present in the starting material.
      This radioactivity does not correspond only to the
      labelled RNA contaminating the DNA preparation. In fact
      COMINGS (1965) has observed that uridine could be in-
      corporated into the DNA via the metabolic pathway of
      deoxycytidine. In normal conditions, with mammalian
      cells, about 2% of the acido precipitable radioactivi-
      ty is found in the DNA. In these conditions, the amount
      of RNA present in the DNA solution is lower than 1%.

   B. Agarose preparation (7B)

      The DNA prepared by filtration on sepharose 4B has
      about the same specific radioactivity and could thus
      be contaminated by similar amounts of RNA.
      This result is in good agreement with those obtained
      by LOEB and CHAUVEAU (1969) preparing rat liver or,
      calf thymus DNA by the same method.

2. *B. subtilis* GSY 267 try$^-$ ilva$^-$, ^{3}H DL-valine treated
   cells (fig.8).

   A. CsCl preparation (8A)

      The DNA has a specific radioactivity of 400 dpm/µg.
      This corresponds to a contamination of 0.03% in terms
      of amino-acid or 0.1 to 1% in terms of proteins.

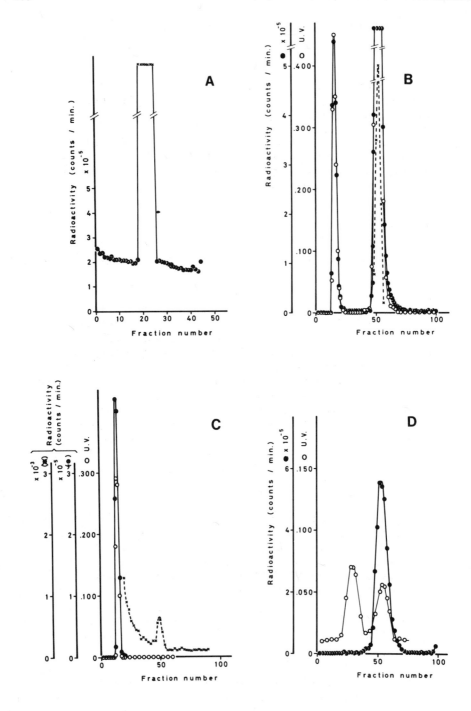

Fig.7

Preparation of radioactive DNA from *B. subtilis* 168 wild type
cultured in presence of ^{3}H-5-uridine.

The pellet has been treated as indicated in fig.2 except that
after pronase digestion, the nucleic acids were precipitated
by ethanol and after redissolution in dilute SSC, a treatment
with RNase (50 μg/ml) and a second digestion with pronase
(2 mg/ml) have been performed before addition of CsCl or NaCl
crystals.

A. by isopycnic centrifugation
   The conditions of centrifugation are those described in
   figure 4. Fractions were pooled when drops appear visquous.

B. by filtration on agarose 4B.
   The conditions are those described in figure 2.

In C we have analysed by filtration on sepharose 4B the DNA
prepared by isopycnic centrifugation. It can be seen that almost all radioactivity is excluded from the gel, with the DNA,
a small peak near the fraction 50 represents 0.1 to 0.2% of the
total radioactivity put on the column.
(note the scale change necessary to show this little peak).

In D we have analysed by ultracentrifugation in CsCl gradient
the DNA prepared by filtration on agarose 4B.
All radioactivity is associated with the *B. subtilis* DNA. No
radioactivity higher than the normal value of the background
is found outside the U.V.peak.
Non labelled *Streptomyces coelicolor* DNA (d = 1.730 g/cm^3) was
added as density marker.
O—O—O : U.V. absorption
●—●—● : radioactivity : X—X—X

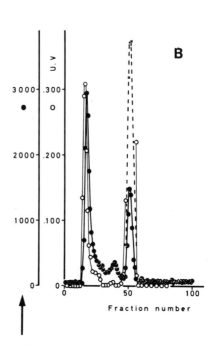

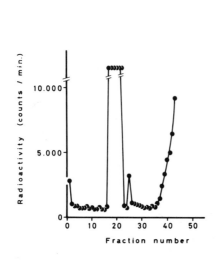

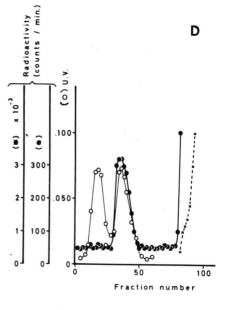

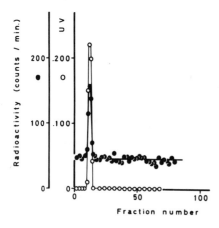

Fig.8

Preparation of DNA from *B. subtilis* GSY try⁻, ilva⁻ cultured
in the presence of ^{3}H DL-valine.
The pellet has been treated as indicated in fig.7.

A. by isopycnic centrifugation.
   The conditions of centrifugation are those described in
   figure 4. Fractions were pooled when drops appear visquous.

B. by filtration on agarose 4B.
   The conditions are those described in figure 2.

in C the DNA prepared by isopycnic centrifugation was analysed
   by filtration on sepharose 4B.

in D the DNA prepared by filtration on agarose 4B was analysed
   by ultracentrifugation in CsCl gradient.
   Unlabelled streptomyces coelicolor DNA (d = 1.730 g/cm^3)
   was added as density marker.
   (Most of the radioactivity is found in the upper part of
   the gradient where normally proteins floats - note the
   scale change).

   O—O—O : U.V. absorption
   ●—●—● : radioactivity : X—X—X

B. Agarose preparation (8B)

The elution profile is peculiar. The peak of radioactivity does not exactly correspond to the U.V.
absorption.
The specific radioactivity of the fractions is
different as indicated hereunder :

fraction 14   :   1.200   dpm/microgram
         15   :   1.650   dpm/microgram
         16   :   6.000   dpm/microgram
         17   :   8.700   dpm/microgram
pooled fractions containing DNA : 6.000 dpm/µg.

It seems, in this case, that two kinds of molecules are excluded together.

An aliquot of the pooled fractions containing DNA
has been analysed by centrifugation in CsCl gradient. It can be seen from the fig.8D that while
some radioactivity sediments in the gradient with
the bacterial DNA, the most important part of the
radioactivity is found in the upper part of the
gradient. This radioactivity is excluded from
the gel together with the DNA but shows, in the
CsCl gradient, a density very different from
that of DNA. The estimated specific radioactivity
of the DNA after centrifugation in CsCl is about
360 dpm/microgram, in good agreement with that
found after CsCl preparation.

In conclusion, the DNA prepared by a succession
of the two methods could be considered as relatively pure and clean. It contains very few proteins and traces of RNA.
Agarose filtration does not improve the quality
of the DNA molecules prepared by isopycnic centrifugation. Centrifugation in CsCl gradient purifies
DNA from contaminants co-excluded from the gel.

II. Biological assay

The different preparations were tested for their biological activity.
DNA from the prototrophic strain B. subtilis 168 prepared by
the two methods has a similar biological activity. The frequencies of transformation of a single marker were about 3.10^{-2} .
For the linked markers, the frequencies were similar to that
obtained with DNA prepared by phenol treatment.

III.   Molecular weight.

       DNA molecules are high molecular polymers with characteris-
tic primary and secondary structures. Their molecular weight can
be estimated by viscometry or sedimentation velocity (for instance
in analytical model E ultracentrifuge). The results obtained by
these two methods are in good agreement (Eigner - 1967).

       From table 1 where comparative results are indicated, it can
be said that :
1. the molecular weight of the DNA prepared by isopycnic centrifugation is higher than that of the DNA prepared by gel filtration.

Table 1	Molecular weight (Estimation by viscometry)			
	Centrifugation in CsCl		Filtration on agarose	
	[η]	M.W.: 10^6daltons	[η]	M.W.=10^6daltons
B.subtilis GSY 276	206	62	80	16
B.subtilis 168	130	32	95	20
L929 cells	330	125	140	36
			120	30

The M.W. of L929 cells DNA (CsCl preparation) is 125 x 10^6 daltons, as compared to the 36 x 10^6 daltons obtained in agarose
preparations. Even if we take into account the fact that M.W. of
the sodium salt of DNA is 0.75 that of the caesium salt, the
observed difference is highly significative.
If a sample of DNA prepared by CsCl centrifugation is analysed
by gel filtration an important drop of the M.W. is observed
after passage through the gel. It is probable that elution is
accompanied by shearing.

Comments on centrifugation in CsCl gradients

        Fixed angle rotors are widely utilized not only for DNA
preparation but also for the analysis of DNA molecules.
Fixed angle rotors have a number of advantages over swing-out
rotors so far as isopycnic centrifugation is concerned (Flamm,
Birnstiel and Walker - 1972).
This include :
1. greater tubes and rotor capacities
2. shorter gradient and shorter equilibration time.
3. better separation of DNA from RNA, since RNA sediments faster
   and pellets on the outer wall of the tube.
4. better resolution of mixtures of DNA with different GC contents.

        We tried to determine whether computing molecular weight
from band width was also applicable when DNA was centrifuged at
equilibrium in a fixed angle rotor.

        The molecular weight (M) is related to the concentration
distribution by the expression :

$$M = \frac{RT_\rho}{(d_\rho/d_r)\ \sigma^2\omega^2 r} = \frac{RT_\rho}{(d_\rho/d_r)\ \omega^2 r} \cdot \frac{1}{\sigma^2}$$

                R = the gas constant
                T = the absolute temperature
                d_ρ/d_r = the density gradient

                σ = the standard deviation of the gausian concentra-
                    tion distribution.
                ω^2 = the angular velocity
                r = radius

        The standard deviation can be estimated graphically at
0.607 of the distribution height.

On fig.9 is shown the effect of reorientating the tube after centrifugation at equilibrium in a fixed angle rotor.

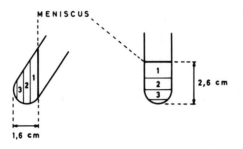

Effect of re-orientation in a fixed-angle centrifuge rotor

At equilibrium the distances 1-2-3 are equal.

After reorientation 1 > 2 > 3

Fig.9

The reorientation produces a constriction of the bands near the bottom of the tube and an expansion of those near the top, the distances between the bands are also affected.
This clearly appear in fig.9.

A given DNA was centrifuged at equilibrium in three different concentrations of CsCl such that the position of the DNA was different in each case (fig.10).

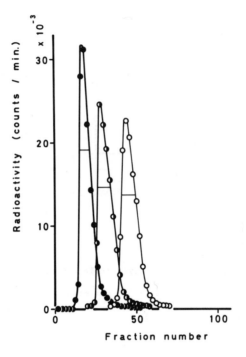

fig.10

Equivalent amounts of Micrococcus sarcina ^{3}H DNA were centrifuged at equilibrium in three different CsCl gradient.
Initial density of the solution :

    1 - 1.690 g/cm^3 n_D = 1.3982   ●—●—●
    2 - 1.708 g/cm^3 n_D = 1.4000   ◖—◖—◖
    3 - 1.728 g/cm^3 n_D = 1.4020   ○—○—○

The standard deviation of the radioactivity distributions was
estimated to 3.0 - 3.75 - 4.25% respectively.
Reorientation produces an expansion of the band width when the
DNA sediments in the upper part of the gradient.

In order to estimate the modifications of the gradient due to
the reorientation of the tube after its centrifugation, 5 DNA's
having different density were centrifuged in the same tube. In
fig.11 it can be seen that the gradient is not deeply disturbed.
Even if it is not perfectly linear, density could be estimated
with an error of ± 2 mg/ml.

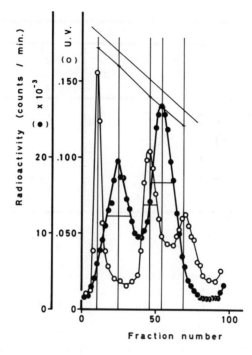

Fig.11

5 DNA's with different densities were centrifuged in the same gradient.

Initial density of the CsCl solution :
$$1.695 \text{ g/cm}^3 \qquad n_D = 1.3991$$

phage 2c DNA	1.742 g/cm
[^{3}H] streptomyces coelicolor DNA	1.730 g/cm
E. coli DNA	1.710 g/cm
[^{3}H] B.subtilis DNA	1.703 g/cm
cl. perfringens DNA	1.691 g/cm

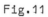 : U.V. absorption
●—●—● : radioactivity

In table 2 are indicated the σ values for DNA's centrifuged at
equilibrium in swing-out or in fixed angle rotor.

Table 2		σ values	
	M.W. 10^6 daltons	After centrifugation in swing-out rotor	After centrifugation in fixed angle rotor.
phage 2c	40.0	1.75	2.0
Cl. perfringens	14.0	3.0	6.5
B.subtilis	7.5	4.0	7.5
St.coelicolor	4.6	5.0	8.5

It can be seen that the estimation of the molecular weight
by the band width is possible when the DNA is centrifuged in
a swing-out rotor but not when it is centrifuged in a fixed
angle rotor.

In order to see whether the method is applicable in a wide
range of molecular weights, we studied the effect of depo-
lymerisation on band width. A DNA of 48 x 10^6 daltons was de-
polymerised by shearing through a needle n° 25 (table 3).

Table 3			σ values	
Number of passage	$[\eta]$	M.W. 10^6 daltons	Centrifugation in fixed angle rotor 2 experiments	From tracing after centrifugation in model E ultracentrifuge
0	170	48	5.0 - 5.0	2.5
1	120	29	4.5 - 5.0	3.0
2	81	16.5	5.2 - 4.7	4.0
4	53	9.0	4.7 - 5.0	5.2
6	41	6.5	7.0 - 8.0	6.5

The molecular weight of the DNA falls rapidly with successive treatments but contrary to what is obtained in analytical ultracentrifuge the band width only varies significantly when the M.W. falls below 9.10^7 daltons, when DNA is centrifuged in a fixed angle rotor.

REFERENCES

Comings, D.E., Incorporation of tritium of ^{3}H-5-uridine into
DNA, (1965), Exp. Cell. Res., 41, 677 - 681

Eigner, J., Molecular weight and conformation of DNA, (1967),
Methods in Enzymology, Vol. XII part B, 386 - 429, eds. L.
Grossman and K. Moldave, Academic Press, New York.

Flamm, W.G., Birnstiel, M.L., Walker, P.M.B., (1972), Iso-
pycnic centrifugation of DNA. Methods and applications,
Subcellular components. Preparation and fractionation, ed.by
G.D. Birnie, Butterworths London, 279 - 310.

Loeb, J.E., Chauveau, J., (1969), Preparation de DNA par
filtration sur gel d'agarose, Biochim. Biophys. Acta, 182,
225 - 234.

Marmur, J., (1961), A procedure for the isolation of deoxyribonucleic acid from micro-organisms, J. Mol. Biol., 3,
208 - 218.

Vinograd, J., Morris, J., Davidson, N., Dove, W., (1963),
The buoyant behaviour of viral and bacterial DNA in alkaline CsCl, Proc. Natn. Acad. Sci. (U.S.A.), 49, 12 - 17.

USE OF MOLECULAR SIEVING ON AGAROSE GELS TO STUDY DNA UPTAKE BY CHLAMY-

DOMONAS REINHARDI

P.F. LURQUIN and R.M. BEHKI*

Department of Radiobiology
Centre d'Etude de l'Energie Nucléaire
CEN/SCK, 2400 Mol, Belgium

Introduction

All the studies so far reported on the uptake and expression of
exogenous DNA in plants have involved the use of whole higher plants
(1-6), callus tissue cultures (7), isolated cells (4,5,8,9) or protoplasts (10-12). Owing to the limitation of our knowledge of these genetic systems and owing to the enormous complexity of higher plants
(13,14), one realizes that the study of foreign DNA uptake and particularly its subsequent expression - if any - in plant systems is extremely difficult.

In order to bypass at least some of these difficulties, we selected the unicellular eukaryotic alga *Chlamydomonas reinhardi* as a model
plant system to investigate the uptake and fate of labelled bacterial
DNA. Two *Chlamydomonas* strains were used in this study; the wild type
137 C(+) strain and the CW 15(+) mutant of Davies and Plaskitt (15)
which makes little or no cell wall. This mutant behaves like a natural protoplast.

The uptake and the fate of the donor DNA were followed by essentially two methods :
1) centrifugation in CsCl density gradients in order to determine the
nature of the labeled DNA inside or outside the cells.

---

*On leave from the Chemistry and Biology Research Institute, Research
Branch, Agriculture Canada, Ottawa, Ontario, Canada.

2) molecular sieving on Sepharose 4B (4% agarose gel, Pharmacia, Uppsala) in order to determine the heterogeneity in size of the donor DNA molecules taken up by the cells.

Preparation of Chlamydomonas DNA

Exogenously supplied thymidine derivatives are not efficiently utilized by *Chlamydomonas* for DNA synthesis (16 and this study). Labeled adenine (^{3}H or ^{14}C) is used for *in vivo* labeling of *Chlamydomonas* nucleic acids; both RNA and DNA are labeled. Since the rate of synthesis and the amount of RNA in the cells are much larger than that of DNA, considerably more radioactivity is incorporated into RNA than into DNA. It becomes difficult, therefore, to obtain DNA, completely free of RNA, by the standard or modified Marmur procedure(17)

To overcome this problem, we developed a method of DNA purification based on the gel filtration on Sepharose 4B at high ionic strength of crude extracts from *Chlamydomonas* labelled with ^{3}H or ^{14}C-adenine. A similar method was independently reported by Heyn et al. (18) to purify DNA from other plant species.
The procedure can be outlined as follows :
- the labeled cells are harvested and washed with cold high salt medium (HSM)(19).
- the cells are resuspended in a small volume of 0.15 M NaCl - 0.1 M EDTA pH 8.0 and sodium sarcosylate is added to a final concentration of 1.5 %. The mixture is then incubated for 5 min. at 37°.
- after lysis, predigested pronase is added to a final concentration of 2 mg/ml and incubation at 37° is performed for another 1 hour.
- solid NaCl is then added to the mixture to a concentration of 2M and the clear solution is poured on top of a Sepharose 4B column equilibrated with 2M NaCl. Elution with the same salt solution is performed at room temperature.

Fig. 1 shows a typical elution pattern with the DNA peak eluting first (excluded from the gel). The second peak, which carries most of the radioactivity consists mainly of acid-soluble compounds together with RNA.
Pigments are well separated (O.D. 665nm). The DNA fractions can be pooled, concentrated and dialysed against 0.15M NaCl. Finally solid CsCl is added to bring the solution to a refractive index of 1.3995 for CsCl density gradient centrifugation.

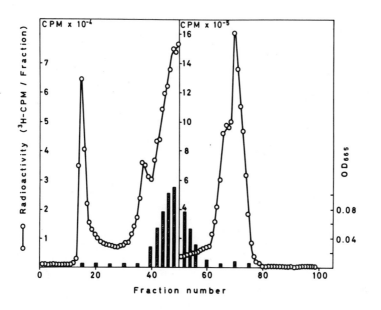

Fig. 1 – *Chlamydomonas WT (+)* cells were labeled for 24 hours with
10 μC/ml ^{3}H-adenine. A total of 10^8 washed cells was resuspended in 5 ml of saline – EDTA and treated as described in
the text. Column dimensions are 2.5 cm x 4.5 cm – 3.2 ml
fractions were collected. ^{3}H-radioactivity, 0 – 0; pigments
(OD_{665}) are represented by hatched bars.

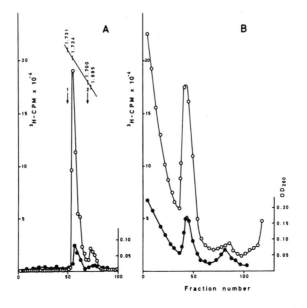

Fig. 2 - A. CsCl density gradient centrifugation of *Chlamydomonas* DNA
            obtained by the agarose procedure - ^{3}H-radioactivity,
            0 - 0; OD_{260} corresponding to unlabelled *Chlamydomonas*
            DNA added as a UV marker, ● - ●. Arrows indicate the
            position of *Micrococcus lysodeikticus* DNA (d = 1.731 g.cm^{-3})
            and ascites cells DNA (d = 1.700 g.cm^{-3}) in parallel runs.
            Centrifugation was done in a SW 60 rotor at 30,000 rpm
            for 63 hours.
       B. CsCl density gradient centrifugation of *Chlamydomonas* DNA
            obtained by the modified Marmur procedure. (see text).
            ^{3}H-radioactivity 0 - 0; OD_{260}, 0 - 0. Centrifugation was
            done in a fixed angle 40 rotor at 33,000 rpm for 63 hours.

Fig. 2A represents the banding pattern of ^{3}H-adenine labeled *Chlamydomonas* DNA in CsCl where nuclear DNA (d = 1.724 g.cm^{-3}) and chloroplast
DNA (d = 1.695 g.cm^{-3}) can be recognized. This DNA preparation, obtained by using molecular sieving on agarose contains no RNA sedimenting
to the bottom of the tube. This is compared in Fig. 2B with the banding
pattern in a CsCl gradient of *Chlamydomonas* DNA obtained by the modified
Marmur procedure (2 pronase treatments, 2 treatments with pancreatic
RNase and 3 alcohol precipitations). This DNA obviously still contains
significant amounts of RNA. In addition, the latter procedure requires
3 days compared to a few hours needed to carry out the molecular sieving

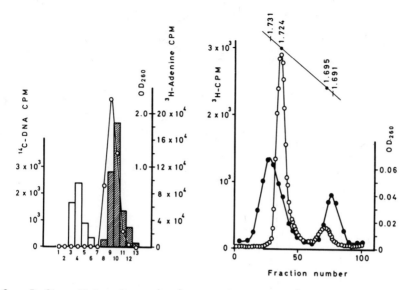

Fig. 3 - Left : Molecular sieving on Sepharose 4B of a mixture of trace
amounts of purified ^{14}C-DNA from *Chlamydomonas*, trace
amounts of ^{3}H-adenine and yeast t RNA. Open area, [14]C-
radioactivity; hatched area ^{3}H-radioactivity; 0 - 0,
OD_{260}

Right: CsCl density gradient centrifugation of ^{3}H-DNA from
Chlamydomonas in a fixed angle rotor showing the excellent separation between nuclear and chloroplast DNA,
0 - 0, ^{3}H-radioactivity; ● - ●; DO_{260} of UV markers
(*M. lysodeikticus* and *Clostridium perfringens* DNA).
63 hours at 33,000 rpm.

on agarose. More details concerning this method will be published elsewhere (20).

Molecular sieving on Sepharose gels offers an additional advantage of separating high molecular weight components from low mol. wt.
ones as seen from the elution pattern obtained and described in
Fig. 3 when purified ^{14}C-DNA of *Chlamydomonas* mixed with ^{3}H-adenine and
yeast transfer RNA was applied to the column. It can be seen that DNA
is eluted from our standardized columns mainly in fractions 3,4 and 5
whereas adenine (or DNA degradation products after treatment with pancreatic DNase) is eluted in fractions 8 to 13. Yeast t RNA is seen to
be a little less retarded than the nucleotides. The figure also shows
the excellent separation of nuclear and chloroplast DNA from *Chlamydomonas* achieved in a CsCl gradient established in a fixed angle rotor.
Thus it became clear that the use of the molecular sieving on agarose

combined with CsCl density gradient centrifugation technique will
allow us to investigate the quality of exogenous DNA taken up by
Chlamydomonas and also its subsequent fate.

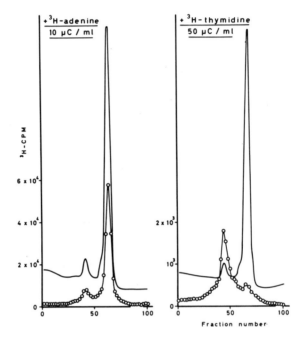

Fig. 4 – Comparison between ^{3}H-adenine and ^{3}H-thymidine uptake by *Chla-*
        mydomonas, 0 - 0,[3]H-radioactivity; solid line, UV absorbance
        of the radioactive DNA monitored with a recorder coupled to
        an ISCO flow cell. The small peak is chloroplast DNA and the
        large peak represents nuclear DNA. The shoulder on the light
        side of the nuclear DNA peak is γ-DNA (d = 1.715 g.cm^{-3}).

Another advantage of the *Chlamydomonas* system for such a study lies
in the fact that these cells cannot use thymine derivatives efficiently for their DNA biosynthesis. Moreover, as shown in fig. 4 exogenously supplied ^{3}H-thymidine almost specifically labels chloroplast DNA
whose specific radioactivity is at least 40 times greater than that of
nuclear DNA under these conditions. Labeling of the cells with [3]H-
adenine results in a much better incorporation of the radioisotope,
the specific radioactivities of both DNA species being comparable.

In other words, the examination of both the quality and the quantity
of label incorporated into DNA would indicate whether the thymidine-
labeled donor DNA is broken down and reused for endogenous DNA synthesis in *Chlamydomonas*. We know of no other system providing such a
salient feature which has been used in DNA uptake studies.

Uptake and fate of bacterial DNA in Chlamydomonas

a) Uptake in log phase

     Polycations (i.e. DEAE-dextran, poly-L-lysine and poly-L-ornithine)
have been used in plant systems to stimulate DNA uptake (8,10,11).
However, these polycations are very toxic to *Chlamydomonas* as seen in
fig. 5. These compounds cause heavy aggregation of the cells which is
followed by partial bleaching, and it is only after an appreciably long

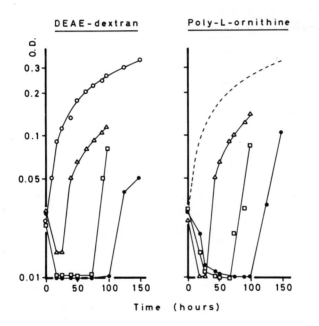

Fig. 5 - Effect of polycations on the growth of *Chlamydomonas* WT (+).
         Growth is monitored with a Beckman C colorimeter (red filter).
         0 - 0, control; ▲-▲, 2 µg/ml; ▫-▫, 5 µg/ml; ●-● 10 µg/ml

lag period that the cells resume growth at a normal rate. A polyca-
tion concentration of 5µg/ml was selected and used in the rest of the
study. The toxic effect of polycations is reduced when exogenous DNA
is also present in the cultures at the same time. This is shown in
fig. 6.

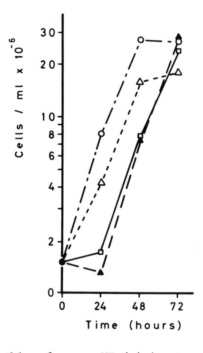

Fig. 6 – Growth of *Chlamydomonas WT (+)* in the presence of 50 µg/ml
   E. coli DNA and 5 µg/ml polycations, 0 - 0, control without polycations; Δ - Δ, with DEAE-dextran, □ - □ with poly-
   L-lysine; ▲ - ▲, with poly-L-ornithine. Cell number was determined by direct counting.

It can be seen that the lag period in the presence of 5 µg/ml polycations and 50 µg/ml *E. coli* DNA does not exceed 24 hours. This reduced
toxicity is understandable in terms of polycations-DNA complex formation which would be less toxic than free polycations. DNA alone up to
100 µg/ml has no toxic effect.

The pattern of DNA uptake was followed 72 hours, a period of time which allows the cells to reach early stationary phase in the presence of polycations starting initially with 2 x 10^6 cells/ml.

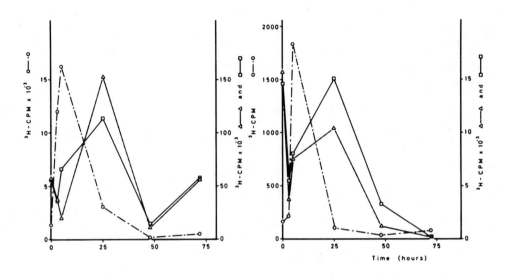

Fig. 7 – Time course of *E. coli* ^{3}H-DNA uptake by *Chlamydomonas* WT (+)
cells.
    Left : the cells are harvested and extensively washed with
           HSM. Aliquots are then precipitated in the cold with
           10% TCA, trapped on Millipore filters and counted in
           Packard Instagel.
    Right: after extensive washing with HSM, the cells are re-
           suspended in 2 ml of HSM containing 10^{-2}M MgCl$_2$ and
           incubated for 15 min at 37° in the presence of
           50 µg/ml pancreatic DNase. After two more washes with
           HSM, they are precipitated with TCA as above.
           0 – 0, control without polycations; Δ – Δ, 5 µg/ml
           poly-L-lysine present, □ – □ , 5 µg/ml poly-L-orni-
           thine present.

Fig. 7 shows that exogenously supplied *E. coli* ^{3}H-DNA (2 x 10^6 dpm/µg,
M.W. = 20 – 40 x 10^6 daltons) appears to become rapidly associated with
the cells in the absence of polycations but gets released after about
5 hours. The phenomenon seems to level off after about 48 hours. A
similar pattern is observed when poly-L-lysine or poly-L-ornithine
are present except that the association is quantitatively much more
pronounced and the peak values are obtained after a lag period   cor-

responding to that observed in fig. 6. It appears that bacterial DNA
is not retained by cells undergoing active division. The right part
of fig. 7 shows the kinetic pattern of DNA uptake when the cells are
also treated with 50 µg/ml pancreatic DNase immediately after the
aliquots are taken and the cells washed with a large excess of HSM.
It is seen that the phenomenon is qualitatively similar to that observed in the absence of DNase treatment. However, about 90% of the
radioactivity is solubilized by the DNase treatment, showing that
to a large extent, donor DNA was simply adsorbed to the cells and
not actually taken up. The large zero values observed in the presence of polycations are probably due to the presence of cell aggregates, as mentioned above, which are not readily accessible to the
DNase action.

Table I

^{3}H-CPM/10^7 cells after 72 hours of incubation in HSM

Donor DNA	Additions	DNase Sensitive	DNase Resistant	AS	% donor
E. coli	None	5,200	790	1520	0.016
	DEAE-Dextran	12,200	740	1700	0.015
	Poly-L-lysine	39,500	1400	1500	0.027
	Poly-L-ornithine	75,000	1860	930	0.038
B. subtilis	None	3,850	430	1190	0.009
	DEAE-Dextran	7,700	520	790	0.011
	Poly-L-lysine	77,000	950	950	0.021
	Poly-L-ornithine	89,000	1200	750	0.027

Acid-soluble counts in medium represent ca. 10-20 % (mean = 100,000
CPM/ml) of donor DNA CPM (initial value at zero time = 0.1 % acid-
soluble CPM in donor DNA).
The DNase treatment of the cells does not affect prelabelled intracellular DNA : TCA precipitable CPM in ^{3}H-adenine labelled cells =
          2.64 x 10^6
          Same after 30 min at 37° with 50µg/ml DNase =
          2.68 x 10^6

Table I summarizes the results obtained after 72 hours of incubation
of *C. reinhardi* with *E. coli* or *B. subtilis* ^{3}H-DNA. It is clear that
polycations stimulate the adsorption of donor DNA considerably. However, irreversible(DNase-resistant) absorption appears to be stimulated by a factor of only 2 - 3 in the best cases. On the other hand,
the presence of polycations seems to protect donor DNA from degradation by endogenous nuclease since the amount of acid-soluble compounds inside the cells is somewhat reduced.

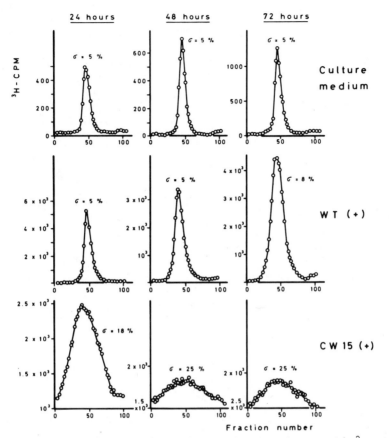

Fig. 8 - CsCl density gradient centrifugation of *E. coli* ^{3}H-DNA supplied to the culture medium, to growing WT (+) cells and to
growing CW 15(+) cells. Considerable widening of the bands
after incubation with the CW 15 (+) mutant indicates heavy
degradation.

The degradation of exogenous DNA in the culture medium was also monitored : Fig. 8 shows the banding properties of *E. coli* DNA in the extracellular medium. It is clear that the culture medium does not degrade DNA since the values of the standard deviations of the gaussian
bands (σ) show no increase with time. It is known that σ is grossly
proportional to the state of the polymerization of DNA.(21)
A similar situation is encountered when the donor DNA is incubated in
the presence of growing WT (+) cells; little increase in σ being observed. On the other hand, CW 15 (+) cells extensively degrade added
exogenous DNA, yielding very broad bands in the CsCl gradients and a
high background of diffusible compounds. This is probably due to mechanical breakage of these fragile cells, and subsequent release of nuclease in the medium.

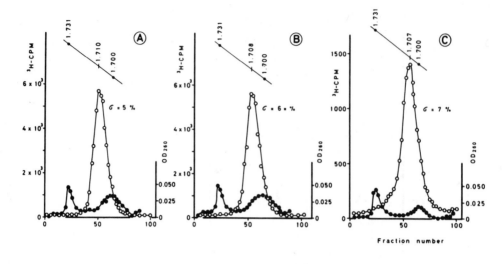

Fig. 9 - CsCl density gradient centrifugation of *E. coli* ³H-DNA.
     A. Donor DNA before incubation with the cells.
     B. Donor DNA adsorbed to WT (+) cells.
     C. Donor DNA adsorbed to CW 15 (+) cells. ³H-CPM, 0 - 0;
       OD$_{260}$ of marker DNA's, ● - ●;

If the DNase treatment is omitted after incubation of the cells with labeled *E. coli* DNA, large amounts of donor DNA are present with the cells (fig. 9). In addition, it can be observed that the cell membrane of the CW 15 (+) mutant is able to adsorb DNA and protect it from exocellular nucleases released under those conditions (compare with fig. 8). This large amount of foreign DNA is apparently aspecifically adsorbed and can be degraded by further incubation with pancreatic DNase at 37° (see table I).

The next step in the study of the nature of irreversibly adsorbed (DNase-resistant) DNA was to examine its heterogeneity. This was done by molecular sieving of extracts of the DNase-treated WT (+) cells on agarose columns.(fig. 10). It is seen that in the absence of polycations no radioactivity is eluted with the void volume in the *E. coli* ³H-DNA treated culture. It thus appears that donor DNA is extensively degraded by WT (+) cells after being taken up. The situation is very different when polycations are added : first, the total radioactivity inside the cells is significantly increased and second, this radioactivity is shown to be carried by compounds distributed over a wide range of M.W. In other words, polycations notably stimulate DNA uptake by WT (+) cells but also protect, at least a part of it, from extensive degradation.

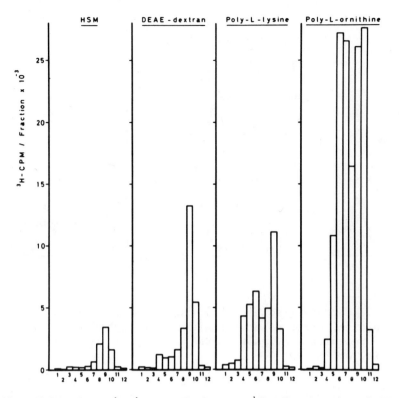

Fig. 10 - Molecular sieving on Sepharose 4B of extracts of DNase-treated *Chlamydomonas WT (+)* cells incubated in log phase for
72 hours with ^{3}H-E.coli DNA.

Three fractions corresponding to the elution diagram of poly-L-ornithine stimulated cells (see fig. 10 above) were dialysed and banded
in CsCl gradients (fig. 11). The results show that, according to the
position of these fractions in the elution diagram, *E. coli* ^{3}H-DNA
showing some degree of polymerization could be recovered from the
cells. However, the radioactive compounds present in fractions
9 - 10 do not band in the gradient although they represent TCA-pre-
cipitable counts and are non-dialysable.

     In conclusion, *Chlamydomonas WT (+)* cells are capable of taking
up *E. coli* DNA but this DNA is degrated to yield degradation products
with a wide spectrum of M.W. The facts that very little radioactivity
is eluted together with the void volume and that there is no incorporation of radioactivity into *Chlamydomonas* endogenous DNA show that
integration of detectable amounts of donor DNA into the recipient genomes (nuclear + chloroplast) does not occur under our experimental
conditions.

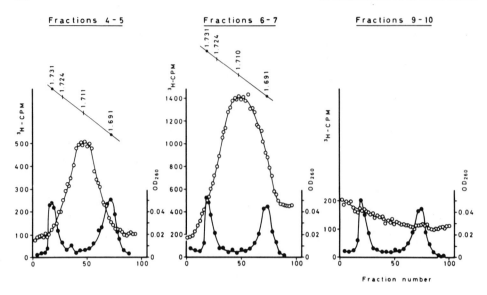

Fig.11 - CsCl density gradient centrifugation of pooled fractions
obtained after molecular sieving on Sepharose 4B of poly-
L-ornithine + *E. coli* ³H-DNA treated *Chlamydomonas* (see
fig.10) ³H-CPM, 0 - 0, OD₂₆₀ of marker DNA's, ● - ●.

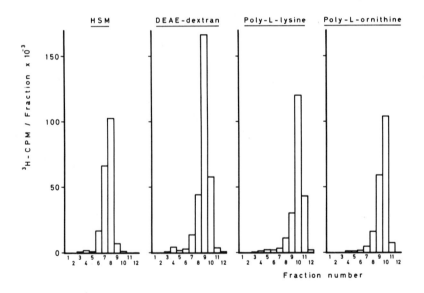

Fig.12 - Molecular sieving on Sepharose 4B of extracts of DNase -
treated *Chlamydomonas WT (+)* cells incubated in early stationary phase for 72 hours with *E. coli* in ³H-DNA.

b) Uptake in early stationary phase

Chlamydomonas cells at a concentration of 1.7 x 10[7] cells/ml were
incubated with *E. coli* ^{3}H-DNA as described above. They were DNase -
treated after extensive washing with HSM. Extracts were then run on
agarose columns in order to determine the M.W. distribution of radioactivity. It was found (fig. 12) that polycations had no stimulatory
effect on DNA uptake by stationary phase cells and that the distribution of radioactivity was not as polydisperse as in the case of log
phase cells. In this case however, due to the larger number of cells,
significant radioactivity (up to 10,000 CPM) was found in the void
volume. When these fractions were banded in CsCl gradients (fig. 13)
as above it was found that radioactivity was located in both the
nuclear and the chloroplast DNA regions of the gradient. However, the
specific activity of chloroplast DNA was much higher than that of
nuclear DNA.

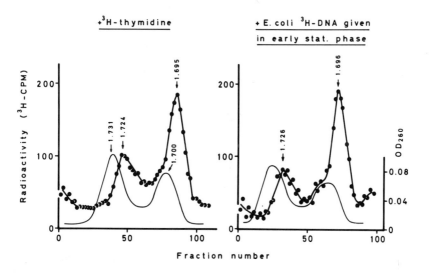

Fig. 13 - Left : Banding pattern in a CsCl gradient of ^{3}H-thymidine
                  labeled *Chlamydomonas* DNA - ^{3}H-CPM, ● - ●; solid
                  line represents OD_{260} of marker DNA's.
         Right : Banding pattern in a CsCl gradient of DNA recovered
                  from *Chlamydomonas WT (+)* cells treated with *E. coli*
                  ^{3}H-DNA for 72 hours in early stationary phase. Same
                  symbols.

Exactly the same banding pattern is obtained if the cells are labeled
with ^{3}H-thymidine (see also fig.4). In conclusion, cells in early
stationary phase break down donor DNA and are able to reuse the [3]H-
thymidine-containing breakdown products to synthesize endogenous DNA.

The same phenomenon might occur in log phase cells but would be masked by the presence of depolymerized donor DNA inside the cells. Little
radioactivity is found to be reutilized by the cells despite the presence of high amounts of DNA breakdown products inside the cells. This
is expected since thymidine is utilized only to a small extent by
Chlamydomonas for DNA synthesis (16 and this study). Furthermore, if
donor DNA is extensively degraded with added pancreatic DNase and
then given to the cells, it is seen (fig. 14) that only little radioactivity is associated with high M.W. *Chlamydomonas* DNA (fractions
3,4 and 5) and most of the degradation products are preserved in
the pool.

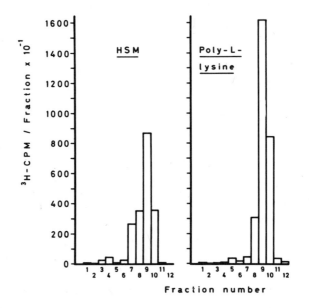

Fig. 14 – Molecular sieving on Sepharose 4B of extracts of *Chlamy-*
        domonas WT *(+)* cells treated for 72 hours in log phase
        with degradation products of *E. coli* ³H-DNA obtained after
        treatment of the **donor** DNA with 50 µg/ml pancreatic DNase
        for 15 min at 37°.

Autoradiographic evidence (V. Kovalinkova, R.F. Matagne and R. Loppes,
unpublished) seemed to support the fact that the *Chlamydomonas* cells
which were labeled after the addition of *E. coli* ³H-DNA to the cultures showed structural abnormalities. In order to investigate whether
dead or dying cells would preferentially take up or bind DNA in stationary phase, degrade it and reutilize it to some extent, the following experiment was done.

Cells in early stationary phase were given *E. coli* ³H-DNA and
incubated for 72 hours. An aliquot was then removed, washed with HSM,
treated with DNase and run through the agarose column. A significant
amount of radioactivity was collected in the excluded fractions (fig.
15) and corresponded to reutilization of donor DNA degradation products.

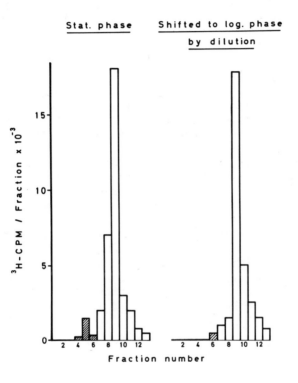

Fig. 15 - Left : Molecular sieving on Sepharose 4B of extracts of
                  Chlamydomonas WT (+) cells treated for 72 hours in
                  early stationary phase with *E. coli* ³H-DNA.
          Right: An aliquot of the stationary phase culture con-
                  taining donor DNA was diluted in fresh HSM in order
                  to bring the cells back to the log phase of growth.
                  Incubation was continued for another 24 hours and
                  an aliquot containing a number of cells equivalent
                  to that in the original aliquot was processed for mo-
                  lecular sieving on Sepharose 4B

However, when an equivalent aliquot of these cells was diluted in
fresh culture medium in order to bring the cells back into log phase,
it is seen that this high M.W. fraction is completely lost. Our inter-

pretation of this phenomenon is that dead or dying cells do indeed preferentially take up and reutilize donor DNA in early stationary phase. But these cells lyse after transfer to fresh medium, which would explain the loss of labeled endogenous DNA. This conclusion is supported by the findings of Howell and Walker (22) who showed that *Chlamydomonas* killed by a toluene treatment is still able to incorporate TTP mainly into chloroplast DNA; this occurs even in the absence of added ATP. It is not unlikely that ^{3}H-TMP or ^{3}H-TdR released after degradation of donor DNA inside the cells could be rephosphorylated and subsequently incorporated into endogenous *Chlamydomonas* DNA.

CONCLUSION

Chlamydomonas reinhardi WT (+) cells are able to take up small amounts of labelled bacterial DNA. This donor DNA appears to be progressively degraded inside the cells and a small fraction of the breakdown products is reutilized for endogenous DNA synthesis. The combination of molecular sieving on agarose gels with the CsCl density gradient centrifugation technique, together with the unique feature of *C. reinhardi* to incorporate ^{3}H-thymidine mainly into its chloroplast DNA allowed us to draw such a straightforward conclusion. No integration of donor DNA sequences could be detected in this system. It is noted that this phenomenon cannot be completely ruled out since calculations show that extremely small (2 x 10^{-3}%* of endogenous DNA), but biologically significant amounts of donor DNA could be taken up and maintained in the cells and still remain undetected for obvious reasons, like the limits of detection and extremely limited total radioactivity of the donor DNA if it does integrate within the host genome.

ACKNOWLEDGEMENTS

We wish to thank Ms. V. Kovalinkova, Drs. R.F. Matagne and R. Loppes (University of Liège) and Dr. A. Kleinhofs (Washington State University, Pullman, U.S.A.) for discussion and advice.

Thanks are also due to Prof. L. Ledoux (CEN/SCK, Mol and University of Liège) for discussion and support.

* This calculation was made assuming a M.W. of 5 x 10^{10} daltons for *Chlamydomonas* nuclear genome and assuming that a piece of donor DNA of 10^6 M.W. is taken up by 10^3 cells in a culture containing 10^8 cells.

REFERENCES

1. Ledoux, L., and Huart, R. - Nature 218, 1256 (1968)

2. Ledoux, L., and Huart, R. - J. Mol. Biol. 43,243 (1969)

3. Ledoux, L., Huart, R., and Jacobs, M. - Eur. J. Biochem. 23,96 (1971)

4. Bendich, A.J., and Filner, P. - Mutation Res. 13, 199 (1971)

5. Hotta, Y. and Stern, H. - Informative Molecules in Biological
   Systems-North-Holland Publishing Cy. Ed. L. Ledoux p.176 (1971)

6. Rebel, W., Hemleben, V. and Seyffert, W.-Z. - für Naturforsch. 28,
   473 (1973)

7. Doy, C.H., Gresshoff, P.M. and Rolfe, B.G. - Proc. Natl. Acad.
   Sci. 70, 723 (1973)

8. Heyn, R.F. and Schilperoort, R.A. - Colloques internationaux C.N.R.S.
   212, 385 (1973)

9. Johnson, C.B., Grierson, D. and Smith, H. - Nature New Biology,
   244, 105 (1973)

10. Ohyama, K., Gamborg, O.L. and Miller, R.A., - Can. J. of Botany
    50, 2077 (1972)

11. Hoffman, F.-Z. Pflanzenphysiol. 69, 249 (1973)

12. Hoffman, F. and Hess, D. - Z. Pflanzenphysiol. 69,81 (1973)

13. Redei, G., This volume

14. Bianchi, F. and Walet-Foederer, H.G. - Acta Bot. Neerl. 23, 1
    (1974)

15. Davies, D.R. and Plaskitt, A. - Genet. Res. Camb. 17, 33 (1971)

16. Swinton, D.C. and Hanawalt, P.C., - J. Cell. Biol. 54, 592 (1972)

17. Marmur, J. - J. Mol. Biol. 3, 208 (1961)

18. Heyn, R.F., Hermans, A.K. and Schilperoort, R.A. - Plant Science
    Letters 2, 73 (1974)

19. Sueoka, N. - Proc. Natl. Acad. Sci. 46, 83 (1960)

20. Lurquin, P., Tshitenge, G. , Delaunoit, G. and Ledoux, L. - Sub-
    mitted for publication

21. Hearst, J.E. and Vinograd, J. - Proc. Natl. Acad. Sci. 43, 581 (1957)

22. Howell, S.H. and Walker, L.L. - Proc. Natl. Acad. Sci. 69, 490 (1972)

MOLECULAR HYBRIDIZATION AND ITS APPLICATION TO RNA TUMOR VIRUS RESEARCH

Michel JANOWSKI

Centre d'Etude de l'Energie Nucléaire, Department of
Radiobiology, B-2400   Mol, Belgium

A. INTRODUCTION

The remarkable fact that, under appropriate conditions, the
two strands of native DNA can be dissociated and reassociated *in
vitro* (Doty et al., 1960 ; Marmur and Lane, 1960) supplied a usefull tool for the examination of genetic homologies. The formation
of hybrid molecules could be demonstrated from the DNA of two different bacterial species (Schildkraut et al., 1961a) or viruses
(Schildkraut et al., 1962). This basic methodology was soon extended to the formation of RNA-DNA hybrid molecules (Hall and Spiegelman, 1960 ; Schildkraut et al., 1961b). In order to prevent the
competition between the hybridization process and the reannealing
of DNA in the reaction medium, techniques were developed for the
immobilization of single-stranded DNA in cellulose (Bautz and Hall,
1962), in agar (Bolton and Mc Carthy, 1962) and on nitrocellulose
filters (Nygaard and Hall, 1964 ; Gillespie and Spiegelman, 1965).
So it became possible to measure the extent of reassociation of
radioactivity labeled single-stranded DNA or RNA with the immobilized DNA.

Reassociation of vertebrate DNA was first observed in 1963
(Hoyer et al., 1963). It had been expected that the enormous dilution of individual nucleotide sequences in the large quantity of
DNA in each cell would result in a very slow reaction, requiring
months for its completion (Huebner and Todaro, 1969). However, si-
zable reactions were produced after quite short times (Hoyer et
al., 1963, 1964). The investigation of this paradox led to the demonstration that some nucleotide sequences are repeated in the DNA
of eukaryotes (Waring and Britten, 1966 ; Britten and Kohne, 1968).
These multiple base sequences reassociate rapidly, but the thermal

stability of the resulting duplexes is much lower than expected
from their guanosine + cytidine content (Martin and Hoyer, 1966),
reflecting various degrees of base pair mismatching.

The elegant and detailed studies of Britten and Kohne (1968)
on the rate of DNA reassociation allowed the development of a new
method for RNA-DNA hybridization (Melli et al., 1971). Hybridization of radioactively labeled RNA in the presence of vast unlabeled DNA excess can be used to analyze any defined fraction of cellular RNA, in terms of reiteration frequencies of the complementary DNA sequences. It became possible, by using this method, to assay homologies between RNA and nonrepetitive deoxyribonucleotide
sequences. Adapting the technique to DNA-DNA hybridization, Gelb
et al. (1971b) could determine directly the number of DNA tumor
virus genomes integrated into the genome of various normal and
virus-transformed cells. The sensitivity of the method was such
that less than one viral genome equivalent per diploid cell could
be detected.

The latest development of the molecular hybridization techniques consists in the use of molecular probes as a new way to
study gene expression. The probes consist of radioactively labeled
DNA, that is synthesized *in vitro* from a specific messenger
(Kacian et al., 1972 ; Verma et al., 1972) or viral (Gelb et al.,
1971a ; Varmus et al., 1972b) RNA with RNA-dependent DNA polymerase (reverse transcriptase : Baltimore, 1970 ; Temin and Mizutani,
1970). Recently, these probes were extensively used in cancer research, to detect RNA tumor virus-specific sequences in the DNA
(Neiman, 1973 ; Varmus et al., 1972b, 1973b) and in various RNA
populations (Benveniste et al., 1973 ; Varmus et al., 1973a) of
infected and uninfected cells or tissues.

B. THE NOTION OF COT

The reassociation of a pair of complementary sequences results from their collision. Therefore, the reaction rate depends
on their concentration. The renaturation kinetics is a second-
order process (Marmur and Doty, 1961 ; Marmur et al., 1963 ; Huebner and Todaro, 1969), and the rate-determining step appears to be
the initial nucleation reaction rather than the subsequent "zippe-
ring" process. The reaction rate is given by the equation :

$$\frac{dC}{dt} = - kC^2$$

in which C is the single-stranded DNA concentration at any time t,
and k the second-order rate constant. It follows that, at any time
after the initiation of the reaction, the fraction of DNA which
remains single-stranded is expressed by :

$$\frac{C}{C_0} = \frac{1}{1+kC_0t}$$

where C_0 is the initial single-stranded DNA concentration, thus the total DNA concentration in the reaction medium. The controlling parameter for estimating the completion of the reaction is Cot. It is expressed in moles of nucleotides times seconds per liter.

The DNA of each organism may be characterized by the value of Cot at which the reaction is half completed under controlled conditions :

$$Cot_{1/2} = \frac{1}{k}$$

Since, for a given DNA concentration, increasing DNA complexity (genome size) results in proportionally decreasing concentrations of homologous sequences, one would expect the $Cot^1/_2$ to be directly proportional to the genome size. This expectation was exactly borne out in all the examined cases (Fig. 1).

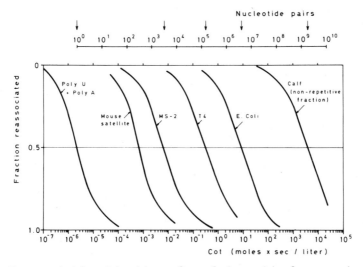

Fig. 1 - Reassociation kinetics of nucleic acids from various sources. Redrawn from Britten and Kohne (15).

However, this fact is only true in the absence of repeated sequences. Actually, the DNA's of higher organisms contain three more or less distinct classes of reiteration : a highly reiterated fraction (frequency of about 10^6) which, in some cases, is sufficiently different in base composition from the bulk of the DNA to appear as a satellite band in a cesium chloride gradient ; an intermediate fraction, which is a heterogenous group of sequences with

reiteration frequencies ranging from 10^3 to 10^5 ; and a nonrepea-
ted (unique) fraction. In the case of mouse DNA, these fractions
represent about 10, 20 and 70 % of the genome, respectively
(Fig. 2).

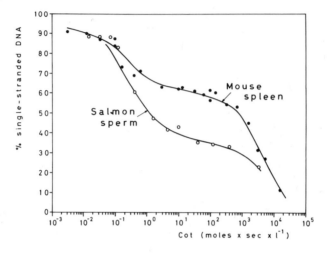

Fig. 2 - Reassociation kinetics of mouse spleen (●) and salmon
         sperm (o) DNA. The proportion of single-stranded and
         double-stranded material was determined by the hydroxy-
         apatite method.

C. CONDITIONS FOR REASSOCIATION. REACTION SPECIFICITY

       The rate of DNA renaturation is determined by the frequency
of collisions between complementary strands (Marmur and Doty,
1961 ; Marmur et al., 1963 ; Huebner and Todaro, 1969). In order
to achieve reproducible reassociation kinetics, one should control
the factors affecting the reaction rate, i.e. ionic strength, temperature, viscosity and DNA fragment size. The reaction proceeds
most rapidly at high ionic strength (Marmur and Doty, 1961 ; Wettmur and Davidson, 1968) and the optimum temperature is about 20
to 25°C below the temperature required for the dissociation of the
resulting double strands (Marmur and Doty, 1961 ; Wettmur and
Davidson, 1968). Therefore, short or highly mismatched complexes,
having a low melting temperature, will not form at the elevated
temperatures optimal for a true, specific renaturation. Nucleic
acids of distantly related organisms thus will associate more readily at lower temperatures (Martin and Hoyer, 1966). Similarly,
optimal temperature for the renaturation of redundant sequences
of eukaryote DNA will be lower than that for the renaturation of

unique sequences (Church and Mc Carthy, 1968 ; Mc Carthy and Mc
Conaughy, 1968). DNA fragment size can be controlled by shearing
the molecules by sonication or by pressure drop through a needle
valve, usually to a length of about 250 nucleotide pairs.

Even at the highest practical concentrations, renaturation
of mammalian DNA may take weeks, with consequent risk of chain
scission and depurination at high temperatures. However, reassociation occurs at much lower temperatures in the presence of some
organic solvents which weaken the hydrogen bonds. In appropriate
conditions, annealing reactions proceed at 37°C in the presence of
formamide, without any loss in specificity (Mc Conaughy et al.,
1969).

Finally, it should be noted that the rate of reassociation
of RNA or DNA fragments with DNA immobilized on an appropriate
support is markedly reduced, compared to the rate in solution (Mc
Carthy, 1967).

D. THE MEASUREMENT OF REASSOCIATION

The relative proportion of single and double-stranded nucleic
acids, at any stage of the annealing reaction, can be measured in
a variety of ways. Double-stranded complexes absorb less ultraviolet light and display a greater degree of optical activity than
single-stranded molecules do. Base-paired RNA is no longer susceptible to the action of ribonuclease (Yankofsky and Spiegelman,
1962a, 1962b). When reassociation of radioactive RNA or DNA is
performed with unlabeled, immobilized DNA strands, unbound radioactive material can be washed away after the required incubation
period (Bolton and Mc Carthy, 1962 ; Gillespie and Spiegelman,
1965).

RNA-DNA hybrids can be physically separated from the parental
molecules by chromatography on methylated albumin-coated kiesel-
guhr (Hayashi et al., 1965) or by equilibrium sedimentation in
cesium salt gradients (Hall and Spiegelman, 1960 ; Giacomoni and
Spiegelman, 1962 ; Goodman and Rich, 1962 ; Yankofsky and Spiegelman, 1962b). Another usefull technique depends on the fact that
single-stranded nucleic acids are eluted from hydroxylapatite at
much lower ionic strength than double-stranded complexes (Bernardi, 1965 ; Miyazawa and Thomas, 1965 ; Walker and Mc Laren, 1965).
Hydroxylapatite chromatography was performed successfully at room
temperature in the presence of formamide (Goodman et al., 1973).

Finally, the S1-nuclease extracted from *Aspergillus oryzae* specifically and completely digests single-stranded RNA and DNA (Sutton,
1971 ; Vogt, 1973). It is, at the present time, widely used for the
measurement of reassociation of homologous nucleic acid sequences.

E. APPLICATIONS TO THE STUDIES ON RNA TUMOR VIRUSES

Tumor viruses fall in two distinct groups : the DNA and the RNA-containing viruses. Oncogenic RNA viruses (also called oncorna-viruses or RNA tumor viruses) are generally divided into three main morphological classes, labeled A, B and C. Most C-type viruses cause, in a large number of animal species, mainly leukemias, lymphomas and sarcomas, all tumors arising in tissues of mesodermal origin. Type B RNA viruses, fewer in number, are primarily associated with breast carcinomas. Type A RNA viruses are only found as intracellular particles and have not been shown to elicit tumors.

Oncornaviruses display the unique property of containing simultaneously a relatively large RNA genome (12×10^6 daltons, sedimentation coefficient of about 70 S) (Duesberg and Robinson, 1966 ; Mora et al., 1966) and an RNA-directed DNA polymerase, or reverse transcriptase (Baltimore, 1970 ; Temin and Mizutani, 1970), an enzyme capable of using the viral RNA as a template to generate a DNA complementary copy. In addition, this copy is converted into a double-stranded form by a DNA dependent DNA polymerase activity (Spiegelman et al., 1970).

After an oncornavirus has entered a cell and shed its protein coat, there is production of a DNA copy of the viral genome by the reverse transcriptase. This intermediate, called provirus, is generally believed to become integrated into the host cell genome to produce a virogene. The virus contains an endonuclease (Mizutani et al., 1971a), an exonuclease (Mizutani et al., 1971b) and a ligase (Mizutani et al., 1971b), all the enzymes required for cleaving cellular DNA, inserting the provirus and mending the break.

1. Evidence for the integration of the viral genome

Highly radioactive, virus-specific DNA can be synthesized *in vitro* by the endogenous reverse transcriptase reaction of partially disrupted virions (Spiegelman et al., 1970). Unlabeled cellular DNA's can be tested for virus-specific nucleotide sequences by their capacity to accelerate the reassociation kinetics of the labeled DNA probe. In all the cases that were examined, viral genomes were shown to be at least partially present in multiple copies in the DNA of both healthy and infected cells and tissues of the natural host (Gelb et al., 1971a ; Varmus et al., 1972a, 1972b; Neiman, 1973) (Fig. 3).

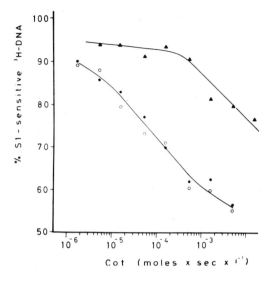

Fig. 3 - Reassociation kinetics of Rauscher leukemia virus-specific
H³-DNA (4.3 ng/ml) in the presence of salmon sperm DNA,
15 mg/ml (▲), normal BALB/c spleen DNA, 15 mg/ml (●),
and leukemic BALB/c spleen DNA, 15 mg/ml (o).

These results were only half surprizing, since it had been known
that leukemia viruses could be induced by nonviral agents from apparently uninfected cells and in apparently healthy animals (Aaronson et al., 1971 ; Lowy et al., 1971 ; Weiss et al., 1971). As a
consequence, the integration of "exogenous" viral genomes upon
infection with an oncornavirus, could not be proved in a natural
system because of the lack of specific markers which could distinguish between exogenous and endogenous viral genes.

However, actual integration was demonstrated in the case of
some heterologous systems, upon infection of duck and mouse cells
with a chicken sarcoma virus (Varmus et al., 1973b).

2. Transcription of the integrated viral genomes

The *in vitro* synthesized, radioactively labeled viral DNA
can be used as a probe to detect virus-specific sequences in any
cellular RNA population. Evidence was obtained that virus-specific
sequences are present in cytoplasmic (Fan and Baltimore, 1973 ;

Varmus et al., 1973a), polyribosomial (Vecchio et al., 1973) and
nuclear (Leong et al., 1972) RNA of transformed cells and of cancer tissues. More direct evidence that the viral RNA transcripts
originate at the level of the integrated genes came from experiments recently performed in our laboratory. It was shown that mu-
rine leukemia virus-specific RNA is present to a much larger extent
in leukemic mouse spleen chromatin than in normal spleen chromatin
(Fig. 4). Moreover, we were able to demonstrate that chromatin
from leukemic spleen serves as a template for bacterial RNA polymerase to synthesize virus-specific RNA *in vitro* (Fig. 5). Whether
the transcription occurs at the level of newly integrated or of
preexisting viral genes cannot be discussed at the present time,
because of the lack of specific markers.

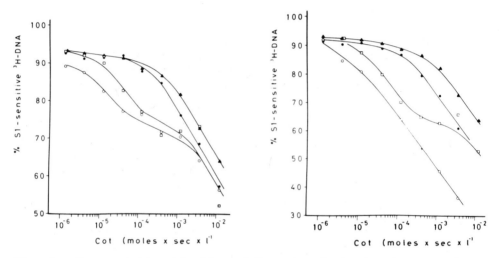

Fig. 4 - Reassociation kinetics of Rauscher leukemia virus-speci-
         fic H3-DNA (7 ng/ml) in the presence of viral RNA, 1.4
         μg/ml (□), endogenous RNA from normal BALB/c spleen chro-
         matin, 200 μg/ml (●), endogenous RNA from leukemic BALB/c
         spleen chromatin, 600 μg/ml (o), and no RNA (▲).

Fig. 5 - Reassociation kinetics of Rauscher leukemia virus-speci-
         fic ³H-DNA (7 ng/ml) in the presence of viral RNA, 2.8
         μg/ml (□), *in vitro* RNA transcripts from normal BALB/c
         spleen chromatin, 1.1 mg/ml (●), *in vitro* RNA transcripts
         from leukemic BALB/c spleen chromatin, 1.3 mg/ml (o),
         and no RNA (▲).

BIBLIOGRAPHY

Aaronson, S.A., Todaro, G.J., and Scolnick, E.M. (1971), Science, 174, 157.

Baltimore, D. (1970), Nature, 226, 1209.

Bautz, E.K.F., and Hall, B.D. (1962), Proc. Natl. Acad. Sci., 48, 400.

Benveniste, R.E., Todaro, G.J., Scolnick, E.M.,and Parks, W.P. (1973), J. Virol., 12, 711.

Bernardi, G. (1965), Nature, 206, 779.

Bolton, E.T., and Mc Carthy, B.J. (1962), Proc. Natl. Acad. Sci., 48, 1390.

Britten, R.J., and Kohne, D.E. (1968), Science, 161, 529.

Church, R.B., and Mc Carthy, B.J. (1968), Biochem. Genet., 2, 55.

Doty, P., Marmur, J., Eigner, J., and Schildkraut, C. (1960), Proc. Natl. Acad. Sci., 46, 461.

Duesberg, P.H., and Robinson, W.S. (1966), Proc. Natl. Acad. Sci., 55, 219.

Fan, H., and Baltimore, D. (1973), J. Mol. Biol., 80, 93.

Gelb, L., Aaronson, S.A., and Martin, M. (1971a), Science, 172, 1353.

Gelb, L.D., Kohne, D.E., and Martin, M.A. (1971b), J. Mol. Biol., 57, 129.

Giacomoni, D., and Spiegelman, S. (1962), Science, 138, 1328.

Gillespie, D., and Spiegelman, S. (1965), J. Mol. Biol., 12, 829.

Goodman, H.M., and Rich, A. (1962), Proc. Natl. Acad. Sci., 48, 2101.

Goodman, N.C., Gulati, S.C., Redfield, R., and Spiegelman, S. (1973), Anal. Biochem., 52, 286.

Hall, B.D., and Spiegelman, S. (1960), Proc. Natl. Acad. Sci., 47, 137.

Hayashi, M., Hayashi, M.N., and Spiegelman, S. (1965), Biophys. J., 231, 1965.

Hoyer, B.H., Mc Carthy, B.J., and Bolton, E.T. (1963), Science, 140, 1408.

Hoyer, B.H., Mc Carthy, B.J., and Bolton, E.T. (1964), Science, 144, 959.

Huebner, R.A., and Todaro, G.J. (1969), Proc. Natl. Acad. Sci., 64, 1087.

Kacian, D.L., Spiegelman, S., Bank, A., Terada, S., Metafora, S., Dow, L. and Marks, P.A. (1972), Nature New Biology, 235, 167.

Leong, J.A., Garapin, A.C., Jackson, N., Fanshier, L., Levinson, W., and Bishop, J.M. (1972), J. Virol., 9, 891.

Lowy, D.R., Rowe, R.P., Teich, N., and Hartley, J.W. (1971), Science, 174, 155.

Marmur, J., and Doty, P. (1971), J. Mol. Biol., 3, 585.

Marmur, J., Rownd, R., and Schildkraut, C.L. (1963), Progr. Nucleic Acid Res., 1, 231.

Marmur, J., and Lane, D. (1960), Proc. Natl. Acad. Sci., 46, 453.

Martin, M.A., and Hoyer, B.H. (1966), Biochemistry, 5, 2706.

Mc Carthy, B.J. (1967), Bacteriol. Rev., 31, 215.

Mc Carthy, B.J.,and Mc Conaughy, B.L. (1968), Biochem. Genet., 2, 37.

Mc Conaughy, B.L., Laird, C.D., and Mc Carthy, B.J. (1969), Biochem., 8, 3289.

Melli, M., Whitfield, C., Rao, K.V., Richardson, M., and Bishop, J.O. (1971), Nature New Biology, 231, 8.

Miyazawa, Y., and Thomas, C.A. (1965), J. Mol. Biol., 11, 223.

Mizutani, S., Boettinger, D., and Temin, H.M. (1971a), Nature, 228, 424.

Mizutani, S., Temin, H.M., Kodama, M., and Wells, R.T. (1971b), Nature New Biology, 230, 232.

Mora, P.T., Mc Farland, V.W., and Luborsky, S.W. (1966), Proc. Natl. Acad. Sci., 55, 438.

Neiman, P.E. (1973), Science, 178, 750.

Nygaard, A.P., and Hall, B.D. (1964), J. Mol. Biol., 9, 125.

Schildkraut, C.L., Marmur, J., and Doty, P. (1961a), J. Mol. Biol., 3, 595.

Schildkraut, C.L., Marmur, J., Fresco, J.R., and Doty, P. (1961b), J. Biol. Chem., 236, PC2.

Schildkraut, C.L., Wierzchowski, K.L., Marmur, J., Green, D.M., and Doty, P. (1962), Virology, 18, 43.

Spiegelman, S., Burny, A., Das, M.R., Keydar, J., Sehlom, J., Travnicek, M., and Watson, K. (1970), Nature, 227, 563.

Sutton, W.D. (1971), Biochim. Biophys. Acta, 240, 522.

Temin, H.M., and Mizutani, S. (1970), Nature, 226, 1311.

Varmus, H.E., Bishop, J.M., Nowinski, R.C., and Sarker, N.H. (1972a), Nature New Biology, 238, 189.

Varmus, H.E., Weiss, R.A., Friis, R.R., Levinson, W.E., and Bishop, J.M. (1972b), Proc. Natl. Acad. Sci., 69, 20.

Varmus, H.E., Quintrell, N., Medeiras, E., Bishop, J.M., Nowinski, R.C., and Sarker, N. (1973a), J. Mol. Biol., 79, 663.

Varmus, H.E., Vogt, P.K., and Bishop, J.M. (1973b), Proc. Natl. Acad. Sci., 70, 3067.

Vecchio, G., Tsuchida, N., Shanmugam, G., and Green, M. (1973), Proc. Natl. Acad. Sci., 70, 2064.

Verma, I.M., Temple, G.F., Fan, H., and Baltimore, D. (1972), Nature New Biology, 235, 163.

Vogt, V.M. (1973), Eur. J. Biochem., 33 , 192.

Walker, P.M.B., and Mc Laren, A. (1965), Nature, 208, 1175.

Waring, M., and Britten, R.J. (1966), Science, 154, 791.

Weiss, R.A., Friis, R.R., Katz, E., and Vogt, P.K. (1971), Virology, 46, 920.

Wettmur, J.G., and Davidson, N. (1968), J. Mol. Biol., 31, 349.

Yankofsky, N.A., and Spiegelman, S. (1962a), Proc. Natl. Acad. Sci., 48, 106.

Yankofsky, N.A., and Spiegelman, S. (1962b), Proc. Natl. Acad. Sci., 48, 146.

DNA-HYBRIDIZATION STUDIES OF THE FATE OF BACTERIAL DNA IN PLANTS*

A. Kleinhofs**

Department of Radiobiology
Centre d'Etude de l'Energie Nucleaire CEN/SCK
2400 Mol, Belgium

INTRODUCTION

Evidence for the uptake and integration of foreign (bacterial) donor DNA into plants, following application of donor DNA to seeds, has been reported in several systems by Ledoux and his collaborators (12,14). In some experiments, radioactive donor DNA is used, while in others, unlabeled DNA is applied and treated plants are subsequently labeled with ^{3}H-thymidine. In both cases, the evidence for covalent joining of donor high buoyant density DNA and recipient low buoyant density DNA is the occurrence of a peak of radioactivity of intermediate density in treated plants. This intermediate peak upon sonication separates into components of approximately donor and recipient buoyant density. These observations are taken as evidence for joining of foreign DNA sequences. However, buoyant density is not a sufficient criterion to identify as donor bacterial DNA the "heavy" component which separates from intermediate density DNA upon sonication. One needs a criterion which identifies base sequences, not just the gross base composition of the DNA. Thus, DNA hybridization measurements are essential to support the model which Ledoux and his collaborators have proposed. This study was undertaken in order to provide such an analysis of intermediate density DNA.

---

*Scientific Paper No. 4322. College of Agriculture Research Center, Washington State University, Pullman, Project 1920.

**On Professional Leave from Washington State University, Department of Agronomy and Soils and Program in Genetics, Pullman, Washington, 99163, U.S.A.

This paper will describe techniques of DNA hybridization as they apply to a study of the fate of exogenous DNA in barley.

DNA/DNA-filter hybridization and DNA/DNA-reassociation in solution will be discussed in detail. RNA/DNA-filter hybridization has already been dealt with (Schilperoort, this volume). For specific studies dealing with the sensitivity of this technique for detection of small amounts of DNA in mixtures see Eden et al. (1).

MATERIALS AND METHODS

DNA/DNA-filter hybridization is a well established technique first described by Denhardt (2). The method is a modification of the RNA/DNA-filter hybridization technique described by Gillespie and Spiegelman (3). For a comprehensive treatment of filter hybridization techniques see Gillespie (4). We use small (6 mm) filters cut out with a paper punch from a large (47 mm) filter. For hybridization the filters are mounted on pins and incubated in small test tubes (10 x 53 mm) with 0.2 ml solution. Techniques for DNA-filter preparation and use (1,5) are summarized in Tables 1 and 2. The amount of DNA bound to the filter was determined by

Table 1

Preparation of DNA Filters for Hybridization (1,5)

DNA Preparation:

1. DNA in 0.1XSSC denatured by NaOH (0.1 N final conc.)
2. Cool and neutralize with 1 M KH_2PO_4
3. Adjust to desired salt conc. (5 x SSC)

Filter preparation:

1. Soak and wash filter with 5 x SSC
2. Load DNA with gentle suction
3. Wash with 5 x SSC
4. Incubate in pre-incubation* mixture (1 hr)
5. Blot dry and punch out 6 mm filters
6. Dry at room temp. (ca. 2 hrs)
7. Bake in oven (65°) overnight
8. Assay for DNA content

*0.2 g/l of Ficoll, Bovine Serum Albumin, and Polyvinyl Pyrrolidone (PVP 360 Sigma) in the same salt solution as used for DNA loading (see Reference 2).

Table 2

Use of DNA Filters for Hybridization

---

1. DNA filters are mounted on pins.
2. Add 0.2 ml hybridization solution containing sheared, denatured labeled DNA in 1XSSC, usually.
3. Overlay with mineral oil to prevent evaporation; cap with aluminum foil.
4. Incubate at appropriate temperature overnight.
5. Wash filters in 3 serial rinses (same salt as hybridization solution) held at incubation temperature.
6. Dry under heat lamp.
7. Drop in toluene based scintillation fluid and count. (The filter is left mounted on the pin during counting.)

---

assaying representative 6 mm filters from each large filter by Burton's (6) diphenylamine procedure (1,5). Radioactivity bound to the filter during hybridization should be checked for reaction specificity by its melting behaviour. This can easily be done by washing the counted filters in toluene to remove scintillants, drying, transferring to 1XSSC and measuring the release of radioactivity during 5' incubations at temperatures ranging from 60-100° C in 5° C intervals (1).

For comprehensive treatment of DNA/DNA-solution hybridization and hydroxyapatite chromatography techniques see Britten et al. (7) and Bernardi (8) respectively. The specific techniques used in our laboratory are those of Chilton et al. (9) and are summarized in Tables 3 and 4. Renaturation kinetics are plotted according to

Table 3

Solution Hybridization

---

1. DNA samples (sheared) are made up in hybridization solution at appropriate concentrations.
2. Take up in capillary tubes at 10-50 μl/sample.
3. Seal both ends in flame.
4. Denature in boiling water bath 5 min.
5. Transfer to water bath at appropriate temperature.
6. Capillaries are removed at desired times and chilled in ice water. Time series should be logarithmic, e.g., 5', 10', 20', 40', etc.
7. Samples are subsequently diluted into 1 ml of 0.15 M phosphate buffer and capillary tube is rinsed several times.
8. Diluted samples may be stored in refrigerator for later assay.

Table 4

Hydroxyapatite Procedure (9)

1. Hydroxyapatite (Biorad HTP) is suspended in 0.15 M PB.*
2. Remove fines by decanting 3 times.
3. Load in columns (5-inch Pasteur pipettes) at 0.5-1.0 ml/column.
    Columns and all solutions must be held at appropriate temper-
    ature (60°-70° C).
4. Wash with 2.0 ml 0.15 M PB.
5. Apply DNA samples. Collect effluent and wash with 2 x 1.0 ml
    0.15 M PB (Single strand fractions).
6. Change collection tubes.
7. Elute duplexes with 2 x 1.0 ml 0.30 M PB.
8. Dilute single strand and duplex fractions to 4.0 ml with H_2O.
9. Add 15.0 ml triton scintillation cocktail. (Triton X-100:
    toluene scintillation fluid, 1:2 V/V.)
10. Mix and count at room temperature.
11. Native and denatured DNA controls must be included.
12. Counts eluted with 0.30 M PB divided by total counts = double
    stranded fraction.
13. Rough data may be corrected as indicated by the native and
    denatured controls.

---

*PB = equimolar quantities of monobasic and dibasic sodium
 phosphates.

Britten and Kohne (10). The Cot value is a product of the DNA
concentration (Co) in moles of nucleotides (assuming 320 g/l =
1 Molar solution) and time (t) in seconds. In some cases it is
advantageous to express Co as the concentration of the labeled
probe DNA only, and is then designated Po according to Chilton
et al. (9).

    DNA samples were sheared by sonication or depurination for 33
min. at 70° C followed by alkali cleavage (11) to approximate
single strand molecular weights of 1.5-2.0 x 10^5 daltons.

    Barley seeds were treated with exogenous DNA as described by
Ledoux and Huart (12). Bacterial contamination was monitored at
each step of the procedure by streaking solutions on nutrient agar
plates. Seed tips cut off prior to incubation in DNA were also
placed on nutrient agar plates. All plates were incubated at 24°
C for a minimum of three days.

    DNA from the various organs was isolated by the Pronase pro-
cedure of Ledoux and his collaborators (12,13) with minor

modifications. Plant parts, frozen with liquid N_2, were homogenized in a mortar and sodium borate (0.05 M) - EDTA (0.01 M) buffer
pH 9.0 was substituted for saline - EDTA. CsCl density gradient
analysis in fixed angle rotors was performed using standard procedures (13 and Charles, this volume). These modifications resulted
in obtaining barley DNA with molecular weight substantially higher
than previously reported (12).

RESULTS

Use of DNA/DNA-filter hybridization to look for integration of
foreign donor DNA

An experiment designed to detect the "intermediate" density
DNA of Ledoux and Huart (12) was performed using Sarcina flava
donor DNA (d = 1.730) and barley cultivars Himalaya, CI 3947 and
Trait d'Union. CsCl analysis of DNA for the Himalaya and Trait
d'Union root DNA samples (Fig. 1) show no unusual density DNA bands.
The peaks of radioactivity appear to correspond exactly to the
peaks of A.260 and are identical to those of the control samples
(not shown). Similar results were obtained with CI 3947 (not shown).
Under these conditions (36 hrs. incubation in H_2O) approximately
one-half of the total radioactivity was expected to be in an
intermediate density peak (see Fig. 7 and 14 in Ref. 12). Since
the high molecular weight of the barley DNA could mask the donor
DNA replicants in CsCl density gradient, a search for the presence
of the bacterial donor DNA was conducted by DNA/DNA-filter hybridization. The radioactive DNA peaks were pooled, sonicated, dialyzed
and hybridized with Sarcina flava DNA filters. It can be seen
(Table 5) that the amount of hybridization by the experimental (DNA-
treated) barley root DNA does not exceed that of the control. A
similar degree of hybridization to filters containing similar
amounts of DNA from an unrelated bacterium (Streptomyces coelicolor)
was also observed.

Taking into account the degree of hybridization between labeled
bacterial DNA and homologous filter bound DNA under identical conditions and with varying inputs, the sensitivity of the assay can
be estimated to be approximately 2%. Addition of 1.8% Sarcina flava
^{3}H-DNA to a control barley root DNA sample resulted in a detectable
increase in the extent of hybridization observed (Table 5). Thus,
it seems fair to conclude that in the experiment reported in Table
5 there can be no more than 2% of the bacterial donor DNA present.

Scutellum DNA samples prepared from the same experiment showed
no unusual density DNA peaks. DNA/DNA-filter hybridization results
(Table 6) show that experimental DNA exhibited very little binding

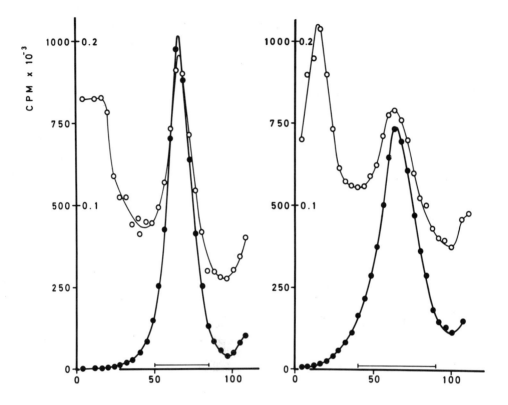

Figure 1. CsCl density gradient DNA analysis of Himalaya (left)
and Trait d'Union (right) root samples. Seeds were peeled, sterilized in 5% $Ca(OCl)_2$ 30 min., incubated in H_2O 11 hrs., Sarcina
flava DNA (1 mg/ml) 12 hrs., H_2O 36 hrs., and ^{3}H-TdR 6 hrs. Centrifugation was performed in a fixed angle rotor for 64 hrs. at
33,000 rpm 25° C. Phage 2C DNA (d = 1.742) was used as marker.
OD_{260} (o), ^{3}H (•).

to the Sarcina flava filters. Control scutellum DNA samples were
not available at 100,000 cpm input, but the control root DNA sample
showed higher binding than any of the exogenous DNA-treated
scutellum samples. Thus, it again seems clear that no large amount
of exogenous DNA has become associated and replicated with the
barley genome.

An experiment using Micrococcus lysodeikticus donor DNA (d =
1.731), cultivar Proctor barley* and 72 hrs. incubation in water

*The Proctor seed used in this experiment was from the same batch
as used by Ledoux and Huart (12). The seed had poor germination,
was old, and somewhat moldy.

Table 5

DNA/DNA-filter Hybridization* with Pooled DNA samples from Fig. 1
and Control DNA

Sample	DNA on filter**	CPM bound (-blank)	% of input***	Difference from highest control
Himalaya roots	S. flava	62	.06	
	S. coelicolor	151	.15	None
	Blank	129	.13	
Trait d'Union roots	S. flava	209	.21	
	S. flava	198	.20	None
	S. coelicolor	146	.15	
	Blank	74	.08	
Control roots	S. flava	214	.21	-
	Blank	116	.12	
Himalaya roots plus 1.8% S. flava (cpm/cpm)	S. flava	316	.31	.10
	Blank	88	.09	

*Hybridization in 2XSSC, 68° C for 18 hrs.
**S. flava = 2.1 μg S. coelicolor = 2.0 μg
***All inputs were ∼ 100,000 cpm

after DNA treatment was performed. The CsCl density gradient analysis of roots from samples sterilized by different techniques show
labeling of only endogenous barley DNA. Under comparable conditions,
Ledoux and Huart (12) showed most of the radioactivity to be in an
intermediate density peak. DNA/DNA hybridization data (Table 7)
were negative. In this case, the inputs were much lower and thus
sensitivity cannot be expected to be as high as in the other
samples.

At this point, it should be noted that the covered seeds
(Trait d'Union and Proctor) were not adequately sterilized by the
procedures used [i.e., hand or H_2SO_4 peeling and 30 min. in $Ca(OCl)_2$].
The naked seeds (Himalaya and CI 3947) were sterilized by the
$Ca(OCl)_2$ procedure.

Several bacterial contaminants were isolated from the Trait
d'Union and Proctor seeds. Single colony samples were grown, DNA
extracted and the buoyant density determined by model E ultracentrifugation. The results showed one sample with d = 1.720,
four with d = 1.714 and one with d = 1.701. Among the four with

Table 6

DNA/DNA-filter Hybridization* with Scutellum DNA Samples from S.
flava Treated Seeds.   Control scutellum DNA was not available at
100,000 cpm input, but compare with control root samples in Table 5

Sample	DNA on filter**	CPM bound (-blank)	% of input***
Himalaya scutellum abnormal	S. flava	110	.10
	Blank	52	.05
Himalaya scutellum	S. flava	146	.15
	Blank	46	.05
Trait d'Union scutellum	S. flava	93	.09
	Blank	41	.04

*Hybridization in 2XSSC, 68° C for 18 hrs.
**S. flava = 2.1 μg
***All inputs were ∼ 100,000 cpm

Table 7

DNA/DNA-filter Hybridization* with Root DNA Samples from M.
lysodeikticus Treated and Control Proctor Seeds

Sample	DNA on filter**	Input CPM	CPM bound (-blank)	% of input
Proctor roots, H_2SO_4 peeled seeds	M. lysodeikticus	16,488	0	-
	Rhizobium H229	16,488	25	0.15
Proctor roots, control	M. lysodeikticus	12,384	0	-
	Rhizobium H229	12,384	34	0.27
Proctor roots, hand peeled seeds	M. lysodeikticus	2,610	0	-
	Rhizobium H229	2,610	23	0.88
Proctor roots, control	M. lysodeikticus	3,456	0	-
	Rhizobium H229	3,456	12	0.35

*Hybridization in 2XSSC, 68° C for 18 hrs.
**M. lysodeikticus - 1.3 μg; Rhizobium H229 - 3.8 μg

d = 1.714, one had a distinctly different phenotype while the other three appeared to be somewhat similar.

A new batch of Proctor seed was obtained* and the above experiment repeated with the following modifications.

1. After the exogenous DNA treatment, the seedlings were fed water and ^{3}H-TdR only through the endosperm. In the previous experiments they were transferred to a film of water and ^{3}H-TdR and allowed to take it up through the roots.

2. After completion of the experiment, the seedlings were sectioned and the various organs (roots, shoots, scutellums, endosperms) stored frozen without alcohol.

Again sterilization was not effective. CsCl analysis of the root and scutellum samples showed an intermediate density (d = 1.715) DNA peak in all samples including controls (data not shown). This and the fact that sonication did not produce heterogeneity in the population indicated that this intermediate density DNA was due to bacterial contamination.

These experiments and more recent ones with sterile seeds [50% H_2SO_4, 2 hrs., room temperature on magnetic stirrer, followed by 5% $Ca(OCl)_2$ for 1 hr.] clearly indicate that no large amounts of exogenous DNA are replicated with the barley genome under these conditions. The nature of the experiments is such that only replicating exogenous DNA would have been detected.

Simultaneously with the above described experiments and under the same conditions barley seeds were also treated with ^{3}H-DNA from Sarcina flava. In these experiments integration in the absence of replication should be detectable. Since no intermediate density DNA peaks were ever observed, it was not possible to check this by filter hybridization techniques.

It is possible to perform filter hybridization experiments which will detect bacterial DNA in plants without the prerequisite of replication. In this case the unlabeled DNA from plants presumed to contain exogenous DNA should be immobilized on filters and hybridized with labeled DNA from the donor bacteria. Sensitivity of such experiments is not good (5) and solution hybridization techniques offer much better opportunity to resolve the question of integration without replication.

---

*Dr. W. E. H. Fiddian, Natl. Inst. Agric. Bot., Cambridge, England.

Use of renaturation kinetic analysis to look for integration of foreign donor DNA

Perhaps the most sensitive techniques yet devised for quantitatively detecting and characterizing small quantities of exogenous DNA are based on renaturation kinetics of probe DNA's in the presence of large excess of test organism DNA (Janowski, this volume). This technique is based on the fact that the rate of reassociation of the probe DNA is dependent upon the concentration of that DNA. If any sequences recognized by the probe DNA are added, then the real concentration is increased and the rate of reassociation accelerated. If only a fraction of the added sequences is recognized by the probe, then a proportional fraction of the renaturation kinetics will be accelerated but not the remainder. This characteristic permits the detection of the presence of partial genomes in test organisms. It also permits the quantitative determination of what fraction of an unusual density DNA peak consists of the donor DNA sequences.

The DNA/DNA solution hybridization technique, although perhaps the best we have today for investigation of the physical parameters of the fate of exogenous DNA in plants, is not without pitfalls (7). Hydroxyapatite chromatography control measurements must be made for each batch and in each laboratory. Reassociation rates are influenced by many parameters other than DNA concentration and thus all other conditions must be kept strictly identical if meaningful comparisons between two Cot curves are to be made. Trace amounts of metal ions can seriously affect reassociation rates, but chelators may disturb hydroxyapatite chromatography. In addition, plant DNA's are difficult to obtain in pure form. Protein and polysaccharide contaminants can seriously change reassociation rates and affect reproducibility of results.

Renaturation kinetic analysis was applied to the study of an intermediate density DNA peak observed on CsCl analysis of a root sample from Proctor barley treated with Micrococcus lysodeikticus DNA (Fig. 2, peak A). The occurrence of this peak was suspected to be due to bacterial contamination; nevertheless, it was pooled and analyzed by solution hybridization techniques. The results (Fig. 3) clearly indicate that addition of donor DNA (Micrococcus lysodeikticus) does not result in the acceleration of the renaturation rate in the region Cot 1/2 = 1. Thus, none of the sequences in the intermediate density peak recognize the donor DNA. The DNA from a suspected contaminant bacteria (BC2Y) was also tested. It can be seen (Fig. 3) that this DNA accelerates the renaturation of about 40% of the intermediate density DNA. Thus, about 40% of that peak must be due to DNA from the contaminating bacteria BC2Y. The remainder is probably due to cross contamination with the adjacent barley DNA peak (Fig. 2, peak B) and from other contaminating bacteria that are not recognized by BC2Y DNA.

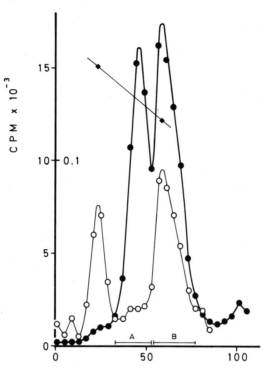

Figure 2. CsCl density gradient DNA analysis of Proctor root
sample. The seeds were hand peeled and sterilized in 5% Ca(OCl)$_2$
30 min. The seeds were then incubated in H$_2$O 11 hrs., <u>Micrococcus</u>
<u>lysodeikticus</u> DNA (1 mg/ml) 12 hrs., H$_2$O 72 hrs., and ^{3}H-TdR 5 hrs.
Centrifugation was performed in a fixed angle rotor for 64 hrs. at
33,000 rpm 25° C. <u>M. lysodeikticus</u> DNA (d = 1.731) was used as
marker. OD$_{260}$ (o), ^{3}H (●).

Use of renaturation kinetic analysis to measure foreign donor DNA
level in the recipient plant

    The following experiment was designed to determine whether
small quantities of exogenous DNA could be found in barley seedlings
after treatment with exogenous DNA and a period of growth. Seeds
from the cultivars Himalaya, Ubamer and CI 3947 (all naked and
easily sterilized) were sterilized and treated with <u>E. coli</u> DNA as
usual. After DNA treatment, the seeds were washed, transplanted
to perlite moistened with nutrient solution (15) and grown for 10

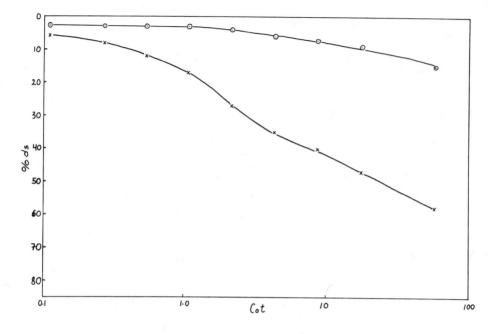

Figure 3. Reassociation kinetics of ^{3}H-DNA from peak A (Fig. 2) in
the presence of large excess <u>Micrococcus lysodeikticus</u> DNA (o) and
BC2Y DNA (x). The Cot value is based on the added DNA concentration.
Reassociation was in 0.15 M PB at 68° C.

days in the dark. The total plant (roots and shoots) DNA was prepared by phenol procedure (16) and further purified by hydroxyapatite chromatography. An <u>E. coli</u> ^{3}H-probe DNA at 0.5 µg/ml was
hybridized with 2 mg/ml barley DNA from the treated samples and one
control sample. Results (Fig. 4) indicate that DNA from all three
barley cultivars exposed to <u>E. coli</u> DNA accelerate the reassociation
of the probe DNA to about the same extent over the control DNA.
Unfortunately, there was not sufficient DNA to determine if this
acceleration of the probe reassociation was proportional to the
added DNA concentration (i.e., would the reassociation rate with
6 mg/ml barley DNA be twice as fast as with 2 mg/ml). A recon-
struction experiment using various concentrations of <u>E. coli</u> DNA
in the presence of 2 mg/ml calf thymus DNA indicates (Fig. 5) that
the increase in reassociation rate is proportional to the added
<u>E. coli</u> DNA.

     It can be estimated that the increase in the reassociation rate
of the probe DNA by the added barley DNA is equivalent to approxi-

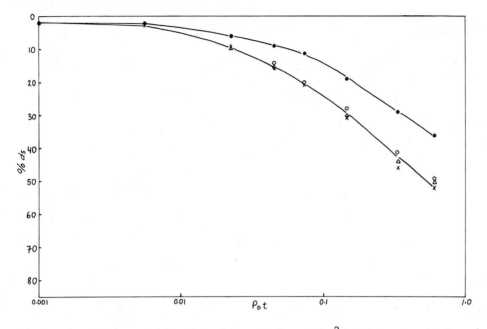

Figure 4. Reassociation kinetics of E. coli ^{3}H-DNA probe (0.5 μg/ml) in the presence of 2 mg/ml barley control (●) or treated (o,Δ, x) DNA samples. Seeds were sterilized in 5% Ca(OCl)$_2$ 30 min., incubated in H$_2$O 11 hrs., E. coli DNA (1 mg/ml) 12 hrs., and grown on perlite in dark at 24° C for 10 days. The Pot value is based on the probe DNA concentration. Reassociation was in 2.0 M sodium perchlorate, 0.033 M PB at 63° C.

mately 0.5 μg E. coli DNA. Thus, the barley DNA preparation appears to contain ca. 0.5 μg E. coli DNA per 2.0 mg/ml barley DNA. This is a ratio of 1/4000. Assuming the barley diploid genome size to be about 7 x 10^{12} daltons (17), the DNA found is roughly equivalent to 1 E. coli genome per 2 diploid barley genomes.

The nature of the experiment is such that it can only be concluded that the E. coli DNA is present after 10 days of germination of the barley seeds. Nothing can be deduced about the state of the DNA or its location.

Network formation as a test of covalent linkage

The question of integration can be examined by techniques based on network formation by eukaryotic DNA. This procedure was

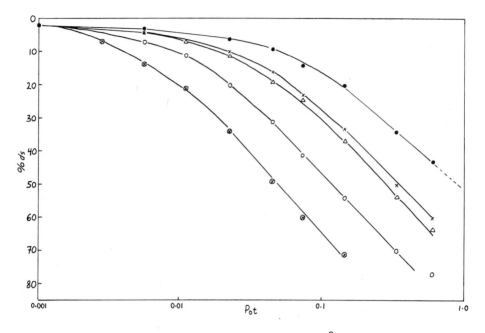

Figure 5.   Reassociation kinetics of E. coli ³H-DNA probe (0.5 μg/ml) in the presence of 2 mg/ml calf thymus DNA and various concentrations of E. coli DNA.   None (●), 0.5 μg/ml (x), 1.0 μg/ml (Δ), 2.5 μg/ml (o), 5.0 μg/ml (⊗).   The Pot value is based on the probe DNA concentration only.   Reassociation was in 2.0 M sodium perchlorate, 0.033 M PB at 63° C.

applied by Varmus et al. (18) to demonstrate the integration of viral DNA in mammalian genomes.   Networks are formed when high molecular weight eukaryotic DNA is incubated to Cot values that permit the reassociation of repetitive sequences, but not unique sequences.   Since the repetitive sequences are interspersed among unique sequences a network is formed that can be collected by centrifugation or other means.

An experiment to test the feasibility of this technique with barley was performed using the procedures of Varmus et al. (18). It can be seen (Table 8) that about 50% of barley DNA enters networks while added E. coli ³H-DNA (0.15 μg/ml) does so only to about 5%.   Thus, although the network formation is not as extensive with barley DNA as with mammalian DNA under these conditions, it is sufficient to differentiate between integrated and free DNA present. Experiments rigorously testing the state of the small amount of exogenous DNA detected in the barley DNA preparations are in progress.

Table 8.

Barley and Added E. coli DNA Found in Pellets
after Network Formation and Centrifugation

Sample	DNA in pellet %	Added E. coli DNA in pellet %
1	44	5
2	47	4
3	55	-

DISCUSSION

The fate of exogenously applied bacterial donor DNA was
examined in detail by several DNA hybridization techniques. At the
outset, this investigation was intended to examine the DNA base
sequence homology patterns of "intermediate density DNA" species
reported to occur in barley by Ledoux and Huart (12,14). In the
course of these experiments, intermediate density peaks were never
observed except when surface sterilization procedures failed and
seedlings were contaminated with bacteria. In this case, the radioactivity in the intermediate density peak was found to have homology
not with donor bacterial DNA but with contaminant bacterial DNA.

DNA/DNA filter and DNA/DNA solution hybridization techniques
provide powerful tools that can be used to study the fate of
exogenous DNA in plants. Filter hybridization techniques provide
a quick and simple qualitative test for the presence of exogenous
DNA in unusual density DNA peaks found after CsCl density gradient
centrifugation. Solution hybridization techniques provide a
quantitative test of these peaks and also permit the detection of
very small quantities of exogenous DNA in plant DNA preparations.
Application of special methods such as network formation, enable
the differentiation between integrated and free exogenous DNA
present.

Application of these techniques to the study of the fate of
bacterial DNA in barley seedlings has provided no evidence for the
presence of large amounts of exogenous DNA as previously reported
(12). It seems possible that these results may be artefacts
produced by bacterial contamination of the barley seeds. Results
presented here do not exclude the integration of small quantities
of donor DNA in the barley genome.

It is of utmost importance that the hybridization methodology
be stringently applied to the question of integration of bacterial

DNA in plant genomes before authoritative claims are made about the existence of bacterial-eukaryotic DNA complexes.

REFERENCES

1. F. C. EDEN, S. K. FARRAND, J. S. POWELL, A. J. BENDICH, M. D. CHILTON, E. W. NESTER, and M. P. GORDON, J. Bacteriol. 119 (1974) 547-553.

2. D. T. DENHARDT, Biochem. Biophys. Res. Commun. 23 (1966) 641.

3. D. GILLESPIE and S. SPIEGELMAN, J. Mol. Biol. 12 (1965) 829.

4. D. GILLESPIE, In: Methods in Enzymology, XII B (1968) 641. (L. Grossman and K. Moldave, Eds., Academic Press, N.Y. and London).

5. S. K. FARRAND, F. C. EDEN, and M. D. CHILTON, In preparation.

6. K. BURTON, Biochem. J. 62 (1956) 315.

7. R. J. BRITTEN, D. E. GRAHAM, and B. R. NEUFELD, In: Methods in Enzymology, XXIX E (1974) 363. (L. Grossman and K. Moldave, Eds., Academic Press, N.Y. and London).

8. G. BERNARDI, In: Methods in Enzymology, XXI D (1971) 95. (L. Grossman and K. Moldave, Eds., Academic Press, N.Y. and London).

9. M. D. CHILTON, T. C. CURRIER, S. K. FARRAND, A. J. BENDICH, M. P. GORDON, and E. W. NESTER, Proc. Nat. Acad. Sci., U.S.A. 71 (1974) 3672.

10. R. J. BRITTEN and D. E. KOHNE, Science 161 (1968) 529.

11. L. GROUSE, M. D. CHILTON, and B. J. McCARTHY, Biochemistry 11 (1972) 798.

12. L. LEDOUX and R. HUART, J. Mol. Biol. 43 (1969) 243.

13. L. LEDOUX and P. CHARLES, In: Uptake of Informative Molecules by Living Cells (1972) 29. (L. Ledoux, Ed., North-Holland Publ. Co., Amsterdam - London).

14. L. LEDOUX and R. HUART, In: Uptake of Informative Molecules by Living Cells (1972) 254. (L. Ledoux, Ed., North-Holland Publ. Co., Amsterdam - London).

15. J. P. MIKSCHE and J. A. M. BROWN, Am. J. Bot. 52 (1965) 533.

16. M. D. CHILTON and A. KLEINHOFS, Unpublished.

17. D. SCIAKY and A. KLEINHOFS, Unpublished.

18. H. E. VARMUS, P. K. VOGT, and J. M. BISHOP, Proc. Nat. Acad.
     Sci.,U.S.A. 70 (1973) 3067.

ACKNOWLEDGEMENT

     The work reported here was performed in Professor Ledoux's
laboratory, Department of Radiobiology, C.E.N./S.C.K., Mol, Belgium,
where the author was a visiting scientist. Sincere thanks are due
to Professor Ledoux and his staff for providing facilities and the
opportunity to do this work. Special thanks are due to Raoul Huart
who participated in the performance of many of the experiments,
and to Dr. P. Charles for the Model E ultracentrifugation analysis.
The contributions and many valuable discussions with Drs. P. Lurquin
and M. Mergeay are also deeply appreciated.

FATE OF EXOGENOUS DNA IN PLANTS

L. LEDOUX

Cell Biochemistry, Radiobiology department,
Centre d'Etude de l'Energie Nucléaire, Mol.
Molecular Genetics, Botany department, Universi-
té de Liège, Belgium

There is now good evidence that higher plant cells can take up
exogenous foreign DNA (1-13).
In general, most of the foreign DNA is broken down and reutilized.
Of special interest are the few cases where this DNA escapes destruction and persists in the plant tissues.
I shall consider two possibilities : either the foreign DNA is
kept free or it becomes bound to the DNA of the recipient cells.
With Proctor barley seedlings that were grown in the dark in
limited humidity after the cut seeds were allowed to stand in the
DNA solution, embryo pointing upward, it was observed that labelled heteropycnic [^{3}H] DNA were rapidly transfered from the
endosperm to the root tip, without much degradation (1-2).
The radioactivity was found associated with DNA of a density intermediate between that of the donor and that of the recipient
DNA, which upon sonication yielded fragments of DNA with densities equivalent to that of exogenous DNA, suggesting a possible
duplex structure for the observed molecules (3-4).

Hotta and Stern (10) obtained similar biochemical results after
X-ray treatment of Hymalaya barley or also using it in low humidity conditions. The authors pointed out that "the formation of
hybrid DNA appeared to be a pathological consequence of physiological mistreatment". Nevertheless, the interesting point was
that such a phenomenon could occur.
In fact, it became clear, later, that the association of foreign
to recipient DNA was an event varying with the conditions of
treatment and (11) limited to some tissues of a few plants only.
In *Arabidopsis thaliana*, for instance, heteroduplexes were mainly found in cotyledons and flowers (4-5). On the other hand,

a screening of several plants (16) such as Helianthus, *Pisum*, *Nicotiana*, *Trifolium*, *Medicago*, *Lycopersicum* and *Sinapis*, indicated that no generalisation could be obtained for the fate of a bacterial DNA in given organs or tissues. Indeed, depending on the plant used, the foreign DNA could be found destroyed, intact and free, or integrated (and released by sonication) in roots, cotyledons, leaves or flowers.

Duplex formation was rare but could be obtained in some cases. With the improvements of the nucleic acid extraction procedures, (see Charles, this book) the molecular weight of the DNA obtainable from plants steadily increased during the last decade, with the consequence that relatively lower proportions of foreign DNA could be found in the larger plant DNA fragments now obtainable, leading to smaller density shifts (in that case, sonication was needed to detect heterogeneity). Reciprocally, the increasing molecular weight of the bacterial [3H] DNA used, could be of importance as it remains to establish how large the foreign DNA has to be in order to be taken up and processed by the plant cells. Experiments are in progress in our laboratory to clarify these points[*].

For a time, it could be considered sufficient to show that the buoyant density of the radioactive DNA recovered from the plant was depending on the density of the labelled DNA used, to prove its exogenous nature (in conditions where [3H] thymidine treated plants (controls) showed purely endogenous DNA labelling). This was particularly true at time when hybridization techniques needed further improvements. Now, that many artefacts of hybridization have been recognised and can be avoided the fate of foreign DNA in barley seedlings can be followed, using a combination of CsCl gradients and hybridization techniques.

A. Kleinhofs indicates elsewhere in this book some of the negative results obtained in six recent assays made in different experimental conditions. In this series, made with high molecular DNA, no integration was observed in the CsCl gradients and consequently no replication was found. The only satellites found were due to bacterial contaminations clearly shown by CsCl gradients, where DNA from both controls and DNA-treated plants appeared similar. No heterogeneity appeared upon sonication and rebanding. Filter hybridization of the contaminant labelled DNA led to positive but incomplete hybridization with the contaminant DNA.

Surprisingly, in conditions where CsCl gradients did not show the presence of foreign DNA, hybridization could detect 1 E.coli genome per 2 plant genomes, in whole seedlings grown in axenic conditions and harvested 10 days after treatment with E.coli DNA. Further experiments are needed to precise these points and also to determine whether some of the parameters described above (molecular weight of the DNA used, method of preparation, etc..)

[*]see note added in proof, page

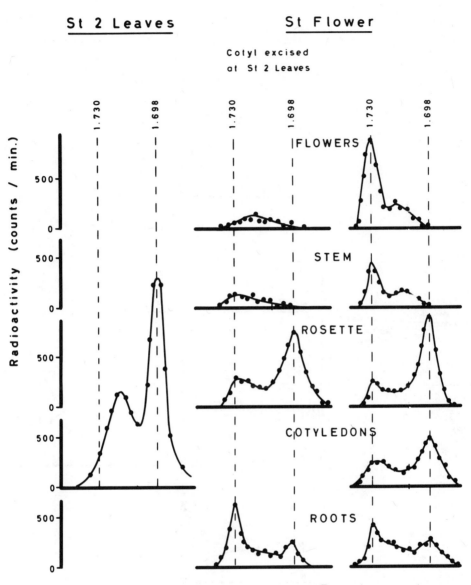

Fig.1 : CsCl gradient centrifugation of DNA isolated from organs
of groups of 80 plants grown from seeds treated for 4
days with S. coelicolor [3H] DNA (d = 1.730 g/cm³).In
one group, cotyledons were excised at the 2-leaves
stage. Density of Arabidopsis DNA = 1.698 g/cm³.

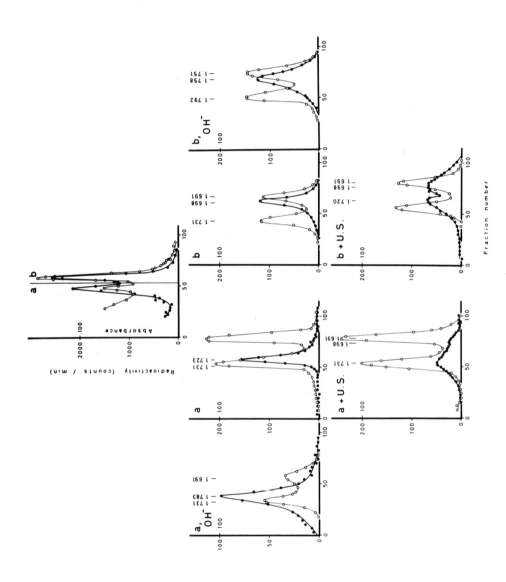

could be responsible for the present observed failures[:].
With *Arabidopsis* convenient experimental conditions appear to be
easier to find. Many seeds can be treated with small amounts of
DNA in physiological conditions and the plants can be grown in
agar test tubes through their entire growth cycle, in stringent
axenic conditions.
With this material, a curious phenomenon was found : when supplied to the seed, different labelled DNA (with differing GC
content) appeared to be stored in the cotyledons and kept there,
rather intact, until the plant flowered. Then, at a time when cotyledons senesce, the foreign DNA appeared to have migrated to
the flowers, where part of it became bound to the recipient DNA
(4-5). The migration of the DNA at the flowering time is exemplified in fig.1, where a comparison is made between the labelling obtained when cotyledons were, or not, excised at an early
stage of the plant development.
No replication of the foreign DNA could be observed in the DNA-
treated seedlings but well in their progeny, in which satellite
DNA were observed. Increasingly important satellite DNA were
found in 3 successive progenies of *Arabidopsis* plants treated
with the same *M. lysodeikticus* DNA (5). This was later confirmed
with J. BROWN in the 4th progeny so obtained (6-9). In that case,
enough material was collected to enable a detection of the absorbance of the satellite DNA. Results are shown in fig.2. It can
be seen that the satellite represents a large proportion of the
DNA actually found and thatsonication produces a striking heterogeneity in the CsCl gradient, leading to the separation of 2 populations with either the recipient or the foreign DNA density.
The appearance of a satellite DNA was accompanied by toxic effects
and by morphological changes of the treated plants (5). Mutants
exhibiting similar phenotypes led to homogenous DNA populations
with D = 1.698 g/cm^3, this density being unaffected by sonication
(6).
As sais before, one of the important features of the*Arabidopsis*
system was that the foreign DNA appeared to be stored in cotyle-

---

Fig.2 : CsCl gradient centrifugation of DNA isolated from F_4ML
        plants treated with [^{3}H] thymidine.
        a, b : pooled fractions, recentrifuged.
        + US : neutral CsCl gradients, after sonication
        OH$^-$: alkaline CsCl gradients
                Radioactivity   Ultraviolet absorption
        Density markers : M.lysodeikticus DNA (d = 1.731 g/cm^3)
                          Mouse DNA (d = 1.700 g/cm^3).

[:] see note added in proof, page 493

dons and despatched from there to the growing tissues during the
entire growth cycle, with a preference for the flowering stage,
when cotyledons senesce.

For this reason, we tried, with G. BERNIER, R. BRONCHART, C.
COUMANNE, R. DELTOUR and J. JACQMARD (16), to analyse the fate
of a bacterial [³H] DNA in *Sinapis alba*, another crucifer, much
used for flowering studies (17, 18). Experiments were made by
incubating sterilised seeds in bacterial [³H] DNA having a high
specific radioactivity (5-10x10^6 dpm/µg). Light and electron microscopy were used to study the autoradiographs obtained from
thick semithin or ultrathin sections. Photos 1 and 2 show the
results obtained. Nuclei and chloroplasts are labelled. [³H] DNA
is also found in the cytoplasmic matrix. Spherosomes, vacuoles
and cell wall are unlabelled.

In other experiments, a labelled *S. coelicolor* DNA was injected
into the stem of a vegetative *Sinapis* (grown in short days), just
below the terminal bud (7). Some plants were kept in short days
while other plants were then permanently transfered to inductive
long days. The growth of the plants is shown in fig.3 and corresponds to the [³H] DNA experiment described below. In fig.4 a summary of the overall picture of the [³H] DNA distribution in the
plant is given.

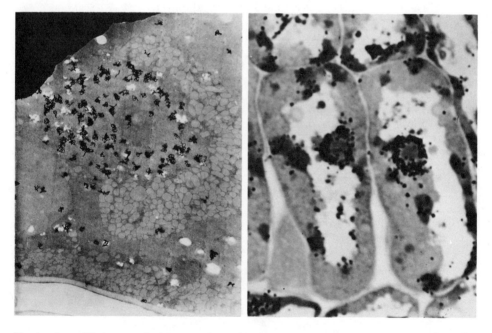

Photo 1 : High-resolution autoradiography of cotyledons of *Sinapis
          alba* treated for 3 days with [³H] DNA.
Photo 2 : Autoradiography of cotyledons of *Sinapis alba* treated for
          3 days with [³H] DNA, then for 3 days with H_2O.

It can be seen that when plants were kept in vegetative conditions
little radioactivity escaped the injection site and migrated in
the plant. Autoradiography of the injection site shows that nuclei
are heavily labelled and that vessels do not contain a significant
radioacitivity at that time (photos 3,4,5).
However, in plants induced to flower by long days, at the flower
stage radioacitivity left the injection site and migrated towards
the influorescence. Fig.4 shows that during flowering the quantity
of radioactivity found below the injection site is not much modified, however that found in leaves is drastically decreased.

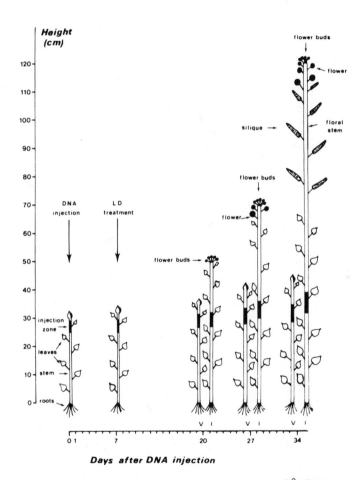

Fig.3 :Schematization of the experiment where [³H]DNA was injected
       in the plant stem, below the terminal bud. Plants were har-
       vested at the given times and dissected.
       The DNA of the different organs was then extracted and
       analysed.

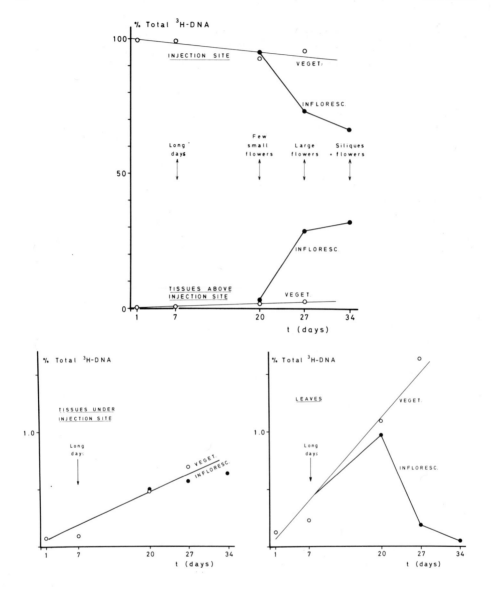

Fig.4 : Overall picture of the [³H] DNA distribution found in
         the plants described in fig.3. The radioactivity found
         in the DNA preparations is expressed in percent of the
         total radioactivity recovered.

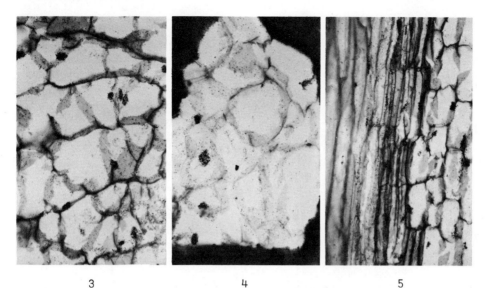

| 3 | 4 | 5 |

Photo 3,4,5 : Autoradiographies of the injection site, 20 days
              after injection of [³H] DNA from S.coelicolor.

Fig.5 summarizes results obtained for stem, leaves, apex, flowers
and pods at different times after the injection. Only results obtained after 1, 20 and 34 days are exemplified here. It can be
seen that much of the radioactivity frequently bands at the density of the foreign DNA used. Labelled recipient DNA can also be
found in leaves, apex and pods.
A comparison of the radioactivity found in leaves 15 days after
injection of [³H] thymidine, *B. subtilis* [³H] DNA,*A.·tumefaciens*
[³H] DNA and *S. coelicolor* [³H] DNA is given in fig.6.
The radioactive molecule recovered band at the density of the
foreign [³H] DNA used.
The leaves obtained from *B.subtilis* [³H] DNA injected plants
were examined by autoradiography.
Photos 6,7 and 8 show results obtained. It is clear that in a
case where only foreign DNA can be recovered from the plants, the
radioactivity is mainly found associated with the nuclei and even
more with chromosomes in all the labelled mitotic figures observed.

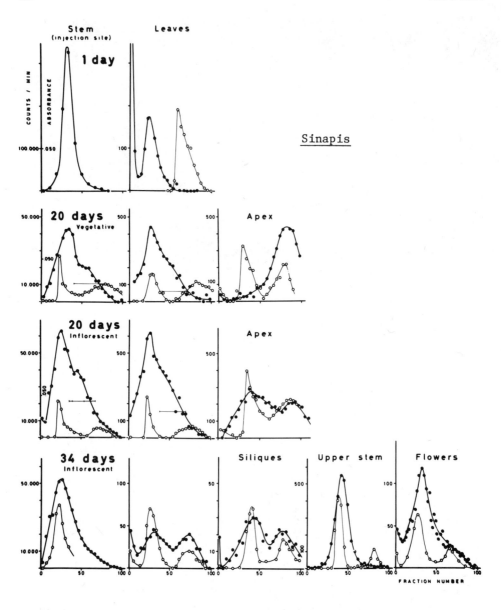

Fig.5 : CsCl gradient analysis of DNA recovered from different
        organs of the plants described in fig.3.
        Plants were injected with [³H] DNA from S.coelicolor
        (d = 1.730 g/cm³)
        ●━━━━━● radioactivity   ○━━━━━○ U.V. Absorbance
        Density marker : M. lysodeikticus DNA (d=1.731 g/cm³)
                         Sinapis DNA (d=1.698 g/cm³).

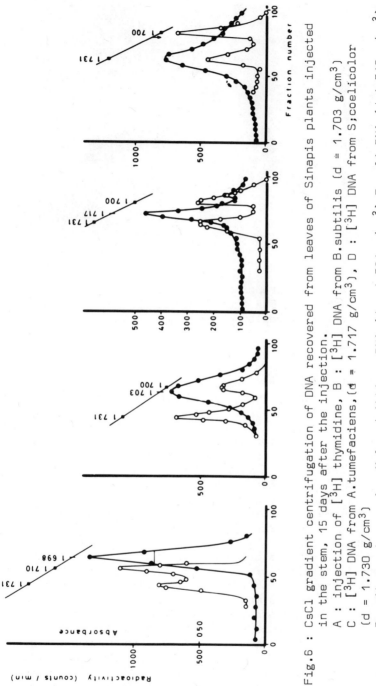

Fig.6 : CsCl gradient centrifugation of DNA recovered from leaves of Sinapis plants injected in the stem, 15 days after the injection.

A : injection of [³H] thymidine, B : [³H] DNA from B.subtilis (d = 1.703 g/cm³)
C : [³H] DNA from A.tumefaciens, (d = 1.717 g/cm³), D : [³H] DNA from S;coelicolor (d = 1.730 g/cm³)

Density markers : A : M.lysodeikticus DNA (d = 1.731 g/cm³),E.coli DNA (d=1.710 g/cm³)
B,C,D : M.lysodeikticus DNA (d = 1.731 g/cm³).

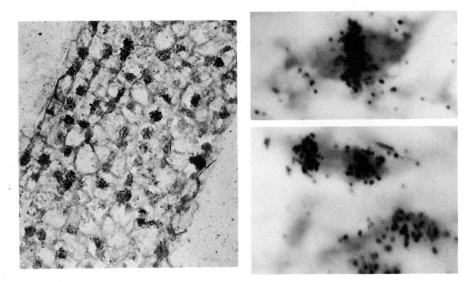

Photos 6 - 8 : Autoradiographies of leaves from plants injected
with [³H] DNA from B.subtilis. Photos show uniformly labelled chromosomes in labelled mitotic
figures.

Once again, this raises the question of the actual state of the
foreign DNA in the plant. Is it really present as free molecules
or is it recovered free due to a fragmentation of the DNA molecules during extraction ? It is impossible as yet to answer this
question. Here too, experiments are in progress to determine the
fate of more or less polymerised foreign [³H] DNA.
Fig.7 shows results of an experiment where [²H-³H] DNA E.coli
(d = 1.730 g/cm³) was injected and the plant tissues collected
after 12 weeks. Seeds were also removed from the siliques and
analysed separately. In siliques and seeds, a radioactive DNA with
d = 1.715 - 1.720 g/cm³ was recovered, which upon sonication
yielded molecules with d = 1.730 g/cm³.
Obviously, further studies are needed to clarify these points
which suggest integration of foreign material in the recipient DNA.
[³H]DNA appears therefore to migrate in *Sinapis* as it does in
Arabidopsis. In both cases most of the migration occurs at the
flowering time. This phenomenon seems to be linked with the
senescence of the plant : indeed at the time when the injected
[³H] DNA starts migrating, the wave of senescence (which starts
from the plant basis) reaches the site of injection. Autoradiography shows that vessels are then heavily labelled (photo 9).
However,as other cells appear also to be labelled, other migration
patterns such as cell to cell transfer cannot be excluded.

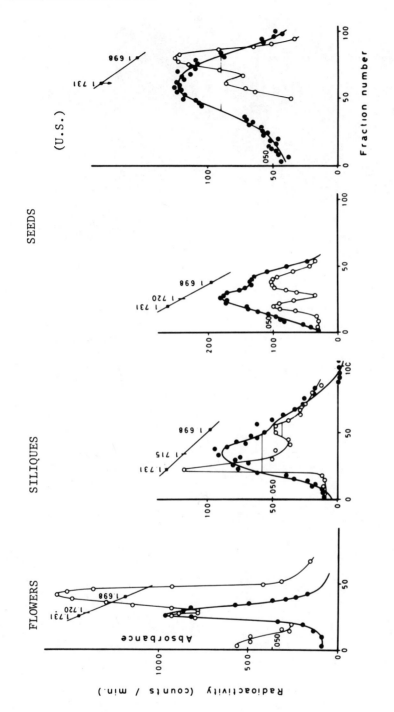

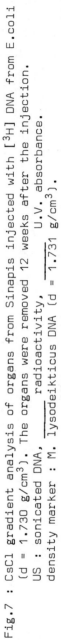

Fig.7 : CsCl gradient analysis of organs from Sinapis injected with [³H] DNA from E.coli (d = 1.730 g/cm³). The organs were removed 12 weeks after the injection. US : sonicated DNA, ———— radioactivity, ———— U.V. absorbance. density marker : M. lysodeikticus DNA (d = 1.731 g/cm³).

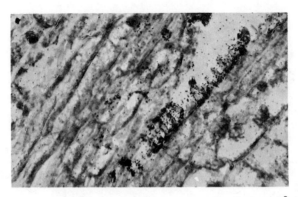

Photo 9 : Autoradiography from plant injected with [^{3}H] DNA
          from B.subtilis and analysed 30 days after the in-
          jection. Important labelling can be found in tracheids
          at that time.

Summing up the informations which have been obtained so far
from different materials, it can be said that in certain instances foreign DNA can be translocated over long distances,
without being necessarily destroyed with time. This DNA is mainly found associated with nuclei. It can become covalently linked
to recipient DNA and can be transmitted to the progeny where it
sometimes replicates together with the recipient DNA.

Thanks are due to the Fonds National de la Recherche Fondamentale Collective and to the Ministère de l'Education Nationale
for their financial help.

Note added in proof :

Experiments were conducted with Proctor barley seeds to determine the optimal conditions necessary for DNA integration and
replication, using *M. lysodeikticus* (M.L.) DNA (ATCC 4698) as
donor DNA. Seeds were peeled after 2 hrs agitation in H_2SO_4
(1/2 conc.), washed several times with H_2O, and soaked for
2 hrs in 5% Ca(OCL)$_2$, followed by washings. A total of about
6 hrs was needed for this sterilization. Seeds were then cut
and placed in 1 drop *M. lysodeikticus* (M.L.) [^{3}H] DNA (1mg/ml)
in spot plates for 2 hrs in the dark and at 24°. The spot
plate was put in a petri dish, on moisted paper and the dish
was sealed with tape. This was repeated at each step of the incubation.
Humidity was kept low, so that root hairs abundantly develop.
The cut seeds were then placed in a drop of ML DNA (1 mg/ml)
for 36 to 72 hrs, [^{14}C] thymidine was sometimes added at the
end of the incubation period. Seedlings were then removed and
dissected. Roots were dissected into meristem and elongation-
differentiation zones, scutellum and coleoptile were removed.
All organs were frozen and kept for DNA preparation, as described
before. Liquid nitrogen was used to help grinding the tissues in
a small mortar. All incubation steps were monitored for microbial contamination as were the cut parts of the seeds.
To check the influence of the DNA size, a ML [^{3}H] DNA with
60×10^6 daltons was prepared. It was then sheared through a
needle nr.25. Samples were taken and their M.W. were determined
by analytical ultracentrifugation. [^{3}H] DNA with 60, 36, 23, 15,
10, 5, 1, .5 $\times 10^6$ daltons were used. After 36 hrs incubation,
DNA were prepared and were analysed in CsCl gradients, with a
density reference. Results showed that maximum uptake of the
foreign DNA occurred for M.W. between 15 and 5×10^6 daltons.
(A recent publication by Levy, J., Kazan, P., and Varmus, H.,
Virology, 61, 1974, 297 – shows that transfection in chicken
fibroblast also depends on the DNA size ; 10^7 daltons, being
adequate).
The quality of the recovered radioactive molecules depended
on the size of the DNA used. At high M.W., only free foreign
DNA was found (mainly in the elongation-differentiation zone).
From 15×10^6 down to 1×10^6 daltons, labelled DNA with d
varying between 1.727 and 1.723 g/cm^3 were recovered. These were
pooled, dialysed, sheared, then denatured and renatured in the
presence of ML or barley DNA at either low or high COT, at 65°
or 78°. The renatured molecules were then run in a CsCl gradient,
without reference DNA. After localisation, they were pooled, dialysed and melted on hydrolapatite, following Y. Miyazawa and C.A.
Thomas, J. Mol. Biol., 11, 1965, 223. Some results are indicated
in figs. 1 and 2.

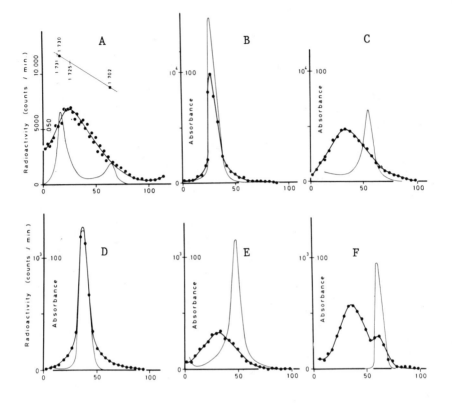

Fig.1 : CsCl gradient analysis of DNA :
    A : [³H] DNA recovered from the elongation-differentiation
        zone of barley roots, after 2 hrs treatment with *M.*
        lysodeikticus (M.L.) [³H] DNA (d = 1.731 g/cm³ - MW =
        10⁷) and 39 hrs with M.L. DNA
    B : ML [³H] DNA sonicated then denatured and renatured in
        the presence of polymerised ML DNA, COT = 100, T = 78°
    C : ML [³H] DNA sonicated then denatured and renatured in
        the presence of polymerised barley DNA, COT = 10.000,
        T = 65°.
    D : [³H] DNA shown in A, sonicated, then denatured and re-
        natured in the presence of polymerised ML DNA, COT =
        100, T = 78°.
    E : [³H] DNA shown in A, sonicated, then denatured and re-
        natured in the presence of polymerised barley DNA, COT=
        100, T= 65°.
    F : [³H] DNA shwon in A, unsheared, denatured and renatured
        in the presence of polymerised barley DNA, COT=10.000,
        T=65°. •————• radioactivity, ————— abondance.

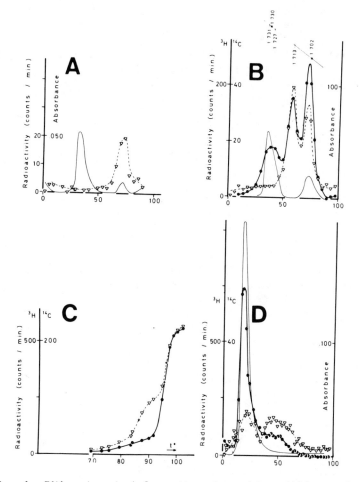

Fig. 2 : A. DNA extracted from the elongation-differenciation
zone of barley roots obtained from seeds treated
for 3 hrs with [^{14}C] thymidine after 48 hrs growth.
B. DNA extracted from the elongation-differenciation
zone of barley roots obtained from seeds treated for
2 hrs with ML [^{3}H] DNA, 46 hrs with ML DNA, then 3
hrs with [^{14}C] thymidine. Fractions 52-65 were
pooled, dialysed sheared, then
C. melted on hydroxylapatite.
D. denatured and renatured in the presence of high molecular ML DNA (at COT = 100, 78°) and analysed in
a CsCl gradient.
●——● ^{3}H radioactivity
▽----▽ ^{14}C radioactivity
——— U.V. absorbance

Fig.2 shows results obtained when [^{14}C] thymidine was added at
the end of the incubation period. In control experiments (fig.2a)
only barley DNA was found labelled.
With barley treated for 2 hrs with ML [^{3}H] DNA, with ML DNA for
36 - 68 hrs, then with [^{14}C] thymidine for   hrs, results similar
to those shown in fig.2b were obtained. Depending on the experiment, the heavy barley component had a density = 1.711 - 1.718
g/cm^{3}.
In the example shown here, fractions 52 - 65 were pooled, dialysed, sheared and melted on hydrolapatite (fig.2c). They also
were sheared,then denatured and renatured in the presence of
high molecular M.L. DNA, at COT = 100, then centrifuged in a
CsCl gradient.
Results show that the [^{3}H] component melts at a temperature close
to that of a sheared ML DNA whilst the [^{14}C] component shows a
biphasic melting curve with Tm of 96° and 86° (close to that of
the sheared barley DNA).
This strongly suggests that the labelled DNA with an intermediate
density contains [^{3}H] ML, [^{14}C] ML and [^{14}C] barley DNA, indicating integration and replication of the foreign ML DNA. Part of
these results was obtained in collaboration with Dr. Y. Hotta.
They will be published in detail elsewhere. Attempts are presently being made to locate the intermediate DNA cytologically and to
precise other parameters of the conditions of incubation.

BIBLIOGRAPHY

1. Ledoux, L., (1965), in Progress in Nucleic acid research and molecular Biology (edit. by J.N. Davidson and W.E. Cohn), Acad. Press., N.Y., 231.

2. Ledoux, L., (1968), L'absorption des DNA par les tissus vivants, Vaillant-Carmanne, Liège, 85pp.

3. Ledoux, L., and Huart, R., (1969), J. Mol. Biol. 43, 243

4. Ledoux, L., Huart, R., and Jacobs, M., (1971), Eur. J. Biochem., 23, 96.

5. Ledoux, L., Huart, R., and Jacobs, M.,(1971), in Informative molecules in biological systems (edit. by L. Ledoux), North Holland Cy., N.Y., 159.

6. Brown, J., Huart, R., Ledoux, L., and Swinnen, J., (1971), Arch. internat. Physiol., 79, 820

7. Coumanne, C., Jacqmard, A., Kinet , J.M., Bodson, M., Ledoux, L., and Huart, R., (1971), Arch. intern. Physiol., 79, 823

8. Ledoux, L., and Huart, R., (1972), in Uptake of informative molecules in living cells, (edit. by L. Ledoux), North Holland Cy., N.Y., 254.

9. Ledoux, L., Brown, J., Cherles, P., Huart, R., Jacobs, M., Remy, J., and Watters, C.,(1972), Adv. in the Biosciences (edit. by G. Raspé), Pergamon Press, 8, 347.

10. Hotta, Y., and Stern, H., (1971J, in Informative molecules in biological systems (edit. by L. Ledoux), North Holland Cy., 176.

11. Bendich,A., and Filner, P., (1971), Mutation Res., 13, 199

12. Ohyama, K., Gamborg, O., and Miller, R., (1972), Can. J. Botany, 50, 2077.

13. Strawn, M., Anker, P., Gahan, P., and Greppin, H., (1971), J. Bacteriol., 106, 634.

14. Johnson, C.B., and Grierson, D., (1974), Curr. Adv. Plant Science, 4, 1

15. Sosson, B., Huart, R., and Ledoux, L., unpublished results.

16. Ledoux, L., Bernier, G., Bronchart, R., Jacqmard, A., Coumanne, C., and Deltour, R., in preparation.

17. Bernier, G., Bronchart, R., and Kinet, J.M.,(1970), in Cellular and Molecular aspects of floral induction, ed. G. Bernier, Longman, Bristol, 51.

18. Bernier, G.,(1969) in the induction of flowering some case histories, edit. L.T. Evans, Mc Millan, 305.

DNA MEDIATED GENETIC CORRECTION OF THIAMINELESS *ARABIDOPSIS*

THALIANA

L. LEDOUX*, R. HUART, M. MERGEAY, P. CHARLES
Section de Biochimie cellulaire, Département de Radio-
biologie, Centre d'Etude de l'Energie Nucléaire
Mol, Belgique
M. JACOBS, Laboratorium voor Plantengenetica, Vrije
Universiteit Brussel, Belgium

Avery's [1] classical experiments showed that it was possible
to influence cell function in procaryotes by the addition of exogenous genetic information. Analysis demonstrated that bacteria
can take up DNA and integrate it into their genome by genetic
recombination (see A. Tomasz, this book).

Until recently, such "cell manipulation" with higher organisms appeared as almost impossible, possibly due to the poverty
of the means available for sound and extensive studies. The
necessary biochemical back-ground had to be obtained : good
methods to prepare nucleic acids and to recognize them in a
population of similar molecules had to be developed. At the genetical level, the scarcity of mutants with defined biochemical
lesions precluded (and still limits) experimentation [2, 3].

Nevertheless, DNA mediated corrections in higher organisms
were reported : with animal cells in tissue culture, by Szybaslka
and Szybalski [4], Glick and Salim [5], Majumdar and Bose [6],
M. Fox et al. [7], Ottolenghi-Nichtingale [8], Borenfreund,
Bendich et al. [9], Roosa [10], Merril et al. [11] Hill and Hillova [12], with *Ephestia* by Nawa, Yamada et al.[13, 14] and
with *Drosophila* by Gershenson [15] and A. Fox, Yoon et al.
[16, 20], with *Petunia* by Hess [21, 24] and with *Arabidopsis
thaliana* by Ledoux, Huart and Jacobs [25, 30[b]].

*also : Génétique moléculaire, Département de Botanique, Univer-
sité de Liège, Sart Tilman, Liège, Belgique.

Finally, phage mediated corrections were reported by Merril et al. [11] with animal cells, by Doy, Gresshoff and Rolfe [31, 35] with haploid tomato callus or *Arabidopsis* haploid cells, and by Johnson et al. with *Sycamore* cells [65] (see P. Gresshoff et al. and H. Smith et al., this book).

On the other hand, an extensive use of the CsCl gradient technique (first applied by Gartler [36] to the problem of DNA uptake by living cells) has led to the astonishing results that foreign DNA can be translocated on large distances, crosses cell membranes [37, 38], and appears to survive several mitotic cycles in different animal or plant systems [2, 37, 39]. In *Arabidopsis thaliana*, it appears to survive at least one round of meiotic division [28, 30b,40]. More surprising was the suggestion that the foreign DNA could become covalently linked to the recipient DNA [26, 28, 30a, 37, 43] as a double stranded material (a phenomenon similar to the incorporation of the λDNA in *E.coli* genome).

Since biochemical and biological data were generally obtained in different laboratories with different materials, the *Arabidopsis thaliana* system appeared to us as a useful one, to try to correlate biochemical and genetical data and to decide whether the biochemical phenomena we observed were a kind of cul-de-sac or whether they had implications for biology and genetics.

As already indicated in preliminary reports [25, 30a, 30b] corrections of nutritional mutants by exogenous DNA were extensively developed in order to build the required statistical analysis; we are presenting here an overall picture of the results so obtained. More extensive genetic data will be presented elsewhere.

Nutritional mutants of *Arabidopsis thaliana*

Among the rare auxotrophs described in *Arabidopsis thaliana*, the thiamine requiring ones are the most frequent. They are obtained by X rays or chemical mutagenesis. They also are conditional lethal mutants with a strict phenotype, whilst other auxotrophs exhibit bradytrophy.

Mutants of one locus (py) control the synthesis of the pyrimidine moiety of thiamine [44, 45], locus tz controls the synthesis of the thiazole half of the vitamin [44] and 2 genes are concerned with some intermediate steps between these two precursors and thiamine. These mutants can be used for strictly genetic studies such as allelic complementation or recombination or reverse mutation because of the built-in selective mechanisms [44].

The mutability of the py locus is apparently the highest [46, 47] and is close to 2×10^{-4}. The frequency of spontaneous reversion of the py locus has been estimated to be lower than 5×10^{-5} [48].

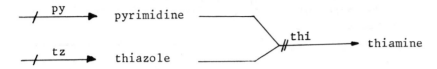

Ethyl methane sulfonate treatment produced apparent reversions at the py locus, at a frequency of about 4×10^{-5} [49].

These revertants were <u>non-homozygous</u> and segregated in the following generations. In test crosses, they also yielded hetero-zygotes and lethal mutants in approximately equal frequencies [50].

The monogenic conditional lethal mutants used here are nor-mally propagated in the presence of thiamine. When sown on mineral medium, the seeds germinate normally and develop their cotyledons which appear normal green. The first leaves progressively bleach out completely and the plant soon dies. Thiamine (10^{-6}M - 10^{-5}M) allows a normal growth of all these mutants.

Mutants used in this study are the following : thi51 and py.er.as. from G. Rédei, thi V447 and py V131 from M. Feenstra, and py 431 and tz 432 from M. Jacobs. They bear the side markers indicated in tables 1 and 3. The only wild type *Arabidopsis* kept in the laboratory is the Wilna gl.

<u>Treatment of the seeds</u>

Seeds are disinfected with a 95 % ethanol and 3 % H_2O_2 mixture (1 : 1) as first used by Langridge [51] or with a 5 % Calcium hypochlorite solution [44].

The seeds are treated for 5 - 8 min and rinsed with a few changes of sterile distilled water. About 50 seeds are then imme-diately placed in a well of a spot plate and immersed in 25 µl of DNA solution (see here-under) or of 0.01 M NaCl. Spotplates are placed in Petri dishes over wet sterile filter paper, to limit evaporation of the solvent. During the course of the 3 following days, 25 µl of the DNA solution are added to the seeds to keep them moistened. Petri dishes are kept at 24°C under continuous illumination for 4 days. Both DNA and NaCl treated seeds germin-ate during the incubation period. After incubation, seedlings are laid out in a) tall Petri dishes, on perlite moistened with the mineral nutrient solution of Jacobs [52] or b) in test tubes containing 5 ml/0.78 % agar dissolved in the mineral nutrient

TABLE 1

Corrections observed in DNA-treated populations, grown in absence
of thamine (nb corrected plants with a progeny / nb germinated
seeds / nb treated seeds)

DNA	Lethal Mutants (+ additional markers)					Total
	thi 51 (gl)	thi V447 (er, gl)	tz 432 gl	py V131 (er, gl)	py 431 (-)	
A.						
E. coli	6/355/685	2/393/525	2/284/550	1/384/400	4/270/477	15/1686/2637
A. tumefaciens	2/182/420	0/100/100	3/230/480	1/100/200	0/130/250	6/742/1450
B. subtilis	0/128/288		3/157/328	0/28/100	0/162/420	3/497/1136
M. lysodeikticus	0/176/450		0/122/120		2/428/705	2/428/1375
S. coelicolor	0/145/274	1/75/75	0/152/272	0/22/100	0/120/410	1/524/1131
B.						
E. coli P678* (thi$_A$)			0/456/500	1/254/350		1/710/850
Phage T7 (E. coli)	0/425/542		0/440/500		0/356/520	0/1221/1562
Phage 2C (B. subt.)	0/189/252		0/182/220			0/371/472
C.						
NaCl 0.01 M	0/695/992	0/233/291	0/795/1020	0/214/262	0/1918/3310	0/3855/5875

*requiring thiazole for growth

TABLE 2

Summary of results of the DNA-treatment

	Treatment		
	NaCl 0.01 M	Phage or E. coli DNA without any thiamine information 0.6 - 1.0 mg/ml 0.01 M NaCl	DNA from thiamine[+] bacteria 0.6 - 1.0 mg/ml 0.01 M NaCl
Nb treated seeds	5.875	2.634	7.729
Nb germinating seeds	3.855	2.048	3.877
Nb growing plants	7	5	73
Nb fertile plants	0	0	27

solution of Miksche and Brown [53]. The tubes are placed in
wooden racks and kept under continuous illumination (6000 lux)
at 24° C. All mutant seedlings on mineral medium die within 15-20
days; they show chlorophyll deficiency in cotyledons and rosette
leaves. Corrected plants grow at a slow rate, with a more or less
normal green colour. About one third of them produce fertile
siliques (*cf.* hereunder). The thiamine concentration necessary
to provide complete growth when seeds were soaked for 3 days,
then washed and allowed to develop in the absence of thiamine,
was found to be about 10^{-3} M.

DNA preparations

A series of DNA used is indicated in table 1. They were prepared from frozen or fresh bacteria (or from isolated and CsCl
purified bacteriophages) by the Marmur technique [54] or by CsCl
gradient preparative ultra-centrifugation, after treatment with
pronase and RNase [55-56]. The DNA was precipitated with 2 vol.
ethanol, kept in 70 % ethanol, and dissolved in sterile 0.01 M
NaCl, just before use. The concentration used was about 0.5-1.0
mg/ml. We successively tried and rejected the use of chloroform
or phenol for deproteinization : both are toxic to the plant.
They also are known to remove the protein or membrane bound molecules from the bulk of the DNA preparation.

Our study of the biochemical fate of labelled DNA in various
systems led us to the recognition that the DNA has to be freshly
prepared, of high molecular weight ($> 10^7$ daltons), very clean
and intact. When single strand breaks in a DNA preparation could
be detected from the depolymerising effects of alkali, the preparation was discarded. Finally, the DNA had to be present during
the first 24 hrs of imbibition (otherwise it was not found integrated into the recipient material (unpublished data).

In general, we used small amounts of seeds per batch of DNA,
and preferred to repeat the treatment with successive freshly
prepared batches. Every time, the DNA batches were used in parallel
in Mol, where plants were grown in test tubes and in Brussels,
were they were sown in perlite. Results were pooled. For some
unknown reason, but supposedly due to the fragmentation of the DNA
molecules during their isolation and purification, some batches of
a given DNA species were ineffective with the mutant plants tested,
whilst others were quite effective. Yet, these DNAs were undiscer-
nable on the basis of the physicochemical methods we used. However,
even if it is tempting to put the blame on the DNA itself, it is
difficult to decide whether these discrepancies were not due to
uncontrolled parameters related to plant growth.

The DNA were prepared from the following strains :

E. coli, K12, wild type; *A. tumefaciens*, B6, obtained from Dr. A. Kurkdjian; *B. subtilis*, 168 T⁻; *M. lysodeikticus*, ATCC 4698; *S. coelicolor*, A3/2 obtained from Dr. H. Hopwood; *E. coli* P678 (thi A); *E. coli* PA371 (thi A, recA) containing the F110 episome (thi⁺) kindly supplied to us by Dr. N. Glansdorff.

Phage T7 (with normal bases) and Phage 2C (with hydroxymethyl uracil replacing thymine) were also used. They were isolated and purified following the technique of May *et al.* [57].

Correction in the DNA-treated populations

When seeds of the different mutant types were treated with different bacterial DNA, corrections could be obtained with a relatively high frequency sometimes comparable to that observed with bacterial transformation (10^{-2} to 10^{-4}). Tables 1 and 2 show an overall picture of the data gathered during the years 1969-1973 with a total of 29 different batches of DNA given to five different mutants. These data include DNA extracted from wild type bacteria, from bacteria with a thiamine deficiency (thiazole requirement) and from phages containing normal or abnormal bases.

Further controls were obtained by treating mutant seeds with 0.01 M NaCl, the solvent used for the DNA assays. After DNA treatment, a few seedlings, which normally die (at the stage 2-4 leaves) within 15 to 20 days after sowing display better growth, form small rosettes and sometimes flower. However, only a few of the flowering ones are fertile (*cf.* table 2). Table 1 only takes into account the restaured plants which produced seeds, thus allowing a study of their progeny. Table 1 also indicates in each case, the number of germinating seeds and the total number of seeds used.

These results indicate that the percentage of correction obtained with the group of DNA from wild type bacteria is similar for all mutants : 0.7 %, 0.85 % and 0.49 % respectively for thiamine, thiazole and pyrimidine requiring mutants. On the other hand, the percentages of correction obtained for five mutants could vary with the source of DNA, *E. coli* being here the more effective one (0.89 %) and *S. coelicolor* the less effective DNA (0.19 %). Results obtained with DNA from phage T7 or phage 2C were negative, with DNA extracted from *E. coli* thi$_A$-, requiring thiazole or thiamine for growth, a pyrimidine mutant but no thiazole mutant was corrected.

When a thi$_A$- bacteria harbours a F' thi⁺ episome, correction can be obtained. In that case, the *E. coli* PA 371 used as a recipient was derived from the P678 strain. It was rec$_A$-, which prevented the episome to recombine with the bacterial genome. The

TABLE 3

Results of treatments with E. coli DNA

	Lethal mutant						Total
Strain	py 431	tz 432	thi 51	py V131	thi V447		
Additional mutation	–	– gl	– gl	er gl	er gl	er as gl	
NaCl 0.01 M							
Nb germinated seeds	1918	795	695	214	233	194	4049
Nb growing plants	3	0	2	0	0	0	5
Nb fertile plants	0	0	0	0	0	0	0
% correction	0	0	0	0	0	0	0
E. coli thi+							
Nb germinated seeds	270	284	355	384	393	282	1968
Nb growing plants	10	5	12	3	5	3	38
Nb fertile plants	4	2	6	1	2	0	15
% correction	1.14	.70	1.69	.26	.51	0	.76
E. coli thi−A							
Nb germinated seeds		456		254		374	1084
Nb growing plants		3		1		2	6
Nb fertile plants		0		1		0	1
% correction		0		.39		0	.09
E. coli thi− + episome thi+							
Nb germinated seeds	239	419	408		94	270	1430
Nb growing plants	46	20	27		2	23	118
Nb fertile plants	6	4	3		0	0	13
% correction	2.50	.95	.74		0	0	.91
E. coli thi− + episome thi+ + DNase							
Nb germinated seeds	193	390	206				789
Nb growing plants	3	1	2				6
Nb fertile plants	0	0	0				0
% correction	0	0	0				0

DNA extracted from such a PA371 + F110 bacteria contained about
95 % PA371 DNA and 5 % episomal DNA, in free form. Table 3 summarizes the results obtained with six mutants and the different
E. *coli* DNA used. Correction is found with the DNA extracted from
the thi A⁻ bacteria harbouring the episome. As the corresponding
bacterial chromosomal DNA was inefficient, the corrections obtained should be due to the episomal information. Upon digestion
by DNase (0.1 mg/ml, 30 min., 37° C) the DNA preparation lost
its correction properties. It should also be noted that in all
cases, the DNA treated plants, growing in the absence of thiamine
show a delay in growth and development, as compared to the wild
type or to mutants supplemented with thiamine (5×10^{-5} M). They
also sometimes show variegations and in several cases, white
segments were apparent on the stems of the treated plants, indicating mosaicism and thiamine deficiency (photo 1).

Analysis of the progenies obtained by selfing the corrected types

Progenies of various corrected types indicated in table 1
and obtained after DNA treatment were sown in perlite soaked with
mineral medium or in soil. The number of F_1 tested plants varied
as a function of the number of seeds present in the pods of the
corrected plant. In a very few cases, thiamine was provided at the
fruit stage to increase the vigor and thus the seed production.
F_2 and F_3 progenies include at least fifty plants for each experiment. For all corrected plants, at least three successive generations were studied and for 5 corrected mutants, fresh and dry
weights were determined (*cf*. table 4).

TABLE 4

Ratios of the weights of F_2 progenies (obtained from 5 corrected
mutants or from the wild type) grown on MM, to the weight observed
after growth on MM + thiamine 5.10^{-4}M (21 days culture) results
MM + thiamine = 100.

Genotype of the treated plants	Correcting bacterial DNA	Phenotype of the corrected plant	Nb of tested plants	Fresh weight	Dry weight
py 431	M. lysodeikticus	light green, variegations	27	102.9	85.4
	M. lysodeikticus	normal green, variegations	13	91.8	73.9
tz 432	E. coli	normal green no variegation	24	78.2	81.5
	A. tumefaciens	light green, variegations	29	43.8	43.8
	B. subtilis	light green no variegation	13	93.5	91.8
wild type		normal green no variegation	22	107.8	105.8

The most striking point of this study concerns the lack of
segregation upon selfing of the progenies of the various corrected
types. All F_1 to F_3 plants originating from each corrected plant
look phenotypically alike and grow reasonably well on mineral
medium. This was also observed in one case where the selfing was
pursued up to the 7th generation. They show however, in most –
but not all – cases, a variegated pattern of chlorophyll pigmentation with light discoloration of the basis of the limb and of
the region along the main vein. Practically in all tested cases,
the average fresh weight (and particularly the average dry weight)
of the corrected types grown on mineral medium, were lower than
those of plants from the same progeny, supplemented with 10^{-4} M
thiamine (37 to 92 %) (table 5). Each of these types thus displays
sensitivity to the addition of thiamine. Other experiments showed
that the corrected "pyrimidine" or "thiazole" mutants specifically
respond to the addition of pyrimidine or thiazole and show an improved growth.

TABLE 5

"Abortive" DNA-treated plants supplemented with thiamine at the
flower stage (nb fertile plant / nb growing plants / nb germinating
seeds / nb town seeds)

Mutant	DNA	Nb plants supplemented	Pooled progeny
py V131	S. coelicolor	1	1/1/50/53
tz 432	E. coli thi$_A$+ episome thi+	3	0/0/201/218
py 431	E. coli thi$_A$+ episome thi+	2	2/6/120/138
thi 51	E. coli thi$_A$+ episome thi+	2	0/0/136/143
as.py.er	E. coli thi$_A$+ episome thi+	2	2/8/116/122

The offspring of mutants corrected in 1970 were again tested
in 1973. Despite a larger number of non germinating seeds, results
were essentially the same and no segregation could be observed
among the growing plants. In selfing experiments, the correction
thus appears to be stable with time. The corrected plants behave
as homozygotes breeding true, in contrast to what is found with
mutagen induced revertants [26]. This is also in contrast to
what is expected in the case of a suppressor mutation introduced
in a homozygous diploïd. Indeed, in the seed, the germline is
represented by two diploïd cells [58-62, cf. also G. Redei, this
book]. These cells, at least should contain the thiamine information to explain the lack of segregation after selfing. In their
immediate progeny the ratio mutants : wild types should vary from
1 : 3 to 1 : 7. The fact that correction ended up with apparently

homozygous seeds suggests that there was a selective advantage
(or a meiotic selection). Indeed, when the selection pressure was
prevented by thiamine supplementation to DNA treated plants
showing signs of abortive flowering, a high percentage of lethal
mutants is observed in the F_1 progeny (table 5).

Analysis of the offspring of crosses

We have analysed, in parallel, the offspring of crosses made
between corrected plants and either the wild or the original
mutant types (back or test crosses). Tables 6 and 7 show the
results obtained in the case of tz⁻, an homozygous "thiazole"
recessive mutant corrected by a treatment with *B. subtilis* DNA.
(Similar data were and are gathered for other corrected types
such as py^c, th^c or tz^c corrected with other DNA. They will be
described elsewhere together with the results of crosses between
mutants corrected with different DNA). The phenotypes presented
by progenies of successive self-fertilization were analysed.

TABLE 6

**Results of reciprocal crosses between tz 432, lethal, corrected by
B. subtilis DNA and the wild type (back cross)**

Cross	Progeny tested		Year	Nb growing plants	Nb ungermin. seeds	% Phenotypes		
						Normal (N)	Leaky (Lk)	Lethal
tz_c x tz^+	X	→ XF_1	1971	11	20	100		
	XF_1	→ XF_2	1971	163	15	90.1	9.2	0.7
	XF_{2N}	→ XF_3	1971	198	5	95.5	2.0	2.5
	XF_{2Lk}	→ XF_3	1971	198	13	21.7	70.2	8.1
	XF_1	→	1973	292	145	80.1	13.0	6.9
	XF_{2N}	→	1973	138	15	84.8	11.6	3.6
	XF_{2Lk}	→	1973	57	11	5.3	17.5	77.2
tz^+ x tz_c	X	→ XF_1	1974	20	30	100		
	XF_1	→ XF_2	1974	91	52	86.8	7.7	5.5

The first generation of the outcrosses do not segregate
(table 6 and 7). The results of the test cross (table 7) implies
that the correction is dominant and that the corrected plants
behave as true homozygotes. On the other hand, reciprocal crosses
between corrected mutants and wild type plants or lethal mutants
(table 8) indicated that the correction can be transmitted through
the male as well as through the female and therefore does not
appear to be due to a maternal or cytoplasmic factor.

TABLE 7

Results of a cross between a tz 432, lethal, corrected by B. subtilis
DNA and the tz 432 mutant (test cross).

Cross	Progeny tested	Year	Nb growing plants	Nb ungermin. seeds	% Phenotypes		
					Normal (N)	Leaky (Lk)	Lethal
tz_c x tz^-	X → XF_1	1971	20	5	100		
	XF_1 → XF_2	1971	116	15	75.8	6.1	17.3
	XF_{2N} → XF_3	1971	131	4	76.3	0	23.7
	XF_{2Lk} → XF_3	1971	202	21	24.7	65.0	10.3
	XF_1 → XF_2	1973	176	251	59.7	12.5	27.8
	XF_{2N} → XF_3	1973	99	3	72.7	19.2	8.1
	XF_{2Lk} → XF_3	1973	109	38	2.8	27.5	69.7

TABLE 8

F_1 progeny of reciprocal crosses between mutants and corrected mutants

Cross	Nb growing plants	Nb ungerm. plants	% Phenotypes		
			Normal	Leaky	Lethal
tz_c x tz	36	4	36	-	-
tz x tz_c	17	5	17	-	-
py_c x py	51	10	51	-	-
py x py_c	15	15	15	-	-
thi_c x thi	184	50	184	-	-
thi x thi_c	49	39	56	-	-

TABLE 9

Results of a cross between the tz 432 mutant and the wild type

Cross	Progeny tested	Year	Nb growing plants	Nb ungermin. seeds	% Phenotypes		
					Normal	Leaky	Lethal
tz^- x tz^+	X → XF_1	1971	15	0	100		
	XF_1 → XF_2	1971	106	7	72.6	0	27.4
	XF_2 → XF_2	1973	63	4	73.0	0	27.0

As exemplified in table 6, the crosses tz^c x tz^+ always lead
to high percentages of non germinating seeds (60 % - 75 %) much
higher than the percentages observed in crosses tz^c x tz^- (15 % -
20 %) or tz^- x tz^+ (0 - 5 %) (table 9). This suggests a sort of
deleterious interaction between the correcting and the original
thi^+ information.

Segregation is observed in the offspring of the tz^c x tz^+
cross. Lethal mutant types are recovered (although in low frequencies) together with plants exhibiting a new phenotype called
here "leaky mutant". This is characterized by a weaker pigmentation, white patches of discoloration on the leaves, sometimes
white sectors on the stem and a relatively poor growth and fertility, in contrast with the normal looking plants of the same
progeny. A whole range of these phenotypes intermediate between
the normal green plants and the lethal chlorophyll deficient
plants were classified under the name "leaky mutants". These leaky
mutants are obtained in crosses between the corrected type and
the wild type, as well as in the crosses between the corrected
type and the lethal mutant (in the latter case, a high frequency
of lethal mutant being obtained) (tables 6, 7). The leaky types
keep their sensitivity to supplementation with thiamine, thiazole
or pyrimidine respectively.

This indicates that the correction has been added to the
mutation and has not been substituted for it. Correction being
dominant, the necessive mutation is not expressed unless the
correction is masked or lost, for instance by crossing with an
uncorrected plant (Photo 2).

When such progenies are tested after two years storage, the
percentages are found to differ considerably ($XF_1 \rightarrow XF_2$, 1973).
The percentage of non germinating seeds is high in both tz^c x tz^+
and tz^c x tz^- crosses. This might be due to the instability of a
genetic factor linked to the correction, rather than to a physiological factor. Indeed, storage of XF_1 seeds from a cross tz^- x
tz^+ does not affect the germination of XF_2 (table 8). It appears
that embryonic lethality could be the reason for his phenomenon.
In fact, these non germinating plants cannot be helped neither
by thiamine nor by yeast extract. Microscopical examination of
the embryos reveals, in some cases, the existence of a growing
but aborting meristeme.

Besides this increased percentage of non germinating seeds,
the percentage of leaky and lethal mutants obtained drastically
increases in the selfed offspring (for both crosses). The phenotypically normal looking plants of the XF_1 progenies do segregate
in their progenies (XF_2N) for lethal and leaky types (XF_2Lk).
Storing the seeds for two years increases the tendency to segre-

gate. It can therefore be concluded that the correction, stable with time in selfing experiments (see above) becomes unstable, with time, upon crossing DNA-corrected plants with normal wild or mutant types. It is thus clear that the cross tz^c x tz^+, conjugating two phenotypically thi^+ partners, leads to an important segregation pattern, never observed when tz^c is self fertilized.

Let us now consider more closely the "leaky mutants" obtained. They are found in equal frequencies in the XF_1 offsprings from tz^c x tz^+ (9.2 %) and tz^c x tz^- (6.1 %). Their selfed offsprings include high frequencies of leaky and lethal types and also normal looking plants. This normal phenotype can be recovered at frequencies (21.7 % and 24.7 %) suggesting that the "leaky mutants" behave as heterozygotes. They should however also segregate into mutant types with similar frequencies. The lower values obtained for the lethal mutants and the reproducibility of the phenotype distributions could be accounted for by various mechanisms.

As said before, we expected that the present study could help correlating genetical and biochemical data. This was in fact the main reason why bacterial DNA was used in the biological studies. We did not use homologous *Arabidopsis* DNA, owing to the difficulty to prepare from this material the clean, high molecular and intact DNA considered by us as a prerequisite for efficient uptake and integration (*cf*. above). On the other hand, the amount of DNA which can be taken up by a cell is limited as are the size of the populations to handle. It therefore seemed reasonable to try to increase the dosage of the interesting gene in the DNA preparation used. This can be achieved by using DNA from transducing phages or episomes. For the time being, there is no phage available for thiamine transfer. In a preliminary attempt to use episomal DNA, we prepared DNA from thiamineless bacteria (ineffective as such for correction) harbouring a F' factor bearing the thiamine information. Next step will be to use purified episomal DNA. This is presently attempted in collaboration with Dr. F. Cannon and results will be described later.

Analyses in CsCl gradients had shown that seeds do accumulate large amounts of heteropycnic foreign DNA. In fact, dry seeds swelling in DNA preparation (mg/ml) absorb about 0.7 ng DNA per seed [38]. The embryo containing about 10^4 cells, with 0.8 pg DNA per cell [64], the amount of foreign DNA taken up by each cell is equivalent to about 20 *E. coli* genomes and corresponds to 1/10 of the actual DNA content of the cell. This huge amount of DNA thus taken up by a diploid cell contains, on the average, 20 thiamine genes. The efficiency of the correction, at the cell level, is indeed very low and the .7 % efficiency observed in our experiments is presumably due to the biological amplification afforded by the system used.

In the embryo, the foreign DNA is mainly stored in the cotyledons and remains associated with the cotyledon DNA for most of
the plant growth. At the flowering time, when cotyledons senesce
the foreign DNA excises and migrates to the flowers from where it
is transferred to the seeds[*]. These results suggest that the
foreign DNA can act as an "episome resembling" DNA, being, at
times, found integrated or free.

Autoradiography, on the other hand, shows that the foreign
DNA becomes associated with cell nuclei, migrates at the flowering
time through the stem vessels and is found associated with pollen
grains (Photo 3). In the flowers of plants treated with *M. lysodeikticus* DNA and ^{3}H thymidine the foreign integrated DNA replicates [28] as it does in the progeny [28, 30a, 40]. At this point,
the biochemical picture could possibly be correlated with the
genetic behaviour of the corrected mutants. Indeed, a *Micrococcus-
Arabidopsis* satellite peak is observed in the progeny of DNA
treated plants (wild type). Its increase upon treatment of successive generations of plants with the same bacterial DNA [30a, 40].
This is accompanied by a series of biological modifications, such
as a drastic decrease of the % germination, a delay or a complete
suppression of the flowering or the appearance of abnormal phenotypes (trichomes, rosula shape of the rosette, browning of the
leaves, white or dark brown seeds, etc...). All these effects point
toward a DNA-induced imbalance of the plant metabolism.

To what type of genetical model do these results lead ?
Different models have been discussed by Fox *et al.* [16-20] to
explain their results showing genetic transformation in *Drosophila*
with homologous DNA. They argue in favour of the exosome model,
also considered by Hess [22] to interprete *Petunia* transformation.
The exosome model (*cf*. fig. 1) is the only one which does not
requires an integration of the exogenous information into the
linear structure of the chromosome. Such an integration is rejected by Fox due to the absence of whole-body transformants in
Drosophila and to the instability of the correction. In the *Arabidopsis* system, the non-autonomous type of biochemical lesion
due to the possible diffusion of thiamine, makes it difficult to
ascertain the predicted mosaic nature of the corrected type. Its
progeny however is easier to analyse. It appears that the offspring of corrected plants behave as homozygotes as they do no
segregate, nor in their offspring (they also do not segregate
1 to 1 in test crosses). The correction being stable in subsequent offspring, it would correspond to a surprisingly stable
form of exosome.

[*] This pattern of DNA release is also found in *Sinapis alba* [63
and L. Ledoux *et al.*, this book]

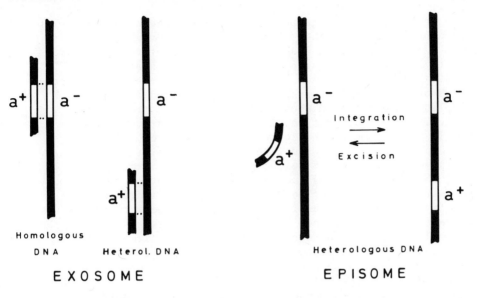

Fig. 1.- Comparison of addition and insertion models (one of two
homologous chromosomes is shown).

In *Drosophila*, transformed by homologous DNA, Fox's exosome
model implies a close association of the foreign gene with its
homologous chromosome locus. This exosome is not integrated but
replicates in step with the chromosome and can be lost or transmitted with it at the time of cell division. Either the exosomal
gene or the chromosomal one is transcribed, leading to phenotypic
mosaicism.

When heterologous DNA is used for correction, as in our case,
the necessity of a close association with the mutated site is less
mandatory and the heterologous exosome could become associated to
another region, where the actual base sequence is in favour of
such an association. Heretoo, the "exosome" could replicate in
step with the chromosome and be lost or transmitted with it at
the time of cell division. The probability of a loss would however
be high due to the imperfect homology.

In the insertion model, the foreign gene is integrated in the
recipient DNA, like and episomal DNA, through the homology of a
few base pairs. Once integrated, it would be hard to lose it, except upon pairing with a chromosome homologous for the rest of the
structure but lacking the inserted foreign piece. Whilst gene
conversion could interfere at that step, chromosome aberration
is an obvious alternative, possibly leading to the loss of the
foreign gene.

The effect of the exogenous DNA appears to be associated with the concerned gene (thiamine, thiazole or pyrimidine loci). This leads to the concept of an association of the bacterial information with the *Arabidopsis* genome. Such a close association is also indicated by the absence of significant differences between progenies of reciprocal crosses implying corrected types : 100 % normal plants are obtained upon crossing either corrected male or female with the mutant type. The thiamine mutation remains present in the genome of the corrected type : by crossing the corrected plants with the wild type, a resurgence of the original mutant type does occur in F_2 although at very low frequencies. In fact, the passage through meiosis for the plants arising from a cross with one of the corrected types seems to increase the instability of the exogenous information. This seems to be the consequence of the appearance of the phenotype "leaky mutant" (which could eventually be considered as functional mosaïcs). Besides, the correction also presents an instability with time : storing F_1 or F_2 seeds resulting from crosses between corrected and mutant or wild types results in the appearance of an increased proportion of mutants; the regularity in the transmission of the genetic information as well as the survival of the mutated site in the corrected plant could be interpreted if we assume that the necessary amount of information has been added to the genome (and not substituted to the mutation) and can be removed by crossing the plant with the wild type or with the mutant but not upon selfing. Maybe difficulties in chromosome pairing, due to the correction present in only one of the two homologous chromosomes forming the bivalent could be responsible for the removal of this correction. Such a picture fits well with the "episomal DNA" type of interpretation (*cf*. fig. 1) emerging from the biochemical analysis. This model also allows an explaination for the variability in the functioning of the bacterial thiamine gene in the recipient plant, possibly related to its relative position.

These differences in the phenotypic expression of the thiamine locus do not appear to be due to a lack of integration but to a change in the gene environment able to influence its genetic transcription and therefore its expressivity.

We thanks J. Swinnen-Vranckx and L. De Mol for their excellent technical help and Drs. Glansdorff and P. Lurquin for numerous fruitful discussions. We are indebted to the Fonds National de la Recherche Fondamentale Collective and to the Ministère de l'Education Nationale for their financial help.

References

1. Avery, O.T., C.M. McLead and M. McCarthy : J. exp. Med. 79, 137 (1944)
2. Ledoux L. : in Progress in Nucleic acid Research and molecular Biology (edit. by J.N. Davidson and W.E. Cohn) 4, 231 (Academic Press, New York, 1965)
3. Bhargava, P.M. and G. Shanmugan : in Progress in Nucleic acid Research and Molecular Biology (edit. by J.N. Davidson and W.E. Cohn) 11, 103 (Academic Press, New York, 1971)
4. Szybalska, E.H. and W. Szybalski : Proc. Nat. Acad. Sci. 48, 2026 (1962)
5. Glick, J.L. and A.P. Salim : J. Cell Biol. 33, 209 (1967)
6. Majumdar, A. and S.K. Bose : Brit. J. Cancer 22, 603 (1968)
7. Fox, M., B.W. Fox and S.R. Ayad : Nature, 222, 1086 (1969)
8. Ottolenghi-Nightingale, E. : Proc. Nat. Acad. Sci. 64, 184 (1969)
9. Borenfreund, E., Y. Honda, M. Steinglas, A. Bendich : J. of Exptl. Med. 132, 1071 (1970)
10. Roosa, R.A. : In Informative Molecules in biological systems (edit. by L. Ledoux) 67 (North Holland Cy, 1971)
11. Merril, C.R., M.R. Geier and J.C. Petricciani : Nature 233, 398 (1971)
12. Hill, M. and J. Hillova : Nature 273, 35 (1972)
13. Nawa, S. and M.A. Yamada : Genetics, 58, 573 (1968)
14. Nawa, S., B. Sakaguchi, M.A. Yamada and M. Tsujita : Genetics, 67, 221 (1971)
15. Gershenson, S.M. : Genet. Res. 6, 157 (1965)
16. Fox, A.S. and S.B. Yoon : Genetics, 53, 897 (1966)
17. Fox, A.S., W.F. Duggleby, W.M. Gelbart and S.B. Yoon : Proc. Nat. Acad. Sci. 67, 1834 (1970)
18. Fox, A.S. and S.B. Yoon : Proc. Nat. Acad. Sci. 67, 1608 (1970)
19. Fox, A.S., S.B. Yoon and W.M. Gelbart : Proc. Nat. Acad. Sci., 68, 342 (1971)
20. Fox, A.S., S.B. Yoon, W.F. Duggleby and W.M. Gelbart : in Informative molecules in biological systems (edit. by L. Ledoux) 313 (North Holland Cy, 1971)
21. Hess, D. : Z. Pflanzenphysiol. 60, 348 (1969)
22. Hess, D. : Z. Pflanzenphysiol. 68, 432 (1973)
23. Hess, D. : Naturwissenschaften, 58, 366 (1971)
24. Hess, D. : Naturwissenschaften, 59, 348 (1972)
25. Ledoux, L. and M. Jacobs : Arch. internat. Physiol. Biochim. 77, 568 (1969)
26. Ledoux, L. and R. Huart : in Barley genetics (edit. by R.A. Nilan) 2, 254 (Washington Univ. Press, 1970)
27. Ledoux, L., R. Huart and M. Jacobs : Arch. Internat. Physiol. Biochim. 78, 591 (1971)
28. Ledoux, L., R. Huart and M. Jacobs : in Informative molecules in biological systems (edit. by L. Ledoux) 159 (North Holland Cy, 1971)

29. Ledoux, L., R. Huart and M. Jacobs : in the Way ahead in plant breeding (edit. by F.G. Lupton, G. Jenkins and R. Johnson) 165 (Adlard & Son, Dorking 1972)
30a. Ledoux, L., J. Brown, P. Charles, R. Huart, M. Jacobs, J. Remy and C. Watters, in : Advances in the Biosciences (edit. by G. Raspé) 8, 347 (Pergamon Press, 1972)
30b. Ledoux, L., R. Huart and M. Jacobs, Nature 249, 17 (1974)
31. Gresshoff, P.M. and C.M. Doy : Planta 107, 161 (1972)
32. Doy, C.H., P.M. Gresshoff and B.G. Rolfe : Search, 3, 447 (1972)
33. Doy, C.H., P.M. Gresshoff and B.G. Rolfe : Proc. Nat. Acad. Sci. 70, 723 (1973)
34. Doy, C.H., P.M. Gresshoff and B.G. Rolfe : in The biochemistry of gene expression in higher organisms (edit. by J. Pollak and J. Wilson Lee) 21 (Australia and New Zealand Book Co, 1973)
35. Doy, C.H., P.M. Gresshoff and B.G. Rolfe : Nature, 244, 90 1973
36. Gartler, S.M. : Bioch. Biophys. Res. Comm. 3, 127 (1960)
37. Ledoux, L. and Huart, R. : in Uptake of informative molecules by living cells (edit. by L. Ledoux) 254 (North Holland Cy, 1972)
38. Ledoux, L., R. Huart and M. Jacobs : Eur. J. Biochem. 23, 96 (1971)
39. Ledoux, L. and P. Charles : in Uptake of informative molecules by living cells (edit. by L. Ledoux) 397 (North Holland Cy, 1972)
40. Brown, J., R. Huart, L. Ledoux and J. Swinnen-Vranckx : Arch. Internat. Physiol. Biochim. 79, 820 (1971)
41. Hotta, Y. and H. Stern : in Informative molecules in biological systems (edit. by L. Ledoux) 176 (North Holland Cy, 1971)
42. Fox, M. and S.R. Ayad : in Uptake of informative molecules by living cells (edit. by L. Ledoux) 295 (North Holland Cy, 1972)
43. Laval, F. and E. Malaise : in Bacterial transformation (edit. by L.J. Arches) 387 (Academic Press, 1973)
44. Rédei, G.P. : Bibliographia Genetica, 20, 20 (1970)
45. Rédei, G.P. : Genetics, 45, 1007 (1960), 47, 979 (1962)
46. Rédei, G.P. : Arabid. inf. Serv. 5, 36 (1968)
47. Feenstra, W.J. : Arabid. inf. Serv. 2, 25 (1965)
48. Rédei, G.P. : personnal communication
49. Van den Berg, B.I., J. Heyting and W.J. Feenstra : Arabid. inf. Serv. 4, 46 (1967)
50. Feenstra, W.J. and B.I. Van den Berg : Proc. XII Int. Cong. Genet. 1, 26 (1968)
51. Langridge, J. : Nature, 176, 260 (1955)
52. Jacobs, M. : Arabid. Inf. Serv. 1, 36 (1964)
53. Miksche, J.P. and J.A.M. Brown : Ann. J. Botany : 52, 533 (1965)
54. Marmur, J. : J. Mol. Biol. 3, 208 (1961)
55. Charles, P. : in Uptake of informative molecules by living cells (edit. by L. Ledoux) 10 (North Holland Cy, 1972)

56. Ledoux, L. and P. Charles : in Uptake of informative molecules by living cells (edit. by L. Ledoux) 29 (North Bolland Cy, 1972).

57. May, P., E. May, P. Granboulan, N. Granboulan and J. Marmur, Ann. Inst. Pasteur : $\underline{115}$, 1029 (1968)

58. Langridge, J. : Austral. J. Biol. Sci. : $\underline{11}$, 58 (1958)

59. Li, Sl and G.P. Rédei ; Rad. Bot. $\underline{9}$, 125 (1969)

60. Nikolov, C.V. and V.I. Ivanov : Genetika, $\underline{5}$, 166 (1969)

61. Ivanov, V.I. : Arabid. Inf. Serv. $\underline{8}$, 29 (1971)

62. Relichova, J. : Arabid. Inf. Serv. $\underline{9}$, 28 (1972)

63. Coumanne, C., A. Jacqmard, J.M. Kinet, M. Bodson, L. Ledoux and R. Huart : Arch. Internat. Physiol. Biochim. $\underline{79}$, 823 (1971).

64. Bennett, M.D. : Proc. R. Soc. Lond. B. $\underline{181}$, 109 (1972)

65. Johnson, C.B., D. Grierson, and H. Smith : Nature, New Biology, $\underline{244}$, 105 (1973)

UPTAKE OF DNA AND BACTERIOPHAGE INTO POLLEN AND GENETIC MANIPULATION

Dieter Hess

University of Hohenheim, D-7000 Stuttgart-70

Emil-Wolff-Str. 25

Among higher plants protplasts, tissues cultures and plant embryos are currently being discussed as systems of genetic manipulation (Review: Hess,1974). The first successes have already been attained on tissue cultures (Doy et al.1973 a, b, c; Johnson et al. 1973) and plant embryos (Review: Hess,1972; Ledoux et al.,1974), whereas the first successes on protoplasts are at least being heralded (Review: Chaleff and Carlson,1974). I confess that I too, like so many others, succumbed at first to the fascination of the protoplast system introduced mainly by Cocking (Power et al.,1970; Review: Cocking 1972). However, once one has regenerated some hundreds of petunias from isolated protoplasts (Hess and Potrykus, 1972; Hess et al.,1973; Donn et al., 1973), one knows that protoplasts do not offer only advantages. Regenerating a large number of plants from isolated protoplasts is coupled with a comparatively high expenditure of time and technology. In order to be able to carry on genetic manipulations with a chance of success, however, large numbers are necessary. Another, serious disadvantage of protoplast systems may be -must not be- that too many colleagues in too many laboratories are also working on protoplasts. Thus, it appeared advisable to look for another, perhaps more favorable system of genetic manipulation. What I intend is not to give you a review. What I am being to do is to give you insight into the first and still fragmentary steps of the experimental examination of an idea: one could use pollen for genetic manipulation under two different aspects, considering only the introduction of exogenous genetic material:

first, one could introduce exogenous DNA into very
young, isolated pollen and then raise them to possibly
genetically altered haploid plants. An important prerequisite for such experiments, the regeneration of
normal plants from pollen in fully synthetic media, has
been provided by Mrs.Nitsch (1974).

second, one could introduce exogenous DNA into older
pollen, capable of germinating. If this DNA would be
maintained, it might be brought into the zygote at fertilisation. In this way too, one might possibly arrive
at genetically altered plants (Hess, 1974).

Our colleagues in Gif-sur-Yvette are more competent in attaining the first possibility. We concerned
ourselves with the second possibility, that of using
pollen as "vector" for exogenous DNA within the range
of natural fertilisation. The advantages of this method
are obvious: since one hasn't removed himself very far
from the natural situation, one ought to obtain a large
amount of seed material in a very simple manner. This
could then be tested for possible genetic alterations,
for example, using appropriate nutrient media.

Before I discuss the corresponding experiments, a
short reminder of the sexual reproduction of angiosperms
which I believe I owe the colleagues who are not professional botanists. On the male side pollen grains with
two cells, the microgametophytes, develop at first from
the gones of the meiosis. These two cells are the vegetative and generative cell. If the pollen has been
carried to an appropriate stigma, it germinates with the
formation of a pollen tube, which emanates from the vegetative cell. The generative cell sooner or later divides
into two sperm cells. These are then transported via the
pollen tube to the ovules where they carry out the so-
called double fertilisation. On the female side as a
rule only one of the four gones of the meiosis develops
into a macrogametophyte of which only the egg cell and
the diploid secondary embryo sack nucleus are of interest here. During the double fertilisation just mentioned
one sperm cell fuses with the egg cell to form the zygote from which the new plant grows via mitotic divisions.
The second sperm cell unites with the secondary embryo
sack nucleus to form the triploid endosperm nucleus from
which the development of the endosperm proceeds the latter usually servin as nutrient tissue.

The description of the course of gametophyte development and fertilisation clearly shows under what prerequisitions pollen may be utilized as DNA carrier:
the pollen must take up and maintain DNA, they must develop into pollen tubes and carry out the fertilisation

in spite of the DNA treatment and, finally, they must
carry the exogenous DNA into the zygote by fertilisation.

DNA TREATMENT, POLLEN GERMINATION, POLLINATION, FERTI-
LISATION AND SEED SET

      I was simple but time consuming to clarify some
of the prerequisitions just mentioned. Experiments on
Petunia hybrida and Nicotiana glauca showed that pollen
can germinate in DNA solutions. Only DNA concentrations
higher than 100 γ /ml impaired germination of Nicotiana
glauca, while Petunia hybrida showed itself to be less
sensitive.
      The methodology of DNA incubation and pollination
is described using Petunia as an example (fig.1). An=
thers are collected 24 hours before anthesis, squashed
in pollen germination medium containing the exogenous
DNA and then incubated with shaking on a 25°C water
bath for 5 hours. The incubation preparations were
either sterile or contained 50γ/ml each of cloxacillin

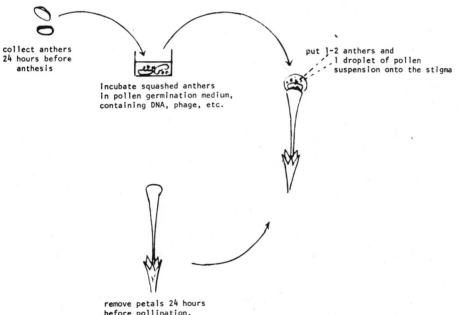

Fig.1. DNA treatment of pollen material and "wet" pollination in the case of Petunia (scheme).

and ampicillin as antibiotics ore were both of them.
The antibiotics mentioned don´t injure our plant material: we succeeded in regenerating normal petunia plants
from protoplasts kept from their isolation in media
containing cloxacillin and ampillin (Hess, unpublished
results). 24 hours before anthesis anthers and petals
were removed from receptor blossoms (removing the petals prevents rotteness if a drop of pollination liquid accidentally rolls down along the style). One to
two anthers and an additional drop of the pollen suspension were then put onto each style.- Nicotiana was
pollinated in the same way, only that removing the petals proved to be unnecessary. Besides, pollen previously from the anthers were incubated as a rule here. It
should be noted that, of course, pollen and anther wall
were separated in the case of Petunia as well if DNA
from pollen was supposed to be re-isolated.
  Normal seeds capable of normal germination were
obtained using such wet pollinations. The amount of
seeds is less than that obtained with dry pollination,
this resulting less from damage than from the smaller
number of pollen brought onto the stigmata via wet pollination.

UPTAKE OF EXOGENOUS GENETIC MATERIAL

  After these first positive findings,it no longer
seemed absolutely unreasonable to attack now the next
big problem, that of the uptake of exogenous genetic
material.

DNA uptake

  The uptake of DNA was investigated first (Hess et
al.,1974 a). Autoradiographic investigations served to
give the initial orientation. Pollen from Nicotiana
glauca were incubated with 14C-labelled DNA from Rhizobium leguminosarum, among others. Before autoradiogra-
phing the pollen were thoroughly washed and treated with
DNase to remove any externally attached DNA. Radioactivity could be detected within germinated and ungerminated
pollen as well as in the region of the cytoplasm emerging after an occasional bursting of the pollen material
during preparation (fig.2). No DNase activity was found
in the incubation medium. Thus, the autoradiographic results are consistent with a DNA uptake, but, as usual,
cannot give a definite proof thereof. In particular,
no statements regarding the fate -decay or not- of the
uptaken exogenous DNA can be made.

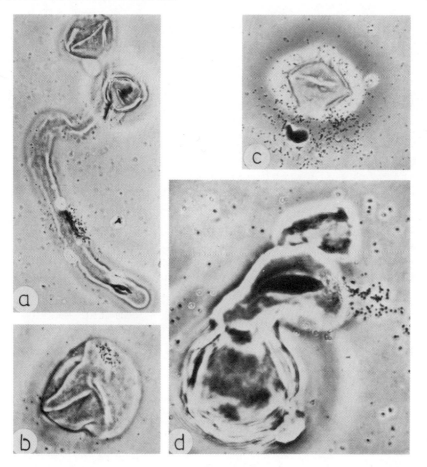

Fig.2. a. Pollen of Nicotiana glauca incubated for 3
hours in germination medium containing 100 /ml 14C-la-
belled Rhizobium DNA. Radioactive labelling in the position of one of the pollen nuclei.- b. Pollen of N.glau-
ca incubated for 3 hours in germination medium containing 300 /ml 14C-labelled Rhizobium DNA. The germination
is blocked by the high DNA concentration. Radioactive
labelling in the position of one of the pollen nuclei.-
c. Pollen of N. glauca incubated for 2 hours in germination medium containing 100 /ml 14C-labelled Rhizobium
DNA. Radioactivity could be detected preferentially
where the pollen was burst during preparation.- d. Pollen of N. glauca incubated for 3 hours in germination
medium containing 50 /ml 14C-labelled Rhizobium DNA.
Location of radioactivity as in c.- Magnification a.
560x, b.900x, c.900x, d.1760.For details see Hess et al.,
1974 a.

Using 3H-labelled bacterial DNA a clarification was attempted in experiments in which the labelled DNA was re-isolated from the pollen after incubation and then separated in the CsCl density gradient. A procedure for obtaining native DNA from pollen had to be worked out first since the methods used to date were much too coarse to even be considered for our objectives. After repeated washings, DNase treatment and renewed washings, cold ethanol was used for a pre-extraction which especially removed lipids and exine pigments that might disturb. Subsequently, the exine was softened by treating with detergents. Several detergents were tested. To this the pollen were incubated in the detergent and then put onto a slide. Then, a slight pressure was exerted with the cover glass and the result microscopically evaluated. Triton X-114 and Triton X-100 proved to be the most appropriate; subsequently we used Triton X-100 routinely (fig.3). A slightly modified Marmur procedure and then the separation in the density gradient followed the Triton treatment.

With Petunia younger pollen, but already in the 2-cell stage, were used. They had not yet germinated in the time of the incubation. The pollen were incubated with 3H-labelled DNA from a strain of E.coli which

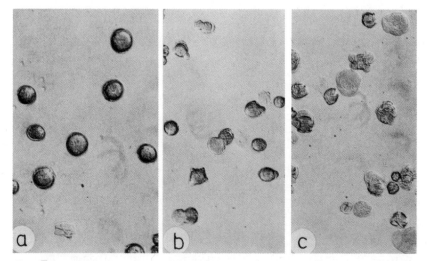

Fig.3. Treatment of pollen grains with Triton X-100. Pollen of Petunia treated for 5 min. with Triton 1%. No pressure with the cover glass (a), slight pressure (b), stronger pressure (c). For details see Hess et al., 1974 a.

carried an R-factor for kanamycin resistance. After incubation and re-isolation of the DNA from the pollen,
the DNA of the pollen could be identified from its extinction, while that from E.coli from its radioactivity. The E.coli DNA gave two peaks of which one represented the chromosomal DNA and the other the R-factors
(fig.4). The radioactivity values are low, but statistically significant and reproducible.

        With Nicotiana older pollen which germinated to
80% during the incubation period in a medium developed
by us were incubated with 3H-labelled DNA from Rhizobium leguminosarum. After re-isolating the DNA from the
pollen, the DNA of the pollen could once again be localized in the density gradient by its extinction, the
bacterial DNA by its radioactivity (fig.5). As expected,
the DNA uptake of germinating pollen was greater than
that of the non-germinating Petunia pollen.

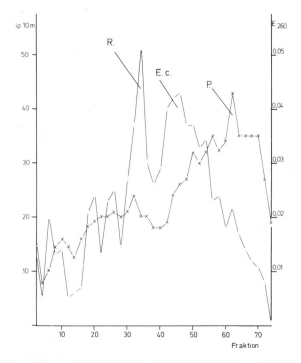

Fig.4. CsCl gradient centrifugation of DNA isolated from
unripe pollen grains of Petunia. The pollen material was
incubated with 3H-labelled DNA from E.coli, strain R_1
drd 16, carrying an R-factor against kanamycin. x-x-x:
extinction 260 nm; .-.-. : radioactivity. R = plasmid
DNA; E.c. = chromosomal DNA of E.coli, P = Petunia DNA.
For details see Hess et al., 1974 a.

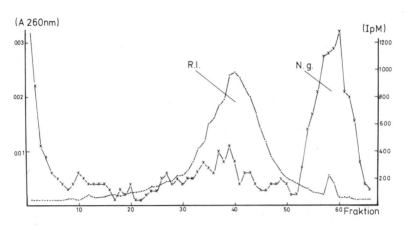

Fig.5. CsCl gradient centrifugation of DNA isolated from germinated pollen material of Nicotiana. The pollen was incubated with 3H-labelled DNA from Rhizobium leguminosarum. x-x-x: Extinction 260 nm; .-.-. : radioactivity. R.l. = Rhizobium DNA, N.g. = Nicotiana DNA. For details see Hess et al., 1974 a.

     A possibility for deception could consist in the reisolation of externally attached DNA or DNA which penetrated between exine and intine. The details of the isolation procedure, especially the DNase and Triton treatment seem to allow to eliminate this possibility.

Uptake of protein and phages

     The chances of the succes of a genetic manipulation increase if one adds the genes of interest at as high a concentration as possible. This may occur in the form of isolated plasmids like the R-factor just mentioned, for example. Bacteriophages as carriers of bacterial genes offer probably even more advantages, as results on animal and plant cells in culture indicated (Review: Merril and Stanbro,1974) since they have in addition a protective protein coat -an advantage, however, only when the protein coat can be removed in the receptor cell. For that reason we checked the possibility of an uptake of phages into-swelling and germinating Petunia pollen (Hess et al., 1975).

First information was obtained on a model system.
Pollen were incubated in FITC-labelled bovine serum albumin and afterwards observed under a fluorescence microscope. Non swollen pollen did not show fluorescence
in their interiors, whereas 50 % each of the swollen
and germinated did (fig. 6). Fluorescence of the exine
can clearly be differentiated from the FITC-fluorescen-
ce of the pollen content, especially at higher magnifi-
cations. In older pollen tubes the fluorescence often
concentrates in the tip region rich in cytoplasm (cf.
also fig. 7). In pollen tubes the fluorescing particles
may be transported by the cytoplasmic streaming -addi-
tional proof that they are actually inside the pollen.
Extracting incubated pollen onto proteins and separating
the protein extracts with the help of polyacrylamid gel
electrophoresis, resulted in fluorescing zones of the
same mobility as with FITC-serum albumin.

After these positive experiments on the model system, phages lambda gal+ were labelled with FITC. After
incubating pollen with such phages, the same fluorescence pattern as in the case of FITC-serum albumin resulted (fig. 7). However, at least part of the fluorescence

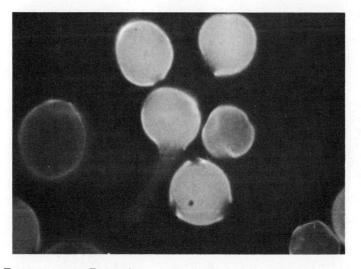

Fig.6. Pollen of Petunia after 5 hours incubation in
germination medium containing 1 mg/ml FITC-bovine serum albumin. Four pollen have taken up FITC-bovine serum albumin, one of them has germinated. The other pollen show only the fluorescence of the exine. For details
see Hess et al., 1975.

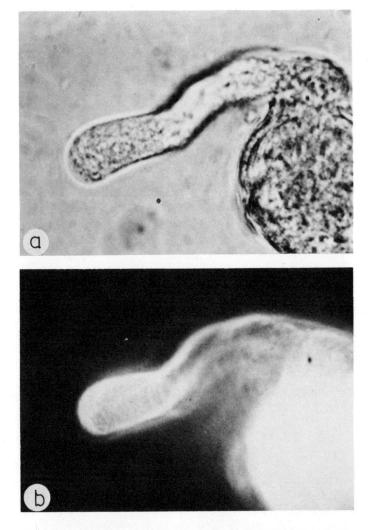

Fig. 7. Germinated pollen of Petunia after 6 hours incubation in germination medium containing FITC-labelled
bacteriophage lambda. a. light field, b. induced fluorescence. Not only the pollen grain itself but also the
growing region at the tip of the pollen tube show extensive fluorescence. For details see Hess et al.,1975.

may originate from FITC-labelled bacterial proteins
still present in the phage preparations. But there now
existed the further possibility of a re-isolation of the
phages from the pollen and a subsequent plaques-test for
biological activity. Petunia pollen (approximate titer
1.5×10^6/ml) were incubated with phages lambda gal+
(approximate titer 5×10^8 pfu/ml). The phages were
subsequently re-isolated. As with the DNA isolation,
this phage re-isolation included a treatment with ethanol and Triton X-100. Ethanol destroys the biological
activity of the phages. Since the pollen were in contact with ethanol for 10 minutes and the ethanol pene-
trates in this time also between exine and intine, all
phage activity after re-isolation must result from phages taken into the pollen. The plaques-tests showed that
one active phage particle could be recovered on every
tenth pollen grain. But this does not mean that only
every tenth pollen grain had picked up a phage since
one must consider that according to the fluorescence
patterns only about 50 % of the viable pollen take up
proteins, and, thus, proteids like phages, that with
the procedure used only 50 % of the pollen are broken
on the average, that phages may be denatured by the
extraction and, finally, that phages already inside the
pollen could be decomposed into their DNA and protein
components. Thus, the uptake of the phages ought to be
greater than the abovementioned numbers indicate.

BIOLOGICAL EFFECTS

Bacterial DNA, including episomes, and phages, can,
as we have seen, be taken up by swelling and germinating
pollen of higher plants. Investigations have been initiated in which the behaviour of the uptaken exogenous
genetic material in the germinating pollen shall be
checked in detail. Let's jump over this gap and ask,
wether a fertilisation via pollen which have been treated with exogenous DNA can induce biological effects on
the resulting descendants. The designation "biological
effects" should be chosen because a phenomenon that
might appear must not necessarily result from an activity of the exogenous DNA. Further extended investigations
are required here.

DNA treatment of Nicotiana glauca pollen

Now to biological effects after treating the pollen
with total DNA. As is known, the hybrid Nicotiana glauca
x langsdorffii develops genetic tumors. This tumor formation also ought to appear after a successfull DNA

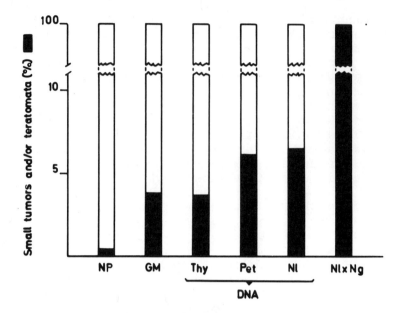

Fig.8. Biological effects of treatments of Nicotiana
glauca pollen on the descendants. Treatments: NP = normal pollination, GM = pollen germinated in germination
medium, then wet pollination, Thy = pollen incubated
in germination medium containing calf thymus DNA, Pet =
pollen incubated in germination medium containing Petunia
DNA, Nl = pollen incubated in germination medium containing Nicotiana langsdorffii DNA. In any case the DNA
was tested in a range of concentrations. Because there
were no significant differences between the concentrations
of a given DNA, the respective values were taken together to one column. Nl x Ng = hybrid Nicotiana glauca
x langsdorffii. Thy and GM are statistically significant different from NP and from Pet and Nl.

transfer between the two. Since Nicotiana glauca shows
a slight innate tendency to tumor formation it was used
as DNA receptor. N. glauca pollen were allowed to germinate in DNA of various origins and different concentrations. N. glauca was then pollinated with this pollen. The young plants resulting from this fertilisation were injured by making a cut in the transition region sprout - root at an age of 6 to 10 weeks. After 2

additional months small tumor formations, easily distinguishable from callus, and teratomic sprout and leaf
formation were found in the area of the former cut (fig.
8). It was already obvious in these first investigations how careful one had to be since the wet pollination with the pollen medium alone let the rate of abnormal growth symptoms increase, while Petunia and N.
langsdorffii DNA did even more so (Hess et al., unpublished results). Now without any doubt, N. glauca reacts
particularly sensitive, but in the following we will
come across the same basic phenomenon, namely, a certain reaction in control groups too.

Treatment of Petunia pollen with R-factors

All further investigations were carried out on
Petunia hybrida. First a look at the initial experiments
with plasmids. Petunia seeds were laid out to germinate

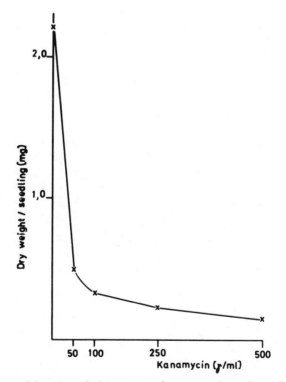

Fig. 9. The effect of kanamycin on the development of
Petunia seedlings (cf. the text).

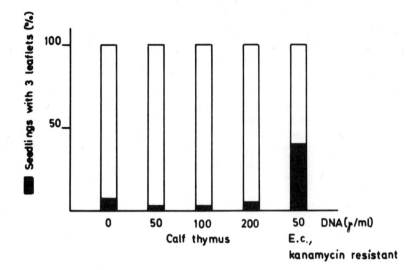

Fig. 10. Development of seedlings on kanamycin agar in
dependance from the treatment of pollen. The seedlings
were 14 days old. Abscissa: treatment of the pollen.
0 = wet pollination with germination medium.

on agar media (Rangaswamy and Shivanna, 1967, modified
according to Wagner and Hess, 1973) that contained antibiotics. Kanamycin impaired the development of the petunia seedlings the most of several antibiotics tested
(fig.9). As a result thereof, pollen were incubated in
total DNA of E.coli containing R-factors against kanamycin or in isolated R-factors. The resulting seeds were
then laid out on agar media with 50 or 100 µ/ml kanamycin. Up to now not much more can be said than that the
development of one portion of the treated seedlings is
less disturbed than that of control seedlings (fig.10;
Hess, unpublished results).

Treatment of Petunia pollen with phages

        Investigations using phages lambda gal are some-
what further advanced. After appropriate incubation of
the pollen, seeds were obtained and laid out to germinate on galactose containing agar. 1 % galactose acts
extremely toxic. The survival rate of the seedlings
from 1 % galactose having previously treated the pollen

Tabl. 1. Biological effects of fertilisations with
lambda phage incubated pollen material

Pollination and fertilization of <u>Petunia hybrida</u> with pollen of
<u>Petunia hybrida</u>, incubated with λ gal+ or λ gal-. The resulting
seeds were tested on Rangaswamy medium containing 1% galactose.

Incubation with gal+	Incubation with gal-
Number of seeds: 1858	Number of seeds: 1669
Seeds germinated: 1471	Seeds germinated: 1413
Seedlings surviving after 6 weeks on 1% galactose: 19	Seedlings surviving after 6 weeks on 1% galactose: 7

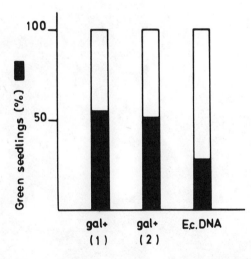

Fig.11. Biological effects of treatments of pollen with
phages lambda gal on the descendants. Ordinate: green
surviving seedlings after 6 weeks on 0,1 % galactose
agar.Abscissa: treatments of the pollen. 1,2 = experiment 1 and 2. The E.coli DNA used was of commercial
origin.

with gal+ is higher than after a control treatment with
gal- (tab.1). Correspnding results were obtained when
the seeds were tested on 0,1 % galactose agar. Here too
the number of green, viable seedlings was greater after
treating the pollen with gal+ than in a control group
treated with total DNA from the wild strain of E.coli
(fig. 12). It should be mentioned that after treating
the pollen with gal- and with Petunia DNA the survival
rate also lies within the range of the E.coli controls.
That the DNA of the wild strain of E.coli doesn´t exert
any effect may depend from the much lower concentration
of the gal+ -genes or from their better protection in
the phage particles.

Further experiments were carried out with phages
lambda lac+ . Petunia seedlings are also disturbed in
their development on lactose containing agar media,
though considerably less than on galactose containing
media. The inhibitory effects become most noticeable in
darkness, especially in the root area. Unfortunately,

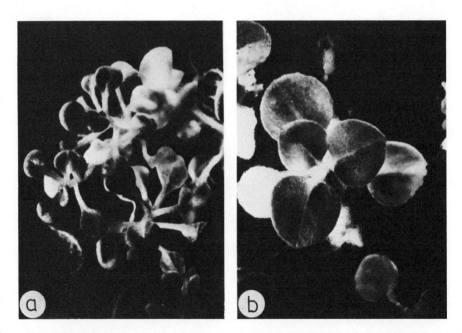

Fig.12. Biological effects of treatments of pollen with
phages lambda lac+. The Petunia seedlings shown were
grown for 6 weeks on 1 % lactose agar. a. normal appear-
ence of the seedlings. b. one of the stronger seedlings.

etiolated seedlings are so weekend that till now without exception they did not survive. For this reason we
were forced to raise the embryos in light were the damage is considerably less under the influence of photosynthesis which is now possible. Petunia pollen were
now incubated with phages lambda lac+ and the resulting
seeds were put out to germinate on agar with 1% lactose.
Among 612 seedlings of a first experiment, 10 showed
particularly strong growth (fig.12). Six weeks after
sowing, the fresh weight of their first primary leaflet was 3.5 times that of the smaller seedlings. The
ß-galactosidase activity determined by the ONPG test·
was twice as high as in the primary leaflets of the
seedlings that remained small (fig.13). In a repeti-
tion of this experiment we found among 652 seedlings
7 of these stronger seedlings.

Untreated control groups and control groups treated with calf thymus DNA or with Petunia DNA corresponded to the smaller seedlings regarding the properties
mentioned. Control groups that had been treated with
phages lambda gal- and with colicinogenic factors are
under investigation. The larger seedlings as well as

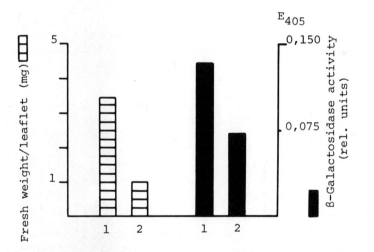

Fig.13. Biological effects of treatments of pollen with
phages lambda lac+ on the descendants. Seedlings were
grown for 6 weeks on 1 % lactose agar. Most of them remained small (2), some grew stronger (1). The stronger
seedlings showed a higher fresh weight of, for example,
their first primary leaflet and a higher ß-galactosidase
activity. cf. the text.

some control seedlings have, in the meantime, been
transferred from agar to soil in order to be able to
raise descendants.

CONCLUDING REMARKS

So much for some biological effects that ought
to result from the respective preceding treatment of
the pollen. We want to remind here only of the control
groups to make it clear that the respective biological
effect falls at least partly within the range of the
species specific reaction norm and has nothing to do
with a becoming effective of the exogenous gene material. As in corresponding experiments on animal cell
cultures as for instance the transfer of resistance to
certain antibiotics or nucleic acid antimetabolites,
the differences are mainly of a quantitative nature.
This makes further analysis in the direction of eventual genetic alterations difficult. We are currently
raising and testing as described above descendants of
experimental and control plants in all cases. It is
obvious that genetically altered plants eventually may
not be identified in view of the spot-test character
of this breeding. The lac+ -system appears to be most
favorable, at least at present, since the number of
altered seedlings is reasonable low, since there was
no background in the controls and since the ß-galactosidase can be easily tested. Furthermore it may be
usefull that the ß-galactosidase from E.coli can be
differentiated from the plant ß-galactosidase with the
help of specific antisera (Doy et al.,1973 b).

Instead of reporting on the uptake of DNA in protoplasts   -something on which we have been working for
quite a while and still will continue to do, so that a
secure basis could already be established (Hess et al.,
1973; Hoffmann and Hess, 1973; Hoffmann, 1973), I have
reported about subjects that are still in a state of
fluxe. But then to me, the purpose of such a meeting
appears to be not only to teach what is already known
ex cathedra, but also to discuss what is new. That this
concerns -possibly still- uncertain territory becomes
especially clear when one attempts a short summary: the
advantages of the pollen system for genetic manipulation
are obvious, the disadvantage is only that in spite of
several positive indices we still do not know wether it
will also function.

References

Chaleff,R.S., and P.S.Carlson: Ann.Rev.Genetics 8, in press (1974).

Cocking,E.C.: Ann.Rev.Plant Physiol.23,29 (1972).

Donn,G., D.Hess und I.Potrykus: Z.Pflanzenphysiol.69, 423 (1973).

Doy,C.H., P.M.Gresshoff and B.G.Rolfe: Proc.Austral. Biochem.Soc.5, 3 (1972).

Doy,C.H., P.M.Gresshoff and B.G.Rolfe: in Pollack and Lee (eds.), The Biochemistry of Gene Expression in Higher Organisms, p. 21 (1973 a).

Doy,C.H.,P.M.Gresshoff and R.G.Rolfe:Proc.Nat.Acad. Sci. USA 70, 723 (1973 b).

Doy,C.H.,P.M.Gresshoff and R.G.Rolfe: Nature New Biology 244, 90 (1973 c).

Hess,D.: Naturwissenschaften 59, 348 (1972).

Hess,D.: Biol.Rdsch. 12, in press (1974).

Hess,D., I.Potrykus, G.Donn and F.Hoffmann: Colloques internationaux C.N.R.S. 212, 343 (1973).

Hess,D., H.Lörz und E.Weissert: Z.Pflanzenphysiol.74, in press (1974).

Hess,D., P.M.Gresshoff, U.Fielitz and D.Gleiss: Z.Pflanzenphysiol. in press (1975).

Hoffmann,F.:Z.Pflanzenphysiol.69, 249 (1973).

Hoffmann,F., and D.Hess: Z.Pflanzenphysiol.69, 81 (1973).

Johnson,C.B., D.Grierson and H.Smith: Nature New Biology 244, 105 (1973).

Ledoux,L., R.Huart and M.Jacobs: Nature 249, 17 (1974).

Merril,C.R., and H.Stanbro: Z.Pflanzenphysiol.72, 371 (1974).

Nitsch,C.: C.R.Acad.Sci.Paris,Serie D,278, 1031 (1974).

Power,J.B., S.E.Cummins and E.C.Cocking: Nature 225, 1016 (1970).

Rangaswamy,N.S., and K.R.Shivanna: Nature 216, 937 (1967).

Wagner,G., and D.Hess: Z.Pflanzenphysiol.69,262 (1973).

THEORETICAL AND COMPARITIVE ASPECTS OF BACTERIOPHAGE

TRANSFER AND EXPRESSION IN EUKARYOTIC CELLS IN CULTURE

PETER M. GRESSHOFF

UNIVERSITÄT HOHENHEIM

STUTTGART, WEST GERMANY

I. Introduction:

There have been numerous reports of experiments demonstrating genetic manipulation of plant cells using intercellular gene transfer between related (same species) and unrelated (different genera) organisms. Due to the relative ease of isolating bacterial DNA, most emphasis was placed on the uptake, fate and expression of prokaryotic DNA in plant cells. Several reviews give an adequate survey and synopsis of the work (Merril, 1974; Merril and Stanbro, 1974; Johnson and Grierson, 1974; Heyn et al, 1974; Chaleff and Carlson, 1974).

Many of the phenomena described have been termed 'transformation' because of analogy to the bacterial system, in which isolated donor DNA has been used to confer a new phenotype to a recipient cell. However, none of the prokaryote-eukaryote gene transfer systems have been investigated extensively enough to justify the use of a precise term which certainly carries delineated connotations of mechanism and mode of action. For this reason the term 'transgenosis' - meaning simply the transfer and subsequent expression of genetic material from one cell to another - was proposed by Doy, Gresshoff and Rolfe (1972). The term contains no implication of mechanism and is not restrictive.

The experimental findings of the phage-mediated

539

transgenosis of the lactose and galactose operon of
<u>Escherichia coli</u> to cultured cells of <u>Lycopersicon</u>
<u>esculentum</u> (tomato) have been described and discussed
previously (Doy, Gresshoff and Rolfe, 1972, 1973 a,
b, c).

In this presentation I wish to discuss some
general aspects of intercellular gene transfer. The
discussion will touch upon the biological and physical
state of the donor gene material, its mode of
application, its subsequent entry into the cell and
its survival from nuclease digestion to finally allow
phenotypic expression (via successful RNA polymerase
recognition, transcription, termination, translation
and finally function within the new cellular
environment). The status of inheritance and the
maintenance of the transgenotic state are also
discussed.

II. <u>How the donor genes are presented to the host</u>
     <u>cell</u>:

Isolated genetic material has been presented to
plant cells in four basic classes. The DNA was either
isolated by conventional techniques and was thus
'naked' (Ledoux et al, 1971, 1974; Hess 1972; Ohyama
et al 1972; Bendich and Filner 1971; Rebel et al 1973;
Hoffmann 1973), or as a plasmid (Ledoux et al, 1974).
The DNA can also be packaged in a membrane envelope
(as an organelle, like a nucleus or chloroplast (for
uptake of these organelles see Potrykus 1973 and
Potrykus and Hoffmann 1973)) or as a whole cell
(plant cell protoplast - for an overall review of
fusion biology see Cocking 1974 this volume). The
final alternative of presenting the gene material to
the recipient is to wrap it in a protective protein
sheath of a bacteriophage (Doy et al, 1972; Carlson,
1973; Johnson et al, 1973).

Two major considerations govern the selection of
the appropriate type of DNA delivery. First, there
is the gene titre which for obvious reasons should be
high for the specific gene or gene cluster to be
transferred. Secondly, there is the survival chance
of the gene material (DNA) to the digestion by
nucleases in the extra and intracellular environment.

Isolation of total DNA from bacteria and plants
gives low specific gene titres. As the process of
gene transfer is concerned with the correction or

addition of a new specific gene to the recipient
genome, and since this process is thought to be rare,
one should use the highest gene titre possible. This
condition is neither met by total DNA extractions nor
by organelle and protoplast fusions. Other non-
relevant genes may have undesired effects by causing
deleterious interactions in finely balanced control
functions of the host cell. This holds especially
true if the donor and recipient cell are widely
separated by evolution.

     The second point concerns the stability of the
DNA in the extra and intracellular environment.
Nucleases there destroy the DNA long before efficient
entry, possible expression and/or integration. High
DNAase activities hampering gene transfer experiments
have been reported to interfere with DNA uptake and
integration in a cellwall-less mutant of Chlamydomonas
reinhardi (CW15, Lurquin, 1974 this volume) and in
cultured tobacco cells (Bendich and Filner, 1971).
The use of freely digestible gene material in such a
situation would clearly eliminate any chance of
success. In converse, nuclease resistant or
protected DNA may have an increased chance of entry
and subsequent function. The use of polyions (Aoki
and Takebe, 1969; Ohyama et al, 1972) and DEAE-dextran
(Hoffmann, 1973; Hoffmann and Hess, 1973) should
possibly be extended in principle to facilitate
greater DNA stability prior to uptake and integration.
Possible protection may also stem from the use of
basic or neutral proteins which would interact with
the DNA thus hopefully masking it from nuclease
digestion.

     A further problem regarding nucleases comes from
within the cell. Host cell recognition and restriction
is critical in the transformation of E. coli K12
(Cosloy and Oishi, 1973 a, b; Oishi and Cosley, 1974)
and of other bacteria (see Tomasz, 1974 this volume).
Similar restriction functions are certain to exist
within plant cells as a natural type of 'immune-
system' against gene transfer in nature. It may
soon be clear that these factors have to be
investigated and understood before intercellular
gene transfer becomes a technique which will serve
directly as a tool for plant genotype manipulation
and improvement. In the context of stability it
should also be mentioned that DNA circularity or the
potential for it may serve as a stabilising factor
against exonuclease digestion. Circular DNA also

has the advantage that it can exist as an autonomously replicating plasmid. Hence the need for integration as a prerequisite for function can be eliminated.

Another problem of DNA isolation and the subsequent feeding of it to a plant cell in the hope of a gene transfer is the biological competence of the DNA. Does the method of isolation alter the DNA? Can it still be transcribed? These are important questions which are seldomly answered.

Taking all these factors into consideration the experimental potential of the specialised transducing phage becomes apparent. Titres of 10^{13} plaque forming units (pfu) per milliliter can be obtained by relatively simple techniques; undesired gene material is kept at a minimal (up to 50 extra genes); protein coat and potential circularity provide increased protection from nuclease digestion and finally phage particles and their DNA are known to have complete biological activity. Additionally one finds that phage are easily assayed, thus providing an empirical basis of comparison for gene titre.

III.   The Mode of Application:

The methods for adding exogenous genetic material to a recipient plant cell are essentially similar. Isolated DNA or phage is applied in a solution designed to inhibit nuclease activity (SSC) to various parts of a plant; a certain time is allotted to allow uptake after which, the phenomenon is studied by a variety of experimental approaches. Intercellular gene transfer has been initiated with seedlings, callus cells, suspended callus cells, protoplasts, pollen grains and ovules. All these modes of application of the exogenous genome did not intentionally foster an increased uptake by means other than a more or less passive mechanism. As yet there is no published record of an attempt which tries to overcome this barrier of passive uptake. Utilisation of plant viruses, micro-injection and/or alterations in the environment to increase uptake (e.g. by pinocytosis) have not been attempted or have failed to provide publishable results. The use of a hybrid DNA molecule, for example between a DNA-plant virus (like cauliflower-mosaic virus) and a specialised transducing phage or a specific bacterial episome could possibly breakdown existing barriers to highly efficient intercellular gene

transfer. Such altered plant viruses may prove to be
efficient 'gene-shuttles' between plant cells.

IV. Gene Uptake:

The uptake of exogenous genetic material was
demonstrated experimentally in several systems. Major
experimental tools have been radioactive uptake
experiments, reisolation of total DNA followed by
isopycnic centrifugation, autoradiography, phage
reisolation and electron microscopy. The above
techniques have provided a spectrum of data to
substantiate the claim for exogenous DNA or phage
uptake into plant cells of a wide variety of species
and cell types.

For long the plant cellwall was thought to
restrict and possibly eliminate the uptake of DNA,
however, experimental findings do not verify this
assumption. Plant cell protoplasts may have their
future uses in the direct manipulation of genotypes
but for many gene transfer experiments their cellwall-
less state is not essential.

The experimental basis and discussion of the
evidence for DNA uptake and integration is presented
by Ledoux (1974, this volume) and Kleinhofs (1974,
this volume). As yet there have been few attempts
to illustrate the entry of whole phage into plant
cells. Future emphasis may have to be given to the
investigation of that point in order to understand
and control phage-mediated transgenosis to a larger
extent. However, the answers may have to await the
development of a synchronous phage-plant cell system,
so that the to be observed effect can be studied on a
larger cell population, rather than on the small cell
numbers, which are transgenosised presently and then
subjected to a selection. In other words, early
processes cannot be studied if the event is rare and
can only be seen after a period of selection. If
synchrony can be established, as in a protoplast
system like that of Carlson (1973) or the fibroblast
system of Merril et al (1971), then the early
functions of uptake and initial fate of the exogenous
gene material can be investigated.

V. Transcription and Translation within Plant Cells:

Bacterial gene transcription, translation and
product function have been demonstrated in human

galactosemic fibroblasts by Merril and co-workers
(Merril et al, 1971, 1972; Geier and Merril, 1972).
A complete study has not been performed on a plant
system as yet. Stroun and co-workers reported the
transcription of bacterial DNA in young plant shoots
following treatment with whole bacteria or isolated
DNA (Stroun, 1971 a, b). However, care should be
taken in the interpretation of results which stem
from experimental systems in which the chance of
contaminating organisms is large. Many data derived
by various workers investigating whole plants or
plant organs may be artifacts introduced into the
system by closely associated fungi and/or bacteria
(see Sarrouy-Balat et al, 1973; Delseny, 1974, this
volume). The use of aseptic tissue cultures
eliminates many of the difficulties encountered in
whole plant work. Cultures in several laboratories
are routinely monitored for intercellular microorganisms. In general these are conspicuous during
normal culture.

Otherwise the evidence for transcription of
foreign DNA within plant cells stems from the
assumption that a specific biological function must
have been preceded by successful transcription and
translation. Biological function (and thus the
assumed translation) has been reported in the following
gene transfer systems examined in plants: (i) the
DNA-mediated correction of thiamine auxotrophs of
Arabidopsis thaliana (Ledoux et al, 1971, 1974, also
this volume), (ii) the transfer of genes controlling
the anthrocyanin biosynthesis and leaf-shape in
Petunia hybrida (Hess, 1969, 1970, 1972, 1973), (iii)
fd phage synthesis and modification of host-range in
tobacco leaves treated with isolated fd phage DNA
(Sander, 1964, 1967), (iv) limited growth and survival
of lambda-gal$^+$ treated tomato cells on a galactose
medium (thus overcoming the inability to utilise this
sugar as the sole source of carbon) (Doy et al, 1973
a, b), (v) growth on lactose and presence of an
immune-specific bacterial ß-galactosidase activity
within specialised transducing phage treated tomato
callus cells (Doy et al, 1973 a,b,c), (vi) cellular
deterioration and subsequent death of haploid and
diploid callus of A. thaliana and L. esculentum
(tomato) after the exposure to phage coding for a
nonsense suppressing transfer-RNA(supF$^+$) (Doy et al,
1973 a,b), (vii) S-adenosylmethionine cleaving enzyme
and RNA polymerase in phage T3 infected barley protoplasts (Carlson, 1973), and (viii) the survival and

growth of lambda-lac[+] treated sycamore suspension
cultures on lactose as the only carbon source (Johnson
et al, 1973; Smith, 1974, this volume).

The question is, what is similar between the above
intercellular gene transfer data. First, they fall
into two distinct classes, one concerned with whole
plants, the other with cultured plant cells. The
whole plant systems have been genetically analysed
and provide data which seem to be best explained by
the 'exosome model' (for a detailed discussion see
Fox and Yoon, 1970; Hess, 1973). In all cases the
new trait was inherited and passed on through mitosis
and meiosis.

The data from cultured cells show the following
similarity. All phage effects appeared to be present
very shortly after phage infection and they were
temporal. The phage functions were usually found
within 2 to 7 days; this mimics the data of phage
transcription and enzyme appearance of Merril et al
(1971, 1972). Clearly phage entered the cells, was
transcribed and translated quickly, and thus altered
the life-style of the host cell for a short period.
Several authors have then reported a decrease of the
phage-induced phenotype (Smith, 1974, this volume,
Carlson, 1973). Additionally data from supF[+] treated
tomato and Arabidopsis cells support this model of
early expression (Doy et al, 1973 a). Within one
week after phage inoculation cellular death and
cessation of cell growth were noticed.

Totally in contrast stand the data of Doy et al
(1973 a,b,c) which showed that the time required after
initial phage infection to demonstrate the phenotypic
response of the tomato cells to the Ø80plac[+] was up
to 6 weeks. Bacterial specific ß-galactosidase
activity was also demonstrated after an identical
phenotypic time lag. Cell growth generally was
concentrated in specific areas of the callus, arguing
that not all cells have been transgenosised initially.
Thus selection and survival depending on the celltype
occurred. Bacterial ß-galactosidase activity
oscillated as did the growth rate over several subcultures. An explanation of this oscillation is
difficult and premature, but it may reflect incom-
patibilities between excessive phage genome
transcription and the balanced plant household.
Clearly not only bacterial genes carried on the phage
were expressed. Possibly other phage specific messages

were present – these interfered or exhausted the
biosynthetic potential of the plant cell, thus causing
a decrease in growth and general callus appearance.
Perhaps a double amber mutation in the N gene of the
phage (lambda) blocked in phage specific transcription
when in a non-suppressor background (such as the
plant cell) would allow controlled expression only of
bacterial genes.

The question of phenotypic lag in the lactose
system remains. Clearly an early period of expression
as noted by Smith, Carlson and Merril might have
occurred in that system too, but it was not detected.
Successful gene transfer took place in only a limited
number of callus cells which (i) were exposed to the
phage through cellular injury and/or intercellular
plasmodesmeta, or (ii) have the 'proper' physiological
state of competence to accept and express foreign
DNA. Within a callus of 20–40,000 cells enough
variability in cell properties would be expected to
satisfy the above prerequisites for transgenosis.
However, this early phage effect was not capable of
completely altering the plant cell metabolism. The
phage function decreased and the plant cell being
under physiological stress exhausted its stored
carbon (i.e. as starch) and thus deteriorated.
Suspension cultured cells deteriorate quicker than
solid grown cells. The inhibitory effect of poly-
phenols and other substances like nucleases and
proteases released from dying and bursting cells is
minimalised in callus culture due to a lack of free
diffusion. Thus callus culture may allow the phage
genome to survive for much longer and eventually to
interact with the plant cell at a later stage, when
the physiological readiness for successful bacterial
gene function is more optimal than previously.

VI. Concluding Remarks:

Information regarding integration and inheritance
of foreign DNA within plant cells is limited to the
data derived from whole plants (Ledoux et al, 1971,
1974; Hess, 1972). Work on cultured plant cells has
not developed far enough to allow the application
of sophisticated techniques of molecular biology.

Three possibilities exist for the mode of
inheritance. Firstly, the exogenous genome is
integrated into the eukaryotic genome, thus falling
under the host's replication control. A single or
double recombinational event (depending on the type

of donor genome used) in a region of homology would
suffice to covalently integrate the foreign gene
material. Inheritance would thus be ascertained
with a stable gene dose remaining within each cell
of the progeny. The second alternative involves
failure of integration, however, the donor genome
is maintained as a cytoplasmic plasmid. Only few
classes of foreign DNA would have this potential
of circularity. If no autonomous replication control
is located on the plasmid, or if an existing one
cannot function within the host cytoplasm, or if the
host replication system has no specificity for the
exogenous DNA, then the gene transfer will be
abortive. A dilution effect of the donor function
and a final loss of the transgenotic state will
characterise the system. In this third form of
'inheritance' the exogenous DNA entered, had a
temporal function, but due to lack of integration or
autonomous existence was lost. In other words, the
transgenotic state is temporal.

As yet it is too early to comment on the precise
mode of 'inheritance' of foreign DNA in cultured plant
cells. However, at present, most data support the
latter alternative of temporal gene transfer. Perhaps
modification of the plant genome may allow integration
and subsequent inheritance. Unfortunately such
pretransfer genetic manipulation of the recipient cell
are beyond present day plant cell technology.

Thus the lack of mutability or the absence of
appropriate selection systems for such mutants hampers
the future development of more efficient gene transfer
systems. This host cell modification not only includes
the establishment of the appropriate cellular
environment for the exogenous gene material to
function in but also involves the isolation of biochemical lesions (auxotrophs) which could be corrected
by the appropriate bacterial gene or gene clusters.
Such mutations, of course, would need to express
their phenotype in tissue culture (a condition not
always met by existing plant mutants). Such mutants
are totally absent from the present repertoire of
recipient cell lines. Biochemical auxotrophs would
supply an ideal recipient system to study the uptake
and expression of foreign genes, since the transgenosised cell and resulting cell clone could easily
be isolated by complementation. Experiments up to
now have centred on the transfer and selection for a
new metabolic capability to the plant cell. Many

unforseen problems may arise, for seldomly one can
transfer a complete biochemical pathway and the
recipient cell systems, which lack only one enzyme,
are limited and not extensive enough to allow a full
investigation of the problem. The future development
of precisely characterised biochemical mutants in
cultured plant cells thus becomes a major prerequisite for the successful extension of intercellular gene transfers. After all, it was through
the advent of biochemically defined mutations of the
prokaryotes, that that system gained its present day
complexity and potential.

Acknowledgement:

I thank Drs C.H. Doy and B.G. Rolfe with whom
the work on phage mediated transgenosis was done.
The Alexander von Humboldt Stiftung is also thanked
for its support during 1974.

Literature cited:

Aoki, S. and I. Takebe: Virology 39, 439 (1969)
Bendich, A.J. and P. Filner: Mutation Research 13,
    199 (1971)
Carlson, P.S.: P.N.A.S. 70, 598 (1973)
Chaleff, R. and P.S. Carlson: Ann. Review of
    Genetics 8 (1974)
Cosloy, S.D. and M. Oishi: P.N.A.S. 70, 84 (1973 a)
 ---- and ---- : Molec. gen. Genetics 124, 1
    (1973 b)
Doy, C.H., P.M. Gresshoff and B.G. Rolfe: Search 3,
    447 (1972)
 ----, ---- and ----: P.N.A.S. 70, 723 (1973 a)
 ----, ---- and ----: in The Biochemistry of Gene
    Expression in Higher Organisms (edit. by Pollak, J.
    and Wilson Lee, J.), 21 (Australia and New Zealand
    Book Co.) (1973 b)
 ----, ---- and ----: Nature New Biology 244, 90
    (1973 c)
Fox, A.S. and S.B. Yoon: P.N.A.S. 67, 1608 (1970)
Geier, M. and C.R. Merril: Virology 47, 638 (1972)
Hess, D.: Z. Pflanzenphysiol. 61, 286 (1969)
 ----   : Z. Pflanzenphysiol. 63, 461 (1970)
 ----   : Z. Pflanzenphysiol. 66, 155 (1972)
 ----   : Z. Pflanzenphysiol. 68, 432 (1973)

Heyn, R.F., A. Rörsch and R.A. Schilperoort:
    Quarterly Reviews of Biophysics 7, 35 (1974)
Hoffmann, F. and D. Hess: Z. Pflanzenphysiol. 69,
    81 (1973)
Hoffmann, F. : Z. Pflanzenphysiol. 69, 249 (1973)
Johnson, C.B. and D. Grierson: Current Advances in
    Plant Sci. Feb. (1974)
Johnson, C.B., D. Grierson and H. Smith: Nature New
    Biology 244, 105 (1973)
Ledoux, L., R. Huart and M. Jacobs: Europ. J. Biochem.
    23, 96 (1971)
----, ---- and ----: Nature 249, 17 (1974)
Merril, C.R., M. Geier and J. Petricciani: Nature
    233, 398 (1971)
----, ---- and ----: Advances in the Biosciences
    8, 329 (1972)
Merril, C.R.: Transactions of the N.Y. Academy of
    Sci. 36, 265 (1974)
Merril, C.R. and H. Stanbro: Z. Pflanzenphysiol. 72,
    371 (1974)
Ohyama, K., O. Gamborg and R. Miller: Can. J. Botany
    50, 2077 (1972)
Oishi, M. and S.D. Cosloy: Nature 248, 112 (1974)
Potrykus, I. and F. Hoffmann: Z. Pflanzenphysiol.
    69, 287 (1973)
Potrykus, I.: Z. Pflanzenphysiol. 70, 364 (1973)
Rebel, W., V. Hemleben and W. Seyffert: Zt. für
    Naturforschung 28, 473 (1973)
Sander, E.M.: Virology 24, 545 (1964)
----   : Virology 33, 121 (1967)
Sarrouy-Balat, H., M. Delseny and R. Julien: Plant
    Sci. Letters 1, 287 (1973)
Stroun, M. : B.B.R.C. 44, 571 (1971 a)
----   : FEBS Letters 13, 161 (1971 b)

STUDIES ON THE USE OF TRANSDUCING BACTERIOPHAGES AS VECTORS FOR THE TRANSFER OF FOREIGN GENES TO HIGHER PLANTS

H. SMITH, R.A. McKEE, T.H. ATTRIDGE and D. GRIERSON

DEPARTMENT OF PHYSIOLOGY AND ENVIRONMENTAL STUDIES
UNIVERSITY OF NOTTINGHAM, SCHOOL OF AGRICULTURE
SUTTON BONINGTON, LOUGHBOROUGH, LEICS., U.K.

Many plant scientists throughout the world are currently attempting to introduce new genes into higher plants by the use of purified DNA. Such attempts are clearly highly ambitious and the difficulties are likely to be formidable. The successful introduction of foreign genetic material into a higher plant in such a way as to modify the plant's heritable characteristics necessarily involves four highly complex processes:

    (i)   DNA uptake
    (ii)   DNA conservation
   (iii)   DNA replication
    (iv)   expression of the genetic information.

Of these four essential prerequisites, we shall only be concerned here with the uptake and expression of foreign DNA.

The ideal experiment to test for the expression of foreign genetic material within plant cells would be to use DNA containing the information for only one structural gene, together with an unambiguous assay for the final gene product. Such an experiment is not yet possible since very few single genes have as yet been isolated, for example, ribosomal-RNA genes from *Xenopus* (1) and the *lac* operon from *E. coli* (2) and the techniques involved do not allow for the production of large amounts of DNA. A more practical method is to use DNA containing only a limited amount of genetic information, and lisogenic transducing bacteriophages, as first used by Merril (3) are useful here. The theoretical aspects of the use of transducing bacteriophages as vectors for the artificial transfer of foreign genetic information into plant cells are discussed in the preceding paper by Gresshof; here we shall be concerned with the practical results achieved so far.

We have used the *lac* transducing phage λp*lac* 5, constructed by
Ippen *et al* (4), as a donor for the gene coding for the *E. coli*
β-galactosidase, and have investigated the properties of cell
suspension cultures of sycamore (*Acer pseudoplatanus*) treated with
the phage. The *lac* genes represent about 2% of the genetic information coded for by the λp*lac* 5 DNA. Although this means that there
is a 50 fold excess of experimentally irrelevant DNA, it nevertheless
represents a considerable enrichment when compared with whole *E. coli*
DNA, where the *lac* genes comprise only about 0.02% of the total with
a 5,000 fold excess of irrelevant DNA. The phage does not contain
the whole of the *lac* operon and portions of the *a* and *i* genes are
missing; however, the *z* gene, which is the structural gene for
β-galactosidase, is present. The strategy of the experiment
therefore was to cause the sycamore cells to take up large amounts
of the λp*lac* 5 phage, and then to assay immunologically for the
presence of bacterial β-galactosidase in extracts of the plant cells.
Sycamore cell suspension cultures were used for this purpose since
it was known that the particular line of cells was not able to
assimilate and grow on lactose. Thus, the ability to grow on
lactose in λp*lac* 5 treated cultures could be used as a selection
procedure for cells containing functional *lac* genes.

RESULTS

Growth of sycamore cell suspension cultures

The pattern of cell division in suspension cultures of *Acer
pseudoplatanus* is shown in Figure 1a. With sucrose as carbon source
cell number rapidly increases over a period of 10 - 20 days. The
growth rate of the cultures depends on the stage of growth of the
cells when subcultured and the size of the initial inoculation. In
rapidly growing cultures the doubling time is approximately 36 - 48
hours and cell number may increase several hundred fold to a final
density of approximately 3×10^6 cells/ml, but at low initial cell
densities division occurs more slowly. Figure 1b shows that in
complete contrast cell division does not occur when cultures are
in oculated into a medium containing 2% lactose in place of sucrose
(it should be noted that cell number is plotted on a linear scale in
Figure 1b).

Phage treatment

In view of the fact that sycamore cells are unable to utilise
lactose as a carbon source it was of interest to see whether they
could grow on lactose after pre-treatment with λp*lac* 5 phage.
Cells grown in sucrose medium were treated for two days with the
phage and the cells were then washed several times and inoculated
into fresh medium containing lactose in place of sucrose. In early

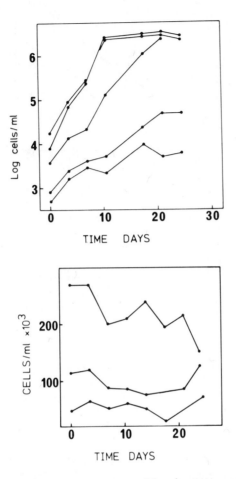

Figure 1. The growth of sycamore cells in suspension culture.

Sycamore cells were grown in 250 ml flasks on an orbital shaker
at 25°C in a medium containing mineral salts, and 2% sucrose
(Fig. 1a) or 2% lactose (Fig. 1b). Flasks were inoculated
at different initial cell densities and growth monitored over
a period of several weeks. Cell numbers were determined on a
haemocytometer slide after treating the cells with 15% chromic
acid for five minutes at 70°C followed by mechanical shaking
for five minutes. Cell numbers are plotted on a log scale in
Fig. 1a, and a linear scale in Fig. 1b.

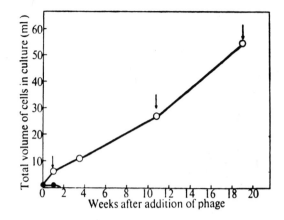

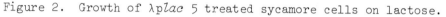

Figure 2.   Growth of λp*lac* 5 treated sycamore cells on lactose.

        Cultures in log phase were incubated in λp*lac* 5 phage
(10^{11} p.f.u. per ml) for two days in 2% sucrose medium (open
circles).   Control cultures were treated in the same way but
without phage (closed circles).   Both cultures were washed in
2% lactose medium and transferred to 2% lactose medium.
Culture growth was determined by measuring packed cell volume
after sedimentation under gravity for one hour.   Arrows represent points of sub-culturing.

experiments cell growth was measured by the increase in volume of
the cultures after sedimentation of the cells for two hours.   The
results (Fig. 2) showed that although control cells did not grow on
lactose those treated with λp*lac* 5 were capable of a substantial
increase in cell volume (5).   In later experiments we measured
directly the increase in cell number in the cultures.   From the
results shown in Figure 3 it is clear that although untreated cells
and those treated with λ$^+$ phage do not divide, the λp*lac* 5 cells
may undergo several rounds of cell division.   The rate of cell
division is very low compared to cultures grown on sucrose and there
is a certain amount of variability in the timing of the response.
Generally it occurs between four and eight weeks after placing the
cells on lactose (compare Figures 3 and 4).   The cell divisions
observed in the λp*lac* 5 cells are not sustained however and over a
further period of several weeks the cell number may actually fall.
Subculturing the cells into fresh medium at intervals during

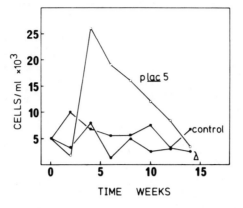

Figure 3.   The growth of phage-treated cells in lactose.

Phage λ⁺ and λ*plac* 5 were grown up on the *E. coli* lac deletion
strain ED914, harvested, and passed through a 0.45 μ nitrocellulose filter.   Sycamore cells (1.8 x 10⁵/ml) grown in 2%
sucrose were treated with either λ⁺ or λ*plac* 5 phage at a final
concentration of 10⁹ p.f.u./ml for two days.   The cells were
then washed in and transferred to 2% lactose medium and changes
in cell number measured over a period of several weeks.   Cell
numbers are plotted on a linear scale.

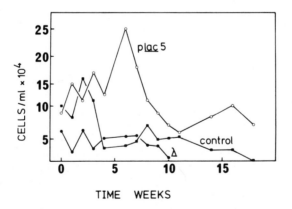

Figure 4.   The subculturing of phage-treated cells grown in lactose
   medium.

Cells were treated as described in the legend to Fig. 3 except
that they were transferred to fresh 2% lactose medium after two,
four, six, eight and ten weeks.

incubation on lactose does not stimulate division of the λp*lac* 5
treated cells (Figure 4).

There may be several different reasons why the increased rate
of cell division after λp*lac* 5 treatment is not maintained: (a) the
phage DNA may not be conserved within the cells; (b) the phage DNA
may not replicate at a rate equal to the cell division rate;
(c) the presence of the phage DNA in the cells may have deleterious
effects due to the expression of other phage genes; and (d) the
accummulation of galactose due to lactose hydrolysis may reach a
toxic level. We have not yet been able to obtain data on the conservation and replication of phage DNA within the cells, but we
have attempted to investigate the other two possibilities.

If phage treated cells are maintained on sucrose, instead of
being transferred directly to lactose, a transient inhibition of
cell division occurs (Fig. 5). This is most marked with the λp*lac* 5

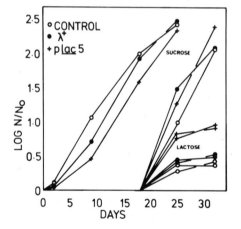

Figure 5.   Growth of phage treated cells on sucrose.

Cells treated with λ⁺, or λp*lac* 5 phage, and untreated controls
were transfered back to 2% sucrose and growth estimated.   At
the stated point, cultures were diluted again onto 2% sucrose,
or onto 2% lactose (two replicates) and subsequent culture
growth measured.

treated cells, although similar effects are observed with the λ^+
phage. At the point of maximum difference, the ratios of the rates
of cell division were control: λ^+, 1.64:1, and control: $\lambda plac$ 5,
2.5:1. Thus there is some suggestion here that phage treatment
reduces the subsequent capacity of the sycamore cells for cell
division. This effect is quickly lost, however, and by 25 days,
when the cultures are approaching the end of log phase, the growth
rates are very nearly equal. If the cells are diluted into fresh
sucrose medium at 18 days (i.e. during log phase) all three
cultures continue growing at similar rates for at least a further
14 days. Thus, there appears to be no long-lived deleterious effect
of the phage on cells growing on sucrose. It is, however,
appreciated that long-lived effects may only become noticeable
during growth on lactose where phage-containing cells would be
selectively maintained for some time.

There are indications, on the other hand, that the $\lambda plac$ 5
treated cultures used in the last experiment still contained
functional lac genes after 18 days growth on sucrose. When samples
from each line were diluted onto lactose, those that had been
previously treated with $\lambda plac$ 5 showed almost a ten fold increase
in cell number in the subsequent 14 days, whereas the controls only
increased two to three fold during that period. This effect was
observed in two separate experiments, both sets of data being
presented in Figure 5.

On the question of the accumulation of galactose, cultures
which had not been treated with phage were inoculated into media
containing various concentrations of glucose and galactose (Fig. 6).

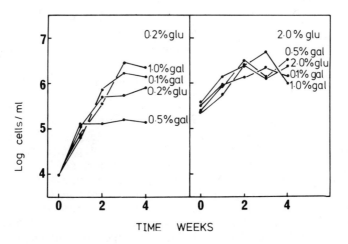

Figure 6.   The growth of sycamore cells in mixed cultures of
glucose and galactose.

Although the data are somewhat variable, there is no indication
that galactose, even at relatively high concentrations is significantly inhibitory to cell division in the presence of glucose. No
cell division occurs on galactose alone.

Fate of the λp*lac* 5 phage

When sycamore cells are treated with phage particles the
number of plaque forming units that can be recovered from the
culture steadily declines over a two day period (Figure 7).

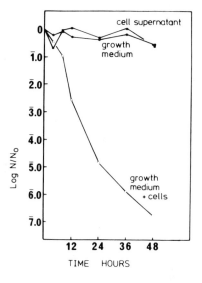

Figure 7. The disappearance of phage during incubation with
     sycamore cells in culture.

Five ml aliquots of λp*lac* 5 phage in nutrient broth was added
to 15 ml of sycamore cells in sucrose medium giving a final concentration of 5 x 10^5 sycamore cells and 10^9 p.f.u./ml. A similar concentration of phage was added to fresh medium and to the
supernatant from a stationary phase cell culture. At intervals
over a two day period the number of phage particles in the medium was determined by the agar layer plating method. Samples
of the sycamore cells were withdrawn after 0, one and two days,
washed, ground in liquid nitrogen, resuspended in phage buffer
and assayed for phage. No phage were detected in the cell
extracts.

Control experiments show that this only occurs when intact sycamore
cells are present and is not due to inactivation of the phage by
some component of the culture medium. This suggests that the phage
particles are either inactivated, or taken up by the sycamore cells,
and although the mechanism is not known the results in Figure 7
suggest that this is a comparatively slow process. For every cell
present at the start of the two day incubation approximately 10
phage particles are lost. At intervals during the incubation period
samples of the treated cells were removed, washed and ground with
liquid nitrogen and aliquots of the extract tested for the presence
of phage. No infective particles were recovered. One possible
explanation of this result is that the phage particles although
present are inactivated during the extraction or by the cell homogenate. This possibility was examined by mixing infective phage
with sycamore cells and immediately breaking the cells by a number
of different methods. The results in Table 1 show that phage
particles are not substantially inactivated by these procedures.

Table 1. The survival of phage during different cell extraction
          procedures.

	Number of phage recovered per ml	
	log phase cells	stationary phase cells
sand	8.0×10^{7}	2.5×10^{7}
liquid nitrogen	9.5×10^{7}	6.0×10^{7}
homogeniser	6.0×10^{5}	–
control	4.1×10^{8}	3.3×10^{8}

Half ml samples of λp*lac* 5 phage were added to 5 ml samples of
log phase and stationary phase sycamore cells. The suspensions were
then ground by hand in a mortar and pestle with acid washed sand or
liquidised nitrogen for five minutes or homogenised at maximum speed
with a Silverson homogeniser for five minutes. Cell debris was
removed by centrifugation and the extracts assayed for phage.
Controls represent the number of p.f.u. recovered from 0.5 ml of the
λp*lac* 5 preparations used.

β-galactosidase acitivity in sycamore cells

After treatment with phage λp*lac* 5 carrying the *z* gene for
β-galactosidase, sycamore cells are temporarily able to grow on

lactose. One explanation of this result is that the genes for
lactose utilisation are taken up and expressed by the plant cells
and one way to test this hypothesis is to measure the β-galactosidase
activity in the cells. Figure 8 shows that untreated cells and those
exposed to phages λ$^+$ and λp*lac* 5 all contain enzymes capable of
hydrolysing p-O-nitrophenyl-β-D-galactopyranoside, the substrate
commonly used for β-galactosidase assay. There is a transient
increase in the enzyme activity of the cells when they are transferred to lactose. This reaches a maximum after about eight days
and the greatest activity is found in cells pretreated with phage
λp*lac* 5. It should be noted that this increase is observed several
weeks before the burst of cell division shown in Figures 2 and 3.
It seems clear from these results that β-galactosidase activity is
not confined to those cells able to grow on lactose. Both animal
and plant cells are known to contain glycosidases with specificity
towards β-galactosides and recently it has been shown that there
are two β-galactosidases in *E. coli* K12 (6). Strains in which the
z gene is deleted are unable to grow on lactose although they

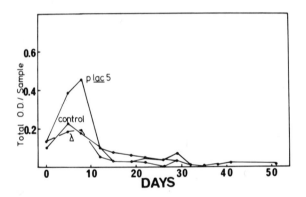

Figure 8. β-galactosidase activity in control and phage-treated
   cells grown in lactose medium.

Sycamore cell cultures were treated for two days with phage
λ$^+$ or λp*lac* 5 and the cells transferred to lactose medium. At
intervals, samples of the cells were filtered and ground after
freezing with liquid nitrogen. One ml of 0.1 M phosphate buffer
pH 7.2 was added and β-galactosidase activity measured with
o-nitrophenyl-β-D-galactopyranoside as substrate. (8)

contain β-galactosidase II. This enzyme is induced by lactose but
has very little lactase activity. A similar situation may exist in
control sycamore cells for the β-galactosidase detected here is
apparently induced by lactose. The failure of the cells to grow
suggests that this enzyme does not metabolise lactose.

The question remains as to whether any enzyme coded for by the
z gene is present in the λplac 5 treated cells. The obvious way to
test this possibility is to use specific properties of the bacterial
β-galactosidase such as antibody reactions, physical properties and
specific inhibitors to differentiate between the bacterial and the
plant enzymes. A specific inhibitor of β-galactosidase is
β-phenylthiogalactoside. Table II shows the effect of this substance
on enzyme extracted from phage-treated and control cells at a concentration which inhibits the bacterial enzyme by 50%. It is quite
clear that there is no specific inhibition of the galactosidase
activity in the extracts treated with λplac 5.

Table II.   Lack of inhibition of sycamore cell β-galactosidase by
             the specific inhibitor β-phenylthiogalactoside.

Source of enzyme	Percent Inhibition	
	Sucrose Medium	Lactose Medium
Control cells	7.7	–
λ$^+$ treated cells	17.8	12.5
λplac 5 treated cells	0	0
E. coli		50.0

We have raised antisera to bacterial β- galactosidase but as
yet have been unable to obtain positive evidence for the presence of
the bacterial enzyme within the plant cells. The antisera reacts well
with the purified bacterial enzyme, but no precipitin reactions
have been observed with extracts from λplac 5 treated plant cells
whether by Ouchterlony plate immuno-diffusion, or by immunoelectro-
phoresis. Furthermore, we have not obtained any heat protection of
the plant β-galactosidase by the antibody. These experiments,
however, are still in a rather preliminary state and a firm
negative conclusion cannot yet be made.

DISCUSSION

The aim of these experiments is to investigate whether plant cells can take up phage particles and utilise the genetic information, and if this is the case to establish whether this information can be incorporated into the cells in a stable manner. The sycamore cells do not normally grow on lactose. This provides a favourable situation for selecting cells that may have acquired the genes for lactose utilisation from the *lac* transducing phage.

The criterion of growth on lactose is not sufficient evidence in itself to conclude that uptake and expression of the *lac* genes is taking place, particularly as the treated cells grow only very slowly and growth is only a transient phenomenon. The results shown in Figure 7 suggest that intact sycamore cells render the phage incapable of infecting *E. coli*. This could occur, for example, if the phage particle was disrupted or more simply if the adsorption site was made inoperative. It is not known whether the phage particles enter the plant cells during this process although the use of radioactive phage labelled in the DNA and the protein coat should answer this question. No factors responsible for phage inactivation can be detected in the culture medium or in cell homogenates.

The critical question that remains is whether there is any acceptable evidence that foreign DNA can be expressed within plant cells. If expression is defined as the production of a recognisable and functional gene product, it must be said that the available evidence is extremely slight. Carlson (7) has reported that when protoplasts of *Hordeum vulgare* are exposed to phage T3, there is a rapid (i.e. within 24 hours) synthesis of phage-specific RNA-polymerase and S-adenosylmethionine cleaving enzyme. Unfortunately, this work has only been reported in the barest outline, and the author does not provide enough information for its soundness to be judged. In our experiments there is no conclusive evidence as yet that the *E. coli* β-galactosidase is synthesized in the sycamore cells. Experiments conceptually similar to ours have also been carried out by Doy and his colleagues (8, 9). They have used haploid callus cultures of *Lycopersicon esculentum* and *Arabidopsis thaliana* treated with phage Φ 80 *lac*+ and λpgal+. In these experiments they claim to have shown the synthesis of the *E. coli* β-galactosidase using the antibody heat-protection assay for the enzyme. However, they were not able to obtain a positive precipitin reaction between the antibody and the plant extracts. Thus, the concept of foreign genes being expressed within plant cells rests, at present, on two as yet unconfirmed reports. On this basis, a substantial degree of caution should be exercised when discussing the potential of genetic engineering for the 'improvement' of crop species.

REFERENCES

(1) Birnstiel, M.L., Speirs, J., Purdom, I., Jones, K., and
     Loening, U.E. *Nature* 219 (1968) 454.

(2) Shapiro, J., MacHattie, L., Eron, L., Ihler, G., Ippen, K.,
     and Beckwith, J.R. *Nature* 224 (1969) 768.

(3) Merril, C.R., Geier, M.R., and Petricianni, J.C. *Nature* 233
     (1971) 398.

(4) Ippen, K., Shapiro, J.A., and Beckwith, J.R. *Journal of
     Bacteriology* 108 (1971) 5.

(5) Johnson, C.B., Grierson, D., and Smith, H. *Nature New Biology*
     244 (1973) 105.

(6) Hartl, D.L., and Hall, B. *Nature* 248 (1974) 152.

(7) Carlson, P.S. *Proceedings of the National Academy of Sciences
     U.S.A.* 70 (1973) 598.

(8) Doy, C.H., Gresshof, P.M., and Rolfe, B.G. *Proceedings of the
     National Academy of Sciences U.S.A.* 70 91973) 723.

(9) Doy, C.H., Gresshof, P.M., and Rolfe, B.G. *Nature New Biology*
     244 (1973) 90.

A uvr MUTATION THAT ENHANCES THE TRANSFORMATION FREQUENCY BY INTERGENETIC DNA IN Bacillus subtilis

K. Matsumoto, H. Takahashi, and H. Saito

Institute of Applied Microbiology

University of Tokyo, Tokyo, Japan

Transformation frequency by heterologous or intergenetic DNA is usually less than that of homologous transformation. The reduction of frequency seems to be ascribed, at least in a part, to the heterodupulex degradation as a function of the recipient.

When Bacillus subtilis mutant strain S-1, selected as UV sensitive, was used as recipient, the transformation frequency by intergenetic DNA of B.megaterium 203 transfered in B.subtilis was appreciably enhanced. The enhancement phenomenon has almost no choice to the intergenotic DNAs of various length. The result suggests that the possible mechanism of heteroduplex degradation seems to have low specificity on the base sequence.

STUDIES ON PROTEASE SENSITIVE TRANSFECTING DNA OF BACILLUS PHAGE

Hideo Hirokawa

Laboratory of Genetics, Faculty of Science
University of Tokyo
Hongo, Bunkyo-ku, Tokyo, Japan

The results of physical analysis of DNA indicated that transfective DNA of Bacillus phage ϕ29 bound a protein (1). This DNA-protein complex was further analyzed with labelled DNA (^{3}H)-protein (^{35}S of ^{14}C). The profile of density distribution of this complex gave a single peak in CsCl density centrifugation. When the DNA was separated into single stranded molecules, a protein was still bound to both strands. The peak of the DNA in CsCl centrifugation shifted to heavy positions either by trypsin or by S1 (single-endonuclease) treatment. Thus treated DNA lost their transfecting actibity. Sedimentation patterns of the DNA in sucrose density centrifugation did not alter at the main peak before and after trypsin treatment (1).

These results, combined with evidence reported previously (1), suggest that a protein is bound to a terminal of both single stranded DNA.

The test of protease sensitivity is an adequate technique to find DNA-protein complex among transfecting DNAs. In addition to ϕ29, transfective DNAs of ϕ15, ϕ105, and SP02 were protease sensitive. Recently, DNA of GA-1 was found to be also trypsin sensitive DNA-protein complex (2). Thus, a borad existence of transfective DNA-protein complex is becoming obvious among Bacillus phages.

(1) Hirokawa, H. 1972. Proc. Nat. Acad. Sci. U.S.A. 69: 1555.
(2) Arwert, F. and G. Venema. 1974. J. Virology 13: 584-589.

GENETIC CONTROL OF D-AMINO ACID METABOLISM IN GRAM-NEGATIVE
BACTERIA

W. Walczak, J. Wild, K. Krajewska-Grynkiewicz, and
T. Klopotowski

Institute of Biochemistry and Biophysics
02-532 Warsaw, Poland

We have previously shown that mutations dhuA which increase
histidine transport enable his auxotrophs of Salmonella typhimurium
to utilize D-histidine. Oxender has demonstrated that other mutations in Escherichia coli increase leucine transport and enable leu
auxotrophs to grow on D-leucine. On the other hand, no mutation is
required for met mutants of either S. typhimurium or E. coli to use
D-methionine as an L-methionine substitute.

These observations indicate that the gram-negative bacteria
have an enzyme system for converting D-amino acids into L-amino
acids. We have shown that D-amino acid dehydrogenase, a structure-
bound enzyme of S. typhimurium and E. coli deaminates most of D-
isomers of the natural L-amino acids and catalyses the first step
of the racemization process. We have isolated mutants dadA of S.
typhimurium which are unable to utilize D-histidine and D-methionine
and lack the deaminating activity toward any D-amino acids with the
only exception of D-serine.

Synthesis of D-amino acid dehydrogenase is inducible by alanine
and repressible by glucose. In our mutants dadR, isolated in S.
typhimurium, the synthesis is no longer under catabolite repression,
but still is inducible by alanine. They map at one-gene distance
from dadA, the structural gene for the dehydrogenase. The dadR
mutants have increased ability to utilize D-histidine, D-methionine
and D-trypotophan. The D-tryptophan utilization resembles that of
dadR mutants isolated in E. coli by another selection procedure by
Kuhn and Somerville.

In the second step, the keto acids produced by D-amino acid dehydrogenase are transaminated to L-amino acids. We have shown that imidazolepyruvate can be transaminated by either imidazole acetol phosphate aminotransferase, coded by the gene hisC, or by aminotransferase A, but keto product of D-methionine deamination is converted to L-methionine by other enzymes.

These results suggest that the two-step process can be used by gram-negative bacteria to make any L-amino acid from its D-amino acid precursor, but racemases specific for alanine or arginine were described by other authors in E. coli.

REGULATION OF DEVELOPMENT IN FISSION YEAST

James H. Meade

The University of Texas at Dallas

Dallas, Texas

In the Yeast <u>Schizosaccharomyces</u> <u>pombe</u>, copulation and meiosis appear to be regulated by the mating-type genes, <u>mat1</u> and <u>mat2</u> (Leupold, Cold Spring Harbor Symp. Quant. Biol. 23: 161, 1958). A <u>mat2</u> gene mutant, <u>meI1</u>, has been reported which is normal with respect to copulation but defective with respect to meiosis. From homothallic strains, we have isolated new <u>mat2</u> mutants representing three additional groups: 1) mutants unable to self-copulate but still able to turn on the mating-type auxiliary gene <u>map1</u> and still normal with respect to the meiosis function; 2) mutants unable to self-copulate as they cannot turn on <u>map1</u>, but still normal with respect to the meiosis function; and 3) mutants which are non-functional both with respect to self-copulation and to meiosis. Furthermore, we have found a new group of genes which appear to regulate the activity of the <u>mat1</u> and <u>mat2</u> genes. Homothallic h^{90} colonies normally exhibit a homogeneous black color after exposure to iodine vapors (non-sporulating colonies turn yellow). The mutants found in h^{90} strains were neither homogeneously black nor yellow but rather were mottled in appearance. Further studies hint that this group of at least four genes may act as specific mutator genes for the mating-type region, changing the region from an active <u>mat1</u>--inactive <u>mat2</u> to an inactive <u>mat1</u>--active <u>mat2</u> and vice versa.

IN VITRO GROWTH & POLYPHENOL PRODUCTION BY TISSUE CULTURES OF DATURA AND CASSIA

A. Mehta, K. Venkatasubbaiah, and R. Shah

Department of Botany, The M. S. University of Baroda

Baroda, India

In many instances it has been shown that the qualitative and quantitative performance of the tissues in forming the secondary plant products may be greatly influenced by the cultural conditions. In the present studies experiments were conducted to examine if the polyphenol content can be altered in the cultured tissues by manipulating the nutritional status and hormonal supplement to the medium.

Callus tissues derived from the anthers of Datura metel L. and Cassia fistula L. were grown on a completely defined Murashige and Skoog's medium. The polyphenol production as influenced by various sugars and different concentrations of sucrose, 2, 4-D, kinetin and gibberellic acid, in presence and absence of light, was examined in the cultured tissues. Of the different sugars tested, sucrose proved to be the best carbon and energy source for the growth of the tissues as well as for the polyphenol synthesis. Further, increase in sucrose concentration enhanced polyphenol accumulation in both the tissues. Raising the auxin level delayed the initiation of polyphenol synthesis; incorporation of kinetin, however, reduced the delaying influence of 2,4-D.

Progressive changes in the patterns of peroxidase and phenylalamine ammonia-lyase (PAL) enzyme systems were also investigated to examine any relationship between the activities of the enzymes and polyphenol synthesis in the tissues. The results obtained will be presented and discussed in the light of recent findings.

PROPERTIES OF 5-BROMODEOXYURIDINE-RESISTANT LINES OF HIGHER PLANT CELLS IN LIQUID CULTURE

Kanji Ohyama

Prairie Regional Laboratory
National Research Council of Canada
Saskatoon, Saskatchewan S7N 0W9

5-Bromodeoxyuridine (BUdR)-resistant cells were obtained from N-methyl-N'-nitro-N-nitrosoguanidine (NTG)-treated soybean protoplasts and cultured in liquid nutrient medium containing BUdR (20 µg/ml) and uridine (100 µg/ml). Addition of uridine to the medium improved growth of the BUdR-resistant cells.

The growth of BUdR-resistant cells was partially inhibited when hypoxanthine, aminopterine, glycine and thymidine were added to the medium. Both BUdR-resistant and BUdR-sensitive cells exhibited thymidine kinase activity.

CsCl density gradient analyses showed that the DNA of BUdR-resistant cells, which were cultured in the presence of BUdR, had a buoyant density of 1.703 g/ml, while the DNA of the parental soybean cells grown without BUdR had a buoyant density of 1.692 g/ml.

Uptake of ^{3}H-thymidine or ^{14}C-BUdR by the cells occurred in both BUdR-resistant and BUdR-sensitive cells. CsCl density gradient patterns of labelled DNA also demonstrated that ^{14}C-BUdR and ^{3}H-thymidine were incorporated into the DNA of BUdR-resistant cells as well as into that of BUdR-sensitive cells.

A colony reisolated from BUdR-resistant cells was subcultured in liquid BUdR (100 µg/ml) medium without presence of uridine. The properties are being investigated.

References: K. Ohyama, Properties of 5-bromodeoxyuridine-resistant lines of higher plant cells in liquid culture. Expt. Cell Res., 1974, in press.

RESPIRATION AND NITROGEN NUTRITION OF CARROT CALLUS CULTURES

G. H. Craven

Agronomy Department

Stellenbosch University, South Africa

The use of stable, karyotypic normal callus or cell suspension lines of important agronomic plants should enable scientists to routinely develop cultivars with increased biological efficiency by using the techniques or modified techniques of microbial genetics.[1] This approach should be particularly attractive to those who are trying to obtain genotypes of C_3-plants in which the enzymes of photorespiration have been rendered inoperative. Attempts to grow plant cells autotrophically in culture have been successful[2,3,4], but knowledge about selection techniques for and factors affecting the CO_2-exchange of suitable cell variants in vitro is at present still scanty.

The accompanying figure shows typical respiratory tracings obtained in an experiment with carrot callus explants grown aseptically in a medium containing White's basal medium plus coconut milk (CM) and sucrose as carbon source, supplemented with either NO_3-N or NH_4-N (both at 10mM)[5]. The rates of CO_2 release, as measured in light and in darkness, in air and in N_2 gas, show that most CO_2 was produced via fermentative pathways, that endogenous CO_2 refixation probably took place in the light and that CO_2 exchange was qualitatively and quantitatively markedly affected by inorganic nitrogen nutrition, especially NH_4-N. The implications of this "nitrogen effect" should be borne in mind in any work involving the CO_2 exchange of undifferentiated or differentiated plant tissue.

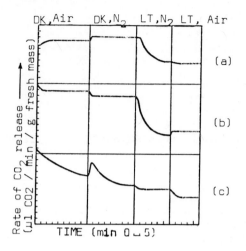

Fig. 1. CO_2 release by cultured carrot explants in light (LT) and
           dark (DK), in air and in nitrogen, as affected by their
           prior conditions of growth:
           (a) = Basal (B) + CM
           (b) = B + CM + KNO_3
           (c) = B + CM + NH_4Cl

1) Carlson, P.S. Science, 180: 133 (1973).   2) Hanson, A.D., and J.
Edelman. Planta, 102: 11 (1972).   3) Chandler, M., N.T. de Marsac,
and Y. de Kouchkovsky. Can. J. Bot., 50: 2265 (1972).   4) Neumann,
K.H., and A. Raafat. Plant Physiol., 51:685 (1973). 5) Craven, G.H.
Ph.D. Thesis, Cornell Univ. (1972).

QUANTITATIVE MUTAGENESIS IN SOYBEAN SUSPENSION CULTURE

Z. R. Sung, J. Smith, and E. R. Signer

Dept. of Biology
Massachusetts Institute of Technology
Cambridge, Massachusetts 02139

Soybean suspension cultures were grown in side-arm flasks and shaken on a rotary shaker at 28°C. Growth rate was conveniently measured with a Klett Summerson photometer by determining the turbidity through the side-arm. Within a given range, the turbidity of the cell suspension was directly proportional to the culture density determined by direct cell counting.

Mutagenesis was investigated quantitatively in terms of the effect of mutagen, EMS, on the growth rate and the mutation frequency. Cell growth was inhibited by EMS and the degree of inhibition was proportional to the EMS concentration. Thus, the number of survivors could be estimated from the amount of growth reduction. For mutants selection, 3×10^8 cells were mutagenized, washed and resuspended in growth medium. Control cells were processed similarly. After the number of survivors were determined from the growth curve, cells were plated on selective medium, 0.5 mM 5-methyl tryptophan (5-MT), at a concentration of 10^7 cells per plate to isolate 5-MT resistant cells. While most of the cells failed to grow, resistant clones grew up in 1-2 months. At this point, mutation rate was estimated as number of resistant clones per number of survivors. In the case of diploid soybean suspension culture, induced mutation resistant to 5-MT was produced at a rate of about 10^{-7}; however, no spontaneous mutants were found in a population of 3×10^8.

These techniques allow determination of survival curve, mutagenesis curve and the relationship of cell killing to mutagenesis of a specific mutagen on plant cell culture.

PROTOPLAST ISOLATION FROM LEAVES OF C_3, C_4 AND CAM PLANTS AND BIOCHEMICAL ACTIVITIES

Maria Gutierrez, S. B. Ku, and G. E. Edwards

University of Wisconsin

Madison, Wisconsin 53706

Leaf protoplasts have been isolated from a number of plants by enzymatic digestion with 2% cellulase (Onozuka R-10, All Japan Biochem. Co.) and 0.1% pectinase (1). Leaf segments less than 1mm wide were incubated in the isolation medium for 3 hours at 30°C. The protoplasts released were purified in a liquid-liquid two-phase system using dextran T20 and polyethylene glycol 6000. Intact mesophyll protoplasts were collected at the interphase. Bundle sheath strands from C_4 plants were collected by filtration techniques through nylon sieves of different porosity. For microscopy observations isolated protoplasts and bundle sheath cells were suspended in 0.5% Evans Blue. The exclusion of the dye was used as an indication of the intactness of the preparation. Comparative studies on the photosynthetic activities by mesophyll protoplasts from C_3 and Crassulcean Acie Metabolism plants further showed the viability of the isolated cells. C_4 plants, such as maize, sugarcane and _Panicum miliaceum_, are characterized as having two types of chlorophyllous cells, the mesophyll and the bundle sheath cells, and two carboxylating enzymes, PEP carboxylase of the C_4-dicarboxylic acid pathway and RuDP carboxylase of the ribulose pentose phosphate pathway. PEP carboxylase and other enzymes of the C_4 pathway were almost exclusively localized in mesophyll protoplasts while RuDP carboxylase and phosphoribulose kinase were localized in bundle sheath cells. Enzyme distribution, photochemical activities and CO_2 fixation have been studies in relation to the compartmentation of photosynthetic carbon metabolism (2,3).

1) Kanai, R., Edwards, G.E.: Plant Physiol. 51, 1133 (1973).
2) Gutierrez, M., Kanai, R., Huber, S.C., Ku, S.B., Edwards, G.E.: Z. Pflanzenphysiol. 72, 305 (1974). 3) Ku, S.B., Gutierrez, M., Kanai, R., Edwards, G.E.: Z. Pflanzenphysiol. 72, 320 (1974).

ANTHER DERIVED PLANTS FROM DIGITALIS PURPUREA

G. Corduan and C. Spix

Lehrstuhl für Pflanzenphysiologie, Ruhr-Universität

Bochum, 463 Bochum, Gebäude ND, Germany

The aim of our work is to raise the level of secondary compounds in plants, which are important for medicine and the chemical
synthesis of which is either unpracticable or uneconomical. One of
these plants we are interested in is Digitalis purpurea producing
cardenolides. To raise the level of these products we frist tried
to get haploid tissues and plants, which can be treated with different mutagens.

We cultured Digitalis anthers on different media and under different conditions after treatment at 5°C for 24 hours. Callus formation on an auxin-containing medium was observed after a culture
period of several weeks. Two criteria indicate that the callus
derived from the anthers is of generative origin: 1) the chromosome number of the callus, 2) the dependence between callus formation and the stage of microspore development.

Depending on the auxin used for callus formation a great number of regenerates was observed under conditions of continuous light
and an auxin-free medium. When anthers were cultured in the dark
diploid plants were obtained. By careful cytological experiments
we were able to show that regeneration starting from haploid callus
leads to a higher degree of ploidy and finally to diploid plants.
Callus from anthers, which were cultured in light, regenerated to
tetraploid plants. Regenerated plants flowered and fruited normally under greenhouse or field conditions. The high frequency of regenerates enables us to propagate a distinct genotype to a nearly
unlimited number of plants.

If the callus was cultured on a medium supplemented with kinetin, plants regenerated only under photoperiodic conditions. These plants had smaller leaves and a different flower morphology as compared to the starting material.

MUTATIONS OBTAINED FROM ANTHER DERIVED PLANTS OF HYOSCYAMUS NIGER

G. Corduan

Lehrstuhl für Pflanzenphysiologie, Ruhr-Universität

463 Bochum, Gebäude ND, Germany

Plants of Hyoscyamus niger (a tropane alkaloid-producing species) used for mutagenic treatment were obtained from another culture by 2 different methods. By the first method plantlets develop directly out of the anther within 6-8 weeks under photo-periodical conditions on an auxin-free medium. About 25% of these plants were found to be haploid. By the second procedure anthers were cultured on an auxin-containing medium in the dark. The callus, which developed under these conditions, was able to produce large numbers of plants under photoperiodic conditions. Of these plants two thirds were haploid. Plantlets derived directly from anthers were treated with UV and x-rays, callus was subjected to treatment with cehmical mutagens.

More than 1,500 of these plants were analyzed for morphologi-cal variations and alkaloid content. A number of morphological abnormalities was found, which were never observed in the control plants, and the alkaloid content of some plants exceeded that of the controls by a factor of five.

Some of these modifications, observed in the M_1-generation were checked for their genetic stability in the M_2-generation. We were able to detect a mutant with roundish leaves and an increased chlorophyll content. Another plant having a tripled alkaloid con-tent was found to be recessive in the M_2-generation. We are now testing the M_3-generation of those plants, which had a higher alkaloid content in the M_2-generation.

RIBONUCLEIC ACID SYNTHESIS IN PLANTS

Donald Grierson

Department of Physiology and Environmental Studies
University of Nottingham, School of Agriculture
Sutton Bonington, Loughborough, Leics., Gt. Britain

The two large RNA components of the ribosomes of the plant cytoplasm have molecular weights of 1.3 and 0.7 x 10^6. These molecules are synthesized in the nucleolus as part of a poly- cistronic precursor which is subsequently methylated and cleaved in a number of processing steps to produce functional rRNA (1). Polyacrylamide gel electrophoresis of pulse-labelled RNA from the nuclei of aseptically grown Phaseolus aureus seedlings shows that the rRNA precursors and processing intermediates have molecular weights of approximately 2.6, 1.45, and 1.0 x 10^6. The precursors have a similar base composition to rRNA and competitive hybridi- zation experiments show that the large precursor contains sequences for both the 1.3 and 0.7 x 10^6 molecular weight rRNAs (2). Satura- tion hybridization experiments between rRNA and nuclear DNA shows that 0.6 - 0.9% of the DNA codes for rRNA. This represents several thousand cistrons per diploid nucleus. These genes have a higher buoyant density (1.703) than the bulk of the nuclear DNA (1.695) and can be detected by hybridizing radioactive rRNA to DNA fractions from a caesium chloride gradient.

In the blue-green alga Tolypothrix distorta no polycistronic precursor accumulates and the rRNAs (molecular weights 1.1 and 0.56 x 10^6) are formed by the processing of separate precursors: $1.22 \rightarrow 1.1$ and $0.76 \rightarrow 0.68 \rightarrow 0.56$ (3). It remains possible that the rRNA genes are initially transcribed as one molecule which is cleaved by a processing enzyme during or immediately after syn- thesis. The mechanism of synthesis of chloroplast rRNA is less clear. A processing pathway similar to that observed in blue- green algae may operate but chloroplasts from Phaseolus aureus also contain molecules of 2.9 and 0.48 x 10^6 daltons (2). It is

not known whether the large RNA is involved in rRNA synthesis.
The other RNA molecule (0.48 x 10[6] daltons) does not appear to be
a breakdown product of chloroplast rRNA (4). The fact that it is
synthesized very rapidly suggests that it serves some other function.

When cultured cells of Acer pseudoplatanus are labelled for
30 minutes with 5-^{3}H uridine only the rRNA precursors and polydisperse RNA became labelled. There is a lag period before the
precursors are processed to form mature rRNA. This affords the
opportunity to study the properties of the messenger RNA associated with the polyribosomes because the mRNA reaches the cytoplasm more rapidly than the rRNA. About 40% of the total polydisperse RNA associated with the polyribosomes contains poly
adenylic acid judged by affinity chromatography on oligo(dT)
cellulose and hybridization to ^{3}H poly uridylic acid. The
simplest interpretation of this result is that only about 40% of
the rapidly labelled mRNA contains poly(A) and that a substantial
proportion of the mRNA is lost during purification by procedures
that depend on poly(A) content.

1. Grierson, D., Rogers, M.E., Sartirana, M.L., and Loening, U.E.
   (1970) Cold Spring Harbor Symp. Quant. Biol. 35, 589-598.
2. Grierson, D. and Loening, U.E. (1974) Eur. J. Biochem. 44,
   501-507.
3. Grierson, D. and Smith, H. (1973) Eur. J. Biochem. 36, 280-285.
4. Grierson, D. (1974) Eur. J. Biochem. 44, 509-515.

FATE OF HOMOLOGOUS DNA IN SEEDLINGS OF MATTHIOLA INCANA

Vera Hemleben

Department of Biology II of the University of Tübingen
74 Tübingen, Auf der Morgenstelle 28
W. Germany

To study the fate of homologous DNA in a recipient system a specific labelling procedure is necessary. We use a ^{3}H-adenine/BrdU labelled donor DNA from <u>Matthiola</u> seedlings (buoyant density: 1.741 g/cm^3) and intact seedlings grown in water as recipient plants (DNA buoyant density: 1.698 g/cm^3).

Seven-day old seedlings were incubated under sterile conditions with 100 µg ^{3}H-adenine/BrdU DNA (specific activity: 5 x 10^6 cpm/mg DNA) and unlabelled adenine and thymidine 1 mg each per ml citrate buffer. After 16 hours of incubation the seedlings were treated several times with DNase and pronase to remove the exogenous DNA from the surface and then the DNA was isolated.

The profile of buoyant density of the DNA separated on a neutral caesiumchloride gradient shows the following result: Two main peaks of radioactivity appear at the position of 1.741 and 1.727 g/cm^3, very little radioactivity coincides with the peak of UV absorbance of the recipient DNA at 1.698 g/cm^3. Because under the incubation conditions described the recipient plants produce only "light" stranded DNA, it must be concluded that large fragments of the density labelled donor DNA enter the plants cells and probably form an intermediate fraction ("hybrid", ρ = 1.727 g/cm^3) with the recipient DNA.

DNA SYNTHESIS AND BACTERIAL CONTAMINATION IN PALNTS

Michel Delseny

Attaché de Recherche CNRS
Laboratoire de Physiologie Végétale, ERA n°226 du CNRS
Centre Universitaire de Perpignan
F 66000, Perpignan, France

A GC rich satellite DNA is detected in many plant DNA preparations. This satellite is rapidly labeled either with 32-P or 14-C uridine, but, in contrast with bulk DNA, it does not incorporate 14-C thymidine. Its synthesis is triggered very early during seed germination, and is also detected in a variety of circumstances such as hormonal treatments, temperature shifts and wounding. Therefore, it has appeared to be of special significance in the regulation of cell differentiation. Unfortunately, this satellite DNA turns out to be bacterial in origin. Indeed, though seeds were thoroughly surface sterilized before soaking and allowed to germinate on sterile wet filter paper, satellite DNA can be washed off with 2% Na-hypochloride, provided that seed coats were removed. Furthermore, DNA with high specific activity, similar in buoyant density to satellite can be recovered from the radioactive incubation medium. Evaluation of bacterial contamination in hormone treated seedlings reveals that higher is the growth stimulation, higher are the bacterial counts. Some of the contaminant bacteria of radish and broad bean seeds were isolated. Isopycnic centrifugation and preliminary reassociation kinetic data indicate that their DNA and the so-called satellite DNA are very similar, in contrast with true satellite DNA. Most of the isolated bacteria are resistant to currently used antibiotics such as penicillin, chloramphenicol, or colimycin. Streptomycin and tetracyclin efficiently prevent bacteria, but disturb normal germination. Differential labelling is explained by the inability of bacteria to use thymidine, and the size of the phosphate pools in plants. Bacteria were observed between the seed coat and the tissues. Upon germination, they proliferate in the hair root region, where they appeared embedded in mucilageneous compounds, and sticking closely to the cell wall. These observations account for most of the striking features of rapidly labelled plant satellite DNA.

MITOCHONDRIAL NUCLEIC ACIDS FROM PARTHENOCISSUS TRICUSPIDATA CELLS

F.VEDEL, F.QUETIER and J.M.GRIENENBERGER

Laboratoire de Biologie Moléculaire Végétale, Bat. 430

Université Paris-Sud - 91405 - ORSAY (FRANCE)

The growth pattern of suspension cultures of *Partheno-cissus tricuspidata* cells has been studied. A nutritive medium derived from that of Heller gives a high yield of metabolically active cells. The cell number, fresh and dry weights, DNA and RNA contents have been followed over a subculture cycle (14 days in defined conditions). A doubling time of 36 hours has been estimated.

Mitochondria have been prepared from *Parthenocissus tricuspidata* cells and purified by several cycles of centrifugation and a linear sucrose gradient. The mitochondria have been observed by electron microscopy.

mt DNA extracted from DNase treated mitochondria gives a sharp and symetrical band when analysed by analytical CsCl gradient centrifugation with a buoyant density of 1 706 g/ml.

mt rRNA extracted from mitochondria purified by 6 washings and a sucrose gradient has been analysed by polyacrylamide gel electrophoresis. mt r RNA appears as $0.84 \ 10^6$ and $0.42 \ 10^6$ species corresponding to about 21 S and 13 S. The mt RNA migrates as stable bands even in EDTA buffer and under denaturing conditions. In spite of the intensive purification used, a contamination by cytoplasmic rRNA cannot be avoided.
The synthesis of mt rRNA is inhibited by BET and is insensitive to actinomycine D, as shown by ^{32}P labelling.

Higher plants show a unique situation since they contain specific rRNA in the cytoplasm (25 S, 18 S), the chloroplasts (23 S, 16 S) and the mitochondria (21 S, 13 S).

INVOLVEMENT OF NUCLEIC ACIDS AND MICROTUBULES IN CILIOGENESIS:

IMPLICATIONS FOR CYTOPLASMIC INHERITANCE

Joanne Keene Kelleher

Department of Biology, Boston University

Boston, Massachusetts 02215

The ciliated protozoan, <u>Stentor</u> <u>coeruleus</u>, undergoes a process of oral development which occurs when cells prepare to divide or when the oral area is artificially removed. This process involves the production of thousands of new cilia and basal bodies in an eight hour period. A location on the cell cortex, the stripe contrast zone, defines the site of ciliogenesis. The data indicate that DNA synthesis is not required. RNA and protein synthesis are required during early stages of regeneration. At late stages a limiting factor is assembly of microtubule protein as demonstrated by sensitivity to the drugs colchicine and podophyllotoxin. A regulatory model based on the polymerization-depolymerization equilibrium of microtubule protein is offered which explains both these results and classic experiments involving grafts between two cells at different stages of regeneration. Such grafts regenerate synchronously (the older cell is retarded and the younger accelerated until they reach the same stage). This result may be expected if cells at different stages have unequal pools of cilia percursors and if these pools mix when cells are grafted together. The polarity of proteins in the cell cortex is thought to determine cortical patterns and basal body location. Assembly of proteins on these basal bodies would be determined by the cilia precursor protein pool. This model does not require involvement of the cell cortex, nuclear-cytoplasmic ratio, or specific cortical nucleic acids in the regulation of morphogenesis. (Supported by USPHS Grant CA5060 from NC1).

METHYL 4-CHLOROINDOLYL-3-ACETATE IN PEA AND BARLEY

K.C. Engvild

Danish AEC, Risø

DK-4000 Roskilde, Denmark

Immature seeds of pea and barley were harvested on plants grown in solutions containing $^{36}Cl^-$, but no other chlorides. Autoradiography of two dimensional thin layer chromatograms (silicagel) of butanol extracts of freeze-dried seeds showed the presence in both species of several radioactive compounds besides Cl^-. One compound, present in pea and probably in barley, cochromatographed with a mixture of 4- and 6-chloroindolyl-3-acetic acid methyl esters. Another, detected in pea, but probably not in barley, cochromatographed with a mixture of 4- and 6-chloroindolyl-3-acetic acids.

Physiologia Plantarum, in press.

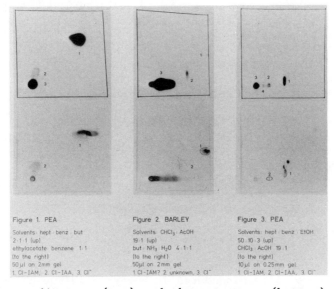

Figure 1. PEA

Solvents: hept : benz : but
2 : 1 : 1 (up)
ethylacetate : benzene 1 : 1
(to the right)
50 µl on 2mm gel
1. Cl-IAM, 2. Cl-IAA, 3. Cl⁻

Figure 2. BARLEY

Solvents: CHCl₃ : AcOH
19 : 1 (up)
but : NH₃ : H₂O 4 : 1 : 1
(to the right)
50µl on 2mm gel
1. Cl-IAM? 2. unknown, 3. Cl⁻

Figure 3. PEA

Solvents: hept : benz : EtOH
50 : 10 : 3 (up)
CHCl₃ : AcOH 19 : 1
(to the right)
10 µl on 0.25mm gel
1. Cl-IAM, 2. Cl-IAA, 3. Cl⁻

Autoradiograms (top) and chromatograms (bottom).

EVIDENCE FOR A PROPOSED FUNCTION OF DNA AS TRANSDUCER ACTING AT THE CELL SURFACE

B.L. Reid

Queen Elizabeth II Research Institute

University of Sidney, Australia

Evidence was presented at the 1970 Summer School for the presence of DNA in filaments projected from the cell wall of certain animal cells during the familiar process of amoeboid movement. It was suggested that such DNA may have an antenna function aiding in subsequent cell differentiation.[1]

Observations and experiments in the interim have shown that the DNA involved differs from the DNA of the whole cell in regard to its melting profiles, buoyant density in caesium chloride gradients and ultrastructural morphology on cytochrome C.[2] Some of these properties suggested that the surface DNA was enriched in polynucleotide of a more homogeneous base composition than that of the bulk of DNA. It was speculated that such a property would enhance its function as an antenna permitting the DNA to form networks at the cell surface. DNA doesnot usually form networks on conventional films but such structures can be readily prepared for and visualised in the electron microscope by using films of polystyrene.[4] In vivo such networks form the scaffold of the mucoid coat which surrounds actively growing cells of the type under notice.[3] It was speculated that substances in the cell environment are able to enhance the production of cell surface DNA by causing its release from the nucleus.[1] The use of the polystyrene film techniques showed that proteins were potent in withdrawing DNA from aqueous solution on to the film. Amongst proteins the histones were highly effective more especially those rich in arginine.[4]

It was therefore decided to test the capacity of histone proteins in the living cell. Amounts of 100 µgm of histone upon addition to rat thymus cells, incubated in buffered saline culture

medium for two hours at pH 712 causes the appearance of a dense
mucoid coat around the cell. Such a coat entraps the cells resulting in agglutination. The effect of histone can be abolished
by prior incubation of the cells in deoxyribonuclease and by any
factor which reduces the cell motility such as lowering the incubation temperature or incubation in medium in which deuterium oxide
replaces water. It is speculated that the histone is able to bind
to cell surface DNA which in turn causes increased amounts of DNA
to be withdrawn from its reservoir in the nucleus. It is further
speculated that filamentous systems in plant cells may contain DNA
which acts as a sensory network near the plasma membrane.

1. Reid, B.L. and Blackwell, P.M. Nuclear extensions of cultured
    cells: a possible mechanism of cellular differentiation in
    Informative molecules in Biological Systems. Ed. L. Ledoux,
    Nth.Holland, Amsterdam, p. 285, 1971.

2. Reid, B.L. and Blackwell, P.M. Aust. J. med. Technol. 3, 121,
    1972.

3. Reid, B.L. Biosystems 5, 207, 1974.

4. Reid, B.L. and Blackwell, P.M. Aust. J. med. Technol. 4, 168,
    1973.

GENOME ACTIVATION DURING SEED GERMINATION

M. Dobrzańska-Wiernikowska

Institute of Biochemistry and Biophysics

Warsaw, Poland

Transcriptional events were found to be activated in a step-wise manner when mature wheat seeds were exposed to the optimal germination conditions. Immediate-early, and late transcription products could be distinguished from each other by differences in their nucleotide composition. The immediate-early transcripts appeared in the seed already within the first 3 hours of imbibition and were unusually rich in UMP /65 mol%/. The early transcripts could be characterized as U+G rich. The late transcripts began to appear 12 hours after germination starts and had nucleotide composition similar to that of the total RNA.

It is suggested that the early transcripts belong to a class of pre-mRNA, whereas rRNA sequences are predominant among the late transcripts. The first transcription products seem to result from a selective and asymmetric transcription of dA:dT rich sequences of the genome. THE UMP-rich clusters would serve as programming sequences of the newly-synthesized pre-mRNA.

PARTICIPANTS

Dr. Karl N. Angerbauer
D-8 Munchen 19
Mana-Wardstrasse 19
Germany

Dr. Fred Ausubel
Dept. of Botany
Univ. of Leicester
Leicester LEI 7RH
England

Dr. S. Baroncelli
Instituto de Genetik
Via Matteotti
IA Pisa, Italy

Dr. Ralf Beiderbeck
Botanisches Institut der
  Universität
Hofmeisterweg 4
6900 Heidelberg, Germany

Dr. R. Bekhi
C.E.N.
2400 Mol
Belgium

Dr. A. Belayew
Chemin du Grand Maître, 25
4040 Tilff
Belgium

Dr. A. Bennici
Institute of Genetics
Via Matteotti 1A Pisa
Italy

Prof. G. Bernier
Botanic Department
Sart Tilman
4000 Liège, Belgium

Dr. J. Bohacek
Institute of Biophysics
Czechoslovak Academy of Sciences
Brno 12, Kralovopolska 135
Czechoslovakia

Dr. M. Branchard
10, Allée des Bathes
F-91400 Orsay
France

R.W. Breidenback
Dept. of Agronomy and Range Sci.
University of California Davis
Davis, Calif. 95616 U.S.A.

Dr. D. Broeckaert
Fakulteit der Genoeskunde
Laboratorium voor Fysiologische
  Chemie
9000 Gent, Belgium

Prof. R. Bronchart
Département de Botanique
Sart Tilman
4000 Liège, Belgium

Dr. J.A.M. Brown
Victorian Wheert Research Institute
Piwate Bag 260 P.O.
Horsham Victoria
3400 Australia

589

Dr. B. Bude
Plant Biochemistry
Monsanto Co.
800 N. Lindbergh
St. Louis, MO 63166 U.S.A.

Dr. John Burrows
Woodstock Agricultural Research
    Center
Sittingbourne, Kent
Great Britain

Dr. H. Caboche
Laboratoire de Génétique
    cellulaire
Cehmin de Borde-rouge 31
Auzeville, Toulouse
France

Dr. F. Cannon
University of Sussex
Sussex,
United Kingdom

Dr. R.S. Chaleff
Department of Biology
Brookhaven Natl. Laboratory
Associated University Inc.
Upton L.I.
N.Y. 11973 U.S.A.

Dr. P. Charles
C.E.N.
2400 Mol
Belgium

Dr. D.K. Choudwary
Institut für Botanik und
    Mikrobiologie
Postfach 365
517 Julich
Deutschland

Dr. E. Cocking
Dept. of Botany
University Park
Nottingham, NG7 2 RD

Dr. Milton J. Constantin
Department of Biology
Brookhaven National Laboratory
Associated Universities, Inc.
Upton, L.I., N.Y. 11973 U.S.A.

Dr. G. Corduan
Plant Physiology
Gebäude ND 463 Bochum
Fed. Rep. Germany

Dr. G. Craven
University of Stellenbosch
P.O. Box 306
Stellenbosch, South Africa

Dr. John W. Cross
California Institute of Technology
Division of Biology
Pasadena, California 91109   U.S.A.

Dr. Joachim Daum
Sekt. Biochem. Mikrobiol.
D 1000 Berlin 10
Max-Dohrn-Strasse, Germany

Dr. P.C. Debergh
R.U.G.
Coupure Li, ks 533
9000 Gent
Belgie

Dr. Xavier Delannay
Institut Carnoy
Vaartstraat, 24
3000 Louvain, Belgie

Prof. De Ley
Rijksuniversiteit Gent, 35
K.L. Ledeganckstraat, 9000 Gent
Belgium

Dr. M. Delseny
Centre Universitaire de Perpignan
Equipe de Recherch Associée au
    CNRS 2
Avenue de Villeneuve
66000 Perpignan, France

Dr. R. Deltour
Département de Botanique
Sart Tilman
4000 Liège, Belgium

M. F. Deprez
Département de Botanique
Sart Tilman
4000 Liège, Belgium

M. Dobrzanska
Institute of Biophysics
Warsaw, Poland

Dr. R.E. Drew
The Univ. of Newcastle Upon Tyne
Department of Genetics
Claremont Place
Newcastle Upon Tyne
NEI 7RU, England

Dr. J. Dubois
5, rue du Cordia
5800 Gembloux
Belgium

Dr. J.L. Durand
Physiologie Pluricellulaire
C.N.R.S.
91190 Gif-sur-Yvette, France

Dr. A. Dutrecq
K.U.L.
3000 Leuven
Belgium

Dr. Kjeld Engvild
Danish Atomic Energy Commission
Research Establishment 5150
DK-4000 Roskilde, Denmark

Dr. G. Fraselle
Ecole de Santé Publique
1200 Bruxelles, Belgium

Prof. E. Fredericq
Institut de Chimie, Sart Tilman
4000 Liège, Belgium

M. Fredj
Institut de Botanique Générale
Laboratoire de Phsyiologie Végetale
Université de Genève
Genève 4, Suisse

Dr. Jacquelyn G. Furman
4012 N. 35th Street
Arlington, Virginia 22207 U.S.A.

Dr. G.G. Gavazzi
University of Milan
Via Celor
Milan, Italie

Dr. Steven M. Gendel
University of California Irvine
Dept. of Developmental and Cell
     Biology
Irvine California 92664 U.S.A.

Prof. J.M. Ghuysen
Département de Botanique
Sart Tilman
4000 Liège, Belgium

Dr. KL Giles
Plant Physiologie Division
Private Bag
Palmerston North NZ, England

Dr. Frank Gillingham
615 Market
Oxford, Pennsylvania U.S.A.

P. Godard

Dr. Cl.D. Goldwaite
Department of Biochemistry
Albert Einstein College of Medicine
1300 Morris Park Ave.
Bronx, N.Y. 10461 U.S.A.

Dr. Medina Gonzalez
Vaarstraat, 24
3000 Louvain, Belgium
Belgium

Dr. N.R. Gore
Department of Biochemistry
University of St. Andrews
Irvine Building
North Street
St. Andeus, KYIG 9 AL
FIEE, Scotland

Sister Veronica Govelitz
Georgian Court College
Lakewood, N.J.   U.S.A.

Dr. Gradman-Rebel
Dept. of Biology 11
D-74 Tubingen
Auf der Morgenstelle 28
Deutschland

Dr. Christ Graf
University of Frankfurt Main
Gunderrodestrasse, 23
6000 Frankfurt Main
Deutschland

Dr. P. Gresshoff
Research School of
    Biological Sciences
R.S.B.S. Aust. Nat. Univ.
Canberra A.C.I., Australia

Dr. D. Grierson
Dept. of Physiology and
    Environment Studies
Sutton Bonington
Loughborough, LE12 5 RD
Great Britain

Dr. M. Guttierrez-Moguera
Horticulture Dept.
University of Wisconsin
Madison, Wis. 53706 U.S.A.

Dr. V. Hemleben
Institut für Biologie der
    Universität Tubingen auf der
    Morgenstelle, 1
7400 Tubingen, Deutschland

Prof. D. Hess
Lehrstuhl für Bot. Entwicklungsph.
    Universite
D 7000 Stuttgart,
BRD Germany

Dr. H. Hirokawa
Laboratory of Genetics
Faculty of Science
University of Tokyo
Tokyo, Japan

Dr. R. Huart
C.E.N.
2400 Mol, Belgium

Dr. M. Jacobs
Vrije Universiteit Brussel
Brussel, Belgium

Dr. A. Collette-Jacqmard
Departément de Botanique
Sart Tilman, 4000 Liège
Belgium

Dr. M. Janofsky
C.E.N.
2400 Mol, Belgium

Dr. EG Jaworski
Monsanto Commercial Products Co.
Agricultural Division
800 N. Lindbergh Boulevard
St. Louis, MO 63166 U.S.A.

Dr. L. Johansson
Murarg. 10B
75437 Uppsala
Sweden

Dr. A. Johnston
125 College Road
Norwich, Great Britain

Joanne Kelleher
Department of Biology
Boston University
2 Cummington St.
Boston, MASS 02215 U.S.A.

Dr. Hartmut Kern
Institut für Botanik und
    Mikrobiologie der Kern-
    forschungsanlage
Julich GMBH
517 Julich

Dr. A. Kleinhofs
C.E.N.
2400 Mol, Belgium

V. Konvalinkova
C.E.N.
2400 Mol, Belgium

Dr. R. William Krul
Plant Hormone & Regulator Lab.
B.A.R.C. West
Bettsville MD 20705 U.S.A.

Dr. J.J. Kummert
Faculté des Sciences
    Agronomiques de l'Etat
5800 Gembloux, Belgium

Dr. B. Leber
Dept. of Biology II
D74 Tubingen
Auf der Morgenstelle 28
Deutschland

Prof. L. Ledoux
Département de Botanique
Sart Tilman
4000 Liège, Belgium

Dr. Ming Chin Liu
Taiwan Sugar Research Inst.
54 Sheng Chan Road
Tainan Taiwan
Republic of China

Dr. R. Loppes
Département de Botanique
Sart Tilman
4000 Liège, Belgium

Dr. Horst Lorz
7000 Stuttgart 70
Steckgeldstrasse, 77
Deutschland

Dr. Wolfgang Lotz
Institut für Mikrobiologie
Universitat Erlangen Nurnberg
Friedrichstrasse, 33
852 Erlangen

Dr. P. Lurquin
C.E.N.
2400 Mol, Belgium

Dr. P. Mahlberg
International Congress
Dept. Plant Sciences
Indiana University
Bloomington, Indiana 47401 U.S.A.

Dr. Morton Mallin
O.N.U. ADA
Ohio 45810 U.S.A.

Dr. A. Maretzki
Physiology Biochemistry
Hawaiian Sugar Planters
1527 Keeaumoku Street
Honolulu, Hawaii 96882 U.S.A.

Dr. R. Matagne
Département de Botanique
Sart Tilman
4000 Liège, Belgium

Dr. K. Matsumoto
Institute Applied Mikrobiology
University of Tokyo
Bunkyo-Ku, Tokyo, Japan

Dr. R.A. McKee
School of Agriculture
Sutton Bonington
Loughborough LE 12 5 RD
England

Dr. J.H. Meade
Box 688
Richerdson, Texas 75080 U.S.A.

Dr. M. Mergeay
C.E.N.
2400 Mol
Belgium

Dr. A. Metha
c/o Prof. H.E. Street
Barsda
Leicester, England

Dr. George Michalopoulos
Brookhaven Natl. Lab.
Upton L.I., N.Y. 11973 U.S.A.

Dr. P. Miedema
Instituut de Haaf
Postbus 117
Stichting voor Plantenveredeling
Wageningen, Nederland

T. Moijica-A
C.E.N.
Mol, Belgium

Dr. M. Nasrallah
801, Triphammer Rd.
Ithaca, N.Y. 14850 U.S.A.

Dr. M. Nys-Dewolf
Kennedy Park 17
3300 Tienen
Belgie

Dr. C. Nitsch
C.N.R.S. Physiologie
    Pluricellulaire
F 91190 Gif-sur-Yvette, France

Dr. K. Ohyama
110 Gymnasium Rd.
University Campus
Saskatoon 57N 0W9
Saskatechewan, Canada

Dr. F. Oostindier Braaksma
P.O. Box 14
Haren (GN) The Netherlands

Dr. L. Owens
Plant Physiology Institute
Beltsville, MD 20705   U.S.A.

Dr. M. Patillon
27, rue de Poissy,
F-75005 Paris, France

Prof. J.R. Postgate
University of Sussex
Brighton, Sussex BN 19Q7
United Kingdom

Dr. A. Powling
775 Konstanz
Fachbereich Biologie der
    Universitat Bundesrepublik
Deutschland

Dr. D. Raveh
Plant Genetics
The Weizmann Institute of Science
Rehovot, Israël

Prof. G. Redei
College of Agriculture
Department of Agronomy
117 Curtis
Columbia, MO 65201 U.S.A.

Dr. M. Reekmans
4108 Rotheux-Rimère
Belgium

Dr. Bevan L. Reid
The University of Sidney
Dept. of Obstetrics and
    Gynaecology
Sidney 2006
New South Wales, Australia

Dr. Robert Rennie
17 Gramge Court
Gramge Rd.
Bowdon, Great Britain

Dr. H.P. Roggen
P.O. Box 16
Wageningen, Nederland

Dr. Irwin Rubenstein
Dept. of Genetics and Cell Biol.
University of Minnesota
St. Paul, Minn. 55101 U.S.A.

Dr. Marcella Schablik
4027 Debrecen Nyar U.
8/2 A., Hungaria

Prof. J. Schell
Laboratorium voor Genetics
Ledeganckstraat, 35
9000 Gent, Belgium

Dr. L. Schilde
Max Planck Institut für Biologie
Abil. Melchers
74 Tobingen
Deutschland, Corrensstrasse 41

Dr. R.A. Schilperoort
Department of Biochemistry
Leiden State Univ.
Wassenaarsweg, 64,
Leiden, The Netherlands

Dr. O. Schimert
Département de Botanique
Laboratoire de Génétique
Sart Tilman
40000 Liege, Belgium

Dr. F. Schwind
V.U.B.
Laboratoire de Génétique
1850, Chaussée de Wavre
1160 Bruxelles, Belgium

Dr. H. Schremph
Gesellschaft für Molekular-
   biologische Forschung MDH
D 3301, Stockheim über
   Braunschweig
Mascheroder Weg 1
West Germany

Dr. P. Scoarnec
Institut Botanique
Montpellier, France

Dr. G. Selzer
Université de Genève
Département de Biologie
   Moléculaire
Sciences II, 30,
   quai Ernest Ansermet
CH-1211
Genève, Suisse

Dr. J. Shen-Miller
Argonne National Laboratory
Argonne, Illinois 60439 U.S.A.

Dr. W.F. Sheridan
University of Missouri
College of Arts and Scineces
205 Curtis Hall
Columbia, MO 65201 U.S.A.

Prof. C. Sironval
Département de Botanique
Sart Tilman
4000 Liège, Belgium

Dr. H. Smith
University of Nottingham
Dept. of Physiology and Env.
   Studies
Sutton Bonington
Loughborough LE12 5 RD
England

Dr. Wolfgang Springer
Institut für Mikrobiologie and
   Molecular Biologie der
   Universität Hohenheim
7000 Stutgart, Hohenheim
Kirschnerstrasse 30, Deutschland

Dr. H.E. Street
Botanical Laboratories
School of Biological Science
University of Leicester
Leicester, England

Dr. Gary R. Stringam
Research Branch Agriculture Canada
University Campus
Saskatoon, Saskatchewan S7N OX2
Canada

Dr. Z. Reneé Sung
Massachusetts Institute of Tech.
Cambridge, MASS 02139 U.S.A.

Dr. Kawai Takeshi
Division of Genetics
National Institute of Agric. Sci.
Hiratsuka, Kanagawa-Ken 254, Japan

Dr. E. Tarantowicz-Marek
IBB PAN
36 Rakowiecka
02532 Warsawa, Poland

Dr. A. Tomasz
The Rockefeller University
New York, N.Y. 10021 U.S.A.

Mr. G. Tschitenge
Département de Botanique
Sart Tilman
4000 Liège, Belgium

Dr. J. Van Assche
Labo voor plantenbiochemie
Vaarstraat, 24
300 Leuven, Belgie

Dr. C. Van de Walle
Département de Botanique
Sart Tilman
4000 Liège, Belgium

Dr. A. van Gool
F.A. Janssenlaboratorium
    voor Genetika
Kardinaal Mercierlaan, 92
3030 Heverlee, Belgie

Dr. A. van Laere
Kortrykstraat, 13
3202 Linden, Belgie

Dr. F. Vedel
Batiment 430
Faculté des Sciences
91405 Orsay, France

S. Venketeswaran
Biology Dept.
Univ. of Houston
Houston, Texas 77004   U.S.A.

Dr. Baldev K. Vig
Department of Biology
University of Nevada
Reno, Nevada 89507 U.S.A.

Dr. Sara von Arnold
Inst. of Physiological Botany
75335 Uppsala, Sweden

W. Walczak
Institute of Biochemistry and
        Biophysics
Warsaw, Poland

Dr. F. White
Brigham Young University
Provo, Utah U.S.A.

Dr. John L. Wray
c/o Dr. P. Ficner
MSU/AEC Plant Research
    Laboratory
Michigan State University
E. Lansing, Michigan 48824 U.S.A.

Dr. Elisabetta Wurzer-Figurelli
Biochemische Lab.
Wassenaarseweg, 64
Leiden, Nederland

Dr. S.K. Zelcer
Plant Genetics
Weizmann Institute
Rehovot, Israel

S. Zilkali
Department Plant Genetic
Weizmann Institute
Rehovot, Israel

SUBJECT INDEX

Acetylene test, 120
Acridine orange, 93
Actinomycin D, 363
Agrobacterium, 50, 135, 141, 163
Arabidopsis thaliana, 183, 265, 329, 483, 499
S-adenosylmethionine, 203
Agarose, 429
Alcohol dehydrogenase, 246, 251
Amino acid metabolism, 567
Anther culture, 297, 576
Antibiotic, 4, 5, 48, 83
Antigenicity, 353
Antimetabolite, 186
Autolysin, 28, 34, 37, 38
Autoradiography, 255, 399, 487, 490, 522
Aza uracil, 186
Azotobacter, 109, 124, 252

Bacillus subtilis, 5, 15, 20, 113, 122, 142, 154, 397
Back mutations, 247
Bacterial contamination, 461, 493, 582
Bacteriocines, 83, 88
Bacteriophages, 8, 155, 206
Bacteroids, 216
Barley (Hordeum), 254, 275, 461
Bromodeoxyuridine, 198, 243

5-Bromouracil, 124

Callus culture, 212, 269, 285, 357, 545
Carrot (Daucus carota), 245, 280
Cells association, 245
    burst, 180, 183
    culture, 211, 231, 245, 552
    fusion, 138, 245
    wall, 31, 35
Chimeral tissues, 249
Chlamydomonas, 80, 429
Chloroplasts, 184
Chromatin, 391
    components, 392
    structure, 395
Chromatography, 21, 255, 401
Chromosome, 5, 45, 59
    Q banding, 402
    structure, 391, 399
    stability, 263, 278
Cistron, 77
Clusters, 133
Colicines, 83, 93
Colicinogenic factors, 48, 531, 547
Competence, 28, 31, 36
Complementation, 10, 18, 68, 77, 83, 193, 200
Complement fixation, 54

Computer aided simulation, 39,
    47
Continous cultures, 218
Conjugation, 2, 5, 92
Cotransduction, 8, 9
Cotransfer, 7
Crossing over, 116, 237, 243,
Crown gall, 141, 163, 229
CsCl gradients, 19, 29, 111,
    262, 295, 404
        artefacts, 33, 308
Cytotoxic effects, 356

Density transfer, 15
Deletion, 5, 63
Differenciation, 183, 248
Diplococcus pneumonial, 3, 27,
    113, 147, 397
Diploidy, 7, 18, 62
DNA
    adsorption, 429
    binding, 37, 40
    biological assay of, 420
    biological effects, 499, 529
    breakdown, 429, 461
    circular, 54
    CsCl gradients, 19, 29, 111,
    262, 295, 404, 422, 429, 461,
    481
        artefacts, 33, 308
    cytoplasmic, 583
    DNA hybridization, 135, 449,
    461
    helper, 151, 157
    integration, 14, 483, 493
    intermediate density, 125, 261,
    265, 268, 303, 311, 394, 405,
    483, 493
    molecular sieving, 429
    molecular weight, 421, 493, 503,
    plasmid, 52
    preparation, 405, 493
    protein interaction, 348

    purity, 415
    replication, 483, 493
    sonication, 493
    surface, 586
    thermodenaturation, 495
    uptake, 27, 311, 429, 461, 479,
        493, 529, 581
    viral, 449
DNase, 28
Dominance, 14
Drug resistance factors, 4, 96,
    131, 138, 571

Eclipse period, 115
Electron microscopy, 22, 73, 170
Electropheresis, 53
Embryogenesis, 233
Endocytosis, 278
Endonuclease, 188
Episomes, 95
    transfer, 144
Epr spectroscopy, 114
Escherichia coli, 1, 9, 10
Esterases, 252
Evolutionary changes, 131
Exonuclease, 109
Extrachromosomal inheritance, 45

F-primes, 59
    deletion, 63
    gal, 61
    generation, 61
    lac, 61
    transduction, 63
    transposition, 64
    fusion, 65
Fertility agent, 50
Flowering mutants, 195
Flower color mutants, 249
Fungi, 235

Gene
  conversion, 19, 236
  dosage, 85
  duplication, 133
  labeling, 2
  linkage, 202
  mutator, 194
  operator, 93
  promotor, 63, 67, 74, 77, 80
  recombination, 137, 150, 167,
    172, 198
  regulator, 94
  transcription, 543
  translation, 545
Genetic correction, 499
        recombination, 137, 150,
        167, 172, 198
        regulation, 89
Genetic transfer
        intergeneric, 11
        episomal, 47
β-galactosidase, 544, 559
Genome structure
  bacteria, 5, 7, 11, 14
  fungi, 18
  virus, 16, 17
Germination, 588

Haploid cells, 7, 18, 236, 297
Haplopoppus, 278
Hemophilus influenzae, 99, 113,
    142, 147, 189
Heterocaryons, 18
Heterocyst, 125
Histones, 393
Hormone action, 241, 247
Host restriction, 12
5-Hydroxymethyl cytosine, 204, 207
Hydroyurea, 321
Hydroxyapatite, 449, 461

Immunity, 67, 94
Immunodiffusion, 54
Immunofluorescence, 54
Isopycnic centrifugation, 19, 29,
    111, 262, 295, 404
Isozymes, 365
  acid phosphatase, 371
  alcohol dehydrogenase, 368, 380
  catalase, 370
  in Arabidopsis thaliana, 386
      Datura stramonium, 383
      Drosophila melanogaster, 385
  lactate dehydrogenase, 368
  leucine amino-peptidase, 370

Kanamycin resistance, 531
Klebsiella, 111

Leakage, 33, 34
Leaky mutants, 245, 511
Leghaemoglobin, 218
Lilium, 263, 281
Linked markers, 2
Lycopersicum esculentum, 264, 540
Lymphoma cells, 295, 318
Lysogeny, 59
Lysosomal apparatus, 284
Lysozyme, 12

Marker efficiency, 6, 8, 116, 119
        frequency, 15
Meiosis, 235
Melanoma cells, 340
Methylation, 191, 208
Micrococcus luteus, 145
Minicells, 62

Modification phenomena, 23, 185
Mössbauer spectroscopy, 114
Mucopeptide, 102
Mutagenesis, 3, 237, 329, 574, 578
  Site specific, 4, 5
Mutants
  Higher plants, 352, 499

Negative interference, 238
Neisseria, 146
Neuraminidae, 381
Neurospora crassa, 20, 80
Nitrate reductase, 219
Nitrogenase, 108, 254
Nitrogen fixation, 107, 123,215, 217
Nodulation, 216
Non-histone proteins, 394
Nopaline, 151, 177
Nucleases, 541

Octopine, 151
Operon, 74, 96, 134

Parasexual cycle, 19
Penicillin enrichment, 4
Permeability barrier, 36
Petunia, 524
Phage
  expression, 529, 551
  λ , 1, 47, 532
  survival, 559
  temperate, 16, 46, 150, 164
  transfer to eukaryotic cells, 539, 551
  uptake by pollen, 519, 529
Phytohormones, 241, 247, 277
Pinocytosis, 277

Plant bacterial association, 252
Plant regeneration, 264
Plasmids, 45
  cryptic, 51
  DNA, 52
  expression, 499, 531
  incompatibility, 51, 59, 65
  in crow-gall formation, 163
  uptake, 531
Plastome, 190
Pleiotropy, 242
Ploidy, 263
Polarity, 240
Pollen, 297, 519
Polyphenol, 570
Polyploidy, 235
Prophage, 46
Protein uptake, 527
Protoplasts, 35, 311, 575
Pseudomonas, 352

Radioimmunoassays, 55
Reassociation kinetics, 449, 461
Recombinants, 12, 13
Recombination, 17, 45
  Rec mutants, 62
Regeneration, 311
Repair mechanisms, 116, 122, 205, 313
Replication point, 15
Repressor, 63, 69
Resistance Transfer Factors, 48
Respiration, 572
Restriction, 12, 66
Rhizobium, 146, 212, 252
Ribosomes, 87
Rice (oryza sati va), 275, 355
RNA, 579, 588
RNase, 28
Root nodule, 126

Saccharomyces, 19, 20, 98
Salmonella typhimurium, 1, 9, 10, 11, 196
Sedimentation analysis, 115
Selection of mutant cell lines, 240
Sexual cycle, 18
Sex Factor, 6, 48, 49
    F-prime, 15, 49, 59
    Hfr, 15, 62
Sex pili, 50
Shigella, 131, 203
Shoot bud initiation, 232
Sinapis alba, 484
Single cell cloning, 238
Spermine, 382
Spheroplasts, 151, 206
Starch synthesis mutants, 249
Streptococcus, 142
Streptomyces, 6
Sucrose gradients, 4
Sycomore (Acer pseudoplatanus), 219, 552
Symbiosis, 218, 245

Tobacco (Nicotiana), 146, 236, 247, 265, 297, 311, 352, 385, 522.
Taxonomy, 141
Teichoic acids, 102
Tetrads, 236
Thiazole, 5
Three-point Cross, 9, 10

Thymine, 5
Thymine starvation, 93
Tomato (lycopersicum), 60, 63, 64, 66, 70, 76
Transduction, 2, 7, 8, 93, 232
Transfection, 29, 566
Transfer, 7
Transformation, 2, 14, 27, 141, 145, 220, 223, 230, 258, 338, 341, 499, 565
    models, 326, 347, 523
Transgenosis, 539
Translocation, 254, 397
Transposition, 2
Trisomic analysis, 185
Tumorization, 220

U.V. irradiation, 95

Velocity sedimentation, 17
Virulence, 71
Viruses, 132
Viscosimetry, 17

X-rays, 242, 314

Zygote germination, 233